PREFACE

This book is written for the young otolaryngologist who is already acquainted with the field through recent formal residency training, as well as for other physicians who are interested in concise descriptions of otolaryngologic conditions.

It is not the intent of the authors to write a complete review of otolaryngology, much less a textbook of otolaryngology. It is a discussion of many current concepts in the field. The materials in this book came from numerous sources. The first edition was compiled from the editor's notes for his own Board Examinations, with contributions from authorities in the field. This revised second edition has been updated, as well as expanded, to make it more useful to medical students and physicians in other specialties.

It is hoped that the reader will freely refer to the list of references for more in-depth dissertations.

KJL

ACKNOWLEDGMENTS

My appreciation goes to Dr. Howard W. Smith, Director, New Haven Ear, Nose, Throat and Facial Plastic Surgery Group, Associate Clinical Professor of Otolaryngology, Yale University School of Medicine, and Dr. John A. Kirchner, Professor of Otolaryngology, Yale University School of Medicine, for their guidance and moral support. I am also very grateful to Dr. Harold F. Schuknecht, Walter Augustus Lecompte Professor of Otology and Laryngology, Harvard Medical School, who very generously contributed the photomicrographs of the temporal bone sections in Chapter 1. My thanks also to all my teachers, including Dr. Harold F. Schuknecht, Dr. Daniel Miller, and Dr. William W. Montgomery, whose lectures became the cornerstone of this book.

My colleagues have been more than kind in spending many valuable hours revising chapters for this publication. I am indebted to the numerous authors of textbooks, monographs and articles whose writings are indispensable in such a preparation.

Finally, I am thankful for an understanding wife, who in the midst of chauffeuring the children and household chores, did the medical illustrations, proofed the manuscript and indexed the book.

K.J. Lee, M.D.

ESSENTIAL OTOLARYNGOLOGY

Second Edition

A BOARD PREPARATION AND CONCISE REFERENCE

Edited by

K. J. LEE, M.D., F.A.C.S.
New Haven Ear, Nose, Throat and
Facial Plastic Surgery Group
Assistant Clinical Professor,
Yale University School of Medicine
Attending,
Hospital of St. Raphael, New Haven
Attending,
Yale-New Haven Hospital
Staff,
New Haven Hearing and Speech Center
Staff,
New Haven Cleft Palate Center
Consultant,
Backus Hospital
Norwich, Connecticut

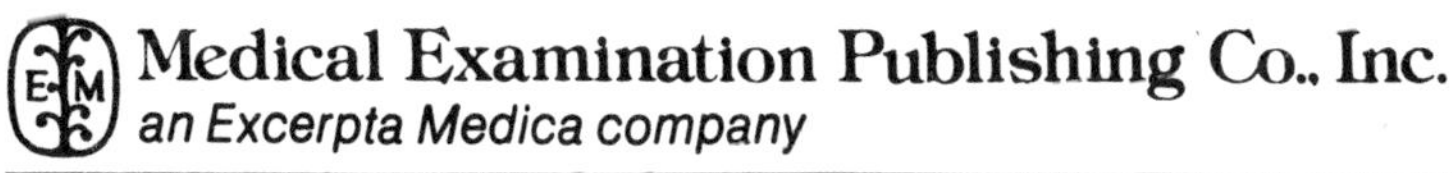
Medical Examination Publishing Co., Inc.
an Excerpta Medica company

969 Stewart Avenue • Garden City, New York 11530

notice

The editor(s) and/or author(s) and the publisher of this book have made every effort to ensure that all therapeutic modalities that are recommended are in accordance with accepted standards at the time of publication.

The drugs specified within this book may not have specific approval by the Food and Drug Administration in regard to the indications and dosages that are recommended by the editor(s) and/or author(s). The manufacturer's package insert is the best source of current prescribing information.

Library of Congress Card Number
77-80104

ISBN 0-87488-313-X

August, 1977

Printed in the United States of America

CONTRIBUTING AUTHORS

EIJI YANAGISAWA, M.D., F.A.C.S. New Haven Ear, Nose, Throat and Facial Plastic Surgery Group; *Associate Clinical Professor,* Yale University School of Medicine; *Attending,* Hospital of St. Raphael, New Haven; *Attending,* Yale-New Haven Hospital; *Staff,* New Haven Hearing and Speech Center; *Staff,* New Haven Cleft Palate Center.

DOUGLAS W. BELL, M.D., LCDR/MC *Staff Otolaryngologist,* Naval Regional Medical Center, Philadelphia; *Clinical Assistant Professor* of Otolaryngology, Hahnemann Medical School, Philadelphia.

DOUGLAS A. FARMER, M.D., F.A.C.S. (Deceased) *Chairman,* Department of Surgery, Hospital of St. Raphael, New Haven; *Clinical Professor of Surgery,* Yale University School of Medicine; *Consultant,* Griffin Hospital, Derby, Connecticut.

PAUL T. GAUDET, M.D. *Senior Resident,* Section of Otolaryngology, Yale University School of Medicine.

ISAAC GOODRICH, M.D., F.A.C.S. *Staff,* Neurosurgical Associates of New Haven, P.C.; *Attending,* Hospital of St. Raphael, New Haven; *Attending,* Yale-New Haven Hospital.

DAVID S. GREEN, PH.D. *Professor* of Speech and *Director* of Audiology and Deaf Education, Southern Connecticut State College.

JONATHAN D. KATZ, M.D. *Assistant Professor* of Anesthesiology, Yale University School of Medicine.

KIRKLAND LEWIS *Morphologist,* Biomedical Research Incorporated.

WOODROW W. LINDENMUTH, M.D., F.A.C.S. *Clinical Professor* of Surgery, Yale University School of Medicine; *Consulting Physician,* West Haven VA Hospital.

DAVID L. McPHERSON, PH.D. *Director,* New Haven Hearing and Speech Center; *Audiologist-in-Chief,* New Haven Ear, Nose, Throat and Facial Plastic Surgery Group.

DAVID D. ROBERTS, M.D. *Resident,* Section of Otolaryngology, Yale University School of Medicine.

ROBERT S. ROSNAGLE, M.D., F.A.C.S. New Haven Ear, Nose, Throat and Facial Plastic Surgery Group; *Assistant Clinical Professor,* Yale University School of Medicine; *Attending,* Hospital of St. Raphael, New Haven; *Attending,* Yale-New Haven Hospital; *Staff,* New Haven Hearing and Speech Center; *Staff,* New Haven Cleft Palate Center.

CLARENCE T. SASAKI, M.D. *Assistant Professor* of Otolaryngology, Yale University School of Medicine; *Attending,* Yale-New Haven Hospital; *Consultant,* West Haven VA Hospital.

HOWARD W. SMITH, M.D., D.M.D., F.A.C.S. *Director,* New Haven Ear, Nose, Throat and Facial Plastic Surgery Group; *Associate Clinical Professor,* Yale University School of Medicine; *Chief* of Otolaryngology and Maxillo-Facial Surgery, Hospital of St. Raphael, New Haven; *Attending,* Yale-New Haven Hospital; *Director,* New Haven Cleft Palate Center; *Consultant,* Meriden Hospital, Backus Hospital, Highland Heights Hospital, High Meadows Hospital and Windham Community Hospital; *Staff,* New Haven Hearing and Speech Center.

GORDON STROTHERS, M.B.B.S., F.R.C.S. New Haven Ear, Nose, Throat and Facial Plastic Surgery Group; *Assistant Clinical Professor,* Yale University School of Medicine; *Attending,* Hospital of St. Raphael, New Haven; *Attending,* Yale-New Haven Hospital; *Staff,* New Haven Hearing and Speech Center; *Staff,* New Haven Cleft Palate Center.

WILLIAM WILSON, M.D. *Assistant Professor* of Otolaryngology, Harvard Medical School; *Attending Staff,* Massachusetts Eye and Ear Infirmary.

ROBERT P. ZANES, M.D. *Chief,* Hematology, Hospital of St. Raphael, New Haven; *Assistant Clinical Professor* of Medicine, Yale University School of Medicine; *Attending,* Yale-New Haven Hospital; *Attending,* Hospital of St. Raphael, New Haven.

ESSENTIAL OTOLARYNGOLOGY

SECOND EDITION

CONTENTS

Chapter

Chapter

Chapter

NOTE: This volume is the second edition of a book which was previously entitled: Lee, K. J.: The Otolaryngology Boards: A Preparation Guide.

CHAPTER I

ANATOMY OF THE EAR

1. The temporal bone forms part of the side and base of the skull. It constitutes two-thirds of the floor of the middle cranial fossa and one-third of the floor of the posterior fossa. There are four parts to the temporal bone:

a) Squamosa
b) Mastoid
c) Petrous
d) Tympanic

2. The following muscles are attached to the mastoid process:

a) Sternocleidomastoid
b) Splenis capitis
c) Longissimus capitis
d) Digastric
e) Anterior, Superior, Posterior, Auricular

(The temporalis muscle attaches to the squamosa portion of the temporal bone and not to the mastoid process)

3. The auricle (Figure 1-1) is made of elastic cartilage, the cartilaginous canal of fibrocartilage. The cartilaginous canal constitutes 1/3 of the external auditory canal (whereas the eustachian tube is 2/3 cartilaginous); the remaining 2/3 is osseous.

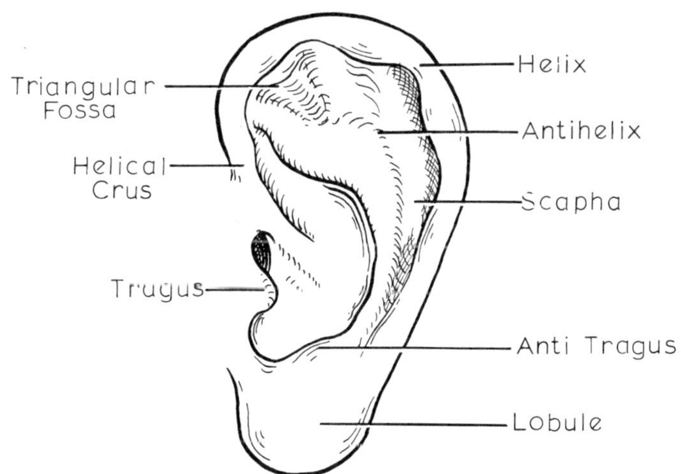

FIG. 1-1. The Auricle

4. The skin over the cartilaginous canal has sebaceous glands, ceruminous glands, and hair follicles. The skin over the bony canal is tight and has no subcutaneous tissue except periosteum.

5. Boundaries of External Auditory Canal:

Anteriorly:	Mandibular Fossa
	Parotid
Posteriorly:	Mastoid
Superiorly:	(Medially) Epitympanic recess
	(Laterally) Cranial Cavity
Inferiorly:	Parotid

The anterior portion, the floor and part of the posterior portion of the bony canal are formed by the tympanic part of the temporal bone. The rest of the posterior canal and the roof are formed by the squamosa.

6. Boundaries of the Epitympanum:

Medially:	Lateral semicircular canal and VII nerve
Superiorly:	Tegmen
Anteriorly:	Zygomatic arch
Laterally:	Squamosa (Scutum)
Inferiorly:	Fossa incudus
Posteriorly:	Aditus

7. Boundaries of the Tympanic Cavity:

Roof:	Tegmen
Floor:	Jugular wall and styloid prominence
Posteriorly:	Mastoid, stapedius, pyramidal prominence
Anteriorly:	Carotid wall, eustachian tube, tensor tympani
Medially:	Labyrinthine wall
Laterally:	Tympanic membrane, scutum (latero-superior)

8. The auricle is attached to the head by:
   a) Skin
   b) An extension of cartilage to the external auditory canal cartilage
   c) (1) anterior ligament (zygoma to helix and tragus)
      (2) superior ligament (external auditory canal to the spine of the helix)
      (3) posterior ligament (mastoid to concha)
   d) (1) anterior auricular muscle
      (2) superior auricular muscle
      (3) posterior auricular muscle

9. Notch of Rivinus is the notch on the squamosa, medial to which lies Shrapnell's membrane. The tympanic ring is not a complete ring, giving a dehiscence superiorly.

10. Meckel's Cave is the concavity on the superior portion of the temporal bone in which the Gasserian Ganglion (V) is located.

11. Dorello's Canal is between the petrous tip and the sphenoid bone. It is the groove for the VI nerve.

(Gradenigo's Syndrome is characterized by:
   a) Pain behind the eye
   b) Diplopia
   c) Aural discharge
It is secondary to petrositis with involvement of the VI nerve).

12. The suprameatal triangle of Macewen's triangle is posterior and superior to the external auditory canal. It is bound at the meatus by the Spine of Henle, otherwise called the suprameatal spine. This triangle approximates the position of the antrum medially. Tegmen mastoidi is the thin plate over the antrum.

13. Trautman's Triangle is demarcated by the bony labyrinth, the sigmoid sinus and the superior petrosal sinus or dura.

Citelli's Angle is the sino-dural angle. It is located between the sigmoid sinus and the middle fossa dura plate. Others consider the superior side of Trautman's Triangle to be Citelli's Angle.

Solid Angle is the angle formed by the three semicircular canals.

Scutum is the thin plate of bone which constitutes the lateral wall of the epitympanum. It is part of the squamosa.

Mandibular Fossa is bound by the zygomatic, squamosa and tympanic bones.

Canal of Huguier transmits the chorda tympani out of the temporal bone anteriorly. It is situated lateral to the roof of the protympanum.

Foramen of Huschke is located on the anterior tympanic plate along a nonossified portion of the plate. This is near the Fissures of Santorini.

Porus Acousticus is the "mouth" of the internal auditory canal. The canal is divided horizontally by the crista falciformis.

14. There are three parts to the inner ear (Figure 1-2):
   a) Pars superior: vestibular labyrinth (utricle and semi-circular canals)
   b) Pars inferior: cochlea and saccule
   c) Endolymphatic sac and duct

15. There are four small outpocketings from the perilymph space:
   a) Along the Endolymphatic duct
   b) Fissula ante fenestrum
   c) Fossula post fenestrum
   d) Periotic duct

16. There are four openings into the temporal bone:
   a) Internal auditory canal
   b) Vestibular aqueduct
   c) Cochlear aqueduct
   d) Subarcuate fossa

17. The ponticulum is the ridge of bone between the oval window niche and sinus tympani.

18. The subiculum is a ridge of bone between the round window niche and sinus tympani.

19. Koerner septum separates the squamosa from the petrous air cells.

20. Only one-third of the population has a pneumatized petrous portion of the temporal bone.

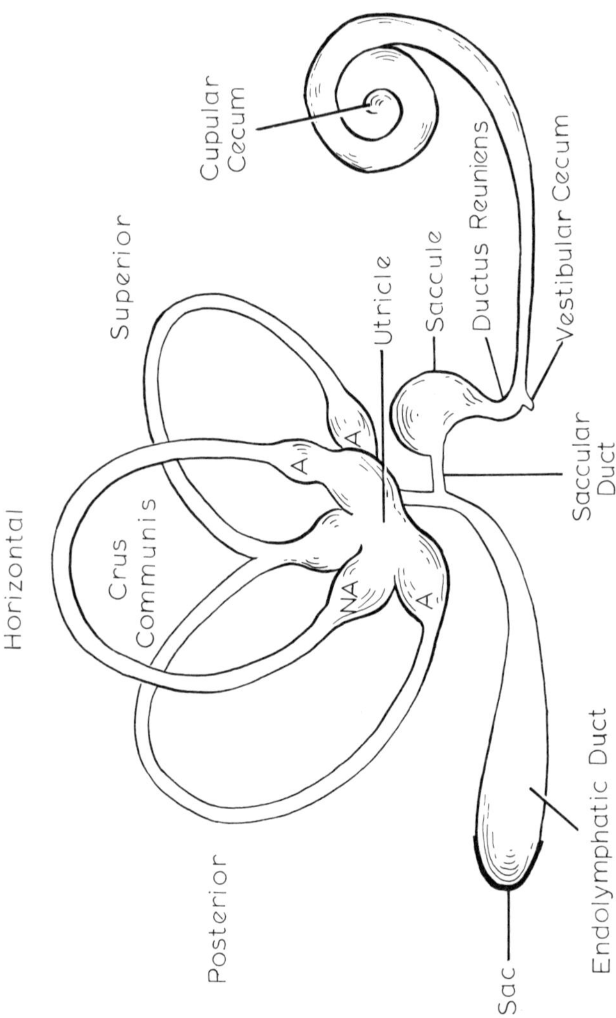

FIG. 1-2. Membranous Labyrinth
(A=Ampulated end, NA=Non-ampulated end)

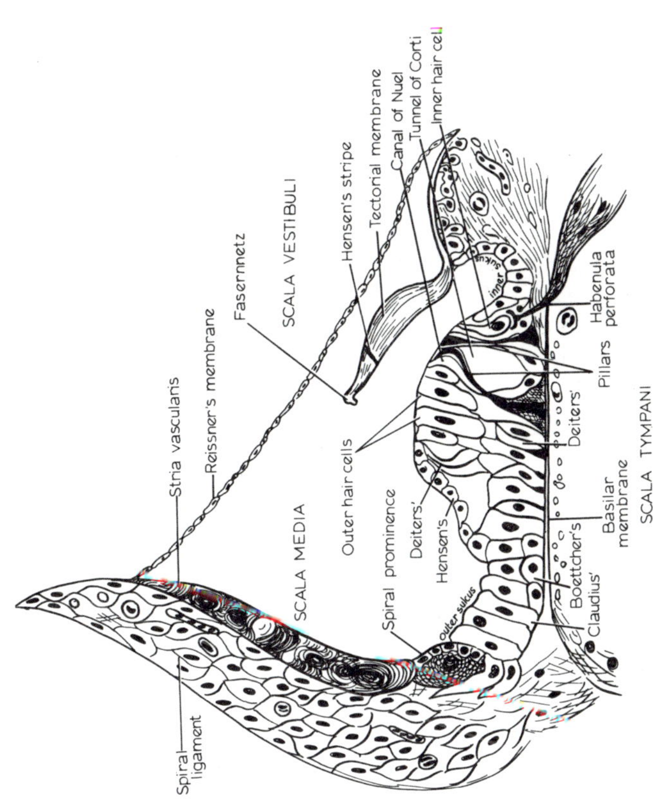

FIG. 1-3. Organ of Corti (Diagrammatic Representation)

21. Scala communis is where scala tympani joins scala vestibuli. The helicotrema is at the apex of the cochlea where the two join. (Figure 1-3)

22. Petrous pyramid is the strongest bone in the body.

23. The upper limits of the internal auditory canal diameter is 8 mm.

24. The cochlear aqueduct is a bony channel connecting the scala tympani of the basal turn with the subarachnoid space of the posterior cranial cavity. The average adult cochlear aqueduct is 6.2 mm long.

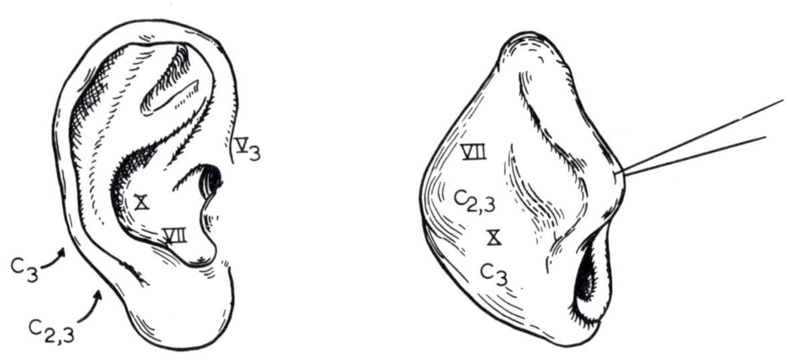

Fig. 1-4. Sensory Innervation of the Auricle
C_3 via Greater Auricular Nerve — V_3 Auriculotemporal Nerve
$C_{2,3}$ via Lesser Occipital Nerve — VII Sensory Twigs
X Auricular Branch

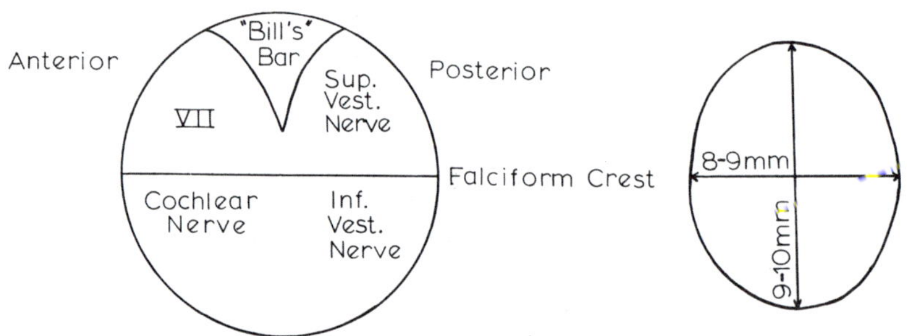

Fig. 1-5. Cross-Section of Internal Auditory Canal

Fig. 1-6. Measurements of the Tympanic Membrane

Sensory Innervation of the auricle is illustrated in Figure 1-4.

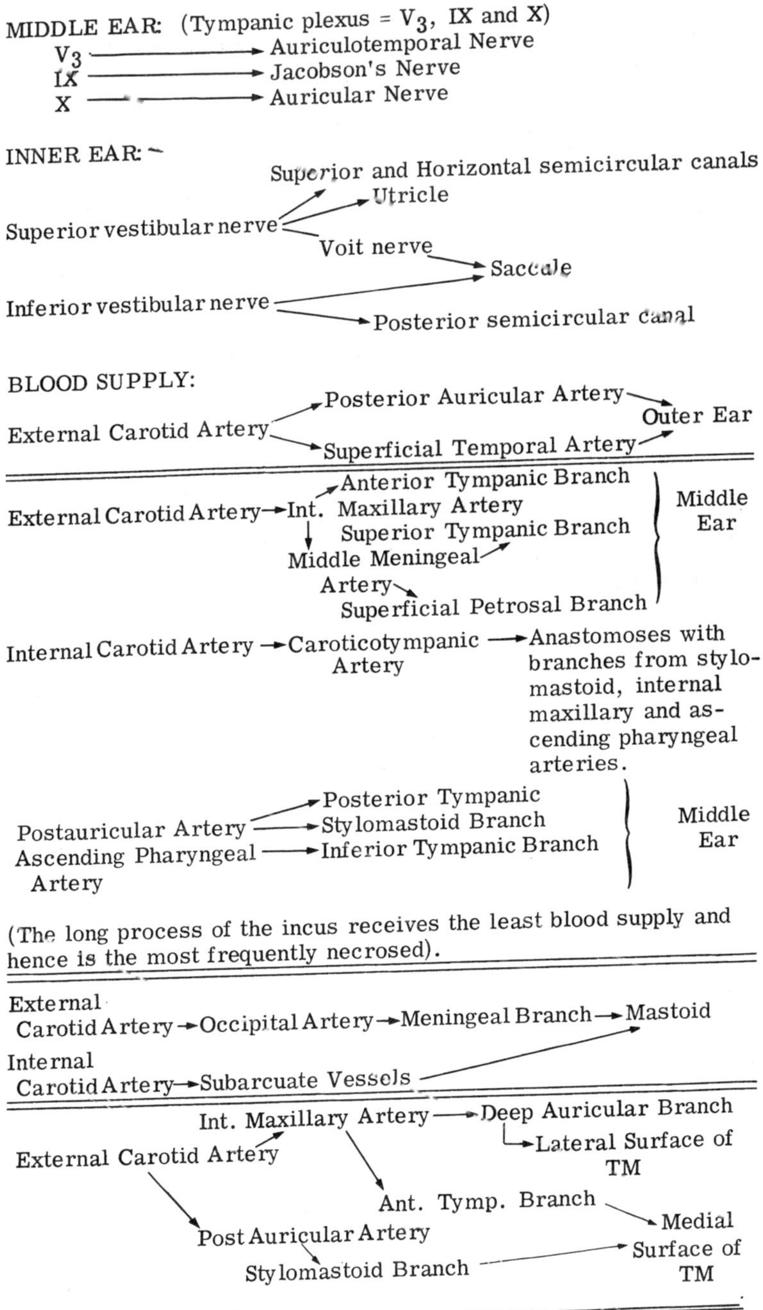
MIDDLE EAR: (Tympanic plexus = V3, IX and X)
V3 → Auriculotemporal Nerve
IX → Jacobson's Nerve
X → Auricular Nerve
INNER EAR:
Superior vestibular nerve
Superior and Horizontal semicircular canals
Utricle
Voit nerve
Saccule
Inferior vestibular nerve
Posterior semicircular canal
BLOOD SUPPLY:
External Carotid Artery
Posterior Auricular Artery
Superficial Temporal Artery
Outer Ear
External Carotid Artery → Int. Maxillary Artery
Anterior Tympanic Branch
Superior Tympanic Branch
Middle Meningeal Artery
Superficial Petrosal Branch
Middle Ear
Internal Carotid Artery → Caroticotympanic Artery → Anastomoses with branches from stylomastoid, internal maxillary and ascending pharyngeal arteries.
Postauricular Artery
Ascending Pharyngeal Artery
Posterior Tympanic
Stylomastoid Branch
Inferior Tympanic Branch
Middle Ear
(The long process of the incus receives the least blood supply and hence is the most frequently necrosed).
External Carotid Artery → Occipital Artery → Meningeal Branch → Mastoid
Internal Carotid Artery → Subarcuate Vessels
Int. Maxillary Artery → Deep Auricular Branch
Lateral Surface of TM
External Carotid Artery
Ant. Tymp. Branch
Medial Surface of TM
Post Auricular Artery
Stylomastoid Branch

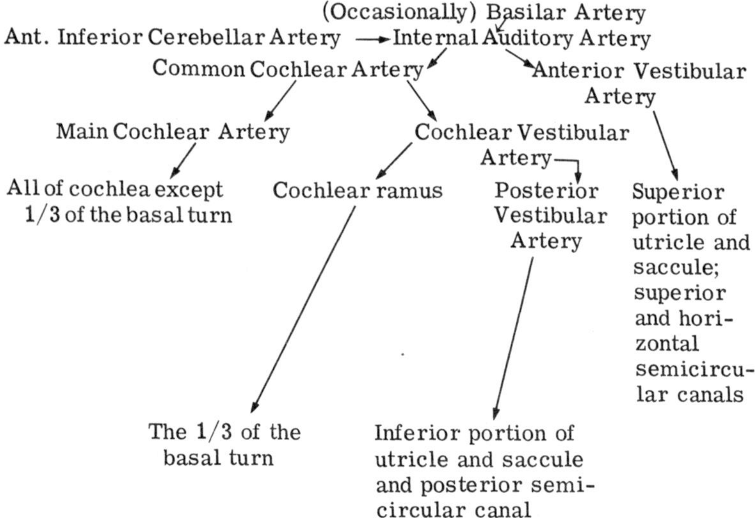

TYMPANIC MEMBRANE HAS FOUR LAYERS:

1. Squamous epithelium
2. Radiating fibrous layer
3. Circular fibrous layer
4. Mucosa layer

Average total area of tympanic membrane = 70-80 sq. mm.
Average vibrating surface of tympanic membrane = 55 sq. mm.

VENOUS DRAINAGE

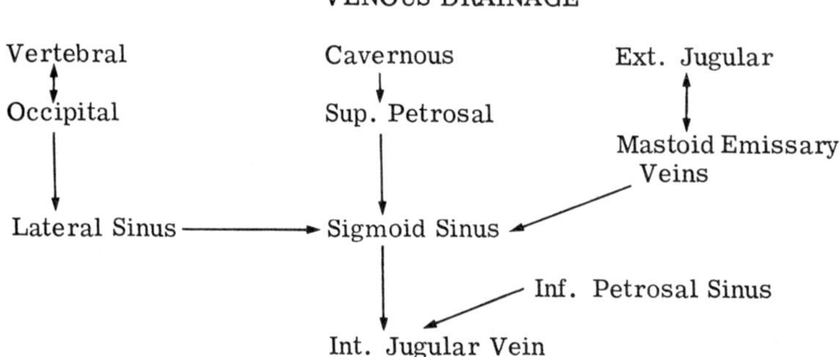

OSSICLES:

	Malleus	Head
		Neck
		Manubrium
		Anterior process
		Lateral or short process
	Stapes	Head
		Posterior crus
		Anterior crus
		Footplate (avg. 1.41 mm x 2.99 mm)
	Incus	Body
		Short process
		Long process (Lenticular process)

LIGAMENTS

MALLEUS:

1. Sup. malleal ligament (head to roof of Epitympanum)
2. Ant. malleal ligament (Neck near anterior process to sphenoid bone through the petrotympanic fissure).
3. Tensor Tympani (Medial surface of upper end of manubrium to cochleariform process).
4. Lateral malleal ligament (Neck to tympanic notch).

INCUS:

1. Superior incudal ligament (Body to tegmen)
2. Posterior incudal ligament (Short process to floor of incudal fossa)

STAPES:

1. Stapedial Tendon (Apex of the pyramidal process to the posterior surface of the neck of the stapes).
2. Annular ligament (Footplate to margin of vestibular fenestrum).

Malleal - Incudal joint is a diarthrodial joint.
Incudo - Stapedial joint is a diarthrodial joint.
Stapedial - Labyrinth joint is a syndesmotic joint.

MIDDLE EAR FOLDS OF SIGNIFICANCE: (In total there are 5 malleal folds and 4 incudal folds).

Anterior Malleal Fold - Neck of the malleus to anterosuperior margin of the tympanic sulcus.

Posterior Malleal Fold - Neck to posterosuperior margin of the tympanic sulcus.

Lateral Malleal Fold - Neck to neck in an arch form and to Shrapnell's membrane.

Anterior Pouch of von Tröltsch - Lies between the anterior malleal fold and the portion of the tympanic membrane anterior to the handle of the malleus.

Posterior Pouch of von Tröltsch - Lies between the posterior malleal fold and the portion of the tympanic membrane posterior to the handle of the malleus.

Prussak's Space (Figure 1-7) is bound:

1. Anteriorly by the lateral malleal fold.
2. Posteriorly by the lateral malleal fold.
3. Superiorly by the lateral malleal fold.
4. Inferiorly by the lateral process of the malleus.
5. Medially by the neck of the malleus.
6. Laterally by Shrapnell's membrane.

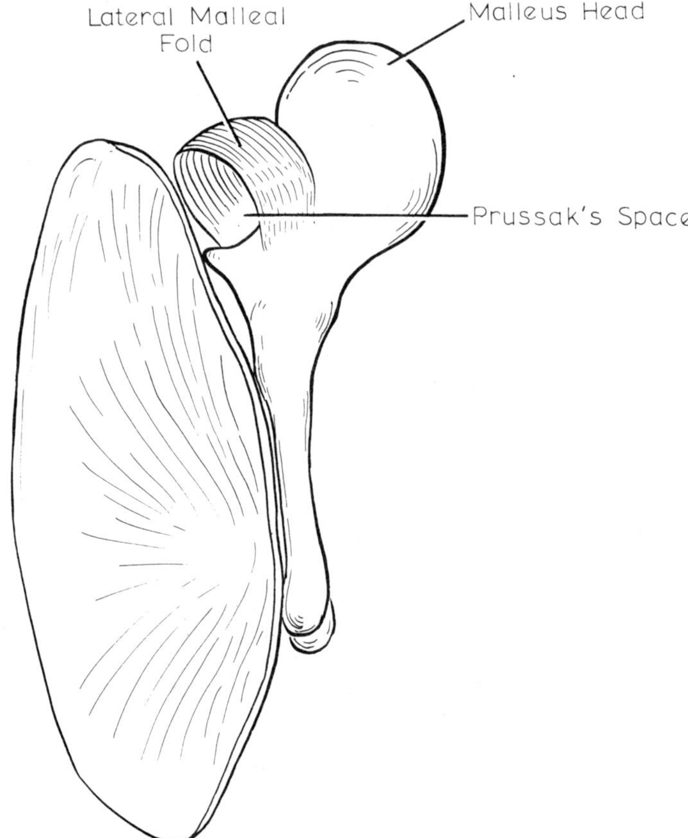

FIG. 1-7. Prussak's Space (Diagrammatic Representation)

The oval window sits in the sagittal plane.

The round window sits in the transverse plane and is protected by an anterior lip from the promontory. It faces postero-inferiorly as well as laterally.

The Tensor Tympani inserts from the cochleariform process onto the medial surface of the upper end of the manubrium. It supposedly pulls the tympanic membrane medially, thus tensing it. It also draws the malleus medially and forward. It raises the resonant frequency and attenuates low frequencies.

The stapedius muscle attaches most frequently to the posterior neck of the stapes. Occasionally it is attached to the posterior crus or head and rarely to the lenticular process. It is attached posteriorly at the pyramidal process. It pulls the stapes posteriorly, supposedly raises the resonant frequency of the ossicular chain and attenuates sound.

EUSTACHIAN TUBE

1. It is 17 to 18 mm at birth and grows to about 35 mm in adult life.

2. At birth the tube is horizontal and grows to be at an incline of 45° in adult life. Thus the pharyngeal orifice is about 15 mm lower than the tympanic orifice.

3. It can be divided into an antero-medial cartilaginous portion (24 mm.) and a postero-lateral bony (11 mm.) portion. The narrowest part of the tube is at the junction of the bony and the cartilaginous portions. (Reminder: the external auditory canal is 1/3 cartilaginous and 2/3 bony).

4. The cartilaginous part of the tube is lined by pseudostratified columnar ciliated epithelium but is lined by ciliated cuboidal epithelium towards the tympanic orifice.

5. It opens by the action of the Tensor Palati (innervated by the 3rd division of the V nerve) acting synergistically with the levator veli palati (innervated by the vagus). In children the only muscle that works is the tensor palati because the levator palati is separated from the eustachian tube cartilage by a considerable distance. Therefore, a cleft palate child with poor tensor palati function is expected to have eustachian tube problems until the levator palati starts to function.

6. In a normal individual a pressure difference of 200 mm. H_2O to 300 mm. H_2O is needed to produce air flow.

7. It is easier to expel air from the middle ear than to get it into the middle ear (reason for more tubal trouble with descent in an airplane).

8. -30 mm. Hg. for 15 minutes or lower can produce a transudate in the middle ear. A pressure differential of 90 mm. Hg. or greater may "lock" the eustachian tube preventing opening of the tube by the muscles. This is called the "critical pressure difference".

9. If the pressure differential exceeds 100 mm. Hg. the tympanic membrane may rupture.

10. Valsalva generates about 20-40 mm. Hg. pressure.

11. The lymphoid tissues within the tube have been referred to as the tonsil of Gerlach.

12. The tympanic ostium of the tube is at the anterior wall of the tympanic cavity about 4 mm. above the most inferior part of the floor of the cavity. The diameter of the ostium is 3-5 mm. The size of the pharyngeal ostium varies from 3 to 10 mm. in its vertical diameter and 2 to 5 mm. in its horizontal diameter.

Figures 1-8 (A) through (O) are temporal bone horizontal sections from Dr. H. F. Schuknecht's Research Laboratory at the Massachusetts Eye and Ear Infirmary.

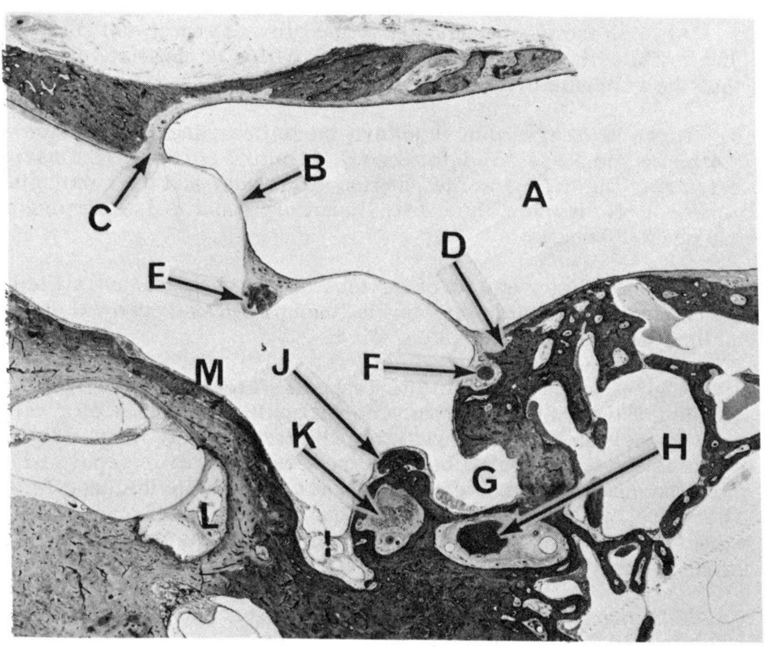

FIG. 1-8 (A).

A = External auditory canal
B = Tympanic membrane
C = Fibrous annulus
D = Tympanic sulcus
E = Malleus handle
F = Chorda tympani
G = Facial recess
H = Facial nerve
I = Sinus tympani
J = Pyramidal process
K = Stapedius muscle
L = Round window
M = Promontory

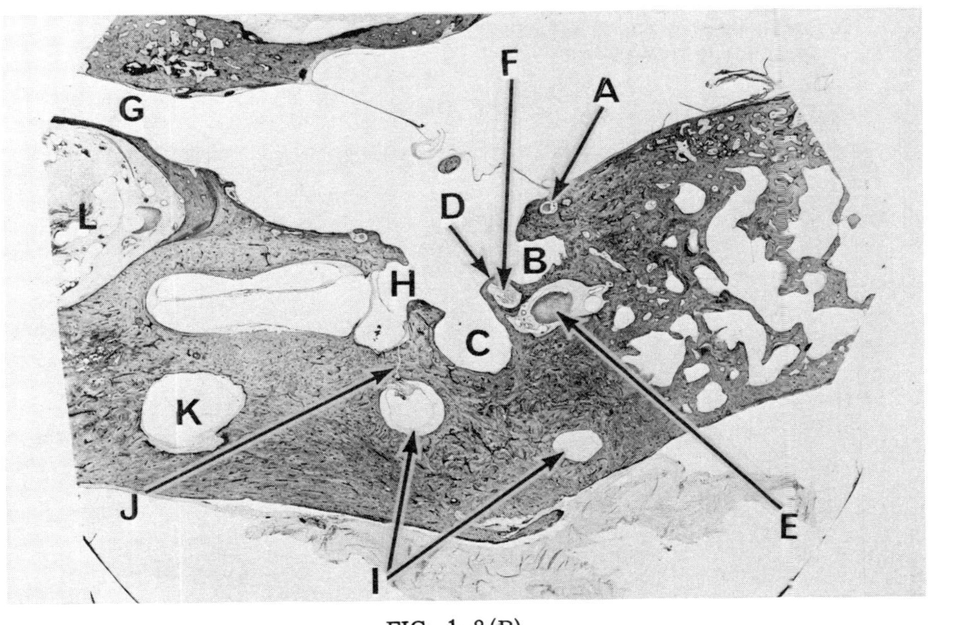

FIG. 1-8 (B).

A = Chorda tympani
B = Facial recess
C = Sinus tympani
D = Pyramidal process
E = Facial nerve
F = Stapedius muscle
G = Eustachian tube
H = Round window niche
I = Posterior semicircular canal
J = Hurtle's fissure
K = Internal auditory meatus
L = Carotid canal

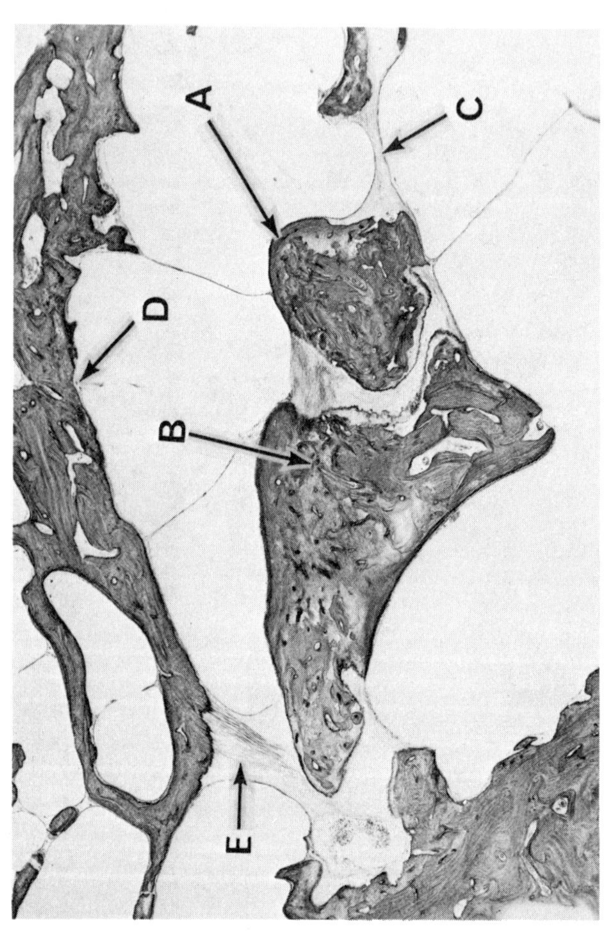

FIG. 1-8 (C).

A = Malleus head
B = Incus body
C = Anterior malleal ligament
D = Lateral wall of the attic
E = Posterior incudal ligament

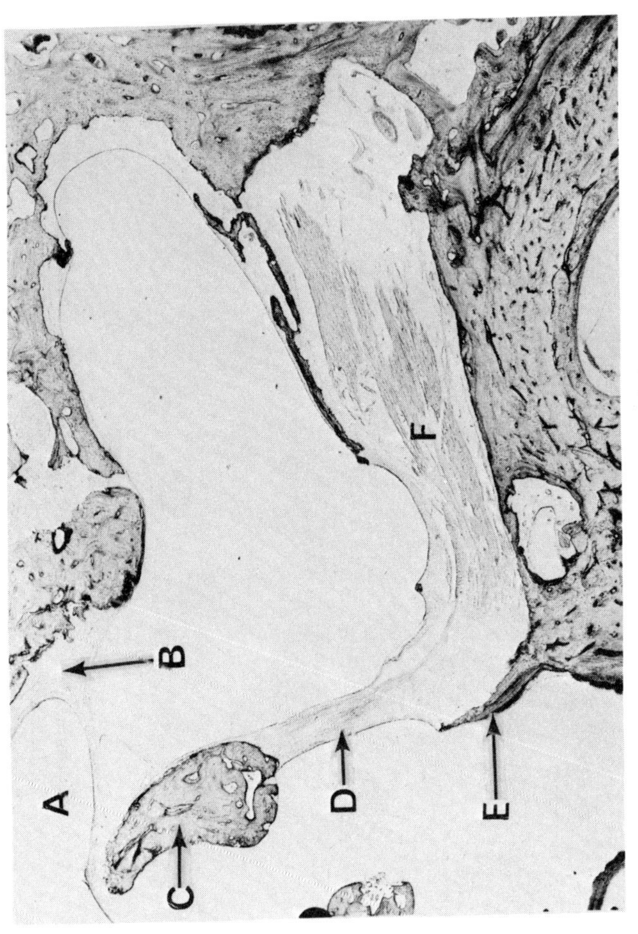

FIG. 1-8 (D).

A = External auditory canal
B = Fibrous annulus
C = Malleus
D = Tendon of tensor tympani
E = Cochleariform process
F = Tensor tympani muscle

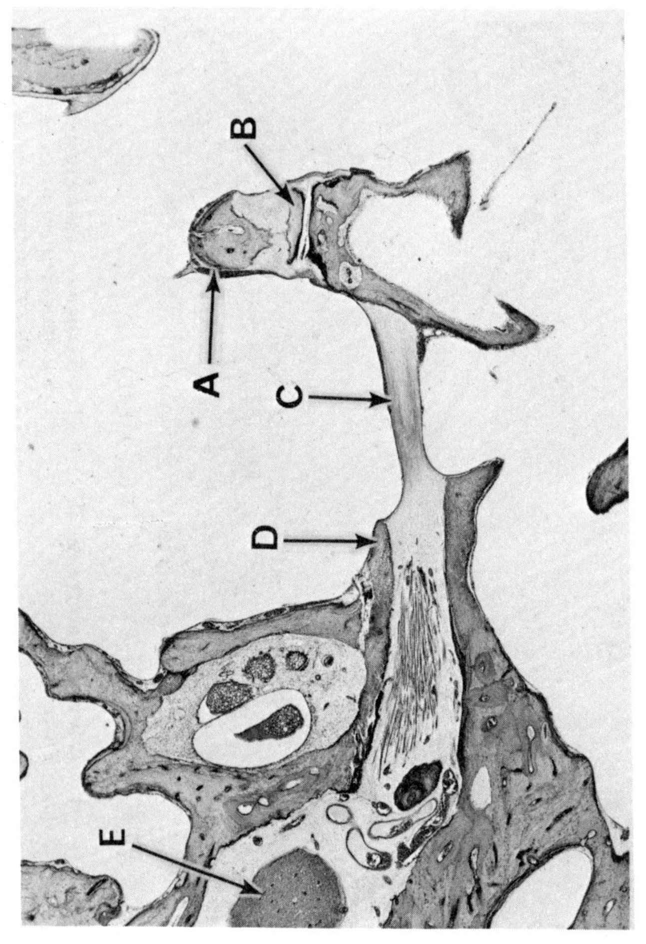

FIG. 1-8(E).

A = Incus
B = Lenticular process
C = Stapedius tendon
D = Pyramidal process
E = Facial nerve

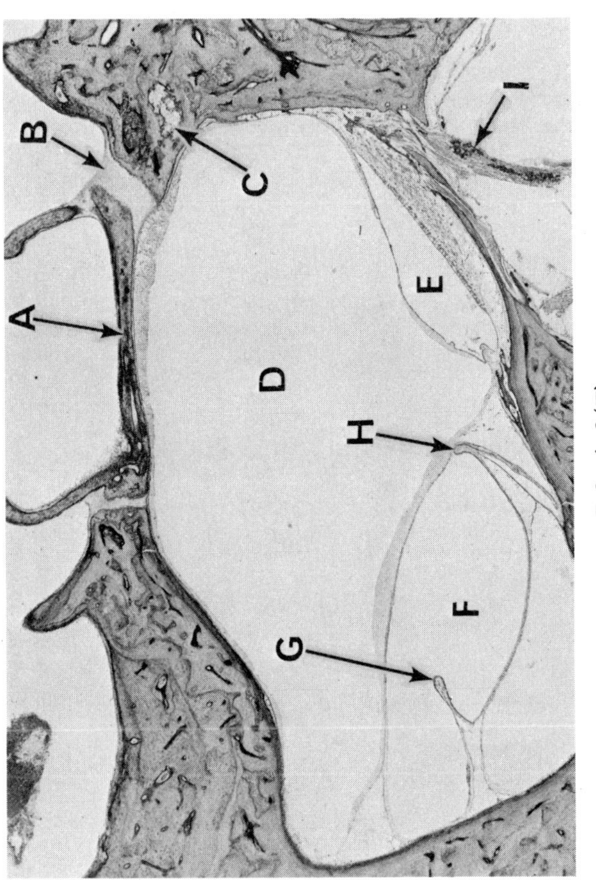

FIG. 1-8 (F).

A = Stapes footplate
B = Annular ligament
C = Fissula ante-fenestrum
D = Vestibule
E = Saccule
F = Utricle
G = Inferior utricular crest
H = Utriculo-endolymphatic valve
I = Saccular nerve

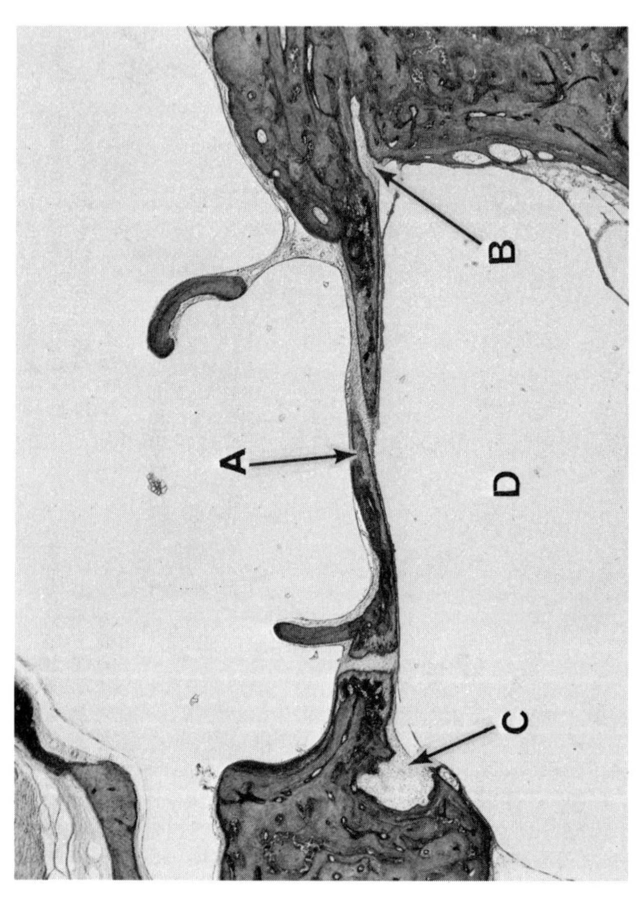

FIG. 1-8 (G).

A = Stapes footplate
B = Fissula ante-fenestrum
C = Fossula post-fenestrum
D = Vestibule

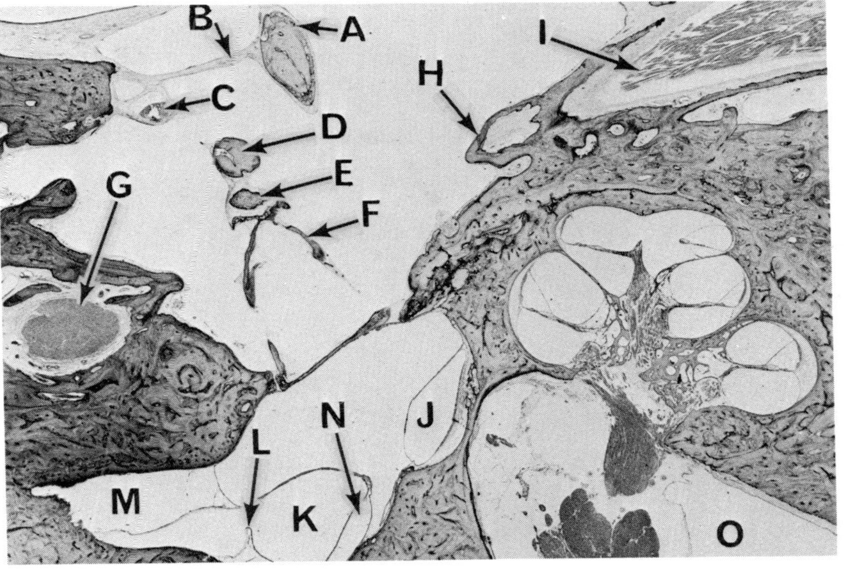

FIG. 1-8 (H)

A = Malleus
B = Tympanic membrane
C = Chorda tympani
D = Incus
E = Lenticular process
F = Stapes
G = Facial nerve
H = Cochleariform process
I = Tensor tympani
J = Saccule
K = Utricle
L = Inferior utricular crest
M = Lateral semicircular canal
N = Sinus of endolymphatic duct
O = Internal auditory canal

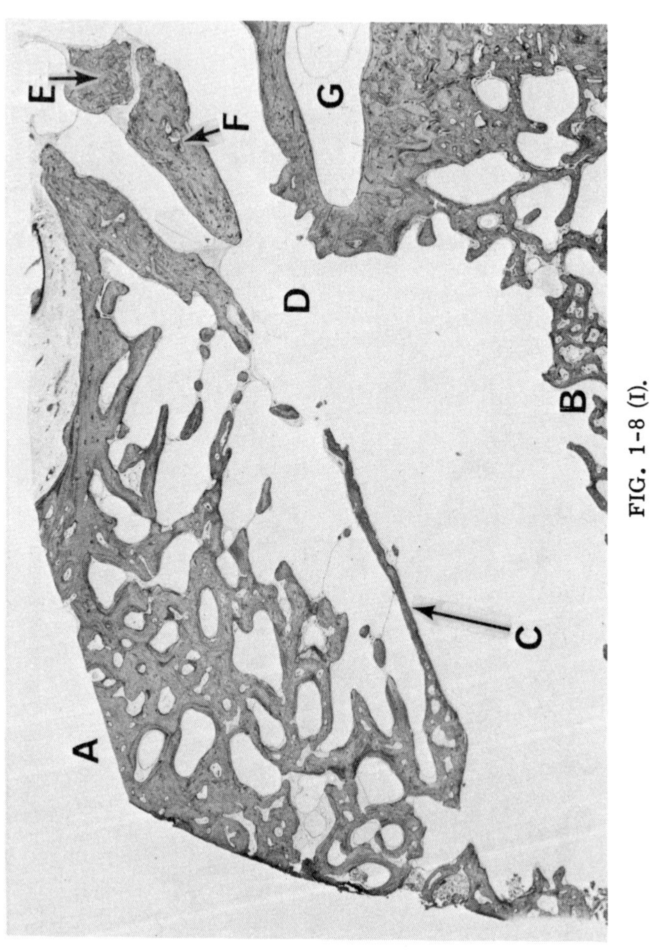

FIG. 1-8 (I).

A = Squamosa part of the temporal bone
B = Petrous part of the temporal bone
C = Koerner's septum
D = Aditus
E = Malleus
F = Incus
G = Lateral semicircular canal

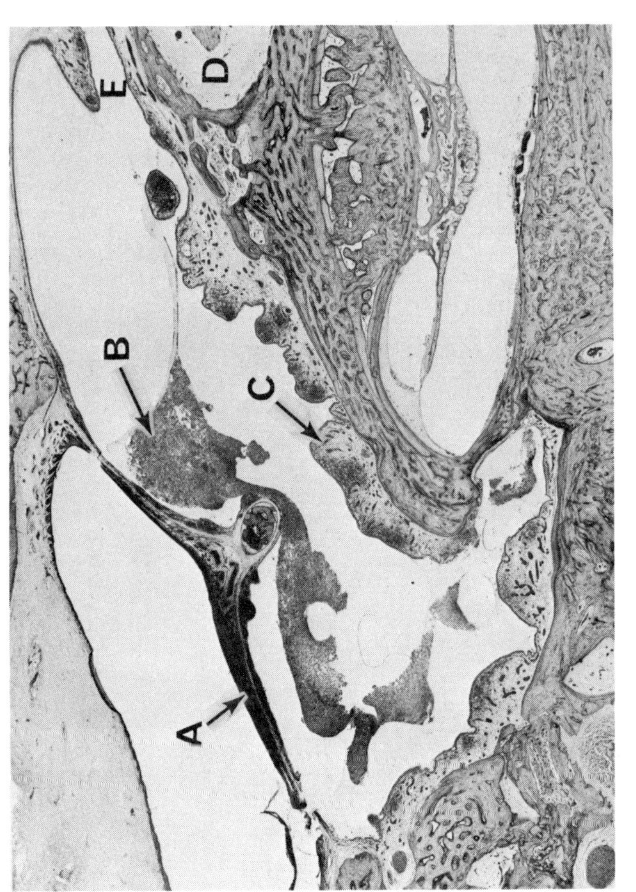

FIG. 1-8 (J). Acute otitis media

A = Tympanic membrane
B = Purulent material
C = Thickened middle ear mucosa
D = Carotid
E = Eustachian tube

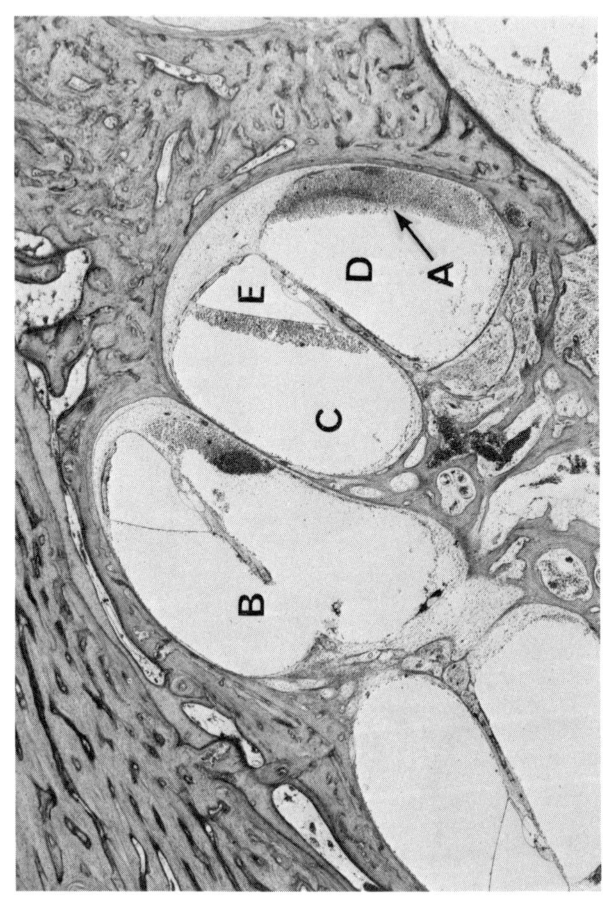

FIG. 1-8 (K). Acute labyrinthitis

A = Leukocytes
B = Helicotrema
C = Scala vestibuli
D = Scala tympani
E = Scala media

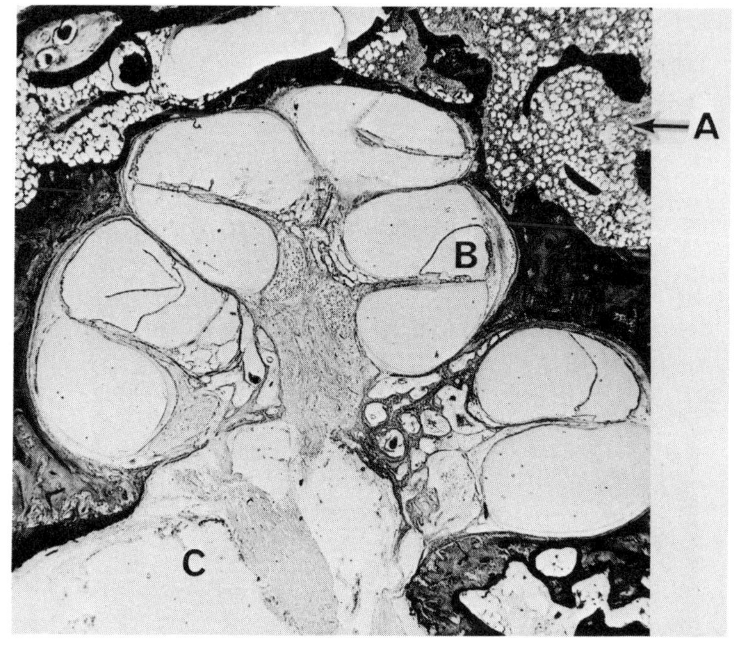

FIG. 1-8(L). Congenital syphilis

A = Luetic changes in the otic capsule
B = Endolymphatic hydrops
C = Internal auditory canal

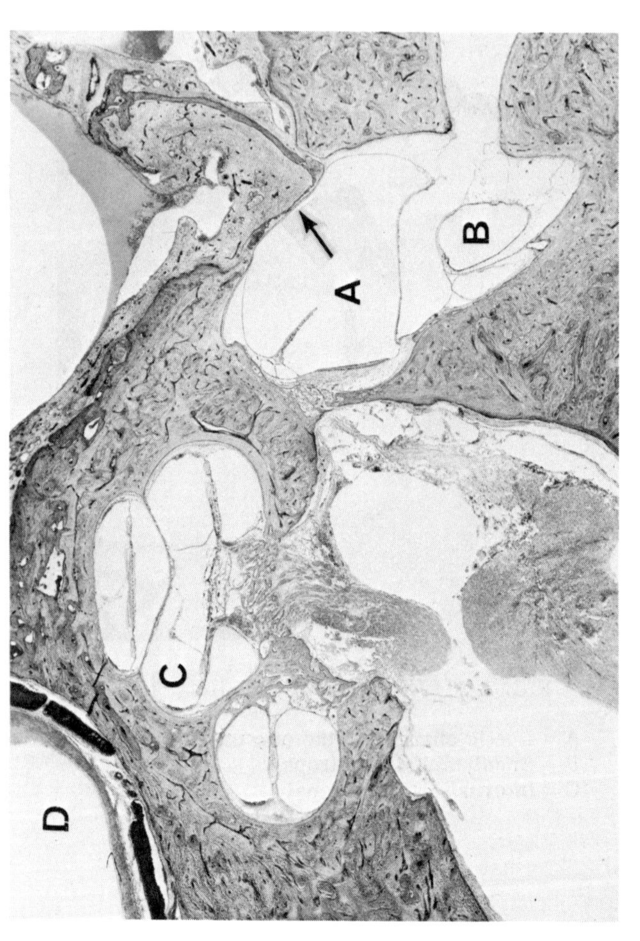

FIG. 1-8 (M). Ménière's Disease

A = Enlarged saccule against footplate
B = Utricle
C = "Distended" cochlear duct
D = Carotid artery

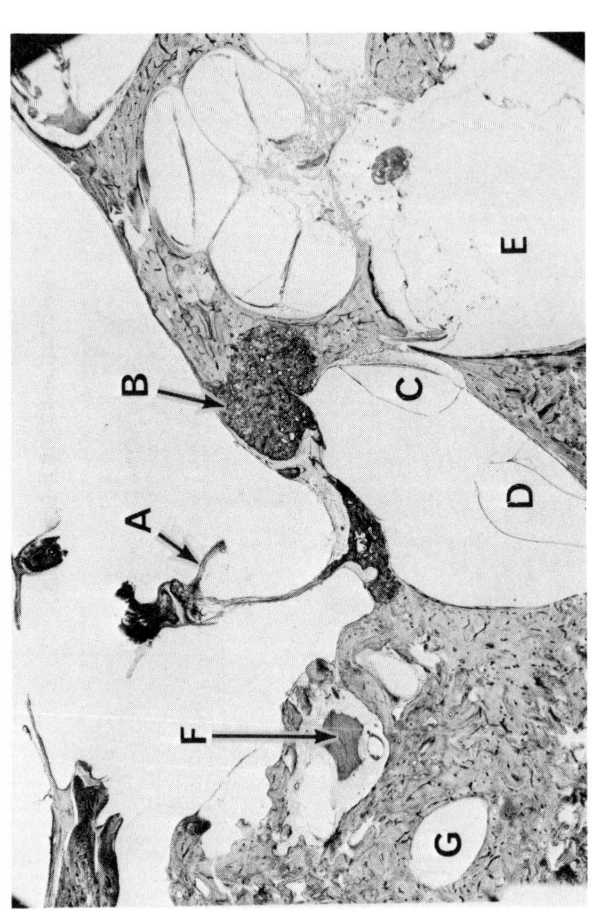

FIG. 1-8 (N). Otosclerosis

A = Stapes
B = Otosclerotic bone
C = Saccule
D = Utricle
E = Internal auditory canal
F = Facial nerve
G = Lateral semicircular canal

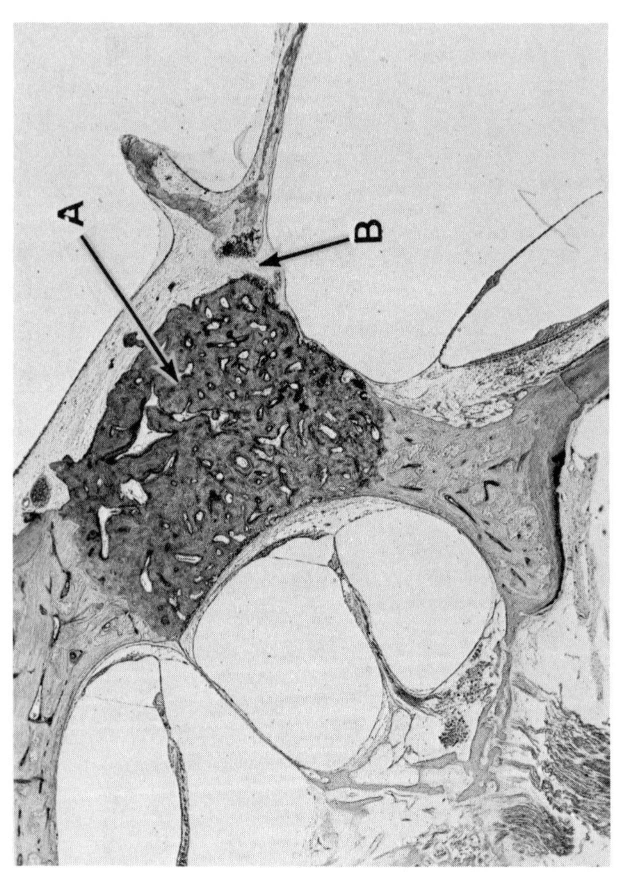

FIG. 1-8 (O). Otosclerosis

A = Histologic otosclerosis without involving the footplate
B = Annular ligament

EMBRYOLOGY OF THE EAR

THE AURICLE: On the 6th week of gestation, condensation of the mesoderm of the 1st and 2nd Arches occurs to give rise to 6 hillocks called the Hillocks of His. The first 3 hillocks are derived from the 1st Arch while the 2nd Arch contributes to the last 3. (Figure 1-9).

1st Arch:	1st Hillock →	Tragus (1)
	2nd Hillock →	Helical crus (2)
	3rd Hillock →	Helix (3)
2nd Arch:	4th Hillock →	Anti-helix (4)
	5th Hillock →	Anti-tragus (5)
	6th Hillock →	Lobule and Lower helix (6)

On the 7th week	formation of cartilage is in progress.
On the 12th week	the auricle is formed by fusion of the hillocks.
On the 20th week	it has reached adult shape although it does not reach adult size till one is 9 years old.

The concha is formed by 3 separate areas from the first groove (ectoderm). (See Figure 1-9)

a) middle part of the 1st groove: concha cavum
b) upper part of the 1st groove: concha cymba
c) lower part of the 1st groove: intertragus incisor

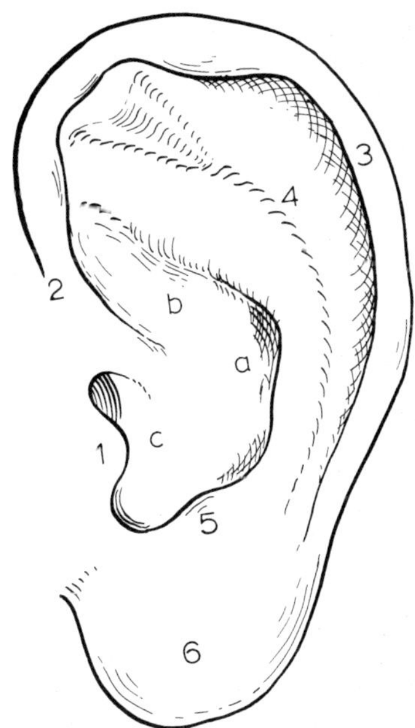

FIG. 1-9. Embryology of the Auricle

THE EXTERNAL AUDITORY CANAL: On the 8th week of gestation, the surface ectoderm in the region of the upper end of the 1st pharyngeal groove (dorsal) thickens. This solid core of epithelium continues to grow towards the middle ear. Simultaneously, the concha cavum deepens to form the outer 1/3 of the external auditory canal. By the 21st week this core begins to resorb and "hollow out" to form a channel. The innermost layer of ectoderm remains to become the superficial layer of the tympanic membrane. Formation of the channel is completed by the 28th week. At birth, the external auditory canal is neither ossified nor of adult size. Completion of ossification occurs around age 3 and adult size is reached at age 9.

THE EUSTACHIAN TUBE AND THE MIDDLE EAR: During the 3rd week of gestation, the 1st and 2nd Pharyngeal Pouches lie laterally on either side of what is to become the oral and pharyngeal tongue. As the 3rd Arch enlarges, the space between the 2nd Arch and the pharynx (1st pouch) is compressed and becomes the Eustachian tube. The "outpocketing" at the lateral end becomes the middle ear space. Because of the proximity to the 1st, 2nd and 3rd Arches, the V, VII, and IX nerves are found in the middle ear. By the 10th week, pneumatization begins. The antrum appears on the 23rd week. However, it is of interest to note that the middle ear is filled with mucoid connective tissue till the time of birth. The 28th week marks the apparition of the tympanic membrane which is derived from all 3 origins.

a) Ectoderm ⟶ Squamous layer
b) Mesoderm ⟶ Fibrous layer
c) Entoderm ⟶ Mucosal layer

Between the 12th and the 28th week, 4 primary mucosal sacs emerge, each becoming a specific anatomical region of the middle ear.

a) Saccus Anticus ⟶ Anterior Pouch of von Tröltsch
b) Saccus Medius ⟶ Epitympanum and petrous area
c) Saccus Superior ⟶ Posterior Pouch of von Tröltsch, part of the mastoid, inferior incudal space.
d) Saccus Posterior ⟶ Round window and oval window niches, sinus tympani.

At birth, the embryonic subepithelium is resorbed and pneumatization continues in the middle ear, antrum and mastoid. Pneumatization of the petrous portion of the temporal bone, being the last to arise, continues till puberty.

The middle ear is well formed at birth and enlarges only slightly postnatally. At age 1, the mastoid process appears. At age 3, the tympanic ring and osseous canal are calcified. The eustachian tube measures approximately 17 mm. at birth and continues to grow to 35 mm. in adulthood.

THE MALLEUS AND INCUS: On the 6th week of embryonic development, the malleus and the incus appear as a single mass. By the 8th week they are separated and the malleal-incudal joint is formed. The head and neck of the malleus are derived from Meckel's cartilage (1st arch mesoderm), the anterior process from the process of Folius (mesenchyme bone) and the manubrium from the Reichert's cartilage (2nd arch mesoderm). The body and short process of the Incus originate from Meckel's cartilage (1st Arch mesoderm) and the long process from Reichert's cartilage (2nd Arch mesoderm). By the 16th week, the ossicles reach adult size. On the 16th week, ossification begins and appears first at the long process of the incus. On the 17th week, the ossification center becomes visible on the medial surface of the neck of the malleus and spreads to the manubrium and the head. At birth, the malleus and incus are of adult size and shape. The ossification of the malleus is never complete so that part of the manubrium remains cartilaginous. (The lenticular process is also known as "Sylvian Apophysis" or "os orbiculare").

THE STAPES: On the 4-1/2th week the mesenchymal cells of the 2nd Arch condense to form the Blastema. The VII nerve divides the Blastema into stapes, Interhyale and Laterohyale. On the 7th week, the stapes ring emerges around the stapedial artery. The lamina stapedialis, which is of the otic mesenchyme appears to become the footplate and annular ligament. On the 8-1/2th week, the Incudal-stapedial joint develops. The Interhyale becomes the stapedial muscle and tendon, the Laterohyale becomes the posterior wall of the middle ear. Together with the otic capsule, the laterohyale also becomes the pyramidal process and facial canal. The lower part of the facial canal is said to be derived from Reichert's Cartilage.

On the 10th week, the stapes changes its ring shape to "stirrup" shape. On the 19th week, ossification begins and starts at the obturator surface of the stapedial base. The ossification is completed by the 28th week except for the vestibular surface of the footplate which remains cartilaginous throughout life. At birth the stapes is of adult size and form.

THE INNER EAR: On the 3rd week, neuroectoderm and ectoderm lateral to the first Branchial Groove condense to form the otic Placode. The latter invaginates until completely submerged and surrounded by mesoderm to become the otocyst or otic Vesicle by the 4th week. The 5th week marks the appearance of a wide dorsal and a slander ventral part of the otic vesicle. Between these 2 parts, the endolymphatic duct and sac develop. On the 6th week, the semicircular canals take shape and by the 8th week, together with the utricle, they are fully formed. Formation of the basal turn of the cochlea takes place on the 7th week and by the 12th week the complete 2-1/2 turns are developed. Development of the saccule follows that of the utricle. Evidently, the pars superior (semicircular canals and utricle) is developed prior to the pars inferior (saccule and cochlea). Formation of the membranous labyrinth without the end organ is said to be complete by the 15th week of gestation.

Concurrent to the formation of the membranous labyrinth, the precursor of the otic capsule emerges on the 8th week as a condensation of mesenchyme precartilage. The 14 centers of ossification can be identified on the 15th week and ossification is completed on the 23rd week of gestation. The last area to ossify is the Fissula ante fenestrum which may remain cartilaginous throughout life. Other than the endolymphatic sac which continues to grow till adulthood, the membranous and bony labyrinth are of adult size at the 23rd week of embryonic development. The endolymphatic sac is the 1st to appear and the last to stop growing.

At the 3rd week, the common macula first appears. Its upper part differentiates into the utricular macula and the cristae of the superior and lateral semicircular canals, whereas its lower part becomes the macula of the saccule and the crista of the posterior semicircular canal. On the 8th week, 2 ridges of cells as well as the stria vascularis are identifiable. On the 11th week, the vestibular end organs complete with sensory and supporting cells are formed. On the 20th week, development of the stria vascularis and the tectorial membrane is completed. On the 23rd week, the 2 ridges of cells divide into Inner Ridge Cells and Outer Ridge Cells. The Inner Ridge Cells become the spiral limbus, the outer ones become the hair cells, pillar cells, Hensen's cells and Deiter's cells. On the 26th week, the tunnel of Corti and Canal of Nuvel are formed.

The Neuro-crest cells lateral to the Rhombencephalon condense to form the Acoustic-Facial Ganglion which differentiates into the Facial geniculate ganglion, superior vestibular ganglion (utricle, superior and horizontal semicircular canals) and inferior ganglion (saccule, posterior semicircular canal and cochlea).

At birth, 4 elements of the Temporal Bone are distinguishable: petrous, squamous, tympanic ring and styloid process. The mastoid antrum is present but the mastoid process is not formed till the end of the 2nd year of life and pneumatization of the mastoid soon follows. The tympanic ring extends laterally after birth forming the osseous canal.

CLINICAL INFORMATION

1. Congenital Microtia occurs about one in 20,000 births.

2. The auricle is formed early. Therefore, malformation of the auricle implies malformation of the middle ear, mastoid and VII nerve. On the other hand, a normal auricle with canal atresia indicates abnormal development in the 28th week, by which time ossicles and middle ear are already formed.

3. Improper fusion of the 1st and 2nd Branchial arches results in a Preauricular Sinus Tract (epithelial lined).

4. Malformation of 1st Branchial Arch and groove results in:
    a) Auricle abnormality (1st and 2nd arches)
    b) Bony Meatus atresia (1st groove)
    c) Abnormal incus and malleus (1st and 2nd arches)
    d) Abnormal mandible (1st arch)

When the maxilla is also malformed, this constellation of findings is called Treacher-Collins Syndrome (Mandibular-Facial Dysostosis):
- a) Outward-downward slanted eyes (anti-Mongoloid)
- b) Notched lower lid

c) Short mandible
d) Bony meatal atresia
e) Malformed incus and malleus
f) Fish mouth

5. Abnormalities of the otic capsule and labyrinth are rare because they are phylogenetically ancient.

6. An incidence of 20-30% dehiscent tympanic portion of the VII nerve has been reported.

7. The incidence of absent stapedius tendon, muscle and pyramidal eminence is estimated at 1%.

8. 20 percent of preauricular cysts are bilateral.

REFERENCES

1. Allam, A.: Pneumatization of the Temporal Bone, Ann. Otol. Rhin. Laryng. 78: 49, 1969.

2. Anson, B.J., Donaldson, J.A.: Surgical Anatomy of the Temporal Bone and Ear, 2nd Ed., W.B. Saunders Co., Philadelphia, 1973.

3. Hough, J.: Malformations and Anatomical Variations Seen in the Middle Ear During the Operation for Mobilization of the Stapes, Laryngoscope: 68: 1337, 1958.

4. Hough, J.V.D.: Malformations and Anatomical Variations Seen in the Middle Ear During Operations on the Stapes, American Academy of Ophthalmology and Otolaryngology Manual, 1961.

5. May, M.: Anatomy of the Facial Nerve (Spacial orientation of fibres in the temporal bone), Laryngoscope 83: 1311, 1973.

6. Pearson, A.A., et al.: The Development of the Ear, American Academy of Ophthalmology and Otolaryngology Manual, 1967.

7. Proctor, B.: Embryology and Anatomy of the Eustachian Tube, Arch. Otolaryng. 86: 503, 1967.

8. Proctor, B.: The Development of the Middle Ear Spaces and Their Surgical Significance, J. Laryng. 78: 631, 1964.

9. Proctor, B.: Surgical Anatomy of the Posterior Tympanum. Ann. Otol. Rhin. Laryng. 78: 1026, 1969.

10. Schuknecht, H.F.: Pathology of the Ear, Harvard University Press, Boston, 1974.

CHAPTER 2

HEARING AND SPEECH

I. THEORIES OF HEARING

The words, "theories of hearing", commonly refer to theories relating to the method by which the ear is able to discriminate pitch. The principal theories are the place theory, the frequency theory, the volley theory, and the traveling wave theory.

THE PLACE THEORY: The place theory is based on the assumption that pitch discrimination is determined by a certain place along the basilar membrane being set into maximum vibration, which in turn excites the sensory nerve fibers at that place. It was presumed that every particular section of the basilar membrane is tuned so that its resonance characteristics will correspond to the frequency of some audible tone. This theory was propounded by Hermann von Helmholtz, who considered the 24,000 or so transverse fibers of the basilar membrane to be tuned like the strings of a piano or a harp. It was thought that when sound waves containing those frequencies were received by the ear, the appropriate fibers would resonate automatically to those pitches thus stimulating the hair cells of the Organ of Corti which rests on those fibers of the membrane. It was assumed that because the transverse fibers at the base of the cochlear are short, they resonate to high pitches. The longer fibers near the apex were thought to resonate to lower pitches. Later exponents of the place theory did not think that the tuning of the basilar membrane was as sharp as Helmholtz had thought, but agreed that a particular region of stimulation in the basilar membrane was responsible for the perception of a particular pitch.

THE FREQUENCY THEORY: This theory explains pitch perception by suggesting that all parts of the basilar membrane are stimulated by every frequency and that the determination of pitch perception is based upon the number of times per second that the fibers of the auditory nerve discharge. For example, this theory holds that an auditory stimulus of 1,000 Hz causes fibers within the auditory nerve to discharge at a rate of 1,000 times per second and that pitch is appreciated in the brain, not in the cochlea. The frequency theory is also known as the "telephone" theory, because displacements along the basilar membrane are in phase with the movements of the stapes, much like a telephone diaphragm. Studies of action potentials of nerve fibers have demonstrated that the maximum rate of discharge of nerve impulses from the peripheral auditory nerve fibers is about a thousand per second. This means that the discrimination of pitches above this frequency could not be explained on the basis of the frequency theory. Rutherford, and more recently Boring, were exponents of this theory.

THE VOLLEY THEORY: This theory combines elements of the place theory and the frequency theory and holds that perception of pitch for frequencies up to 5,000 Hz can be explained on the basis of the frequency of nerve impulses firing in volleys. It holds that the primary explanation for perception of pitch for frequencies in excess of 5,000 Hz is the place of greatest excitation along the basilar membrane. The volley theory is advocated by Weaver.

THE TRAVELLING WAVE THEORY: This is one of the place theories which holds that pitch discrimination is determined when a certain place along the basilar membrane is set into maximum vibration. The place on the membrane where the nerve endings will be stimulated depends upon where the maximum displacement of the travelling wave occurs. Support for the travelling wave theory is contributed by experimentation carried out by George von Békésy. According to Békésy the energy for creating the travelling wave comes from the stapes, but the wave starting at one end, runs along the length of the membrane gradually increasing in amplitude until it gains maximal displacement. The wave travels from the base to the apex of the cochlea and the maximum amplitude occurs at a point along the basilar membrane that corresponds to the frequency of the stimulus. Increasing the frequency of the tone moves the place of maximal vibration toward the base of the cochlea, decreasing the frequency moves it in the direction of the apex.

These four theories of hearing are concerned with how the ear discriminates pitch. Intensity discrimination appears to be dependent upon the number of nerve fibers activated, the total number of impulses per second of all fibers, and the existence of fibers that tend to respond to stimuli which fit a particular category of intensity.

II. THEORY OF BONE CONDUCTION

Air conduction thresholds reflect what is happening in the outer, middle, and inner ear as a package, while bone conduction thresholds provide direct information about the function of the inner ear. Thus, by subtracting bone conduction from air conduction thresholds, the amount of conductive hearing loss when present can be ascertained. For this reason differential diagnostic audiometry relies heavily on the measurement of bone conduction.

The device used for bone conduction measurements is a small vibrator that is usually attached to a headband which holds it firmly against the skull. It is usually positioned behind the ear on the mastoid process of the temporal bone. Sometimes the vibrator is placed on the forehead when bone conduction is tested. When sound vibrations reach an intensity of 40 or 50 dB above the normal air conduction threshhold they may set the skull into vibration and set up pressure waves in the cochlear fluids. At low frequencies the skull vibrates as a unit while segmental vibrations of the skull occur at the higher frequencies. The two different types of vibrational patterns result in two types of transmission of sound, inertial and compressional. For frequencies below 800 Hz when the skull vibrates as a unit, the ossicular chain, the mandible, and the cochlear fluids tend to lag behind the skull due to inertia. The lagging action of the ossicular chain causes movement of the stapes relative to the oval window and stimulates hearing in the same manner as in air conduction stimulation. Compressional bone conduction occurs at frequencies above 800 Hz and is related to the difference in mobility between the round and oval windows. When the compressional forces of the skull are transmitted to the inner ear they act on the noncompressible fluids of the inner ear, vestibule, and semicircular canals, and cause these fluids to move toward or away from the more mobile round window depending upon the phase of the wave. This fluid movement may result in deformation of the basilar membrane sufficient to stimulate the sensation of hearing. While some theorists believe low frequency hearing to be due entirely to inertial factors and high frequency hearing to be due to compressional factors, others feel that both inertial and compressional factors are present in hearing for all frequencies.

III. PHYSIOLOGY OF THE HEARING IN THE MIDDLE EAR

The average surface area of the tympanic membrane = 70 to 80 sq. mm.

Weight of tympanic membrane = 14 mg, elasticity = 4.9×10^{-8} dynes.

The average surface area of the vibrating portion of the tympanic membrane = 55 sq. mm.

The surface of the footplate = 3.2 to 3.5 sq. mm.

The surface area of the round window is 2 sq.mm.

Lever mechanism =

$$\frac{\text{Length of the long process of the malleus}}{\text{Length of the long process of the incus}} = \frac{1.3}{1} \text{ or } 2.5 \text{ dB}$$

$$\text{Hydraulic action} = \frac{\text{Vibrating TM}}{\text{Footplate}} = \frac{55}{3.2} = 17 \text{ or } 25 \text{ dB}$$

Total Transformer ratio = (1.3 x 17) : 1 = 22:1 or 27.5 dB

MISCELLANEOUS:

1. Auditory range of a human being is about 10 cycles per second to about 24,000 cycles per second. The intensity range is from about 0 to 120 dB or 0.0002 dynes per cm^2 to 200 dynes per cm^2.

2. Increase of mass within the middle ear space will produce a high frequency hearing loss. An increase of stiffness within the middle ear space would give a low frequency hearing loss.

3. a) Maximum conductive hearing loss with an intact ossicular chain with no pars tensa is approximately 40 to 45 dB.
   b) Ossicular discontinuity with no pars tensa gives a maximal conductive loss of 40 to 45 dB.
   c) Ossicular discontinuity with an intact tympanic membrane may give a 50 to 55 dB conductive hearing loss.

4. The maximal increase in sound pressure occurs when the applied sound has a wave length 4 times the effective length of the external auditory canal. The resonant frequency of the external auditory canal is 3,000 cycles per second, that of the ossicles and tympanic membrane is about 800 cycles per second.

5. a) Hyperacusis = an unusually low threshold level for hearing. It is not necessarily associated with low tolerance to sound.
   b) Dysacusis = disturbance of discrimination of speech, abnormal tone quality, pitch or loudness.
   c) Hypoacusis = hearing thresholds above the limit of normal.
   d) Paracusis Willisane = a person with a conductive hearing loss hears better in a noisy environment.
   e) Central Hearing Impairment = a defect of hearing due to a lesion within the auditory nervous system but not involving the primary neuron.
   f) Central Auditory Imperception = receptive aphasia (sensory aphasia) in which the patient hears but does not understand.
   g) Monaural Diplacusis = disorder in which pure tones are perceived as impure or noisy tones.
   Binaural Diplacusis = disorder in which the same pitch sounds different in the 2 ears.
   h) Phonemic Regression = the loss of discrimination which leads to an inability to differentiate phonemes. This happens in the elderly who have difficulty understanding in spite of the fact that sentences are presented at proper thresholds. Their discrimination is improved by presenting the sentences slowly. This defect is due to loss of central communicating neurons and axons.

6. When the external auditory meatus of the test ear is occluded, the bone conduction thresholds are improved in normal patients and in those with sensorineural hearing loss. This is not true in patients with conductive hearing loss. (Occlusion effect).

7. Usual Norms:
   - 4-month-old baby = responds to mother's sounds.
   - 6-month-old baby = turns head to a source of sound located three to four feet away.
   - 24-month-old baby = responds to some words and perhaps phrases; able to obtain thresholds with play audiometry.
   - 40-month-old baby = is able to perform a conventional audiogram if cooperative.

8. Any conductive hearing loss greater than 40 dB suggests ossicular problems.

9. "Intensity Difference Limen" = the smallest detectable change in intensity. "Frequency Difference Limen" = the smallest detectable change in frequency.

10. Sono-inversion = the round window is open to the external auditory canal while the oval window is protected.

11. Inter-aural attenuation is estimated to be between 40 and 50 dB by air conduction. Inter-aural attenuation for bone conduction is O dB.

IV. TUNING FORK TESTS

Every otological patient should be tested with a tuning fork before an audiogram is performed. If the responses to the tuning fork do not agree with the audiogram, the situation should be resolved with repeated testing and repeated audiometric studies. Clinically, the most useful fork is the 512. A negative Rinné response to the 512 fork indicates a 25 to 30 dB or greater conductive hearing loss. A 256 fork may be felt rather than heard. Besides, ambient noises are also in the low frequencies, around 250 cycles per second. When striking the fork, it is essential to strike it gently to avoid overtones. The maximum output of a tuning fork is about 60 dB.

WEBER TEST: In this test the tuning fork is placed on a midline structure on the skull. The forehead, the nasal bone, and the incisor teeth are favorite sites. In a normal individual the tone is heard symmetrically in both ears. In a person with a sensori-neural hearing loss, the tone lateralizes to the opposite ear. It lateralizes to the ear with conductive hearing loss. Possible reasons for this are:

a) less masking noise via air conduction from the environment in the ear with conductive hearing loss.
b) an abnormal conductive mechanism prevents escape of energy through the ossicular chain thus enhancing bone conduction.

RINNÉ TEST: This test compares the loudness of the sound perceived when holding the tuning fork next to the external auditory canal with holding it against the mastoid. It is important to place the fork firmly against the mastoid (preferably near the posterior-superior edge of the bony canal) and to hold the tines of the fork about 1 inch lateral to the tragus.

A negative Rinné with a 256 fork implies a conductive deficit of 15 dB or more. However, the 256 fork is not a reliable fork to use for this test. The 512 fork is the most commonly used fork. A negative Rinné with this fork implies a 25-30 dB or more conductive hearing loss. A 1024 fork would give a negative Rinné when a conductive loss is 35 dB or more.

BING TEST: The tuning fork is applied to the forehead and lateralization is noted when present. The external auditory meatus of one side is then occluded. The patient is to indicate whether the intensity of the sound has increased or whether it lateralizes to the occluded side. This is repeated with occlusion of the opposite ear.

In an ear with a normal sound conduction mechanism (i.e., a normal ear or one with sensori-neural hearing loss) occlusion of the meatus would intensify the sound or cause lateralization to that ear. An ear with a significant conductive hearing loss would have no effect from occlusion of the meatus.

GELLE TEST: A tuning fork is placed against the mastoid. The intensity of the sound heard is compared with various amounts of pressure applied against the tympanic membrane. An increase in pressure results in a decrease in intensity of bone conduction if the tympanic membrane and ossicular chain are mobile and intact. When ossicular discontinuity or fixation is present, there is no decrease in intensity with an increase in applied pressure.

LEWIS TEST: A tuning fork is placed against the mastoid. When it is no longer heard, it is placed against the tragus with gentle occlusion of the meatus. The patient is then asked if he hears the tone again. The interpretation of this test is neither simple nor consistent.

SCHWABACH TEST: This test compares the hearing acuity of the patient with that of the tester as transmitted by a vibrating fork applied on the mastoid. (Assuming the tester has normal hearing.)

The tuning fork can also be used to test recruitment and diplacusis between the two ears.

V. AUDIOLOGY

1. The Decibel: In general, the decibel is a measure of the intensity of a sound and may refer to either sound power or sound pressure. In the usual application, the measurement of hearing by audiometry, the decibel refers to sound pressure. Some sources have erroneously stated that one decibel is equal to the smallest "just noticeable difference" that the ear can detect. While this is approximately true, it would be more accurate to say that the just noticeable difference varies as a function of sound intensity. For very faint sounds, the difference must be three or four decibels to be perceived while for very intense sounds the normal ear can detect changes as small as 0.3 dB. A tone that is made 10 dB more intense than another, is likely to be perceived as twice as loud.

To further understand the decibel, it should be noted that intensity is a physical attribute of sound which can be manipulated and measured with appropriate electronic equipment in a laboratory. The psychological correlate of intensity is loudness. The sensation of loudness is related to stimulus intensity but not on a one to one basis. For soft sounds, a relatively small change in absolute intensity units will cause a change in loudness. However, for relatively loud sounds, it is possible to make large changes in absolute intensity units without getting a perceived change in the sensation of loudness. In terms of sound pressure, the loudest sound that the normal ear can tolerate is about 10,000,000 times that of the softest sound it can hear. Since the ear detects differences in loudness by ratios of pressure or power rather than by actual differences, a logarithmic system employing decibels has been adopted by acoustic scientists and engineers.

Technically, the decibel can be defined as the logarithm of the ratio of two sound powers. The formula which relates intensity or sound power to decibels is

$$NdB = \frac{I_1}{I_0}$$

where power is given in watts/cm^2. Since it is a mathematical fact that acoustic pressures are proportional to the square root of the corresponding acoustic powers, it is possible to derive a formula which relates changes in sound pressure to decibels. It has already been noted that for purposes of hearing measurement we usually deal with acoustic pressure. The formula relating changes in sound pressure to decibels is:

$$NdB = 20 \log \frac{P1}{P2}$$

(P1 = the greater pressure in dynes/cm^2
P2 = the lesser sound pressure)

(Remember that we are interested in the ratio of one pressure to another).

Suppose that we would like to know how many dB a tone will increase if we increase the sound pressure one hundredfold. The formula would be applied as follows:

$$NdB = 20 \log \frac{100}{1}$$

(the pressure ratio $\frac{P1}{P2}$ with a one hundredfold increase in pressure would be 100:1)

$$NdB = 20 (\log 100)$$

$$NdB = 20 (2) - 40 \text{ dB}$$

The log of a number is the power to which the base 10 must be raised to give that number. Common log tables are available to make this determination, although when the number under discussion is 1, followed by a number of zeroes, the log of that number can be found by simply adding up the zeroes. For example, the log of 1000 = 3, the log of 10,000 = 4, etc.

Unless otherwise stated, the standard reference pressure is 0.0002 dynes/cm^2. The standard reference for power is 10^{-16} watts/cm^2. When dB are calculated using the standard reference pressure as the denominator of the pressure ratio in the dB formula, it is customary to refer to the results as dB SPL (sound pressure level).

Some common sound pressure levels associated with different sounds are:

SOUND	dB SPL
Leaves rustling in light breeze	20
Whisper at 5 feet	30
Conversational speech at 3 feet	60
Noisy restaurant	70
Shouted speech	90
Thunder clap	120
Riveting gun	130
Jet engine (100 feet)	140
Threshold of pain	140

AUDIOMETRIC REFERENCE LEVELS

SOUND PRESSURE LEVEL (SPL): Stimulus levels in pure tone audiometry may be stated with reference to Sound Pressure Level (SPL), Sensation Level (SL), or Hearing Level (HL). From the discussion of the decibel it may be recalled that the standard reference for pressure is 0.0002 dynes/cm^2 or the standard reference for power is 10^{-16} watts/cm^2. Whenever decibels are discussed in terms of the pressure standard they are given as dB SPL. A 50 dB SPL tone is 50 dB above the reference pressure, 0.0002 dynes/cm^2. Occasionally steady state industrial noise or audiometric masking noise will be specified in SPL.

HEARING LEVEL (HL): Audiometric test tones are specified in HL rather than SPL because the normal ear is not equally sensitive to low and high pitched tones. According to current standards (ANSI, 1969) it takes 39 dB more SPL for the normal ear to barely hear a 125 Hz tone than it does for it to barely hear a 1000 Hz tone. Since it is desirable to have a zero dB dial reading at the point where the normal ear can just barely hear the stimulus, regardless of frequency, the audiometer has been designed to compensate for differences in hearing sensitivity as a function of frequency.

If O dB HL is set on the attenuator dial, the sound pressure generated by the audiometer will automatically change, whenever the frequency selection dial is rotated to select a different test frequency. Table 2-1 shows how many dB SPL is required at each frequency to achieve O dB HL according to current as well as past standards.

TABLE 2-1

FREQUENCY (in Hz)	PRESENT STANDARD (ANSI-1969, same as ISO, 1964) dB re 0.0002 dynes/cm^2	PAST AMERICAN STANDARD ASA - 1951 dB re 0.0002 dynes/cm^2
125	45.5	54.5
250	24.5	39.5
500	11.0	25.0
1000	6.5	16.5
1500	6.5	
2000	8.5	17.0
3000	7.5	
4000	9.0	15.0
6000	8.0	
8000	9.5	21.0

SENSATION LEVEL (SL): Sensation Level (SL) is another way to refer to stimulus intensity. Its reference is the threshold of the individual being tested. Thus, 30 dB SL means 30 dB above the individual's threshold for test stimulus, whether it be tone or some other types of sound.

The term SL is often used to specify the level at which speed discrimination tests are administered. For instance, if an individual's speech reception threshold is 40 dB HL, a speech discrimination test administered at the 30 dB sensation level will be given at a Hearing Level (HL) of 70 dB. If his speech reception threshold was 10 dB HL, the speech discrimination test would have to be given at the 40 dB Hearing Level to meet the condition of a 30 dB SL presentation.

The SISI test, which employs pure tones, is usually administered at the 20 dB Sensation Level.

SUMMARY:

A. O dB SPL is equivalent to a sound pressure level of 0.0002 dynes/cm^2, O dB intensity level is equivalent to 10^{-16} watts/cm^2.

B. O dB HL (audiometric zero) has different sound pressures for different frequencies. This is because the normal ear requires less sound pressure to make a tone audible in the middle frequencies than in the very low or very high frequencies. For example, O dB HL for 250 Hz is 24.5 dB above 0.0002 dynes/cm^2 (24.5 dB SPL), while O dB HL for 2000 Hz is 8.5 dB above 0.0002 dynes/cm^2 (8.5 dB SPL). In order to simplify the appearance of an audiometric curve, the audiometer is set such that O dB for each frequency does not generate O dB SPL (0.0002 dynes/cm^2) but produces the necessary energy to be just audible to the normal subject. Hence, the O dB on the audiometric dial is not O dB SPL or 0.0002 dynes/cm^2 but rather the threshold of normal subjects. For example, a patient whose threshold at 500 Hz is 30 dB has a threshold that is 30 dB higher than that of normal subjects at 500 Hz but not 30 dB higher than 0.0002 dynes/cm^2.

C. Sensation Level (SL) for auditory stimulus is based on the individual's threshold for that stimulus whether the hearing is normal or impaired. The 20 dB SL for a 500 Hz tone in a person who has an audiometric threshold of 50 dB HL for the 500 Hz tone is 70 dB HL.

SPECIAL AUDITORY TESTS

Pure tone air and bone conduction thresholds provide important but limited diagnostic information about an individual's hearing. A number of special tests have been developed which contribute additional and supplementary information. Among these special tests which will be discussed in this chapter are the Alternate Binaural Loudness Balance (ABLB), Short Increment Sensitivity Index (SISI), Tone Decay, Békésy, and PI-PB function. These special auditory tests contribute information about the site of lesion and are most effective when employed as a battery rather than as a single test.

A. ALTERNATE BINAURAL LOUDNESS BALANCE: This is a test for loudness recruitment which was first described by E. P. Fowler. It explores the growth of loudness in a relatively normal ear. The patient is required to determine when tones presented at different levels sound equally loud to both ears. If, as intensity is increased to the pathological ear, the perceived loudness of the signal grows more rapidly than it does in a normal ear, the pathological ear is said to demonstrate recruitment. The presence of recruitment is associated with a cochlear lesion.

The ABLB test for recruitment is commonly used when one ear is within normal limits and the impaired ear is at least 20 dB poorer for the frequency to be tested. Provided that these criteria are met, the ABLB test can be carried out by any audiometric frequency.

For best results, the test requires an audiometer with which the tester can present pulses of a tone of the same frequency but of different intensity level, alternately to each ear of a patient.

(Reger's Test is a monaural balance test comparing the loudness of two frequencies in the same ear. This test is used when the threshold of the frequency is about the same in both ears).

Interpretation: Recruitment is (a) rarely, if ever, associated with middle ear pathology, (b) present in pathologies associated with acoustic insult, ototoxic drugs and Ménière's disease at certain stages, and (c) indicative of a cochlear lesion.

Results of ABLB tests fall into one of four categories -- no recruitment, complete recruitment, partial recruitment, and decruitment, sometimes called "reverse recruitment". The categories may be described as follows:

No Recruitment: equal loudness occurs at equal sensation levels (SLs). For example, if the pathological ear has a 50 dB threshold, 60 dB HL in the impaired ear (10 dB SL) would be judged equal in loudness to 10 dB HL in the normal ear (10 dB SL). By the same token, 80 dB HL, in the poor ear (30 dB SL) would be judged equal in loudness to 30 dB HL in the normal ear (30 dB SL).

Complete Recruitment: equal loudness occurs at equal hearing levels (HLs). For example, even if there is a 50 dB difference between the ears at threshold, at 90 or 100 dB HL, the patient with complete recruitment would perceive the sound in the normal and the impaired ear as being equally loud.

Partial Recruitment: equal loudness occurs somewhere between complete and no recruitment.

Decruitment: equal loudness occurs with 10 dB or greater sensation level (SL) in the poor ear than in the good ear. Decruitment is related to abnormal tone decay and is pathognomonic of a retrocochlear lesion. For example, if there is a 50 dB difference between ears at threshold, a 70 dB HL tone in the poor ear might be judged equally loud to a 10 dB HL tone in the normal ear. In this type of pathology, a large increase in the intensity of the stimulus yields a smaller than usual increase in loudness.

B. SHORT INCREMENT SENSITIVITY INDEX (SISI): This is a test which assesses the ability of a patient to detect one dB intensity increments at the 20 dB Sensation level (20 dB above threshold). The normal patient or a patient with non-cochlear lesion usually does not detect such small increments. A high level of detection is associated with cochlear pathology. The test is administered monaurally through earphones and consists of 20 brief one dB intensity increments superimposed on a sustained tone presented at a sensation level of 20 dB at each test frequency. (Special test apparatus is required to perform the SISI test).

Procedure: The first step is to establish thresholds at all frequencies for the ear to be tested. Then, the test frequency selected is set at the 20 dB sensation level. The patient is instructed to signal each time he hears a "jump in loudness" and he is given an opportunity to practice the task. The SISI test apparatus permits adjusting the size of the intensity increment from zero to 5 dB. The 5 dB increment which should be audible to normal and pathological ears alike, is used to train the patient to perform the task. However, once the patient understands what he is to listen for, the intensity increment is reduced to one dB and the test is begun. The increments come at intervals of one every 5 seconds. 5% is scored for each correct identification. If all 20 intensity increments are correctly identified, the patient scores 100% for the test.

Interpretation: In general, purely conductive losses yield very low SISI scores, while losses presumed to be localized to the cochlea tend to show very high scores. Values between very high and very low appear infrequently. The SISI test scores may be categorized according to percentage correct as follows:

0 - 30% - Normal or non-cochlear
30 - 60% - questionable
60% + - considered positive (cochlear)

C. BÉKÉSY AUDIOMETRY: The clinical application of the Békésy audiometer is based on a comparison threshold obtained using pulsed versus continuous tones. The audiometer used for this test is capable of sweeping from low to high frequencies automatically while the intensity of the stimulus is controlled by a switch held by the patient. The patient's threshold responses are automatically recorded on the special Békésy audiogram paper.

Five Békésy types have been identified on the basis of the comparison of pulsed versus continuous tones in a given ear. They are as follows:

Type I: Threshold traces from pulsed and continuous tones are interwoven across all frequencies. Associated with normal hearing and with middle ear pathology.

Type II: The continuous and pulsed traces interweave from low to middle frequencies, but above 1000 Hz the continuous tone trace shows poor but not more than 20 dB poorer thresholds including a reduction in the amplitude of the trace. Associated with cochlear pathology.

Type III: The continuous and pulsed traces interweave only at low frequencies and then the continuous trace breaks away showing markedly poorer thresholds than shown for the pulsed trace. The difference in thresholds exceeds 20 dB, and in extreme cases, the continuous threshold may exceed the maximum limits of the audiometer. This type is associated with a retrocochlear lesion.

Type IV: The continuous and pulsed traces never interweave. They are separated at low, high, and middle frequencies and the continuous trace is usually more than 20 dB poorer than the pulsed trace. This type is also associated with a retrocochlear lesion.

Type V: The continuous and pulsed traces are separated. However, unlike the separation encountered in the other types, threshold traces obtained with pulsed tones are poorer. Type V is associated with non-organic hearing loss.

D. THE THRESHOLD TONE DECAY TEST: The threshold tone decay test is one of a battery of site-of-lesion tests. It is primarily used to differentiate between cochlear and retrocochlear lesions. The threshold tone decay test measures adaptation to continuous pure tone stimuli at threshold. In an individual who shows threshold tone decay, increased intensities of the stimulus are required to keep the tone audible at threshold. Ears with normal hearing and cochlear pathology may show some degree of tone decay but ears with retrocochlear pathology often show extreme and rapid tone decay. When there is more than 30 dB of tone decay observed in one minute, there is a high probability of a retrocochlear lesion. A number of different tone decay testing techniques have been reported. Several of these stress the importance of requiring the patient to respond to stimuli that have subjective tonality and not to respond to just any audible sound. The loss of subjective tonality for a sustained tone has been called "tone perversion" and is related to abnormal tone decay. Carhart and Rosenberg have described tone decay techniques that are widely used. The Carhart technique involves the search for a tonal threshold which can be maintained for sixty seconds at a given intensity level. The Rosenberg modification of the Carhart test takes sixty seconds for any given test frequency. In both the Carhart and Rosenberg methods, the amount of tone decay is defined as the difference between the initial thresholds and the final threshold for the test tone. The threshold tone decay test can be administered easily and requires only a conventional pure tone audiometer.

E. SUPRA-THRESHOLD ADAPTATION TEST (STAT): The STAT may be used along with threshold tone decay tests to identify retrocochlear lesions. The STAT is based on the hypothesis that symptoms of abnormal auditory adaptation (tone decay) first appear only at the highest testable sound intensities.

Procedure: To administer the STAT, the sustained test signal is presented for 60 seconds at 110 dB SPL. 500, 1000, and 2,000, Hz are the recommended test frequencies. The patient is asked to respond as long as he hears the sound.

Interpretation: If the patient responds for the full 60-second test period, the result is negative. If, however, he fails to respond for the full 60 seconds, the result is considered positive for retrocochlear lesion.

F. BÉKÉSY COMFORTABLE LOUDNESS (BCL) AUDIOGRAM: A variation of conventional Békésy audiometry which is designed to identify retrocochlear lesions is known as the BCL test. It is based on the hypothesis that symptoms of abnormal auditory adaptation (tone decay) first appear only at the highest testable sound intensities.

Procedure: The subject is instructed to carry out the Békésy audiometry procedure and to control the intensity of the stimulus through the use of a manually operated switch. However, instead of being required to respond at threshold levels as in conventional Békésy audiometry, he is told to keep the sound at a "comfortable loudness level", neither too loud nor too soft. Both pulsed and continuous traces are obtained for an ascending sweep, and continuous traces are obtained for a descending test frequency sweep.

Interpretation: Based on the amount of tone decay shown by the continuous traces as compared to the pulsed, the BCL audiograms are classified as either positive or negative. They are, positive when consistent with retrocochlear pathology as shown by large amounts of tone decay in the continuous mode; they are negative when consistent with normal, conductive, or cochlear hearing (little or no differences between pulsed and continuous traces).

G. PERFORMANCE-INTENSITY FUNCTION FOR PHONETICALLY BALANCED WORDS (PI-PB): In this test, phonetically balanced (PB) word lists are used to obtain speech discrimination scores at a number of different sensation levels, instead of at the single level usually used to report speech discrimination scores. It is known that PB scores improve, up to a point, as the intensity level of the stimulus presentation is increased above threshold. At about 40 dB SL most subjects reach a maximum score (PB Max) beyond which further increases in stimulus intensity fail to change the test scores to any significant degree.

In cases of retrocochlear lesions, however, a "roll-over" phenomenon has been observed. After PB Max has been reached, further increases in the intensity of the stimulus cause reduced speech discrimination scores.

Procedure: PI-PB functions are generated by presenting half-lists (25 words) in 10 to 20 dB intensity steps until the shape of the function is clearly defined. Percent correct for each half-list is plotted against intensity level in SPL. In general, the aim is to cover the range from that speech intensity yielding a PB score of approximately 20% up to a maximum speech intensity of 110 dB SPL. Usually 6 levels are sufficient to define the shape of a function.

Interpretation: Results are reported as a) normal or cochlear, b) retrocochlear, or c) questionable. If performance climbs to a maximum and then remains there or declines less than 20% as intensity is increased above the level yielding maximum percent correct, results are reported as normal or cochlear. If performance declines more than 20% when intensity is raised above the level yielding maximum performance, results are reported as retrocochlear. Questionable findings are indicated in those subjects who "roll-over" exactly 20%.

H. GLYCEROL TEST FOR MÉNIÈRE'S DISEASE: Pre-test restrictions: NPO for 6 hours before test; no sedatives, tranquilizers, strong analgesics, anti-vertiginous medications for 48 hours before the test. (Caution should be exercised in patients with cardiovascular disorders, diabetes and gastrectomy surgery).

Dosage: 1.2 ml of 95% glycerin per kg in equal volume of saline with several drops of lemon juice. Audiological Testing consists of Pure Tones (AC & BC), SRT, and PB-Max. (NPO during test)

a) Pre-ingestion of glycerol
b) 1 hour post ingestion
c) 2 hours post ingestion
d) 3 hours post ingestion

Side effects:

Thirst (usual)
Headache (23%)
Nausea (37%)
Emesis (5%)
Drowsiness

Positive test:

15 dB or more improvement at any one frequency
12% or more improvement in PB-Max
10 dB or more improvement in SRT

(The test is inaccurate for minimal loss)

I. SPECIAL TEST FOR FUNCTIONAL HEARING LOSS: A number of different terms exist which describe hearing losses which have no organic etiology. Non-organic hearing loss, functional hearing loss, psychogenic hearing loss, malingering, pseudohypoacusis are all terms relating to this type of hearing loss. In cases where exaggerated hearing loss is present, it is important that the tester determine the organic level of hearing. In order to do this the tester may use a special battery of tests, such as the Stenger, the Lombard, and the Delayed Auditory Feedback (DAF).

THE STENGER TEST: The best test for functional unilateral hearing impairment is the Stenger test. The test can be used not only to determine the presence of non-organic hearing loss, but often leads to a close approximation of the patient's true threshold of hearing. The Stenger test is founded on the principle that when two tones of identical frequency are sounded simultaneously in each ear, an individual with normal hearing or with an equal bilateral hearing loss will be aware of hearing the tone only in the ear in which it is louder. And he will not be aware of hearing it in the ear in which the tone is weaker. To perform the test the tester merely presents a test tone 5 dB above threshold to the normal ear, and at the same time presents the same tone to the ear suspected of non-organic hearing loss. The tester then holds the intensity level to the good ear constant and gradually increases the intensity to the other ear. The test tones are presented to each ear simultaneously while the intensity to the so-called poor ear is increased. The subject is instructed to raise his finger when he hears the tone and to lower it when he cannot hear the tone. If the ear in question is truly deafened, the subject will be aware of perceiving the tone only in the good ear and will continue to respond to it. If the ear in question has a non-organic hearing loss, the tone will eventually be perceived as being only in the poor ear since its intensity will be greater in the poor ear. Since it will appear to the subject that he is hearing only in the so-called poor ear, even though he is actually hearing it in his good ear as well, he will cease responding to the tone. The intensity at which he ceases to respond is closely related to his threshold for the test tone. The Stenger test may also be used with speech stimuli. The same principle holds on the Speech Stenger and is performed in much the same way as the pure-tone Stenger. When speech stimuli are used the test is called the Modified Stenger.

THE LOMBARD TEST: The Lombard test is also called the "voice reflex" test. The Lombard test is based on the principle that a speaker tends to raise his voice when he is speaking in a noisy environment. This is usually done unconsciously and serves to help the speaker regulate his voice so that he is able to hear himself speak.

In the test, masking noise is introduced to both of the subject's ears through earphones while he is reading aloud. If he is deaf, he will not hear the masking noise and his voice will not change in loudness. However, if his hearing loss is feigned, he will hear the loud masking noise in his ears and will automatically increase the loudness of his own voice. A noticeable increase in loudness while the subject is reading aloud in the presence of masking noise, is an indication of non-organic hearing impairment. The Lombard test can be used to detect either unilateral or bilateral non-organic hearing impairment by the use of unilateral or bilateral presentation of the masking noise stimulus.

DELAYED AUDITORY FEEDBACK (DAF): This test is also called the delayed sidetone test and is based on the principle that a disruption of reading fluency will occur if a speaker hears his own voice as an echo after a 2/10ths of a second delay. In this test the subject reads aloud into a microphone which delivers the speech to a tape recorder. The tape recorder plays back the speech through earphones and incorporates a 2/10ths of a second delay. The delay corresponds to about one syllable. When the delayed speech is made loud enough the subject will begin to stutter, drag out his words, and raise the intensity of his voice. If the subject is truly hearing impaired and does not hear the delayed speech, he will suffer no disruption of speech fluency. If the speech dysfluency occurs under the condition of delayed auditory feedback it is an indication that the subject hears his own voice. If the dysfluency occurs at levels below the voluntary threshold for the test ear, the response may be taken as an indication of non-organic hearing loss.

ELECTROPHYSIOLOGICAL TESTS: Occasionally it is desirable to use a hearing test that does not require the voluntary cooperation of a subject. Two such tests are electrodermal audiometry (EDA) and electroencephalic audiometry (EEA). Although these two tests have been called "objective" hearing tests because they do not require voluntary responses, the interpretation of the test results frequently has subjective components.

(1) ELECTRODERMAL AUDIOMETRY (EDA): This test, also called psychogalvanic skin response (PGSR) audiometry, is based on the principle that changes in sweat gland activity result in changes in the resistance of the skin which can be measured with appropriate electrodes. The test involves conditioning the patient to pure tone stimuli. In order to do this a tone that is audible is followed by an electric shock. The electric shock always elicits the sweat reflex which causes a change in the skin resistance that can be measured as a deflection on a meter. After several of the tonal stimuli are paired with shock, the electric shock may be withdrawn and the sweat reflex will be triggered by the tone alone. Thresholds for the tones are then obtained by reducing the intensity of the tones until the sweat reflex is no longer triggered. In this manner thresholds are obtained which are equivalent to voluntary thresholds. EDA is currently used less frequently than in the past with children because of the development of more pleasant and sophisticated techniques. However, it continues to be a valuable procedure to evaluate the hearing of persons suspected of having non-organic deafness, and is also still useful with children in selected cases.

(2) ELECTROENCEPHALIC AUDIOMETRY (EEA): EEA, also known as Evoked Response Audiometry (ERA) is an electrophysiological method of testing hearing. Clinically useful data on hearing thresholds have been obtained through EEA, based on transient changes in the electrical activity of the central nervous system in response to sound stimulation. The resulting electroencephalogram (EEG) can be analyzed to produce the desired information. Before the availability of summing computers the EEGs were analyzed individually by comparing successive recordings resulting from a series of identical stimuli. The current method uses a summing computer to analyze the EEG's electronically. The electroencephalic responses (EERs) to sound represent only a small part of the EEG. To extract this information from the record, short segments of the EEG which follow the stimulus and fall within circumscribed latency periods are summed electronically. The small responses which are timelocked to the tonal stimuli take form as a result of the summing process while the random background information tends to be cancelled out.

Interpretation of EERs requires a high level of training to perform and the equipment is very expensive. The test results with certain types of handicapped individuals, including the multiply handicapped, the mentally retarded, and the aphasic, are frequently ambiguous and difficult to interpret. In selected cases, however, EEA can provide useful supplementary information about hearing.

(3) THE DOERFLER-STEWART (D-S) TEST: This screening test for the detection of bilateral non-organic hearing loss is based on an individual's ability to understand spondee words in the presence of sawtooth masking noise. It is performed binaurally through earphones in which masking noise and spondee words are mixed. In theory, the person with non-organic hearing loss relies on background sound to gauge the level of incoming test stimulus and will not respond to any sound fainter than his self-imposed threshold. Introduction of the masking noise in conjunction with the presentation of spondee words serves to disturb the frame of reference of the patient with non-organic hearing loss and will interfere with his ability to judge the level at which he should no longer be capable of hearing the test words. It has been found that subjects with normal hearing and those with genuine hearing impairment can repeat spondee words when the level of masking noise equals or slightly exceeds the level of the speech signal. However, patients with non-organic hearing loss may cease repeating words when the intensity of the masking noise is 10 to 15 dB less than the level of the spondees. The Doerfler-Stewart test is one of the oldest audiological measures used to detect the presence of non-organic deafness. However, recent investigation suggests that it is not as sensitive a measure as was originally believed.

VI. ACOUSTIC TRAUMA AND NOISE INDUCED HEARING LOSS

TEMPORARY THRESHOLD SHIFT (TTS): When the ear is exposed to loud noise such as heavy machinery, lawn mowers and the shooting of small arms, the ear shows signs of fatigued hearing and the auditory thresholds become raised. The recovery from brief exposure to these noises is usually complete, and for this reason the threshold shift is called temporary. The greatest shift is for tones about one half octave above the exposure tone, but other higher frequencies may be more or less affected as well. Hearing for lower tones is relatively unaffected.

It has been noted that maximum energy at low frequency produces less temporary threshold shift than those whose energy is at high frequencies. Intermittent noise is also much less harmful than steady noise. Recovery from temporary threshold shift usually occurs within the first hour or two; however, a moderate shift may not recover for days or even weeks.

PERMANENT THRESHOLD SHIFT (PTS): Individuals who are exposed to high levels of noise without ear protection, inevitably develop hearing loss, although there are differences in susceptibility. In some individuals, the loss of hearing develops rapidly; in others, more slowly. The amount of PTS depends upon the intensity and duration of exposure. Some investigators have suggested the use of TTS to predict PTS. However, there is conflicting opinion on the efficacy of this procedure.

Two major categories of hearing loss caused by noise have been defined: (a) acoustic trauma and (b) Noise Induced Hearing Loss (NIHL). The term acoustic trauma is usually reserved for a sudden loss of hearing associated with noise from a blast or an explosion. NIHL usually results from exposure to loud noise over longer periods of time, often for many years. In both categories, the audiometric picture is quite similar, and it is not possible to distinguish one from the other on the basis of audiometric data. The typical configuration that occurs as a result of noise exposure is a notch in the hearing at 4000 Hz and evidence of recruitment. It is also of interest to note that a head injury will also produce a similar audiometric pattern. In the case of acoustic trauma, it is usually possible to trace the incident which caused the hearing loss. The resulting hearing loss may be very severe at first but it is usual that a great deal of recovery of function may occur over a period of several months. In contrast, NIHL resulting from long time exposure, demonstrates very little improvement in hearing after the first 48 hours during which noise exposure is eliminated. There is a typical progression of hearing loss that occurs with NIHL. In the beginning, the audiogram is generally normal with a dip at 4000 Hz and a recovery to normal in the higher frequencies. With increased exposure the notch at 4000 Hz is widened and deepened, and the recovery in the higher frequencies diminishes. In the later stages, there is normal or near normal hearing for the low frequencies with sharply dropping hearing for the higher frequencies yielding the typical "ski slope" audiogram.

When it is necessary to test the hearing of an individual who has developed NIHL, and who is no longer working in a noisy environment, it is well to postpone the test for a month. This will allow the recovery of TTS so that PTS may be accurately measured. It has been demonstrated that after one month of quiet, the additional recovery that may be expected is minimal.

Damage Risk Criteria: Although hearing loss from noise is almost completely preventable, either through reduction of the noise or the wearing of ear plugs or ear muffs, millions of industrial workers have developed NIHL. For this reason safety standards have been developed by governmental agencies. According to the Occupational Safety and Health Act of 1970 (OSHA), permissible durations of exposure without ear protection to different intensities of steady state noise have been developed. The noise levels are measured on a sound level meter using the "A" scale and are shown in Table 2-2.

TABLE 2-2

PERMISSIBLE NOISE EXPOSURE

Duration per day Hours	Sound Level dBA
8	90
6	92
4	95
3	97
2	100
1 1/2	102
1	105
1/2	110
1/4 or less	115

The Occupational Safety and Health Act also specifies that exposure to impulsive or impact noise should not exceed 140 dB peak sound pressure level, as measured with an impact meter or an oscilloscope.

2. Ear Protectors: (Table 2-3)

TABLE 2-3

ATTENUATION IN dB IN THE VARIOUS FREQUENCIES

	250	500	1000	2000	3000	4000
Fluid sealed muffs	28	38	39	41	44	47
V-51R Plug	11	13	19	27	30	25
Glass down	11	13	17	29	34	35
Waxed cotton	10	12	16	27	31	32
Dry Cotton	3	4	8	12	14	12

4000 Hz DIP (8 TO 10 MM. REGION OF THE COCHLEAR DUCT): The 4000 Hz sensori-neural dip is one of the principal audiometric features of a hearing loss resulting from excessive noise. There are basically two theories to explain this. One hypothesis is that the area of the organ of Corti responsive to 4000 Hz is highly susceptible to damage. The other view contends that the mechanical stress on the basilar membrane is excessive in the 4000 Hz region due to the mechanics of cochlear action. This latter explanation is based on the asymmetrical distribution of the amplitude of displacement of the basilar membrane. It is believed that the stress is due to the acceleration of the basilar membrane during stimulation. Acceleration of the basilar membrane is greatest at the basal end and becomes progressively less at the apical end. Greater losses for frequencies above 4000 Hz do not occur because there is less auditory sensitivity in that region. The mechanical hypothesis is preferred by a number of investigators since there is evidence from auditory fatigue studies that stimulation by a given level tone caused no greater auditory fatigue at 4000 Hz than at 1500 Hz. It has also been found that the recovery rate for 4000 Hz did not proceed less rapidly than at other frequencies.

VII. HANDICAP IN HEARING

1. TABLE 2-4

Class	Degree of Handicap	Average between 500, 1000 and 2000 Hz in the better ear	Ability to understand speech
A	Not significant	Loss of < 25 dB	No problem
B	Slight	25-40	Difficulty with faint speech
C	Mild	40-55	Difficulty with normal speech
D	Marked	55-70	Difficulty with loud speech
E	Severe	70-90	Can understand only shouted speech
F	Extreme	> 90	Can understand only shouted speech

2. COMPUTATION OF THE PERCENTAGE OF HANDICAP IN THE HARD OF HEARING:

A. <u>Unilateral Loss:</u> 1-1/2% handicap is assigned to each dB exceeding 26 dB (ISO) for the average thresholds at 500, 1000, and 2,000 cycles per second.

B. <u>Bilateral Loss:</u>

$$\frac{\text{(Percentage of handicap in the better ear) x 5 + (percentage of handicap in poor ear)}}{6}$$

= Percentage of handicap for Binaural hearing loss

3. It is estimated that at age 55, 22% of the population with no exposure to noise has significant hearing loss as compared to 46% among the individual working around loud noises. Hence in calculation of VII-2 above, 1/2 dB per year after the age of 40 should be the correcting factor for the average thresholds at 500, 1000, 2000 Hz.

VIII. TABLE 2-5

Enzymes Found in the Organ of Corti and Stria Vascularis
Succinate dehydrogenase
Cytochrome oxidases
Diaphorases (DPN, TPN)
Lactic dehydrogenase
Malic dehydrogenase
Alpha-glycerophosphate-dehydrogenase
Glutamate dehydrogenase

TABLE 2-6

	Serum	CSF	Perilymph S. tymp.	Perilymph S. vest.	Endolymph cochl.	Endolymph vest.	Endo-lymph Sac
Na mEq/L	141	141	157	147	6	14.9	153
K mEq/L	5	3	3.8	10.5	171	155	8
Cl mEq/L	101	126	-	-	120	120	-
Protein mg%	7000	10-25	215	160	125	-	5200
Sugar mg%	100	70	85	92	9.5	39.4	-
pH	7.35	7.35	7.2	7.2	7.5	7.5	-

TABLE 2-7

A. Endocochlear potential — Scala media +80 mV
Endolymph potential — Scala vestibuli +5 mV
Resting potential — Scala tympani 0
DC potential — Hair cell and cortilymph -80mV
Endolymphatic sac (+)
Cells of Hensen and Claudius (-)

B. Action Potential of the nerve
C. Cochlear microphonics (due to stimulation of outer hair cells)
D. Summation potential (due to stimulation of inner hair cell and is more significant in higher frequencies)

(The recording of Endocochlear potential and summation potential requires an intracochlear electrode while the action potential of the nerve and cochlear microphonics can be picked up with a round window electrode).

IX. SPEECH

Speech sounds are generally classified as consonants, vowels or diphthongs. Vowel sounds are produced by a modification in size and shape of the resonating cavities without obstruction or interference with the breath stream. Consonants are speech sounds which are produced with some degree of restriction or obstruction of the breath stream by the organs of articulation. Diphthongs are vowel-like sounds made by gliding two vowels together. The most common diphthongs are: (aI) as in ice, (oI) as in boy, (aU) as in house, (eI) as in bay, (oU) as in hoe. Consonants are often classified according to:

a) Place of articulation
b) Manner of articulation
c) Element of vocalization

The place of the production of sound, that is the locus of the blockage, constriction, or diversion of the air stream may be designated as follows: Labial (p, b, m, w); Labio-dental (f, v); Lingua-dental (voiced and unvoiced th); Alveolar (t, d, n, l); Post-dental (s, sh, z, zh); Palatal (y as in yellow, r as in red); Velar (k, g, ng); Glottal (h).

When classifying consonants according to the manner of articulation, the terms plosive, fricative, affricate, nasal, lateral, glide and semi-vowel are used.

Plosives: Plosives are produced by stopping and then suddenly releasing the stream of breath. The plosive sounds are (p, b, t, k, g).

Fricatives: Fricatives are produced by a partial closure of the articulators which results in the creation of a restricted passage of the breath stream. This may take place as a result of grooving of the tongue or by having other organs of articulation come close together. The fricative sounds of speech are (f, v, voiced and unvoiced th, s, z, zh, and h).

Nasal sounds: Nasal sounds are those which are emitted through the nose rather than the mouth. The nasal sounds in American speech are (m, n, ng).

Affricates: Affricates are blends of two sounds, one of which is a fricative and the other of which is a plosive. The affricates are (ch, dzh).

Lateral Speech: The lateral is produced by having air emitted at both sides of the tongue or the tip of the tongue is in contact with the gum ridge. The only lateral sound in American speech is the (l) sound.

Glide: A glide consonant is characterized by a continuous movement of the articulator or articulators while a sound is being made. The glide consonants include (w, y as in yellow, and r as in red).

Semi-vowel: The semi-vowel is related to the glide in that there is movement involved in its consonant function. The semi-vowels are (w, r, y as in yellow, and l). The element of vocalization as a means of classifying consonants depends upon whether the vocal folds are in vibration when the sound is produced. If they are, the sound is said to be voiced and if it is not, the sound is said to be unvoiced. A labio-dental voiced fricative would describe how the consonant (v) is produced during the three factors of place, manner and vocalization.

Cleft Palate and Adenoidal Speech: Two types of speech problems which are frequently seen by the otolaryngologist are associated with abnormal nasal resonance. The nasality is "hyper" if there is too much and "hypo" if there is too little.

In the case of a normal speaker, the soft palate effectively seals off the nasal cavity for most sounds, but allows the nasal sounds (m, n, ng) to pass through the nose. For the cleft palate speaker who has insufficient velopharyngeal closure, all sounds tend to pass through the nose and the speech becomes hypernasal. Both vowels and consonants are adversely affected. The vowels are given excessive nasal resonance and hence sound distorted. The most common articulatory error is the substitution of some nasal equivalent for the plosive and fricative sounds. The voiceless plosives (p, t) are usually preceded by a sharp nasal puff and a pinching of the nostrils. The velar plosives (k, g) are among the most difficult to make since they require an air pressure build-up behind the tongue. This is virtually impossible without sealing off the nasal cavity. Fricative sounds are usually accompanied by nasal snorts. The nasal snort frequently is substituted for the (s) and (sh). This type of speech may in severe cases be extremely unintelligible. Good test words to show velopharyngeal insufficiency are cool, coca cola, quack quack.

The hypernasality and articulatory problems associated with cleft palate speech also occur when there is no actual cleft of the palate. It may occur with a soft palate that is paralyzed, sluggish, or too short. A child with a short palate may be able to avoid excessive nasality by compensating with hypertrophied adenoidal tissue. However, if the adenoidal tissue is removed surgically, hypernasality may result. For this reason, surgical removal of adenoidal tissue should be given careful consideration prior to this undertaking.

Adenoidal Speech: Hyponasality (or denasality) is often called "cold in the nose" speech. It is primarily a substitution of (b, d, g) for the nasal (m, n, ng). The quality of other sounds is also somewhat affected. Hyponasality is usually associated with some structural pathology such as hypertrophy of the adenoids or polyps.

REFERENCES

1. Boies, L.R., Editor: Hearing Loss--Problems in Diagnosis and Treatment. Otolaryngol. Clin. N. Am., Feb., 1969, W.B. Saunders Co., Philadelphia.

2. Irwin, J.V.: Disorders of Articulation. Bobbs-Merrill Co., Inc., 1972.

3. Jerger, J. and Jerger, S.: A Simplified Tone Decay Test. Arch. Otolaryng. 101:403-407, July 1975.

4. Jerger, J. and Jerger, S.: Diagnostic Value of Békésy Comfortable Loudness Tracings. Arch. Otolaryng. 99:351-360, May 1974.

5. Katz, J., Editor: Handbook of Clinical Audiology. Williams and Wilkins Co., Baltimore, 1972.

6. Kirikae, I.: Physiopathology of the Middle Ear. Refresher Audio-Visual Course (Mexico), Univ. of Tokyo Press, Tokyo, Japan, 1969.

7. Newby, H.A.: Audiology, 3rd Edition, Appleton-Century-Crofts, 1972.

8. Riper, C.V.: Speech Correction, 5th Edition, Prentice-Hall, Inc., 1972.

9. Snyder, J.M.: Changes in Hearing Associated with the Glycerol Test. Arch. Otolaryng. 93:155-160, 1971.

10. Swanson, S.N., et al.: Pre and Post-Glycerol Special Audiometric Tests Battery Results in Endolymphatic Hydrops. Laryngoscope 86: 490-500, 1976.

CHAPTER 3

INFECTIONS OF THE EAR

I. COMMON PATHOGENS FOUND IN INFECTIONS OF THE EAR

ACUTE OTITIS MEDIA:

1. Pneumococci, beta-hemolytic Streptococci and Haemophilus influenzae, are the bacterial species most frequently recovered in acute otitis media.
2. Haemophilus influenzae is the most frequent pathogen recovered from children under five years of age (25% of acute otitis media).
3. Staphylococcus and Pseudomonas aeruginosa isolated in acute otitis media probably represent an overgrowth or contamination of the culture by infection of the external auditory canal.
4. The role of viruses and mycoplasmas in the etiology of acute otitis media has not been proven.
5. The antibiotic therapy for acute otitis media after age five should be directed principally against the Pneumococcus and the group A Streptococcus. For this group penicillin alone should be effective. In the case of penicillin allergy either Erythromycin or Cephalothin is an acceptable alternative.

Under age five, treatment must also be effective against Haemophilus influenzae and, therefore, Ampicillin is the agent of choice. In the event of penicillin allergy, Erythromycin plus sulfonamide can be used.

6. Acute necrotizing otitis media is a virulent form of acute otitis media, nearly always caused by a beta-hemolytic Streptococcus, and seen in children who are acutely ill from a systemic infectious disease such as scarlet fever, measles, pneumonia, or influenza. The pathologic process is true necrosis of the soft tissues and bones of the middle ear and mastoid.

   The disease is characterized by a profuse, purulent, foul-smelling otorrhea, a large tympanic membrane perforation (in contrast to a small perforation seen in the usual acute suppurative otitis media), sloughing of the annulus tympanicus, portions of ossicles, the scutum and the mastoid air cells. Occasionally, naked white bone of the promontory and the antrum may be observed.[45]

CHRONIC OTITIS MEDIA:

1. The bacterial flora found in chronic otitis media varies considerably. The predominating organisms are usually gram negative bacilli.
2. Friedmann found the distribution of bacteria causing chronic otitis media in 1700 patients as follows:
   Staphylococcus aureus 31.7%
   Staphylococcus aureus 12.9% (Penicillin resistant)
   Bacillus proteus 25.4%

Pseudomonas aeruginosa 12.8%
Mixed 8.4%
Escherichia coli 8.1%
Streptococcus pyogenes, hemolytic 7.0%
Streptococcus viridans and Streptococcus pneumoniae 4.6%
No growth 10.6%

3. Tuberculous otitis media is a rare type of infection caused by acid-fast tuberculous bacilli (Mycobacterium tuberculosis), characterized by an incidious and painless onset; scanty thin, odorless discharge; progressive enlargement of the perforation in the pars tensa; multiple perforations with pale granulations; and hearing loss out of proportion to other symptoms. It is usually secondary to pulmonary tuberculosis. Early investigators believed that the portal of entry was the eustachian tube, while others felt that the infection was spread by the hematogenous route. (Proctor and Lindsay). Any caseous focus may be a source from which tubercle bacilli enter the blood stream to reach the temporal bone. Histologically, it is characterized by (1) extensive edema and infiltration of the mucosa and tympanic membrane by round cells and giant cells, (2) formation of numerous tubercles consisting of epithelioid and lymphoid cells and containing characteristic giant cells of Langerhans' type, (3) caseation and ulceration.[39]

   Diagnosis may be made from direct smears, cultures and histological examination of granulation tissue removed from the middle ear or mastoid. Tuberculosis should be suspected when otitis media does not respond readily to ordinary methods of therapy.

   Isoniazid and PAS (para-aminosalicylic acid) are commonly used for initial treatment. Streptomycin may be added in more severe cases.

4. Syphilitic otitis media (rare today) is caused by Spirochaeta pallida (Treponema pallidum). The usual aural manifestation of syphilis is a meningoneuro-labyrinthitis, but occasionally the middle ear cleft is involved by a gummatous osteitis or osteoperiosteitis. The gummatous change may lead to a foul discharge and extensive destruction of the mastoid. Secondary pyogenic infection develops. Diagnosis may be suspected by foul painless otorrhea in the presence of sensorineural deafness and confirmed by specific tests for syphilis: (1) detection of T. pallidum by direct darkfield examination of material obtained from a primary and secondary lesion, (2) Serological tests (Wassermann, VDRL, Kahn and Kline, Kolmer, Rapid Plasma Reagin tests), (3) Treponema pallidum immobilization test (TPI) and (4) the more sensitive fluorescent treponemal antibody absorption test (FTA-ABS). Incudectomy may help the diagnosis (Nodol).[29] Treatment should be both local (removal of sequestra may be necessary) and general (systemic penicillin and steroid therapy). There is some evidence that penicillin alone will not eradicate T. pallidum from the human temporal bone, and that ampicillin may reach higher levels than penicillin in perilymph. However, ampicillin and penicillin, when each is combined with a high

dosage of steroids, seem equally effective in the treatment of syphilitic hearing loss.[22]

5. Late congenital syphilis is characterized by the following: a rather abrupt onset of deafness in apparently healthy young adults; bilateral involvement, which initially may be asymmetrical; family history of lues; periods of exacerbation, i.e., pregnancy, colds; rapid progression even to complete bilateral loss of cochlear and vestibular function in some cases; vestibular symptoms occasionally resembling those seen in Meniere's disease: Tullio's sign (vertigo and nystagmus on stimulation with loud noise); Hennebert's sign: despite an intact drum, a positive fistula test, especially with negative pressure; predominance in females; negative or equivocal blood serology (Wassermann, VDRL, Kahn and Kline, Kolmer tests), with negative spinal fluid serology; positive fluorescent treponenal antibody absorption test (FTA-ABS); and long interval between eye and ear involvement.[22, 33, 34, 39]

One should remember that some diseases may produce false positive reactions to serological tests. These include malaria, infectious mononucleosis, systemic lupus erythematosus and leprosy. Syphilis, both congenital and acquired, can cause sensorineural hearing loss. The incidence of such loss among various forms of syphilis has been estimated at 18 percent for late congenital, 17 percent for early congenital, 25 percent for late latent, 29 percent for asymptomatic neurosyphilis, and 80 percent of symptomatic neurosyphilis.[39]

The histopathology of syphilitic infection is primarily twofold. Firstly, syphilis may cause a meningo-neuro-labyrinthitis as the predominant lesion in early (infantile) congenital syphilis and in the acute meningitides of secondary and tertiary syphilis. Secondly, syphilis may cause an osteitis of the temporal bone as the predominant lesion with secondary involvement of the membranous labyrinth in late (tardive) congenital, late latent and tertiary syphilis. Pathologically, the lesions of congenital and acquired syphilis cannot be differentiated and similarly the hearing loss may be sudden or progressive, with or without vestibular involvement in both congenital and acquired syphilis.[19, 33, 34, 39]

The basic histological feature of bone involvement is an inflammatory rarefying osteitis featured by round cell infiltration, multinucleated giant cells and endarteritis leading to varying degrees of destruction of the bony labyrinth. Mononuclear leukocytic infiltration and obliterative endarteritis are common to all syphilitic lesions, whatever the organ affected. Mild reactions promote proliferation of fibrous tissue leading to an inflammatory fibrosis. Severe reactions result in gummatous lesions which are characterized by lymphocytic infiltration, vascular occlusion and central necrosis.

Other sites commonly involved in congenital syphilis are (1) the nasal cartilaginous and bony framework (snuffles), (2) periosteitis of the cranial bones (bossing of the skull), (3) periosteitis of the tibia (sabre shins), (4) injury to odontogenous tissue (Hutchinson's teeth), (5) involvement of epiphyseal cartilages (reduction in stature), and (6) interstitial keratitis (cloudy cornea).

OTITIS EXTERNA:

1. The usual infecting organism found in localized external otitis (furunculosis) is Staphylococcus aureus.
2. The most common organisms found in diffuse external otitis (swimmer's ear) are Pseudomonas aeruginosa (B. pyocyaneus) and Staphylococcus. Less commonly found are Streptococcus and Proteus vulgaris.
3. The most common organism found in perichondritis is Pseudomonas aeruginosa (B. pyocyaneus).
4. The most common fungi affecting the external ear are Candida albicans, Aspergillus niger, and yeast-like fungi.
5. The most common organism found in impetigo contagiosa of the external ear is Staphylococcus aureus.
6. Bullous myringitis is caused by a virus and generally associated with an acute upper respiratory infection (most commonly influenza). The serous or hemorrhagic blebs on the tympanic membrane and adjacent meatal wall may produce severe pain without fever and hearing loss. Treatment is supportive. The blebs may be opened in the presence of severe pain.
7. Herpes zoster oticus (Ramsay Hunt Syndrome) is a viral infection affecting the geniculate ganglion characterized by facial paralysis, herpetic vesicles in the external auditory canal and cavum conchae, severe ear pain, and impairment of lacrimation, salivation and taste, often with vertigo and a sensorineural hearing loss. Treatment is symptomatic. Facial nerve decompression including the region of the geniculate ganglion may be indicated when electrical excitability is lost or markedly impaired.[10]
8. Malignant external otitis (Chandler)[5] (necrotizing external otitis) is a serious infection of high mortality rate which occurs in the elderly diabetic. The responsible organism is uniformly Pseudomonas aeruginosa.

   It begins insidiously, frequently with a history of minor trauma, and is characterized by progressive pain and purulent discharge from the external auditory canal. The infection begins in the external auditory canal and extends inferiorly into the soft tissues at the junction of the cartilaginous and osseous portions of the external auditory canal or through the fissures of Santorini. The infection thus involves the parotid gland, cartilage, bone, nerves and blood vessels.

   The pathognomonic sign is the presence of active granulation tissue in the external auditory canal at the junction of its osseous and cartilaginous portion. There is pain on movement of the temporomandibular joint and marked tenderness on palpation beneath the external auditory canal. Facial palsy is an ominous prognostic sign and is due to involvement of the facial nerve at its exit from the stylomastoid foramen.

   The infection is resistant to ordinary methods of treatment and, if not arrested, progresses to result in chondritis, osteitis and osteomyelitis of the temporal bone and base of the skull, facial nerve paralysis and other multiple cranial nerve palsies, sigmoid sinus thrombosis, meningitis, brain abscess and death.

Treatment should consist of local debridement and systemic administration of carbenicillin and gentamicin for four to six weeks. Wide surgical debridement, including radical mastoidectomy, total parotidectomy, excision of the condyle and ascending ramus of the mandible, and occasionally sacrifice of the facial nerve, may be necessary for its control. [5]

CHOLESTEROL GRANULOMA: [30, 41]

The cholesterol granuloma does not represent an independent clinical or pathological entity. Rather, it is a term used for the description of a tissue response of the temporal bone to the presence of a particular foreign body, i.e., cholesterol crystals.

Three factors are considered to play an important role in its development: 1) interference with drainage, 2) hemorrhage, and 3) obstruction of ventilation. The cause of the initial hemorrhage may be a hemorrhagic inflammation or diathesis, a trauma, or some other form of vascular disorder. Interference with air exchange and clearance can be caused by: tubal blockage, persistent mesenchyme, polypoid changes, scar formations, tympanosclerosis cholesteatoma, etc.

The cholesterol granuloma may develop in any portion of the pneumatic system of the temporal bone and it can be associated with a variety of middle ear disorders. Its principal precursor is the chronic middle ear effusion or serous otitis media. Its clinical expression and hallmark is the "idiopathic hematotympanum," (Sheehy and Linthicum [40]), the dark bluish discoloration of the tympanic membrane.

Osteitis and bone erosion are manifestations of an unusual, more advanced stage. Resorption of bone, in a rare instance, may lead to extensive destruction of the temporal bone. [30]

II. DEFINITION OF TYMPANOPLASTY AND MASTOIDECTOMY

DEFINITION:

1. Simple Mastoidectomy: (Cortical Mastoidectomy) A complete mastoidectomy with anatomic dissection of all accessible pneumatic cells is indicated for acute mastoiditis with impending or existing complications or acute mastoiditis which does not resolve after appropriate antibiotic therapy and myringotomy drainage.

2. Myringoplasty: An operation in which the reconstructive procedure is limited to the repair of tympanic membrane perforation.

3. Tympanoplasty without mastoidectomy: An operation to eradicate disease in the middle ear and to reconstruct the hearing mechanism, without mastoid surgery.

4. Tympanoplasty with mastoidectomy: An operation to eradicate disease in both the mastoid process and middle ear cavity and to reconstruct the hearing mechanism.

5. Modified radical mastoidectomy: An operation to eradicate disease of the epitympanum and mastoid in which the mastoid and epitympanic spaces are converted into an easily accessible common cavity by removal of the posterior and superior external bony canal walls. In this operation the tympanic membrane and functioning ossicles are left intact. Thus infection is eradicated and hearing preserved.

6. Radical mastoidectomy: An operation to eradicate disease of the middle ear and mastoid in which the mastoid, antrum, and the middle ear are exteriorized so that they form a common cavity with the external auditory canal. In this operation, the tympanic membrane, malleus, incus, chorda tympani and the mucoperiosteal lining are all removed.

7. Mastoid obliteration operation: An operation to eradicate disease when present and to obliterate mastoid or fenestration cavities.

TABLE 3-1: CLASSIFICATION OF TYMPANOPLASTY BY WULLSTEIN

TYPE	DAMAGE TO MIDDLE EAR	METHOD OF REPAIR
I	Perforated tympanic membrane with normal ossicular chain	Closure of perforation, type I same as myringoplasty
II	Perforation of tympanic membrane with erosion of malleus	Closure with graft against incus or remains of malleus
III	Destruction of tympanic membrane and ossicular chain but with intact and mobile stapes	Graft contacts normal stapes; also gives sound protection for round window
IV	Similar to type III, but head, neck, and crura of stapes missing; footplate mobile	Mobile footplate left exposed or graft attaches to mobile footplate; air pocket between round window and graft provides sound protection for round window
V	Similar to type IV plus fixed footplate	Fenestra in horizontal semicircular canal; graft seals off middle ear to give sound protection for round window

Paparella modified Type V tympanoplasty, subdividing it into Type Va (fenestration of the horizontal semicircular canal) and Type Vb (stapedectomy in cases of Tympanoplasty Type IV with stapes fixation). (Figure 3-1). [31, 38]

CLASSIFICATION OF TYMPANOPLASTY BY FARRIOR:[11] Farrior proposed the types of tympanoplasties according to the basic pathological anatomy at the completion of the surgery, rather than classifying them according to the method of reconstruction utilized. He also advocated the grouping of cases according to the preoperative status of the middle ear mucosa, eustachian tube function, and associated diseases of the nose and nasopharynx.

CLASSIFICATION:

Type I: The reconstruction of a new ear drum, intact malleus, incus and stapes.
Type II: The reconstruction of a new ear drum in its natural position.
Type III: The reconstruction of a new ear drum on top of an upright, freely mobile stapes.
Type IV: Reconstruction of a new ear drum and columella on the stapedial footplate.
Type V: Reconstruction of an ear drum either over a fistula in the horizontal semicircular canal or a new ear drum with a secondary fenestration of the horizontal semicircular canal.

TYMPANOPLASTY III (FARRIOR)[11]

Type III	Drum on stapes
Type III IG	Incus graft
Type III IGM	Incus graft to malleus
Type III MR	Malleus repositioned
Type III MG	Malleus graft
Type III BG	Bone graft
Type III SS MS	Stainless steel malleus to stapes, etc.

The best results in tympanoplasty are obtained when the stapes is upright and freely movable, regardless of the type of reconstruction utilized. In classifying tympanoplasty according to basic pathologic anatomy all cases with intact stapedial superstructures are classified under type III with indication of the type of superstructure by initials, as IG incus graft.

TYMPANOPLASTY IV (FARRIOR)[11]

Type IV	No columnella
Type IV IG	Incus graft
Type IV MG	Malleus graft
Type IV BG	Bone graft
Type IV C SS	Cartilage graft with stainless steel
Type IV HG MIS	Homograft drum with malleus, incus and stapes

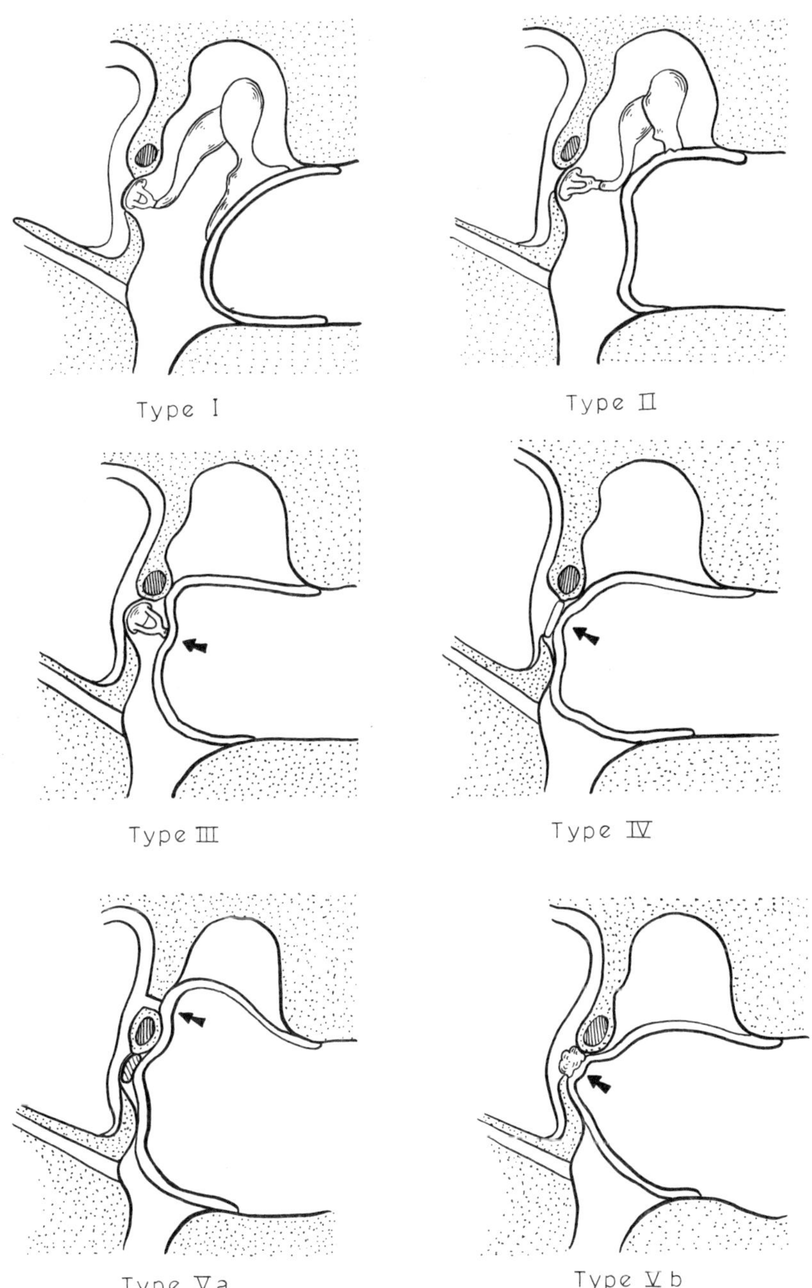

FIG. 3-1. Tympanoplasties

In classifying tympanoplasty according to the basic pathologic anatomy all cases with absent stapedial superstructures are sub-classified under Type IV with indication of the type of superstructure reconstructed as MG-malleus graft.

GROUPING (BELLUCCI):[3]

Group I: A good prognosis being those cases who are relatively free of any associated middle ear or eustachian tube disease.
Group II: A fair prognosis, has a period of quiescence.
Group III: With a poor prognosis, had no period of quiescence.
Group IV: With a very poor prognosis, has persistent disease with associated deformity of the nasopharynx as cleft palate.

III. SYSTEMATIC APPROACH TO EVALUATE AND TREAT CHRONIC OTITIS MEDIA

Systematic preoperative evaluation of patients with chronic otitis media and a brief description of surgical procedures commonly performed for chronic otitis media will be described.

PREOPERATIVE EVALUATION: Preoperative evaluation should include:

A. Careful analysis of symptoms and signs
B. Otologic examination
C. Examination of the upper respiratory tract
D. Audiological evaluation
E. Preoperative preparation

1. CAREFUL ANALYSIS OF SYMPTOMS AND SIGNS: Careful analysis of the symptoms and findings allows the otologist to determine the need for surgery, its urgency (if any) and the anticipated results.

OTORRHEA:

A. Discharge from the ear is the most common manifestation of chronic otitis media. Note should be made of its duration, frequency, character, and odor.
B. Malodorous discharge, at times bloody, of a constant or frequently recurring nature usually indicates significant middle ear and mastoid disease.
C. A central perforation without significant disease is usually accompanied by episodes of mucoid discharge of short duration. This discharge may be initiated by an upper respiratory infection or by introduction of water into the ear.

HEARING LOSS:

A. The extent of hearing impairment in chronic otitis media is dependent primarily on the degree of ossicular disruption.
B. In the absence of cholesteatoma, a conductive loss of 20 dB or less usually indicates that the ossicular chain is intact.

C. Disruption or fixation of the chain results in an impairment of 30 dB or more.
D. It is not unusual to find normal hearing in an ear with an attic perforation and cholesteatoma. This may be an indication of an intact ossicular chain. However, this may indicate that sound transmission is accomplished through a mass of cholesteatoma that has replaced ossicular tissue ("cholesteatoma hearer" or "silent cholesteatoma").
E. A progressive conductive impairment in the absence of active disease suggests ossicular fixation. This may be due to tympanosclerosis or otosclerosis. This is significant because surgery may have to be performed in two stages: one a graft of the tympanic membrane to eliminate disease, the other a revision to perform stapedectomy or Type VB tympanoplasty. The patient should be advised of this possibility preoperatively.

PAIN (OTALGIA):

A. Pain is not a frequent complaint in chronic otitis media unless there is secondary otitis externa.
B. Dull pain, in the absence of otitis externa, particularly when it is severe enough to disturb sleep, is usually an indication of an expanding mass of cholesteatoma or empyema in the antrum. Surgery should not be delayed.
C. Pain may indicate acute exacerbation of infection by upper respiratory infection.
D. Pain may indicate development of complications of chronic otitis media such as petrositis, subperiosteal abscess, lateral sinus thrombosis.

VERTIGO:

A. Minor degrees of postural vertigo are seen frequently in patients with chronic otitis media.
B. Continuous vertigo or postural vertigo of recent onset in a patient with cholesteatoma is usually an indication for immediate surgery. It indicates labyrinthine irritation or a semicircular canal fistula.

FACIAL NERVE PARALYSIS: Facial nerve paralysis occasionally develops in the course of chronic otitis media with cholesteatoma. If and when it occurs, surgery should be undertaken without delay to relieve pressure on the nerve. It is not necessary to "decompress" the nerve in most cases; elimination of the disease is sufficient.

2. EXAMINATION OF THE UPPER RESPIRATORY TRACT:

A. A sound review of the history and careful examination of the upper respiratory tract is mandatory.
B. Gross abnormalities and chronic suppurative sinus disease should be identified and corrected before reconstructive surgery is performed.
C. Patients with histories of "repeated colds" in winter months are not good candidates for tympanoplasty.

3. OTOLOGIC EXAMINATION:

A. Careful inspection of the ear should be the first part of the systemic evaluation. The inspection should include examination under magnification, with an otoscope or preferably with a surgical microscope.
B. Pneumatic otoscopy should be a routine to examine the mobility of the tympanic membrane and malleus and to rule out coexisting chronic serous otitis media. Care must be taken to avoid forceful insufflation. Lethal intracranial complications following air insufflation have been reported.[13]
C. Careful examination of the attic area should be done to identify hidden retraction pockets, perforation, and/or cholesteatoma. It is often necessary to freely change the position of the patient's head and the angulation of the otoscope or microscope.
D. The fistula test should be performed whenever a marginal perforation is present or when there is a history of dizziness.
E. Specific notes should be made regarding the type of perforation, the character of the discharge, the status of the mucosa, and the presence or absence of ossicular tissue.

DISCHARGE (OTORRHEA):

A. The character of the discharge, whether mucoid or purulent, with or without odor, is noted.
B. A mucoid discharge without odor is usually an indication of mucosal disease and/or eustachian tube malfunction, often of a temporary nature.
C. Purulent discharge is an indication of infection. This may be a transient mucous membrane infection by oppotunistic organisms, in which case it should clear rapidly with local treatment. Purulent discharge that does not subside on local treatment is an indication of a resistant organism, irreversible mucous membrane disease, cholesteatoma, or all of these.
D. The presence of odor suggests tissue necrosis. A malodorous discharge is usually found in active cholesteatoma.

PERFORATION:

A. Perforations of the tympanic membrane are generally divided into two types: central and marginal.
B. A central perforation is not usually associated with cholesteatoma although there are exceptions, especially in children. Intermittent discharge of mucoid material, responding quickly to local treatment, is the rule.
C. A marginal perforation is usually associated with a cholesteatoma. Continuous or frequently recurring malodorous discharge is the rule. This may respond only temporarily, if at all, to local treatment.
D. There are two types of marginal perforations: attic and postero-superior marginal. Attic perforations involve the area of the pars flaccida. The pars tensa may at times appear quite normal. As a result, perforations in this area are occasionally overlooked. A small perforation may be covered by dried

crusts. A polyp of granulation tissue may be seen to extrude through the perforation and tends to block discharge. The hearing impairment is negligible at times due to the fact that the cholesteatoma develops external to the ossicles and even may extend into the antrum without producing significant ossicular necrosis.

E. A posterosuperior marginal perforation below the malleolar ligament may or may not be associated with cholesteatoma. When cholesteatoma is present, the hearing impairment tends to be more severe than with attic perforation. The incus, and at times the stapes, is destroyed early in the development of the disease.

STATUS OF THE MIDDLE EAR MUCOSA:

A. Much may be learned regarding the possible outcome of surgery by careful evaluation of the middle ear as seen through the perforation.

B. The character of the mucosa, the status of the ossicles, and the presence or absence of tympanosclerosis are noted.

C. The presence of normal or near normal mucous membrane is a favorable prognostic sign. When squamous epithelium is observed in the middle ear, the status of the tubotympanic recess should be checked.

D. When ossicular necrosis occurs, usually the incus is the first involved. Of prime importance is the status of the stapes. When the stapes superstructure is absent the prognosis for restoration of hearing is usually less favorable. If the malleus handle is also absent, a two-stage operation may be required for hearing improvement.

E. <u>Tympanosclerosis</u> is the term used to describe a sclerotic or hyaline change of the submucosal tissue of the middle ear. It appears to be an end product of recurrent acute or chronic ear infection. Hyalinized connective tissue develops under the mucous membrane superficial to the bone. Calcification and ossification may occur. Its presence may affect the ultimate prognosis for hearing improvement. If there is a progressive hearing impairment, there may be ossicular fixation by tympanosclerosis. A second operation for stapedectomy may be required at times; the patient should be informed of this possibility.[36, 43, 44, 47]

<u>Myringosclerosis</u> (Doyle) is the term applied to describe deposits of hyaline masses with fibrous layer of the tympanic membrane, but it is also generally referred to as tympanosclerosis of the tympanic membrane. It is often necessary to remove these hyaline masses for a successful myringoplasty.

FISTULA TEST: This is a production of vertigo and deviation of the eyes on the application of pressure to the affected ear. This is elicited by increasing the pressure within the ear canal by means of a pneumatic otoscope or Politzer bag with an olive tip, or pressing sharply on the tragus with the thumb. Suction with the Politzer bag may cause the reversal of the labyrinthine symptoms. The significance of this test is that there is a fistula of the labyrinth due to destructive cholesteatoma or infection. Positive fistula test is present in two-thirds of the cases with a labyrinthine fistula.

Positive fistula test despite an intact tympanic membrane may indicate an abnormally mobile footplate of the stapes, and suggests congenital syphilis (Hennebert's sign).

PATCH TEST: When some hearing loss accompanies a central perforation, it is possible to assess the damage of the ossicular chain by placing a small patch of cigarette paper or a Teflon sheet over the perforation. Should the hearing improve with this maneuver, it is assumed that the ossicular chain is intact, and that myringoplasty is likely to succeed in improving the hearing.

EUSTACHIAN TUBE FUNCTION:

A. The eustachian tube function should always be tested by Valsalva and Politzer inflation of the eustachian tube. If these are unsuccessful, it may be tested by catheter inflation.

B. Methods of estimating the pressure required to open the eustachian tube have been devised. Unfortunately, the methods of testing the eustachian tube are not entirely satisfactory and it may be difficult to derive at a quantitative measurement in a clinical situation.

C. Miller[28] developed a method of eustachian tube function test by applying the pressure differential through a catheter sealed in the external auditory canal. The effect of swallowing on this pressure may be easily recorded on a paper writer such as an ECG machine. The necessity of a perforated tympanic membrane has made the determination of normal values difficult, but this is not a problem in clinical practice since most surgical patients have a pre-existing perforation. The application of this method in patients with secretory otitis media requires placing a tube through the intact membrane. In practice the test is carried out by causing a negative pressure of 250 mm H_2O within the external auditory canal and observing the equalization of pressure as the patient swallows. With normal function, the pressure difference is eliminated after several swallows. Four gradations of abnormality have been described, the most severe being in those patients in whom no air flow occurs even with the application of a positive pressure of 250 mm H_2O, indicating complete functional obstruction of the tube.

D. Tympanic cavity clearance test with use of a dye through the intact tympanic membrane or through the tympanic perforation has also been used as a measure of function (Compere 1958).

E. Inflation (Valsalva), although not always accurate, remains the simplest and a most satisfactory method. For practical purposes, if the eustachian tube can be inflated easily by the Valsalva or Politzer method the prognosis for successful tympanoplasty is excellent. If inflation is difficult, requiring repeated attempts or use of the catheter, there may be development of secretory otitis after tympanoplasty, requiring insertion of a polyethylene tube through the tympanic membrane.

F. Tympanometry has become a useful method of eustachian tube function test. (See item 5). Blocked eustachian tube is usually associated with Type B or C tympanogram.

4. AUDIOLOGICAL EVALUATION: Careful audiometric tests should be performed routinely. The findings are confirmed by the otologist using the tuning fork with a Barany noisemaker to mask the opposite ear.

The minimum audiometric test requirements are pure-tone bone air conduction thresholds, speech reception levels, and speech discrimination scores. The audiometric test results should always coincide with those of the tuning fork test.

5. TYMPANOMETRY: The most significant advance in the identification of middle ear disease is the use of a new instrument, the electro-acoustic impedance bridge with which a tympanogram can be obtained.

Tympanometry is a reliable, simple procedure, easily carried out in a short time. To perform tympanometry, a small probe is inserted in the external auditory canal. A tone of fixed characteristics is presented via the probe, and the compliance of the tympanic membrane is measured electronically while the external canal pressure is artifically varied.

As is true for eardrum mobility observed visually with a pneumatic otoscope, acoustic compliance is greatest when pressures are equal on both sides of the tympanic membrane. Thus, a peak is present when the middle ear pressure is normal (Type A). A peak is present in the negative range when middle ear pressure is reduced (Type C). Middle ear effusions are present in most cases in which no impedance peak can be determined (Type B).[4, 21] See Figure 3-2.

For evaluation of chronic otitis media, tympanometry is useful to detect or confirm the following: (Jerger)[21]

a) Otitis media	Type B (43%) or C (47%)
b) Cholesteatoma	Type B (54%) or C (42%)
c) Middle ear fluid	Type B (44%) or C (45%)
d) Scarred or thickened TM	Type A (45%) or C (40%)
e) Ossicular fixation	"Shallow" Type A (reduced peak)
f) Ossicular discontinuity	"deep" Type A (100%) (open high peak) (high compliance)

Tympanometry is also useful (a) as an aid in diagnosis when otoscopy is equivocal or difficult, particularly in children, (b) in conforming otoscopic diagnosis, and (c) as a screening test of ear diseases.

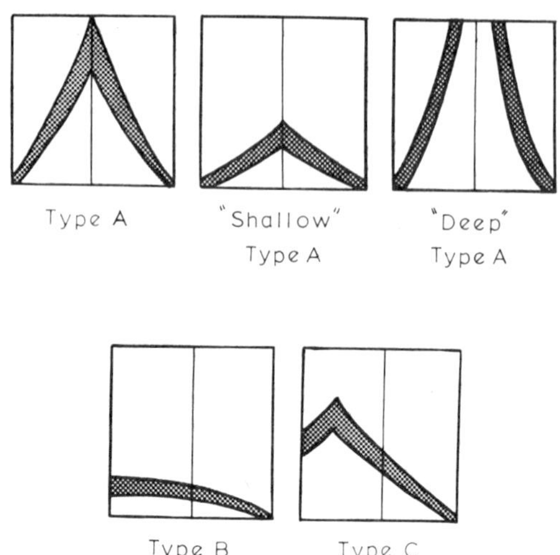

FIGURE 3-2. Diagrammatic Representation of Tympanograms

6. RADIOGRAPHIC EXAMINATION: Mastoid x-rays which are useful for evaluation of chronic otitis media include Law, Schüller, Stenver, and submentovertical. Polytomography may clearly demonstrate bony destruction by cholesteatoma, presence or absence of ossicles, and, in some cases, fistula of the horizontal semicircular canal. (See Chapter 19)

The decision to operate or not to operate is rarely based on the x-ray findings alone. They are helpful, however, in detecting disease not otherwise suspected but which requires mastoid investigation. Occasionally one detects an anatomic variation, eg., a far forward lateral sinus, which allows a better planned approach to the mastoid disease.

7. PREOPERATIVE TREATMENT: Systemic antibiotics are of minimal value in chronic otitis media. Before any drugs are applied to the ear, the ear should be thoroughly cleared of debris and discharge. This can be done in several different ways. Whenever possible, suction should be employed. The ear can be gently cleaned with cotton applicators. Insufflation of boric acid powder may assist in drying the ear. If fungus infection is suspected, an antifungal agent should be used, usually in powder form.

In patients with chronic otitis media with mucoid discharge treatment of coexisting upper respiratory infections must always be a part of the management of otitis media. Exacerbation of the chronic otitis media commonly accompany and are dependent upon infections in the nose and nasopharynx. Any conditions, therefore, such as sinusitis, nasal obstruction or any other causes of recurrent nasal infection must be treated before reconstructive surgery is attempted. This also includes allergic evaluation when indicated.

SURGICAL TREATMENT: Any patient with a perforated tympanic membrane, chronic ear infection, or a defect in the ossicular chain is a potential candidate for surgical treatment. The primary purpose of surgery may be any one or all of the following:

a) Elimination of infection
b) Improvement of hearing
c) Closure of a perforation (prevention of infection)

It should be understood first that the complete erradication of disease is a pre-requisite of all surgical treatment and preservation and restoration of hearing are secondary.

Indications for immediate surgery include:
a) Persistent ear pain
b) Vertigo (continuous)
c) Facial paralysis
d) Threatened intracranial complications

The following are the common operations performed in chronic ear surgery. With rare exceptions, an operation for chronic ear disease can be classified as one of the following. Technical surgical variations peculiar to one or another surgeon do not alter the fundamental classifications (Standard Classification for Surgery of Chronic Ear Infection).[9, 31, 43, 45]

1. Modified radical mastoidectomy
2. Radical mastoidectomy
3. Mastoid obliteration operation
4. Myringoplasty
5. Tympanoplasty without mastoidectomy
6. Tympanoplasty with mastoidectomy

1. MODIFIED RADICAL MASTOIDECTOMY: This commonly performed operation (Bondy's operation) remains the basic operation in most mastoidectomies and tympanoplasties, particularly in the sclerotic mastoid, when the disease extends medial to the facial nerve and into the posterior tympanic recesses. This is frequently used for acquired cholesteatoma and exteriorizes the mastoid antrum to form a common cavity with the external auditory canal. Unlike the radical mastoidectomy the tympanic membrane and functioning ossicles are left intact.

2. RADICAL MASTOIDECTOMY: This operation is performed for cases of chronic otitis media with cholesteatoma which have developed secondary to the marginal tympanic perforation, those beyond the scope of the modified radical mastoidectomy, chronic otitis media with extension into the labyrinth or petrous portion of the temporal bone, chronic otitis media with osteitis or osteomyelitis, and certain neoplasms.

In this operation, the mastoid antrum, mastoid air cells and middle ear space are exteriorized so that they form a common cavity with the external auditory canal. Meatoplasty is always performed. This permits inspection and periodic cleaning in the postoperative period.

Radical mastoidectomy is primarily for eradication of infection with no intention to restore the hearing.

3. MASTOID OBLITERATION OPERATION: This is an operation to obliterate the mastoidectomy cavity, which is created following the radical or modified radical mastoidectomy, using a muscle or other tissue pedicle graft. The purpose of this operation is to restore near normal anatomic contour and avoid the frequent aftercare of the mastoid cavity.[23]

When the disease, either cholesteatomatous or necrotic, has extensive ramifications, and there is the slightest doubt in the surgeon's mind regarding complete removal, obliteration of the cavity is not advisable. Recurrent cholesteatoma behind the muscle may develop.

4. MYRINGOPLASTY: (Type I Tympanoplasty): Myringoplasty is an operation in which reconstructive procedure is limited to the repair of tympanic perforation, utilizing a tissue graft. The ossicular chain is intact and mobile.

Since Zollner (1951) and Wullstein (1952) opened the way to tympanoplasty, there have been many grafting materials used. These include pedicled canal skin (Sooy, 1956), canal skin (House and Sheehy, 1961), vein (Tabb, 1960, Shea, 1960), fascia (Storrs, 1961), fat (Ringenberg, 1962), perichondrium (Goodhill, 1967), heart valves, corneas, gelfoam and more recently, homograft tympanic membranes have been used (Chalat, 1964, Marquet, 1966, Perkins, 1970). Temporalis fascia has become the most widely used of all the grafting materials.

If there has been any discharge from the ear or any moisture in the ear during the previous six months, myringoplasty alone is contraindicated. If there has been recent discharge, the repair should be combined with inspection of the attic, aditus and antrum.

An edema or polyposis of the mucous membrane of the middle ear will render the operation unlikely to succeed. Poor eustachian tube function is also a contraindication.[40, 50]

5. TYMPANOPLASTY WITHOUT MASTOIDECTOMY: This refers to an operation to eradicate disease in the middle ear and to reconstruct the hearing mechanism without mastoidectomy, with or without tympanic grafting.

The cardinal principles of tympanoplasty have been and still are: first control of infection through eradication of disease, and second, reconstruction of the middle ear sound-conducting mechanism.

A. Type I Tympanoplasty: This was previously discussed. Tympanoplasty Type I or Myringoplasty is an operation in which the procedure is limited to repair of the tympanic membrane perforation.

It is a good habit to routinely evaluate the middle ear and ossicles to rule out ossicular fixation or discontinuity. This can be done by elevating the tympanomeatal flap. It is important to prepare the graft recipient site first since it is difficult to denude the drum head after it becomes flaccid. A wide recipient site should be established. In the presence of a total tympanic perforation, this necessitates reflecting the graft up onto the adjacent denuded bony canal wall for at least several mm. It is especially important to position the graft "tightly" in the anterior sulcus where graft failure occurs most commonly as a result of technical error. It is here that the branches of the anterior tympanic and deep auricular artery provide critical blood supply to the graft.

The graft may be placed on the denuded outer surface (overlay graft) or on the denuded inner surface (underlay graft) of the ear drum. In the latter case, the graft is supported by gelfoam in the middle ear.[20, 43]

One of the persistent problems encountered with lateral placement of the graft is lateral migration of the graft away from the handle of the malleus or the anterior sulcus causing a thick blunting or rounding off in this area. Medial placement of the graft avoids this problem. However, when the perforation is total or involves the anterior half of the tympanic membrane, one should be aware that the anterior portion of the medially placed graft may have a tendency to be pulled away from the drum remnant toward the medial wall of the middle ear and may result in postoperative perforation in this area.

B. Type II Tympanoplasty: Type II tympanoplasty consists of a graft placement directly upon the incus. This can result from a destroyed malleus but more commonly it is seen in instances in which wide atticoantrotomy or removal of the posterior bony canal wall with mastoidectomy is done, in which case the graft necessarily rests upon the body of the incus.

C. Type III and Type IV Tympanoplasty: Type III and Type IV tympanoplasty are more often done in association with complete mastoidectomy. It is important to expose the facial recess (suprapyramidal recess) and sinus tympani (infrapyramidal recess) for the removal of the disease.

D. Type V Tympanoplasty: While performing tympanoplasty fixation of the stapes due to either otosclerosis or more commonly to tympanosclerosis may be found.

When tympanosclerotic fixation is found it is best to effect a mobilization by removal of the tympanosclerotic tissue, if possible. If this is not possible, all infected tissues should be removed, a graft applied and the ear observed for at least six months to a year.

Assuming a dry ear with no tendency toward infection, good tubal function and good auditory function in the opposite ear, Type V tympanoplasty can be considered.

The original Type V tympanoplasty consisted of fenestration of the horizontal semicircular canal (Type V a). If anatomical characteristics are suitable, stapedectomy can be performed (Type V b). Surprisingly good hearing may be obtained (Gacek).[16, 31]

Stapes mobilization or stapedectomy at the time of tympanic membrane grafting, even in the dry ear, may result in a sensorineural hearing loss. At least 12 months should elapse between the initial tympanoplasty and secondary stapedectomy.

6. TYMPANOPLASTY WITH MASTOIDECTOMY: The elimination of infection by mastoidectomy is combined with reconstruction of the hearing mechanism.

Intact posterior wall mastoidectomy with tympanoplasty:[42] Intact canal wall technique has been popularized in recent years by many otologists. This procedure prevents a mastoid cavity postoperatively. It should be stressed, however, that the primary objective should always be removal of the disease and not the preservation of the posterior canal wall.

Following a complete mastoidectomy, the antrum and aditus are enlarged so that the incus is readily seen. The epitympanum is inspected through the aditus. The facial recess (suprapyramidal recess) and sinus tympani (infrapyramidal recess) are exposed and are cleared of disease and tympanoplasty is accomplished. If a large area of the posterior superior canal wall is removed, retraction of the tympanic membrane may develop. A silicone rubber sheet is placed to prevent adhesions. This procedure is contraindicated in the following situations (Sheehy):[42, 43]

a) The only hearing ear
b) Labyrinthine fistula when the other ear has cholesteatoma
c) Inadequate exposure due to severely contracted mastoid
d) Extensive canal wall destruction by disease

In these situations, it is "safer" to remove the posterior bony canal, and perform modified radical mastoidectomy combined with tympanoplasty.

7. OSSICULAR RECONSTRUCTION IN TYMPANOPLASTY:[17, 18, 36, 38, 43, 45, 49, 50, 51]

A. The goal of functional reconstruction is to obtain a permanent restoration of hearing with neither conductive or sensorineural hearing loss.

B. When the stapes is normal, a carefully fitted ossicular prosthesis (autograft or homograft) is the procedure of choice. The incus is the most readily available ossicle. The incus (shaped or sculptured) may be placed between the handle of the malleus and the head of the stapes, or it may be placed adjacent to the manubrium. When the stapes capitulum is more deeply seated, the malleus head may be used instead of the incus.

C. The commonest ossicular problem encountered is necrosis of the long crus of the incus.

D. The most common cause of failure is separation of the ossicle from the head of the stapes, followed by fixation of the ossicle to adjacent bony structures. Extrusion of the repositioned ossicle is uncommon.

E. When the suprastructure of the stapes is missing, a shaped incus may be placed between the handle of the malleus and the mobile footplate, or it may be placed adjacent to the manubrium of the malleus. A strut of cartilage may be used instead. Cartilage has advantages; it does not become fixed by bone and it rarely extrudes.

F. When the malleus handle is absent, there is nothing to stabilize the graft. A two-stage procedure may be necessary: at the first stage disease is removed, and Silastic sheet inserted to prevent adhesion and a graft applied; the second stage involves removal of the plastic and insertion of a suitable prosthesis (cartilage). One may use a homograft tympanic membrane en bloc ossicles as a single procedure.

G. The most common cause of ossicular fixation in case of chronic otitis media is tympanosclerosis. It may fix the malleus head and the stapes. When the malleus head is fixed, it should be amputated and the incus repositioned. When the stapes is fixed, disease is removed and the tympanic membrane repaired. At the second operation, a stapedectomy is performed.

H. Plastic and wire prosthesis tends to be extruded. Bone chips tend to resorb in time.

8. OTOLOGIC HOMOGRAFTS: 1, 24, 26, 32, 36, 46, 50, 51

A. Homograft ossicles, mostly obtained from patients when the ossicle must be removed for various reasons, are autoclaved and then stored in 70% alcohol. These ossicles may be used interchangeably with autografts in any situation in which ossicular repositioning is indicated. They are well tolerated and it is difficult to tell microspically a repositioned incus from a homograft incus (Linthicum).[24]

B. The most frequently used homograft ossicle is homograft incus, followed by malleus and stapes. Smith (1957) employs a stapes homograft when there is a loss of the stapedial arch and there is a mobile footplate.[46]

C. Homograft septal and tragal cartilage maintains its shape and structure with the exception of the chondrocyte, which are missing from the lucunae. It is well tolerated and becomes covered with mucosa.[2, 24]

D. Homograft tympanic membranes are now available through the ear bank of Project Hear, Palo Alto, Calif. (Perkins)[32] It was first used by Chalat 1964, then Marquet 1966, later by Brandow 1969 and Perkins 1970.

E. Tympanic membrane ossicles en bloc homografts may be indicated in the following situations (Perkins):

a) Large tympanic membrane perforations with malleus manubrial disease (malleus fixed, retracted, defective, or absent) (Alford).

b) Large tympanic membrane perforations with malleus head and incus disease (attic cholesteatoma).

c) Tympanomastoid reconstruction (radical mastoidectomy cavity)

F. Many techniques to reconstruct the radical mastoidectomy cavity have been proposed. They include:

a) Obliteration procedures with soft tissues (musculoplasty) - soft tissues atrophy but cavity filled with dense fibrous tissues

b) Obliteration with bone (Shea, M.C.)

c) Cartilage reconstruction of the ear canal either with tragal or homograft knee cartilage (Wehrs)

d) Intact posterior canal bone homograft with a homograft tympanic membrane

e) Reconstruction with a homograft dura form and autogenous bone pate (Perkins 1976) using a homograft tympanic membrane with ossicles en bloc for middle ear reconstruction

G. Complications of otologic homografts are absorption, infection, fibrous hyperplasia, extrusion and rejection. They should not be used in an infected cavity.

IV. COMPLICATIONS OF SUPPURATIVE OTITIS MEDIA

FACTORS THAT INFLUENCE THE DEVELOPMENT OF COMPLICATIONS[31, 45]

1. Factors influencing the spread of infection beyond the middle ear space are the type and virulence of the infecting organism, its susceptibility to available antibacterial medication, the adequacy of treatment, the resistance of the host and the presence or absence of associated chronic systemic illness.

2. The Type III pneumococcus has a particular predilection for intracranial extension. The resistance of the host especially to this organism is lowered in infancy, old age and diabetes. Intracranial extension of an acute infection of the middle ear occurs more often in poorly pneumatized than in the well pneumatized temporal bones and in ears with a previous history of recurrent otitis media.

3. The bone-invading types of chronic otitis media that lead to complications are relatively uncommon chronic osteomyelitis of the temporal bone and the much more common cholesteatoma of either the attic retraction or secondary acquired variety.

4. Complications often result from insufficient dosage or insufficient period of administration of the drug or selection of a less effective drug without the benefit of culture and sensitivity tests.

PATHWAYS OF SPREAD OF INFECTION

1. EXTENSION BY OSTEOTHROMBOPHLEBITIS: Infection may pass along the vascular channels through intact bone by the process of osteothrombophlebitis. Complications from this pathway usually occur within 10 days of the original infection.

2. EXTENSION BY BONE EROSION: This is the most frequent manner of spread leading to a complication in case of acute otitis in a well pneumatized temporal bone and it is nearly always the manner of spread in cases of chronic suppurative otitis media.

Complications resulting from this spread of infection usually do not occur for several weeks.

In acute otitis media the bone erosion is the result of a coalescent mastoiditis. In chronic otitis media the bone erosion is usually due to a cholesteatoma, less often due to chronic osteomyelitis. Through bone erosion, infection can spread to the mastoid cortex, the petrous portion of the temporal bone, facial nerve, the labyrinth, the lateral sinus, or the dura. The treatment of a complication by bone erosion is directed toward the complication and always includes surgical removal of the focus of suppuration in the temporal bone.

3. EXTENSION BY PREFORMED PATHWAY: The preformed pathway may be a normal opening in the bony wall such as the oval or round window leading from the middle ear to the labyrinth or the internal auditory meatus, perilymphatic duct, or endolymphatic duct and sac leading from the labyrinth to the meninges. The pathway may be developmental dehiscence of the floor of the hypotympanum or it may be the result of a skull fracture or previous ear surgery such as a fenestration, a stapedectomy, a labyrinthotomy for Meniere's disease or a mastoidectomy in which dura was exposed. Perilymph fistula following partial or total stapedectomy establishes an open pathway for infection to extend into the labyrinth.

Acute infections often spread through a preformed pathway, causing early complications. Extension in chronic ear infection is usually secondary to bone erosion, causing late complications.

TYPES OF COMPLICATIONS: There are two major categories of complications: extracranial and intracranial. Complications can usefully be classified as follows:

EXTRACRANIAL	INTRACRANIAL
1. Subperiosteal abscess	1. Extradural abscess
2. Facial paralysis	2. Subdural abscess
3. Labyrinthitis	3. Brain abscess
4. Petrositis	4. Lateral sinus thrombosis
	5. Meningitis
	6. Otitic hydrocephalus

SUBPERIOSTEAL ABSCESS

1. Postauricular abscess (the commonest type) is formed by pus spreading through the minute vascular channels in the suprameatal (Macewen's) triangle and presents as a swelling between the tip of the mastoid and the Macewen's triangle. The auricle is displaced forward, outward and downward.

2. Zygomatic abscess is formed by pus escaping from the zygomatic cells near the squama. This presents as a swelling above and in front of the ear and may be confused with a parotid swelling. Rarely, the pus may spread downward and forward into the mandibular fossa with a displacement of the mandible toward the normal side so that the teeth no longer meet in occlusion.

3. Bezold's abscess results from the perforation of the tip of the inner aspect of the mastoid by the pus which will track down the sternocleidomastoid muscle and present as a swelling in the posterior triangle of the neck.

4. Sagging of the posterosuperior meatal wall by a subperiosteal abscess may rarely occur as a result of a coalescent mastoiditis. Today, this occurs much less likely in an acute otitis media than in a chronic otitis media with cholesteatoma formation.

5. Parapharyngeal or retropharyngeal abscess may result from an acute suppurative otitis media or mastoiditis. The pus may track from peritubal cells or by formation of an abscess below the petrous pyramid.

6. Treatment of postauricular, zygomatic and Bezold's abscess is simple mastoidectomy, although a Bezold's abscess may require separate additional incision and drainage.

FACIAL PARALYSIS

Direct extension of infection into the facial canal through a dehiscence in the bony covering of the tympanic portion of the nerve or by destruction of the bone overlying the nerve causes facial nerve paralysis.

Immediate surgical decompression is recommended for facial nerve paralysis caused by chronic ear disease. Surgical decompression of the nerve is usually unnecessary for patients with acute otitis media and is offered to those patients who fail to respond to the usual treatment with myringotomy and antibiotics and/or whose nerves undergo degeneration as determined by electrodiagnostic tests.

LABYRINTHITIS

Labyrinthitis is the most frequent complication of otitis media due to extension of infection within the temporal bone. Three types of labyrinthine inflammation may occur as a complication of acute otitis media and mastoiditis. They are, in the order of ascending severity, perilabyrinthitis, serous labyrinthitis, and suppurative labyrinthitis.

1. PERILABYRINTHITIS (LABYRINTHINE FISTULA): This may be surgically produced (simple or radical mastoidectomy, fenestration, labyrinthotomy or stapedectomy) or it may occur spontaneously due to bone erosion by cholesteatoma. Spontaneous fistula usually results from erosion of one of the semicircular canals, especially the lateral semicircular canal.

The most common severe complication from cholesteatoma is fistulization of the horizontal semicircular canal.

The diagnosis of labyrinthine fistula is established by eliciting the fistula sign. This consists of nystagmus and vertigo when positive and negative pressure is applied to the soft tissue covering the fistula. The nystagmus is produced by a movement of endolymph toward the ampulla with inward pressure displacement, with the quick component toward the affected ear. With negative pressure there is outward displacement and a movement of endolymph away from the ampulla, with the quick component of nystagmus toward the normal ear. The absence of the fistula test does not rule out the presence of a fistula. Positive fistula test is present in two-thirds of the cases with a labyrinthine fistula. The presence of a fistula in the horizontal semicircular canal may be demonstrated on the AP polytome x-ray.

The patient with active fistula of the labyrinth often complains of dizziness if he presses against the tragus or manipulates the auricle, or if he turns the head quickly. Rarely he may experience momentary vertigo when exposed to a loud noise (Tullio phenomenon).

A strong positive fistula sign is always an indication for surgical examination of the labyrinth. When erosion is associated with chronic otitis media, a radical or modified radical mastoidectomy must be performed to eradicate the pathologic condition. In this way, spread of infection into the labyrinth can be prevented.

Cholesteatoma matrix can be removed with reasonable safety from most small (less than 2 mm) semicircular canal fistulae. When the matrix is firmly adherent to a large area of membranous semicircular canal, its removal is not recommended in view of high incidence of postoperative sensorineural deafness. When the fistula involves the cochlear wall, the cholesteatoma matrix should not be removed. Its removal carries a high risk of postoperative sensorineural deafness. If the contralateral ear has no auditory function and the ear with the fistula is the only hearing ear, the cholesteatoma matrix over the fistula is best left undisturbed. In such cases, the cavity should be kept open and the patient should be followed closely to determine further active suppuration develops.[15]

2. SEROUS LABYRINTHITIS: This is a diffuse intralabyrinthine inflammation without pus formation, and not followed by permanent loss of auditory and vestibular function. It is, however, a prepurulent condition and potential precursor of suppurative labyrinthitis.

The treatment of serous labyrinthitis secondary to acute otitis media is primarily medical with large dosage of antibiotics. Surgery is mandatory in chronic infections when serous labyrinthitis develops.

3. SUPPURATIVE LABYRINTHITIS (PURULENT LABYRINTHITIS): This is a diffuse intralabyrinthine infection with pus formation and is associated with permanent loss of auditory and vestibular function.

This may occur as a result of direct extension of the purulent process in the middle ear or mastoid into the labyrinth or may result from the spread of meningeal inflammation into the labyrinth through the internal auditory canal or less frequently through the cochlear aqueduct.

Clinical symptoms include nausea and vomiting, intense vertigo, tinnitus, hearing loss and nystagmus.

Treatment should consist of intense antibiotic treatment and surgical drainage of the labyrinth.

PETROSITIS

Petrositis is an inflammation of the petrous portion of the temporal bone characterized by that clinical triad of otitis media, paralysis of the VIth cranial nerve, and pain of the Vth cranial nerve (Gradenigo's syndrome). The symptoms of petrositis depend upon the area of the petrous pyramid affected.

Approximately 30% of the temporal bones past the age of three years have pneumatization in the petrous apex. Even the pneumatized petrous apex has unpneumatized areas containing marrow. This makes this site more susceptible to osteomyelitis. Air cells extend into the petrous pyramid in two main groups: a posterior group from the epitympanum and antrum around the semicircular canals into the base of the pyramid, not infrequently extending to the apex; and an anterior group from the tympanum, hypotympanum and eustachian tube around the cochlea into the apex of the pyramid. The posterior group of cells is present in about 30% of temporal bone whereas the anterior group of cells is present in about 15% of temporal bones.

Additional symptoms of petrositis, though not frequent, include transient facial weakness, mild recurrent vertigo, and fever. If the suppuration extends beyond the petrosa there may be added symptoms of localized and/or generalized meningitis, a cerebellar or a temporal lobe abscess, thrombophlebitis of the inferior petrosal sinus and jugular bulb, or of a lateral pharyngeal, retropharyngeal or deep neck abscess (Bezold's abscess).

Petrositis should be suspected in any patient whose ear continues to drain after surgery for chronic infection or in any patient with ear disease who complains of persistent pain that is otherwise unexplained.

Treatment is by surgical drainage. A systematic search of the common pathways for extension of infection into the petrous area must be undertaken. The easiest and safest surgical approach to infected petrous cells is along the route by which the cells invaded the petrosa. Surgical drainage should always be preceded by a complete simple mastoidectomy for the posterior group of cells and a radical mastoidectomy for the anterior group of cells. Care must be taken to prevent injury to the carotid artery in exploring the anterior cell group.

EXTRADURAL ABSCESS

An extradural abscess is a collection of pus between the dura and bone. Apart from coalescent mastoiditis, this is the most common complication of otitis media. It is usually secondary to bone erosion rather than due to osteothrombophlebitis or via preformed pathways. If the pus lies against the dura of the posterior fossa medial to the sigmoid sinus, it is called an extradural or epidural abscess. If it lies against the split of posterior fossa dura enclosing the lateral sinus, it is called perisinus abscess.

The most common symptom is persistent headache; however, many extradural abscesses are unnoticed prior to surgery. Other symptoms include an unusually severe earache and a malaise with low grade fever. Marked pulsation of the purulent discharge accentuated by compression of the jugular vein is noted. One clinical feature that is somewhat pathognomonic of an extradural abscess is relief of headache by profuse drainage from the ear. The treatment is surgical drainage.

SUBDURAL ABSCESS

Subdural abscess develops when pus accumulates between the dura and the arachnoid. This is uncommon. This may develop as a result of extension of an infection of the middle ear and mastoid through the intact bone and the dura by means of thrombophlebitis of veins or by direct extension with erosion of bone and dura.

The symptoms include headache, malaise, delirious state, focal seizures, and other neurological signs such as hemiplegia, aphasia or hemianopsia. Signs of meningeal irritation are almost always present.

Attacks of Jacksonian epilepsy with hemiplegia developing in association with middle ear infection should be regarded as indicative of subdural abscess until proven otherwise. Treatment is surgical drainage of the subdural space.

BRAIN ABSCESS

Otogenic brain abscess occurs usually in the temporal lobe of the cerebrum (more frequent) or in the cerebellum. It is said to be the most frequent cause of death from otitis media.

The abscess may develop as a result of direct extension of the otologic infection, by means of thrombophlebitis, or along the preformed pathway. It may result from previous skull fracture. An extradural abscess usually forms prior to the development of a brain abscess. Cerebellar abscesses from otitis media usually form through preformed pathways whereas temporal lobe abscess results from seeding through bone erosion. Three clinical stages of brain abscess have been observed:

1. THE FIRST STAGE OF INITIAL ENCEPHALITIS: Elevation of temperature, headache, nuchal rigidity or other meningeal signs are often noted.

2. THE SECOND LATENT OR QUIESCENT STAGE: The symptoms are minimal or absent as an abscess is becoming organized and beginning to expand. This stage may last several weeks. The patient may complain of headache, irritability or lethargy.

3. THE THIRD STAGE OF AN EXPANDING ABSCESS: The symptoms and signs of this stage are due to generalized increased intracranial pressure and localized pressure on brain centers. They include severe and continuous headache (the most constant symptom), projectile vomiting, slowing of the pulse, Cheyne-Stokes respiration, apathy and drowsiness, change in mental activity, disorientation, Jacksonian convulsions, ocular paralysis with pupillary changes, hemianopsia,aphasia, and elevated blood pressure. The most constant signs of increased intracranial pressure occur in the eyeground with blurring of the disc margins, hyperemia or papilledema.

A left temporal lobe abscess in the right handed patient most commonly results in nominal aphasia. The next most common finding is paresis of contralateral face and mouth spreading to the extremities. A right temporal lobe abscess in a right handed patient results in paralysis and numbness of the left side.

Cerebellar abscess usually gives more localizing signs. Among them are:

a) Ataxia (Tendency to fall to the diseased side)
b) Ipsilateral hypotonia and weakness
c) Spontaneous vertical or variable nystagmus
d) Rapid emaciation
e) Dysdiadochokinesia
f) Intention tremor with past pointing

DIAGNOSIS: Otogenic brain abscess is suspected from the characteristic clinical features described above in a patient with a coexisting or pre-existing suppurative otitis media. Definitive diagnosis of brain abscess is made by special neurosurgical procedures which include lumbar puncture, ventriculography, angiography, electroencephalography, brain scanning, computerized tomography and brain puncture. Ultimate diagnosis is made by finding the pus by brain puncture via a burr-hole.

Lumbar puncture shows an increase in cerebrospinal fluid pressure and protein. Lumbar puncture is valuable in differentiating brain abscess from other otogenic intracranial complications. However, it should be noted that lumbar puncture in advanced brain abscess with increased intracranial pressure can be followed by death due to herniation of the brain stem into the foramen magnum. A cerebellar abscess seldom reaches a large size since it is near the respiratory center. Compression of this center results in respiratory arrest and death. A temporal lobe abscess can keep expanding until it ruptures into the fourth ventricle causing fulminating meningitis. The treatment is primarily surgical drainage and an intense course of antibiotics.

LATERAL SINUS THROMBOPHLEBITIS:

Lateral sinus thrombophlebitis usually develops as a consequence of erosion of the lateral sinus plate by coalescent mastoiditis or chronic mastoiditis. First a perisinus abscess is formed. A mural thrombus then develops in the walls of the sinus, and becomes infected and spreads proximally and distally. The lumen of the sinus is eventually occluded by increased thickness of the infected clot and by clotting of the stagnant blood. The ends of the infected clots then soften and infected material continues to escape into the systemic circulation (septicema). Lateral sinus thrombophlebitis can also be caused by infections of the scalp or adjacent bones along the mastoid emissary vein. The usual organisms are hemolytic Streptococci and Pneumococci.

The clinical features vary according to the stage of the infection. When a perisinus abscess develops, headaches and malaise are usually the only symptoms. When the mural thrombus becomes infected within the vessel, septicemia develops with septic fever and chills. The primary symptoms of lateral sinus thrombophlebitis may be a persistent and spiking type of fever ("Picket-fence"). Between bouts of fever the patient is often alert and feels well. Anemia may develop. With occlusion of the lumen of the sinus, interference with cerebral circulation results in headaches, papilledema and increased cerebrospinal fluid pressure. When the thrombophlebitis spreads to the mastoid emissary vein, edema and tenderness may be produced over the mastoid process (Greisinger's sign). When the thrombophlebitis spreads to the jugular bulb and internal jugular vein, it may produce pain in the neck particularly on rotation of the neck. This may simulate neck rigidity of diffuse meningitis. The clot may be felt as a tender cord in the neck. The 9th, 10th and 11th cranial nerves are occasionally paralyzed by the pressure of a clot in the jugular bulb.

The diagnosis is based upon positive blood cultures taken during the febrile phase and the demonstration of lateral sinus obstruction by a Tobey-Ayer or Queckenstedt's test. With the spinal needle in place, digital pressure is applied over the internal jugular vein in the neck. This maneuver on the normal side produces a prompt rise in the spinal fluid pressure, but no increase on the side of the lateral sinus obstruction.

The treatment is always surgical. The sinus should be completely uncovered and the perisinus abscess eradicated. A needle aspiration of the sinus will determine if the sinus is occluded. If the sinus is occluded and there is an intrasinus abscess, it is necessary to open the sinus and remove the infected thrombus. When embolism or cavernous sinus thrombosis appears to be developing, anticoagulation together with intensive antibiotic therapy is recommended. Ligation of the internal jugular vein may be necessary.

Lateral sinus thrombophlebitis has been said to be the second most common cause of death from otitis media.

MENINGITIS

Meningitis is the most common intracranial complication from suppurative otitis media and mastoiditis. There are two types of meningitis: localized and generalized.

1. Localized or circumscribed meningitis (no bacterial organism present in the spinal fluid).

2. Generalized meningitis (bacterial organisms are present in the spinal fluid). The patient suddenly becomes very ill and restless with severe headache, vomiting and pyrexia, but soon loses consciousness. The classical signs of meningitis soon appear: stiffness of the neck, positive Kernig's sign, nausea and vomiting, delirious and confused mental state or coma. In children, convulsions, a low weak cry and bulging fontanelle suggests meningitis until proven otherwise. The cerebrospinal fluid looks turbid and shows an increase in pressure and cell count. Protein concentration is raised but the glucose and chloride are reduced. In generalized meningitis, numerous microorganisms can be found.

Treatment of meningitis is chemotherapeutic. Surgery is indicated in those patients developing meningitis secondary to chronic otitis media when the patient's general condition permits.

OTITIC HYDROCEPHALUS

This is a syndrome of increased intracranial pressure without a brain abscess following several weeks or more of acute otitis media. The condition occurs most often in children and adolescents. The most constant symptom is headache, often with a VIth nerve paralysis on the same side, sometimes with vomiting. Otherwise the patient looks and feels quite well. The most constant findings are papilledema and spinal fluid pressure exceeding 300 mm. of water. Unlike localized meningitis the spinal fluid is clear without increased cell count or protein content. There are no localizing neurological changes. Ventriculography fails to show a space occupying lesion.

The exact mechanism of increased cerebrospinal fluid pressure is not known, but it is assumed to be due to increased production or decreased resorption of cerebrospinal fluid secondary to a previous meningeal inflammation. Treatment is repeated lumbar punctures. Subtemporal decompression may become necessary.

CONGENITAL CHOLESTEATOMA (EPIDERMOID) OF THE TEMPORAL BONE: Congenital cholesteatoma or epidermoids arise from aberrant epithelial remnants and are, therefore, considered blastomatous malformations. Their predilective sites are the intracranial cavity, the diploe of the skull and the spinal canal. In the base of the skull the temporal bone is the most frequent site.

Epidermoids account for about 0.2-1.5 percent of all intracranial tumors. The majority originate in the cerebellopontine angle where they account for 6-7 percent of all tumors. Their age incidence reveals a great scatter from birth to 80 years. The majority are recognized during the third and fourth decades with the onset of clinical symptoms occurring much earlier. They affect males more frequently than females. Their delicate capsule with a whitish mother-of-pearl sheen lends them a typical appearance.

Epidermoids are generally slow growing lesions which may remain asymptomatic for years. The irritative effect of their content, however, can produce symptoms of dysfunction and intense inflammation. Malignant changes occur infrequently. Diploic epidermoids are easily recognized, whereas intradural epidermoids are more difficult to identify.

Epidermoids may arise in the vicinity, on the outer aspect or within the temporal bone. Epidermoids originating in any of these locations have certain characteristic features which may arouse suspicion of their presence. Examples of an epidermoid with origin in the typical locations within the temporal bone and cerebello-pontine angle are discussed to portray their individual characteristics (Laryngoscope 85: suppl. 2, Dec., 1975).

REFERENCES

1. Alford, B.R., et al.: Homograft replacement of the tympanic membrane. Laryngoscope 86:199-208, 1976.

2. Austin, D.F. (Editor): Symposium on Surgery for chronic ear disease. Otolaryng. Clin. N. Am. Volume 5, No. 1, Feb. 1972.

3. Bellucci, R.: Basic considerations for success in tympanoplasty. Arch. Otolaryng. 90:732-741, 1969.

4. Bluestone, C.D. and Shwin, P.A.: Middle ear disease in children, pathogenesis, diagnosis and management, Ped. Clin. N. Am. 21:379-400, 1974.

5. Chandler, J.: Pathogenesis and treatment of facial paralysis due to malignant external otitis. Ann. Otol. Rhin. Laryng. 81:648-658, 1972.

6. Chandler, J.R.: Malignant external otitis. Laryngoscope 78: 1257-1294, 1968.

7. Cody, D.T.R. and Taylor, W.F.: Tympanoplasty: Long term hearing results with incus grafts. Laryngoscope 83:852-864, June, 1973.

8. Cody, D.T.R. and Taylor, W.F.: Tympanoplasty: long-term results. Ann. Otol. Rhin. Laryng. 82:538-546, July-Aug., 1973.

9. The committee on conservation of hearing of the American Academy of ophthalmology and otolaryngology: Standard classification for surgery of chronic ear infection. Arch. Otolaryng. 81:204-205, 1965.

10. Crabtree, J.A.: Herpes zoster oticus. Laryngoscope. 78: 1853-1878, 1968.

11. Farrior, J.B.: Classification of tympanoplasty. Arch. Otolaryng. 93:548-550, 1971.

12. Feldman, A.: Acoustic impedance measurement at the eardrum as an aid to diagnosis. J. Speech Res. 6:315, 1963.

13. Finsnes, K.A.: Lethal intracranial complication following air insufflation with pneumatic otoscope. Acta Otolaryng. 75:436-438, 1973.

14. Friedmann, I.: The pathology of otitis media (III) with particular reference to bone change. J. Laryng. 71:313-320, 1957.

15. Gacek, R.R.: Surgical management of labyrinthine fistulas in chronic otitis media with cholesteatoma. Ann. Otol. Rhin. Laryng. Suppl. 10, Vol. 83, Jan-Feb., 1974.

16. Gacek, R.R.: Results of modified type V tympanoplasty. Laryngoscope 83:437-447, 1973.

17. Glasscock, M.E., III: Ossicular chain reconstruction, Laryngoscope 86:211-221, 1976.

18. Goodhill, V.: Tragal Perichrondrium and Cartilage in Tympanoplasty, Arch. Otolaryng. 85:480-491, May 1967.

19. Goodhill, V.: Syphilis of the ear: a histopathological study. Ann. Otol. Rhin. Laryng. 48:676, 1939.

20. Hough, J.V.D.: Tympanoplasty with the interior fascial graft technique and ossicular reconstruction. Laryngoscope, 80: 1385-1413, 1970.

21. Jerger, J., et al.: Studies in impedance audiometry. III: middle ear disorders. Arch. Otolaryng. 99:165-171, 1974.

22. Kerr, A.G., et al.: Congenital syphilitic deafness. J. Laryng. Otol. 87:1-12, 1973.

23. Lee, K.J. and Schucknecht, H.F.: Results of tympanoplasty and mastoidectomy at the Massachusetts eye and ear infirmary. Laryngoscope 81:529-543,1970.

24. Linthicum, F.H.: The histology of otologic homografts, Trans. Am. Acad. Ophthalmol. Otolaryngol. 80:53-59, 1975.

25. McCandless, G.A. and Thomas, G.K.: Impedance audiometry as a screening procedure for middle ear disease. Trans. Am. Acad. Ophthalmol. Otolaryngol. 78:98-102, 1974.

26. Marquet, J.F.E.: Homograft in middle ear surgery--tenyears of experience. Trans. Am. Acad. Ophthalmol. Otolaryngol. 80:30-36, 1975.

27. Mawson, S.: Diseases of the ear. Williams & Wilkins Co., Baltimore, Md., 1967.

28. Miller, G.F., Jr.: Eustachian tubal function in normal and diseased ears. Arch. Otol. 81:41-48, 1965.

29. Nadol, J.B.: Hearing loss of acquired syphilis: diagnosis confirmed by incadectomy. Laryngoscope 85:1888-1897, 1975.

30. Nager, G.T. and Vanderveen, R.S.: Cholesterol granuloma involving the temporal bone. Ann. Otol. 85:204-209, 1976.

31. Paparella, M.M. and Shumrick, D.A. (Ed.): Otolaryngology, Vol. 2, Ear. W.B. Saunders Co., Philadelphia, 1973.

32. Perkins, R.: Otologic homograft indications, techniques, and anatomic and functional results. Trans. Am. Acad. Ophthalmol. Otolaryngol. 80:41-46, 1975.

33. Perlman, H. and Leek, J.: Late congenital syphilis of the ear. Laryngoscope 62:1175-1196, 1952.

34. Perlman, H.B.: Granulomas and specific diseases of the ear and temporal bone. In Otolaryngology (Paparella and Shumrick), W.B. Saunders Co., Philadelphia, Vol. 2, Chapter 12, 1973.

35. Proctor, B. and Lindsay, J.: Tuberculosis of the ear. Arch. Otolaryng. 35:221, 1942.

36. Pulec, J.J. and Sheehy, J.L.: Symposium on Tympanoplasty. IV. Tympanoplasty: ossicular chain reconstruction, Laryngoscope 83:448-465, 1973.

37. Sahn, S.A., and Davidson, P.T.: Mycobacterium tuberculosis infection of middle ear. Chest 66:104-106, July, 1974.

38. Saunders, W.H. and Paparella, M.M.: Atlas of ear surgery, 2nd ed., C.V. Mosby Co., St. Louis, 1971.

39. Schuknecht, H.F.: Pathology of the ear, Harvard University Press, Cambridge, Mass., 1974.

40. Schuknecht, H.F.: Stapedectomy. Little, Brown & Co., Boston, 1971.

41. Sheehy, J.L. and Linthicum, F.H.: Chronic serous mastoiditis: idiopathic hematotympanum and cholesterol granuloma of the mastoid. Laryngoscope, 79:1189-1217, 1969.

42. Sheehy, J.L.: The intact canal wall technique in the management of aural cholesteatoma. J. Laryng. 84:1-31, 1970.

43. Sheehy, J.L.: Surgery of chronic otitis media. Otolaryngology, Vol. II, Chap. X, Harper and Row, New York, 1972.

44. Sheehy, J.L. and House, W.: Tympanosclerosis. Arch. Otolaryng. 76:151-157, 1962.

45. Shambaugh, G.E.: Surgery of the ear, 2nd ed., W.B. Saunders Co., Philadelphia, 1967.

46. Smith, M.F.W. and Downey, D.: Otologic homograft indications, techniques and anatomic and functional results. Trans. Am. Acad. Ophthal. Otolaryngol. 80:47-51, 1975.

47. Smyth, G.D.L.: Tympanosclerosis. J. Laryng. and Otol. 86:9-14, 1972.

48. Storrs, L.A.: Myringoplasty with the use of fascia graft. Arch. Otolaryng. 74:45-49, 1961.

49. Symposium: Methods of reconstruction in tympanoplasty (5 papers), Laryngoscope 86:173-195, 1976.

50. Symposium: contraindications to tympanoplasty, I-IV, Laryngoscope 86:64-83, 1976.

51. Wehrs, R.E.: The homograft notched incus in tympanoplasty, Arch. Otolaryng. 100:251-255, 1974.

52. Zwislocki, J.: Acoustic measurement of the middle ear function. Ann. Otol. Rhin. Laryng. 70:599, 1961.

CHAPTER 4

NONINFECTIOUS DISEASES OF THE EAR

I. HISTOPATHOLOGY OF OTOSCLEROSIS[34, 36]

This bony disorder of the otic capsule assumes various histopathological characteristics throughout its development. The early state is characterized by bone resorption and loose spongy bone widely interspersed with multiple vascular spaces. The more mature state being denser is characterized by fewer vascular spaces and by redeposition of bone. Otosclerotic bone can involve all three layers of the otic capsule (endosteum, endochondral and periosteal) though it is said to begin at the endochondral layer. The involved endochondral layer lacks the typical "globuli ossei" (islands of ossified cartilage) of normal endochondral bone. Both osteoblastic and osteoclastic activities take place in otosclerosis. It is believed that the otosclerotic process starts with finger-like invasion along blood vessels. On H and E stains, this invasion appears bluish and is thus named the "blue mantle of Manasse". Histological otosclerosis exists in about 8 to 10% of the white race, rarer among Orientals and Blacks. The incidence among East Indians, however, is believed to be comparable to that of the white race. Clinical otosclerosis giving rise to conductive hearing loss is estimated to be 1% in the white population.

The sites of predilection for otosclerotic involvement are:

a) Just anterior to the oval window (80 to 90% of the temporal bone with otosclerosis)
b) The border of the round window (30 to 50%)

The incidence of bilateral involvement is about 75 to 85% among temporal bones with otosclerosis. This disease shows a familial tendency; 60% of the patients with clinical otosclerosis have a positive family history. Some believe it to be transmitted by a monohybrid autosomal dominant gene with 25 to 40% penetrance, others believe that it may be transmitted by an autosomal recessive gene. Among those with hearing loss, a positive family history can be obtained from 50-60% of them. The risk of increasing hearing loss from any one pregnancy in a woman with stapedial otosclerosis is 1 chance in 4. If one parent has clinical otosclerosis, the children have a 20% chance of developing clinical otosclerosis.

Clinically, two eponyms are attached to otosclerosis: Schwartze sign and Carhart's notch. The Schwartze sign is the reddening of the promontory seen through a translucent tympanic membrane. This supposedly represents the increase of vascular spaces in the periosteal layer of the promontory. The Carhart's notch is a depression of the bone conduction threshold, greatest at 1000 or 2000 Hertz. The Carhart's notch is eliminated after a successful stapedectomy suggesting that it is not sensori-neural but is rather due to the impairment of bone conduction by a fixed footplate.

Malleus fixation caused by bony ankylosis between the head of the malleus and the tegmen can give a conductive hearing loss similar to that of stapes fixation. The incidence of malleus ankylosis coupled with stapes fixation by otosclerosis has been estimated to be about 1.6%.

Paget's disease (osteitis deformans) is histopathologically very similar to otosclerosis. The main differences are:

a) Paget's disease has diffuse involvement whereas otosclerosis is limited to the temporal bone.
b) Otosclerosis involves all 3 layers of the otic capsule (endosteal, endochondral and periosteal) whereas Paget's disease involves mainly the periosteal layer.
c) Osteitis deformans seldom involves the footplate or any part of the ossicles.

Osteogenesis imperfecta tarda is a systemic disease in which there is abnormal osteoblastic activity resulting in resorption of bone. This is an autosomal dominant disease and is characterized by the patient with multiple fractures. Forty to sixty percent of these patients also have bluish-colored sclerae together with stapes fixation. This constellation of findings has been referred to as the van der Hoeve-de Kleyn syndrome.

II. COMPLICATIONS OF STAPEDECTOMY

Some of the complications of stapedectomy may indeed stem from inadequate preoperative evaluation and poor selection of the patients for surgery. In order to prevent unnecessary and avoidable complications, some of the suggestions by experienced otologists are as follows: [4, 5, 16, 34, 40]

1. The minimum audiometric test requirements are puretone bone and air conduction thresholds, speech reception levels, and speech discrimination scores. The intelligent use of masking is highly important. The audiometric test results should always coincide with those of the tuning fork test. If they do not, do not proceed with surgery, but search for an explanation for the discrepancy. It may be due to a "shadow curve" from poor masking.
2. A sufficient conductive hearing loss should be confirmed by negative Rinne test for at least two of the three speech frequencies.
3. A careful assessment of discrimination ability is essential. The ear that discriminates better should not be operated upon because of the risk of postoperative sensorineural deafness.
4. Stapedectomy when indicated should be performed in the worse hearing ear first. If a successful result is achieved, the operation on the second ear can be considered 12 months or more later.
5. This operation should never be done in an only hearing ear. [35]
6. The pros, and especially the cons of this operation should be carefully discussed with the patient before surgery. The patient should be advised of the chief risk of the operation, namely postoperative sensorineural deafness, and other possible complications.

7. Patients with otosclerosis rarely complain of vertigo. When there is vertigo and clinical evidence of coexisting labyrinthine hydrops (Ménière's disease), stapedectomy should not be carried out for fear of a "dead ear". The distended saccule which may be in contact with the footplate, may be damaged during stapedectomy.
8. Stapedectomy should never be carried out in the presence of external otitis. The ear canal should be carefully examined the day before the operation and external otitis be ruled out.
9. There is a higher incidence of failure in younger individuals due to activity of the otosclerotic growth. This probably results from stimulation of the otosclerotic growth by stapedectomy.
10. Some otologists feel that stapedectomy should never be done in children because the risk of poststapedectomy sensorineural loss is high, especially if the preoperative bone conduction is poor. Bilateral infantile cases should be advised to wear a hearing aid until older.
11. The risk of prolonged postoperative vertigo is small but should be a consideration for some patients, for example, professional athletes, high construction workers, roofers and other individuals whose livelihood depends on special motor skills.
12. For patients engaged in frequent air travel, underwater sports, or other activities associated with unusual alterations in atmospheric pressure, Schuknecht suggests a use of a large fatty connective tissue graft and a shorter prosthesis.
13. Stapedectomy may result in worsening of speech discrimination. The elimination of stiffness by successful stapedectomy in a patient with a descending pattern of bone conduction thresholds converts the pattern of air conduction thresholds from flat to descending (paralleling the bone conduction) and results in a loss of speech discrimination. This discrimination is caused by the descending gradient of threshold sensitivity, not by morphological changes in the inner ear. (Schuknecht)[34] When this condition has been produced by the first stapedectomy, stapedectomy on the second ear should be discouraged.
14. Large exostoses of the external auditory canal may interfere with the surgical approach. In such cases, it is best to remove the exostoses first and to delay stapedectomy for several months.

COMPLICATIONS ENCOUNTERED DURING STAPEDECTOMY[4,10,34]

Complications encountered during stapedectomy include tears of tympanomeatal flap, dislocation of the incus, fracture of the long crus of the incus, cerebrospinal fluid leak, bleeding, vertigo, depressed footplate and floating footplate. Exostoses, superiorly located jugular bulb, overhanging facial nerve, round window otosclerosis, persistent stapedial artery, malleus ankylosis, congenital anomalies of the stapes and incus and obliterative otosclerosis also present problems during stapedectomy.

TEARS OF THE TYMPANOMEATAL FLAP: A linear tear may require no repair. Most tears can be satisfactorily repaired with fat from the earlobe, temporalis fascia or tragal perichondrium. A flat piece of tissue of suitable size is introduced into the perforation with the graft on the medial surface. The margins of the perforation are approximated as closely as possible.

DISLOCATION OF THE INCUS:
1. Subluxation of the incus consists of a tear of the incudomalleal joint but with sufficient intact capsule to maintain the incus in its normal anatomical position. Although the long process of the incus will be excessively mobile, the operation may be completed and the functional result may be satisfactory.

2. Luxation of the incus is due to a complete disruption of the incudomalleal joint and demands that the incus be removed and a malleus-oval window prosthesis be utilized. Attempts to replace and maintain the incus in its original position usually are not successful. The incus may be accidentally dislocated during curetting of the bony annulus and during extraction of the stapes. The long process of the incus may be accidentally displaced when withdrawing hooked instruments from the oval window niche.

FRACTURE OF THE LONG PROCESS OF THE INCUS: Rare. If the fracture occurs near the tip of the long process, the wire prosthesis still may be placed on the stump. If the stump is too short, a malleus oval window prosthesis should be used. When the lenticular process is particularly long, and close to the promontory, it is advisable to fracture and shorten it to prevent a fibrous adhesion to the promontory.

CEREBROSPINAL FLUID LEAK: In about one in three hundred cases, opening of an oval window results in a sudden profuse flow of clear fluid. These ears apparently have large patent cochlear aquaducts through which cerebrospinal fluid enters the inner ear. The fluid traverses the scala tympani to the helicotrema and then passes through the scala vestibuli to the vestibule to reach the oval window. In these cases, the fat graft technique is preferred and the patient is maintained in a head-elevation position for several days postoperatively. Cerebrospinal fluid flow is more common in cases of congenitally fixed stapes.[8]

BLEEDING: All bleeding from the ear canal should be controlled before the middle ear is opened. Bleeding from the mucous membrane of the oval window usually subsides spontaneously but, if necessary, may be controlled by pressure applied with a cotton pledget or gelfoam soaked with epinephrine. Occasionally there are large vascular channels in the otosclerotic bone which may bleed during footplate removal. Thus, bleeding into the vestibule may be unavoidable. Most otologists prefer to leave the clot in the vestibule untouched to complete the stapedectomy. A blood clot in the vestibule does not compromise the end result.

VERTIGO: Vertigo occurring during the stapedectomy operation is due either to mechanical stimulation of the vestibular sense organs or to cold caloric stimulation. One of the advantages of using local anesthesia is to permit this symptom to be monitored during surgery.

The aspiration of perilymph and its replacement with air results in displacement and collapse of the vestibular labyrinth and is associated with vertigo. Manipulations within the vestibule may cause vertigo. No instrumentation should be performed within the vestibule, and any maneuver which creates vertigo should be avoided. A fragment of footplate or a "broken" instrument which have fallen into the vestibule should be left alone. Attempts to remove it are followed by a high incidence of sensorineural hearing loss.

The introduction of a prosthesis which is too long may cause vertigo. The proper length should be determined by measurement. Before a prosthesis is tightened to the incus, it should be determined if vertigo is ellicited by an inward movement of the prosthesis. This is particularly important when fitting a piston prosthesis.

When perilymph has been removed, the utricle may assume an abnormally superior position in the vestibule. In this position it will be free from possible contact with a prosthesis during surgical procedure, but it will return to its normal position subsequently, as perilymph is reformed. This constitutes an important reason for avoiding loss of perilymph.

The pooling of an anesthetic agent in the round window niche may lead to its resorption into the inner ear and result in vertigo and nystagmus. During the injection procedure, care should be used to avoid anesthetic agent entering the middle ear.

DEPRESSED FOOTPLATE: Every effort should be made to avoid a depressed footplate. A severely depressed footplate or footplate fragment should be left in the vestibule and a gelfoam wire or tissue wire prosthesis introduced in the usual manner. These patients usually experience postoperative vertigo for several weeks and unsteadiness for many months.

FLOATING FOOTPLATE: The two conditions which lead to a floating footplate are previous stapes mobilization and minimal stapes fixation. When these conditions exist, a small opening should be created in the footplate prior to removal of the superstructure. This opening should be large enough to admit a 0.3 mm hook. If in spite of adequate precautions the floating footplate occurs, its removal must be effected through an inferior margin burr hole. A 0.5 mm sharp cutting burr is used to make a notch in the inferior margin of the oval window.

COMPLICATIONS FOLLOWING STAPEDECTOMY:[4, 5, 34, 40]

Postoperative complications following stapedectomy include acute otitis media, suppurative labyrinthitis and meningitis, vertigo, reparative granuloma, perilymph fistula, facial paralysis, fluctuating conductive hearing loss, persistent perforation of tympanic membrane, taste disturbance and dry mouth, postoperative fibrosis, incus necrosis, and delayed sudden deafness.

ACUTE OTITIS MEDIA: To prevent this complication, many otologists prescribe antibiotics. Acute infections should be treated intensively with the appropriate antibiotics as determined by culture and sensitivity studies.

SUPPURATIVE LABYRINTHITIS AND MENINGITIS: The most serious complication of stapedectomy is suppurative labyrinthitis leading to meningitis. Although it is extremely rare, several deaths from this complication have occurred.[3, 34] Presumably the bacterial invasion occurs through a thin membrane or fistula of the oval window. There is a higher incidence of meningitis with a polyethylene strut than with other tissue-wire prosthesis. Patients having had stapedectomy should be counseled regarding the importance of prompt treatment of respiratory infections when they are associated with ear discomfort.

POSTOPERATIVE VERTIGO: Vertigo may occur immediately following stapedectomy, or its onset may be delayed. Immediate postoperative vertigo is a result of perilymph loss, direct surgical trauma, or postoperative serous labyrinthitis, and it usually subsides within a few days. When vertigo or a sensation of unsteadiness persists for longer than a few days, a search for the cause should be made. Possible causes are: depressed footplate, reparative granuloma, excessively long prosthesis, and an oval window fistula. The long prosthesis is readily detected by eliciting the fistula response with the pneumatic otoscope. Exact position of the metallic prosthesis may be demonstrated by polytomography. Surgical intervention may be required, not only for the comfort of the patient but also to preserve inner ear function. Positional vertigo of the benign paroxysmal type (cupulolithiasis) may follow stapes surgery and probably is due to injury to the utricle with release of otoconia. This type of vertigo is usually self-limiting, but it may persist for several months or years (Schuknecht).[33]

REPARATIVE GRANULOMA: Granuloma of the posterior mesotympanum occurs as a complication of stapedectomy in approximately 1 or 2 out of 100 cases. The condition usually becomes manifest between the 7th and 15th postoperative days. Progressive sensorineural hearing loss after an initial hearing gain in the earliest and most consistent symptom. Vertigo, tinnitus and sensation of fullness in the ear may be present. Reparative granulomas are associated with serous labyrinthitis in the early stages and serofibrinous labyrinthitis in the later stages when the inner ear damage becomes permanent (Kaufman, R.S. and Schuknecht).[23]

Examination reveals an edematous thickened tympanic membrane with redness in its posterior half. Audiometric tests show a combined sensorineural and conductive hearing loss worse in the high frequencies and with marked decrease in speech discrimination. Emergency surgical intervention is imperative in these patients. Complete removal of granuloma within the first two poststapedectomy weeks may prevent permanent sensorineural hearing loss (Gacek).[6, 34]

PERILYMPH FISTULA (OVAL WINDOW FISTULA): The incidence of oval window fistula following a stapedectomy varies from 0.3% in 1772 patients (Cody)[4], to 2.5% in 1784 patients (Hemenway).[14] The symptoms of perilymph fistula are similar to those of endolymphatic hydrops. A sudden decrease in hearing often with vertigo and unsteadiness, a sense of fullness in the affected ear and sometimes roaring tinnitus, are common symptoms. Gradual progressive deterioration, but with fluctuation, is the rule in perilymph fistula.

The symptoms of oval window fistula may be evident within a few days or weeks following stapedectomy or may be delayed for weeks or months. The delayed type of fistula is especially common after insertion of a polyethylene tube or Teflon prosthesis. The incidence is higher with wire-gelfoam prosthesis than with wire-tissue prosthesis.

The treatment of perilymph fistula is unsatisfactory in most cases as far as hearing is concerned, but satisfactory for elimination of vertigo and risk of meningitis. Removal of the entire membrane from the oval window and replacing it with a wire-tissue prosthesis usually will stop the leakage of perilymph and the fluctuating symptoms, including vertigo. Early recognition and treatment may recover the hearing to the previous good level.[40]

FACIAL NERVE PARALYSIS: Immediate facial paralysis usually results from the local anesthetic reaching the facial nerve. Recovery of facial function is complete in two to four hours. If immediate paralysis persists, surgical trauma is likely and the nerve should be explored and decompressed within 24 hours. Direct instrument injury to the facial nerve is rare, but extreme caution should be used to prevent this complication. Approximately 50-60% of patients have dehiscence of the inferior aspect of the facial canal. Facial paralysis that begins several days after operation may be assumed to be the result of the edema of the facial nerve.

FLUCTUATING CONDUCTIVE HEARING LOSS: Fluctuating conductive hearing loss is the result of loose linkage of either end of the prosthesis. A faulty linkage characterized by intermittent contact with the oval window membrane causes large fluctuations in hearing, and is corrected by introducing a longer prosthesis. Loose linkage on the incus is characterized by small fluctuations in hearing, and is corrected by either tightening the wire loop or by removing the prosthesis and replacing it with a properly tightened wire look.

Although hearing impairment with perilymph fistula is predominantly of the sensorineural type, a fluctuating or persistent conductive loss may be caused by perilymph fistula (Goodhill).[9] This is considered to be due to the "backsplash" of a leaking vestibular perilymph space.

PERFORATION OF TYMPANIC MEMBRANES: A small postoperative perforation will usually heal spontaneously. Large perforations due to surgical trauma or postoperative infection require later myringoplasty.

TASTE DISTURBANCE AND DRY MOUTH: Stretching, tearing, or cutting the chorda tympani nerve can cause loss of taste on that side of the tongue and dryness of the mouth. Dryness of the mouth may be a particularly disagreeable poststapedectomy complication if both nerves are damaged. It was House's opinion that the patient has fewer symptoms when the chorda tympani nerve is cut than when it is over-stretched, and he advocates cutting it if it is in the way.

The disturbance of taste dryness of the mouth, and numbness of the anterior part of the tongue after trauma or section of the chorda tympani nerve begin to lessen in a month or two and usually disappear after three or four months, but they may persist longer or can be permanent.

POSTOPERATIVE FIBROSIS: A fibrous band from the incus to the promontory is a common cause for incomplete closure of the bone-air gap. The incidence of this complication can be minimized by avoiding surgical trauma to the mucosa of the promontory. Corrective surgery includes removal of the fibrous band and introduction of a Teflon or Silastic disc.

INCUS NECROSIS: Pressure necrosis of the tip of the long process of the incus appears to be caused by direct surgical trauma or by the irritation of the prosthesis. The incidence of this complication is highest with polyethylene tube prostheses in which case the resorption is due to osteitis initiated by foreign body reaction. A loosely crimped wire also can produce a low-grade reaction and local bone resorption. For this reason the loop of the prosthesis must be secured tightly to the incus.

DELAYED SUDDEN SENSORINEURAL HEARING LOSS: This is a rare complication of stapedectomy and may be caused by alterations in atmospheric pressure such as are experienced in an airplane or elevator. It is most common in patients who have had a polyethylene tube prosthesis inserted and is usually accompanied by severe vertigo and profound hearing loss. Presumably in these cases the prosthesis has been displaced into the vestibule.

Sudden profound sensorineural hearing loss, without vertigo and without obvious provocation, may occur some months or years following stapedectomy, particularly after revision procedures (Schuknecht).[34]

III. TRAUMATIC PERFORATION

Traumatic perforation can be caused by blast injury, welding injury, a force striking the auricle thereby occluding the external auditory canal (e.g. a slap with the open palm) and by penetrating injury (e.g. Q-tip injury). There are many ways of treating these perforations and the results are, to a large extent, comparable. Most otologists would agree that, without infection, 85 to 90% of all traumatic tympanic perforations heal spontaneously. However, whenever vertigo is associated with the injury, dislocation of the stapes is suspected, and hence surgical exploration should be performed as soon as possible. Among the above mentioned etiologies, penetrating injury gives the highest incidence of stapes dislocation.

A small traumatic perforation without ossicular dislocation with no foreign body or squamous epithelium embedded in the mesotympanum can be treated expectantly. When no infection is evident antibiotic drops are not necessary. The use of 10% trichloroacetic acid and paper patch (or gelfoam) has been practiced by some otologists.

In the case of a large perforation without ossicular dislocation but with infolding of the edges of the perforation, the mesotympanum should be cleaned of foreign debris and the edges unfurled over a piece of adipose connective tissue or over pieces of gelfoam. A tympanoplasty packing should be applied over this repair. In adults or in cooperative older children, this minor procedure can be performed under local anesthesia.

Whenever there is doubt as to the possibility of ossicular dislocation with a traumatic perforation, exploratory tympanotomy and tympanoplasty should be considered.[2, 44]

IV. SUDDEN DEAFNESS

Sudden deafness is defined as a sensorineural deafness that becomes instantly apparent or one that rapidly develops over a period of hours or a few days. The hearing loss is often noticed on awakening in the morning, or during any of the days' activities such as those involving physical or emotional strain or even while at rest. Some patients do not complain about a hearing loss but may complain of stuffiness or blocked feeling in the ear or tinnitus. The hearing loss may range from mild to total and is typically unilateral although it may be bilateral. There may be an accompanying dizziness or vertigo (50%) but this is usually mild and typically improves over a period of a few days. Males and females appear to be equally affected.

ETIOLOGY

1. Frequently cited predisposing factors include changes in the physical environment such as altitude, and other forms of change in atmospheric pressure, allergic manifestation, use of alcohol, emotional disturbance of the patient, physical exertion, diabetes, arteriosclerosis, pregnancy, use of a contraceptive drug, stress of surgery and general anesthesia.
2. Specific etiologies that are well documented are limited to viral agents. The sites of the viral induced pathological changes are the cochlea ("viral and endolymphatic labyrinthitis") and the components of the 8th cranial nerve ("viral neuronitis and ganglionitis"). The viruses of mumps, measles, influenza and adenoviruses may cause sudden deafness of the viral endolymphatic labyrinthitis type. The viruses of herpes zoster are the sole agents that have been shown to produce viral neuronitis and ganglionitis. The presence of active upper respiratory infection is noted in 25 per cent of patients at the onset of sudden deafness.

3. Vasospasm, thrombosis, embolism, hemorrhage into the inner ear, hypercoagulation and sludging of blood are frequently considered as the most common cause of sudden deafness, but the evidence is lacking.
4. Cerebellopontine angle tumors (retrocochlear tumor) have been demonstrated to produce sudden deafness.
5. Simmons theorized a break in Reisner's membrane as a cause of sudden deafness resulting from sudden pressure changes (getting out of bed, sneezing, coughing, bending, performing a Valsalva maneuver or scuba diving).[45]
6. Goodhill (1971) recognized round window fistula as a cause of sudden deafness.[11] Many reports of labyrinthine window ruptures followed. The anterior part of the oval window is the likelihest area to rupture. The findings of positional nystagmus, a positive Romberg or fistula sign with a sensorineural loss makes the diagnosis of an inner ear window rupture most probable. Tympanotomy is necessary to identify and close the fistula.[11,12,13]
7. Morimitsu (March 1976) reported a new theory and therapy for sudden deafness.[24] He treated 60 cases of sudden deafness with Urografin, injecting 1 ml. intravenously the first day and two ml. injections daily until hearing reached the maximum recovery point.

Twenty-two of those cases have had a complete recovery. Eight have had a "remarkable recovery, meaning that there has been a hearing gain of more than 30 dB in the average threshold of 250, 500, 1000, 2000, and 4000 Hz." Three cases have shown slight improvement with average hearing gains between 10 and 30 dB. The remaining 27 cases have shown either no change or hearing threshold changes within 10 dB.

He noted that there was no improvement with Urografin in patients with vertigo. He also noted that recovery was almost complete in all test frequencies even in the patient treated 43 days after onset. Therefore, he believed that the lesion is probably not in the hair cells "which easily develop irreversible changes," but is a functional change in the cochlea. Based on the pharmacology of Urografin, Morimitsu has deduced that dysfunction occurs in the stria vascularis.

It is well established that both the stria vascularis and the renal tubular epithelium are damaged equally by ototoxic antibiotics and the diuretics, furosemide and ethacrynic acid. Both diuretics deactivate the Na-K-ATPase in the stria vascularis, decreasing the endocochlear DC potential and cochlear microphonics; and the stria vascularis generates endocochlear DC potential.

If one can assume that the hearing loss of sudden deafness is caused by a depression of endocochlear DC potential by whatever cause, then it is easy to understand why the hearing loss occurs so suddenly and recovers so quickly and so very completely.

It is Morimitsu's theory that in sudden deafness of this type the blood cochlear barrier is broken down at the area of the stria vascularis and that the molecular weight and character of Urografin is such that a little of it leaks into the circulation to fill the broken membrane pores and reactivate the Na-pump to produce again normal DC potentials and also normal endolymph.

CLASSIFICATION: Sudden deafness may be classified from the etiological standpoint into two groups (Jaffe):

1. Localized lesions of the temporal bone:
   a) Acoustic neuroma
   b) Cerebellopontine angle tumor
   c) Oval or round window fistula
   d) Aneurysm of anterior inferior cerebellar artery

2. Systemic diseases involving the temporal bone:
   a) Viral infections which are cochleapathic
   b) Accelerated coagulation
   c) Hyperviscosity
      (1) polycythemia vera
      (2) macroglobulinemia
   d) Arteriosclerosis secondary to
      (1) aging
      (2) hypertension
      (3) diabetes
      (4) hyperlipidemia
   e) Collagen diseases
   f) Multiple sclerosis, syphilis and many others

SYSTEMATIC EVALUATION AND MANAGEMENT: The evaluation and management of these patients with sudden deafness must proeeed in a systematic fashion. The protocol shown in Figure 4-1 is suggested by B. F. Jaffe. (Sudden Sensori-neural Deafness, Maico Audiological Library Series, Vol. XI, Report Two).[20]

1. OTOLOGIC EXAMINATION: Sudden deafness may be of a conductive or sensorineural type. These can be differentiated by otoscopic examination, tuning fork tests, and audiometric tests. When the tympanic membrane is normal, sensorineural loss is most likely present. Wax in the external auditory canal and serous or acute otitis media may often present as sudden conductive deafness.

Vestibular function tests should include spontaneous nystagmus, positional test, Rhomberg, gait, caloric test, and electronystagmography when indicated.

2. AUDIOGRAM: The pure tone audiogram with air and bone conduction will confirm the clinical diagnosis of sensorineural loss. Cochlear or retrocochlear (8th nerve and cochlear nuclei) losses can be differentiated by special audiometric tests which include alternate binaural loudness balance (ABLB) short increment sensitivity index (SISI), discrimination scores, tone decay and Bekesy audiometry.

If a cochlea loss is present, proceed to number 3 and 4. If a retrocochlear loss is present, proceed to number 7.

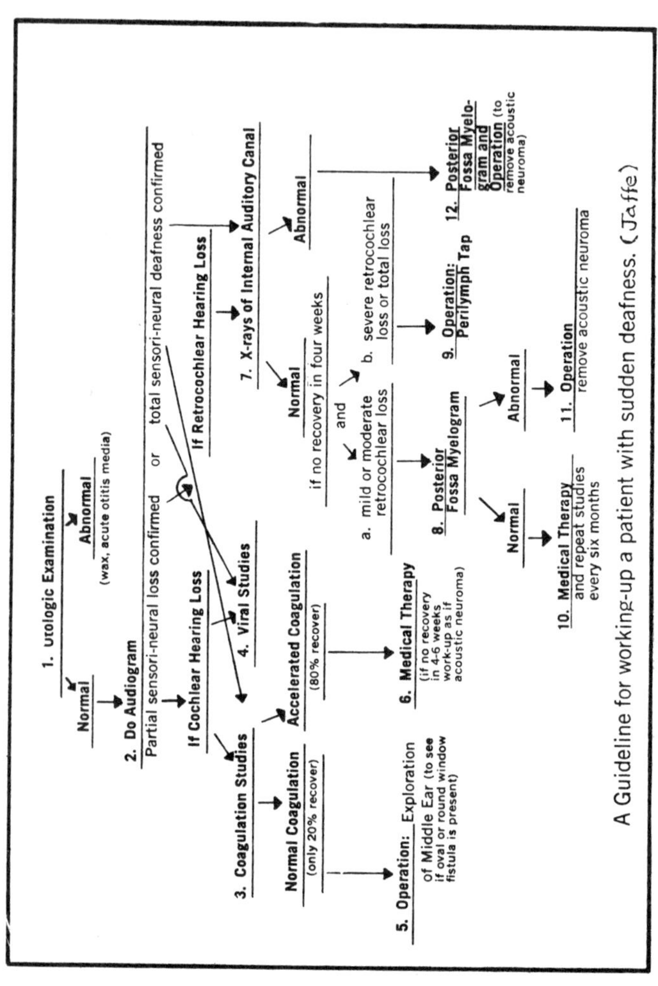

A Guideline for working-up a patient with sudden deafness. (Jaffe)

FIG. 4-1.

3. COAGULATION STUDIES: The sudden nature of sudden deafness suggests a sudden vascular occlusion which could arise from thrombosis of the cochlear vessels. Yet, many of the patients are young, without any evidence of arteriosclerosis, diabetes mellitus, hypertension, hyperlipidemia, and other vascular diseases. Therefore, the possibility of a thrombosis arising from a hypercoagulated state is considered by Jaffe and multiple tests have been utilized to assess the presence of accelerated coagulation. About 40% of the patients have an increase in prothrombin consumption, a test which has proven to be the most sensitive indicator of accelerated coagulation. When the coagulation is normal, only about 25% recover. Other hematological studies include CBC, platelet count, prothrombin time, and partial thromboplastin time (PTT). When the coagulation study is normal, proceed to number 5. When the coagulation is accelerated, proceed to number 6.

4. VIRAL STUDIES: About 25 per cent of patients with sudden deafness have an antecedent upper respiratory infection. The documentation of an acute infection should include virus isolation from swabs of the nasopharynx and four-fold or greater rise of antibody titer when comparing the acute and convalescent sera. Specimens for virus studies should be obtained as early as possible and within 21 days of the onset of deafness. Specimen sources include whole clotted blood, stool, washing from throat or nasopharynx, cerebrospinal fluid, fluid from the middle ear. Jaffe and Maassab and others identified adenovirus types I and III, Mycoplasma pneumoniae, and parainfluenza. About 60% of the patients with viral infections will recover spontaneously. No specific antiviral therapy exists. Medical therapy (Number 6) is indicated.

5. EXPLORATION OF MIDDLE EAR: When the coagulation studies are normal and when there is a history of otologic trauma or physical exertion prior to the onset of sudden deafness, an exploration of the middle ear is indicated to rule out a fistula of the oval window or round window with leakage of perilymph from the inner ear. A plug of gelfoam or fat may be used to seal the fistula.[11, 12, 13]

6. MEDICAL THERAPY:[19, 20, 24, 25, 31, 37, 42, 45, 46, 47] When coagulation studies indicate accelerated coagulation, one should proceed with the medical therapy.

A. Ambulatory care: Vasodilating drugs such as Arlidin, nicotinic acid and roniacol have been used.[19, 37, 42] Suga and Snow showed that nicotinic acid, even in massive doses, has no measurable effect on cochlear blood flow.[46, 47]
B. Hospitalization: (1) Bed rest, (2) Intravenous histamine given as 2.75 mg in 500 ml. normal saline over 30 min. daily for three days with careful monitoring of blood pressure and pulse every five minutes, (3) Low molecular dextran (10%) given intravenously 500 ml. every 12 hours for three days, (4) Heparin given to maintain a clotting time of two to three times normal.[19, 20]
C. Anticoagulants, steroids,[31] Urografin[24] may be effective in some cases.

7. X-RAY STUDIES OF INTERNAL AUDITORY CANAL: When the audiometric studies indicate a retrocochlear loss, radiographic examination of the internal auditory canal should be performed. (See Chapter 19).

If the x-rays are normal, wait for four weeks. If no recovery of hearing occurs and if the retrocochlear hearing loss is mild or moderate, proceed to number 8 (posterior fossa myelogram). If the hearing loss is severe or total, proceed to number 8 and/or number 9 (perilymph tap).

8. POSTERIOR FOSSA MYELOGRAM: If the retrocochlear hearing loss does not recover and if the hearing loss is mild or moderate, one should perform a posterior fossa myelogram. If the posterior fossa myelogram is abnormal, acoustic neuroma is suspected and removal indicated. If the posterior fossa myelogram is normal the patient must be followed every six months with repeat audiograms, repeat posterior fossa myelogram,or repeat diagnostic labyrinthotomy.

9. PERILYMPH TAP: (diagnostic labyrinthotomy [43]) Small acoustic neuromas produce an elevated protein content of the perilymph of the inner ear while cerebrospinal fluid protein remain normal. Because the diagnostic labyrinthotomy may produce a worsening of the hearing loss, it should not be used to evaluate a mild or moderate hearing loss.

For diagnostic labyrinthotomy, under local anesthesia, a tympanomeatal flap is created and the middle ear entered. The footplate of the stapes is identified, cleaned of mucosa and all bleeding controlled with adrenalin. Then a hole is made in the footplate and a capillary tube is placed into the vestibule of the inner ear and perilymph obtained. Analysis of the fluid will be diagnostic of an acoustic neuroma if the protein content is 1,000 mg per cent or greater (1971).

10. REMOVAL OF ACOUSTIC NEUROMA: Three major approaches to the internal auditory canal are available: a) translabyrinthine approach, b) middle cranial fossa approach and c) combined suboccipital and translabyrinthine approach. (See Chapter 4, V).

The translabyrinthine approach destroys hearing so it is used only if severe or total deafness is present or if the discrimination is so poor as to produce a nonfunctioning ear. The middle cranial fossa approach is somewhat more complicated by intracranial complications but it is possible in some cases to remove the tumor, while preserving the hearing and facial nerve function.

PROGNOSIS AND REHABILITATION: [47]

1. Approximately one-third of patients have a return of normal hearing, one-third are left with a 40 to 60 dB speech reception threshold, and one-third have total loss of useful hearing.

2. Spontaneous recovery to normal hearing is more likely to occur if the deafness is not associated with severe vertigo and if the deafness is not total initially.

3. Once recovery of hearing begins, it usually takes place rapidly in a matter of a few days. The longer the delay between the onset of deafness and the onset of recovery, the worse the prognosis for complete recovery.

4. Children who do not recover spontaneously from a unilateral sudden deafness should have preferential seating in school. Adults should be advised of the availability of CROS (contralateral routing of signals) hearing aid.

5. Those patients who do not recover serviceable hearing from bilateral sudden deafness should have speech reading and auditory training. A hearing aid should be tried and utilized when appropriate (Snow).[47]

6. When sudden deafness develops in an only hearing ear, exploration of the middle ear is indicated to rule out a hidden oval or round window fistula.

THERAPEUTIC PROTOCOLS: Therapeutic protocols suggested by the National Registry for Idiopathic Sudden Deafness include:[25]

METHOD A:

1. Bed rest for three days with barbiturate or phenothiazine sedation.
2. Atropine (only if begun within four hours of the onset of deafness) 0.75 mg I.M. or in 250 ml. of 5% dextrose in water I.C. as a single dose.
3. Procaine - 0.2% in 250 ml. of 5% dextrose in water I.V. twice daily for three days.
4. Benadryl - 50 mg. four times daily orally or by injection until the hearing has stabilized for at least three weeks.
5. Nylidrin (Arlidin) - 6 mg. orally four times daily until the hearing has stabilized for at least three weeks.
6. Ascorbic acid (Vitamin C) - 1000 mg. in each I.V. of Procaine.

METHOD B:

1. Bed rest for three days.
2. Histamine phosphate - 2.75 mg. in 250 ml. of 5% dextrose in water I.C. daily for three days. Adjust the rate to produce a flush but not a headache. Do not run at the same time as Dextran as this seems to produce a severe headache.
3. Dextran - 10% (Rheomacrodex) - 500 ml. every twelve hours for three days.
4. Nicotinic acid in a flushing dose (50 to 300 mg.) before meals and at bedtime, until hearing has stabilized for at least three weeks. This is begun in the office when the patient is first seen.

METHOD C:

1. Hospitalization for at least three days.
2. Heparin 200 mgm. (20,000 units) every 12 hours I.M., I.V., or subcutaneously to keep the Lee White Clotting Time between 15 and 20 minutes which is two to three times normal.
3. Coumadin is begun on the second day and then the Heparin is discontinued when the prothrombin time is $2\frac{1}{2}$ to 3 times normal. Anticoagulation is continued for four weeks. Medical consultation should be obtained to manage the Heparin and Coumadin anticoagulation.
4. Procaine - 0.2% in 250 ml. of 5% dextrose in water I.V. twice daily for three days.

METHOD D: Prednisone - 10 mg. three times daily for ten days, then in reducing amounts to nil over 10 days.

METHOD E: Exploratory tympanotomy to seal a perforated round or oval window.

METHOD F:

1. Bed rest for three days or until hearing and/or vertigo is stable.

2. No medication - It is possible that the previously recommended medications have no effect or even an adverse effect on the prognosis. This group would serve as a control.

V. BENIGN TUMORS OF THE EAR

EXTERNAL EAR: Benign tumors of the auricle and the external auditory canal include angioma (capillary hemangioma, cavernous hemangioma and lymphangioma), dermoid tumors, cylindroma, melanoma, Winkler's disease, osteoma, exostosis, adenoma, ceruminoma, chondroma, lipoma, xanthoma, myoma, myxoma, mixed tumors of the salivary gland type, and keratosis obturans.

1. OSTEOMA: Osteoma (cancellous) occurs in the auditory canal as a single large pedunculated tumor near the lateral end of the bony portion on one side only. It arises from the region of either the tympanosquamous suture or the tympanomastoid suture. Hearing loss and discomfort are common symptoms.

Treatment: surgical removal when symptomatic.

2. EXOSTOSIS: Exostoses (dense ivory compact bone) are the most common tumors of the external auditory canal. These are usually bilateral and asymptomatic unless accompanied by accumulation of debris against the tympanic membranes resulting in infection or obstruction. The etiologic factor most likely responsible is prolonged and repeated stimulation of the external auditory canal by cold water. Exostoses are most commonly seen in saltwater swimmers. Other factors which might play a role include chronic irritation from infection, eczema and trauma.

Treatment: surgical excision when symptomatic. Attempts to remove exostoses with a hammer and gauge may produce fractures in the surrounding bone, possibly resulting in facial palsy. Removal should be done with a small cutting burr. In some cases exostoses can be removed through a speculum, raising a flap of meatal skin by an incision external to the exostoses. In others, an endaural or postauricular incision is necessary.

3. CERUMENOMA: This uncommon tumor is an adenoma of sweat gland origin and presents as a smooth intraverted polypoid swelling in the outer end of the meatus. This tumor may become malignant.

Treatment: local recurrence after excision is common. Wide excision including a margin of healthy skin is advised.

4. WINKLER'S DISEASE: This is a rare, painful nodular growth of unknown origin occurring on top of the helix mostly in men. It consists of tiny arteriovenous anastomosis with many nerve endings similar to a glomus body. The small nodule is painfully tender, preventing some patients from sleeping on the ear.

Treatment: surgical excision or injection of Cortisone for the relief of pain.

5. KERATOSIS OBTURANS: This rare condition is also called cholesteatoma of the external auditory canal, and is characterized by an accumulation of large plugs of desquamating squamous epithelium (cholesteatoma) deep in the external auditory canal, and is often associated with chronic pulmonary diseases, sinusitis and bronchiectasis. Pain is the common presenting symptom and results from erosion of the bony canal (destructive or invasive keratitis). Hearing loss is usual.

Etiology: unknown, but probably due to faulty migration of squamous epithelial cells from the surface of the tympanic membrane and adjacent canal.

Treatment: periodic removal of accumulated debris. General anesthesia may be required.

MIDDLE EAR: Benign tumors of the middle ear and mastoid include glomus jugulare tumor, osteoma, neurinoma of the VIIth and VIIIth cranial nerve, intratympanic meningioma, glioma, cylindroma, dermoid cysts, hemangioma, and acoustic neuroma.

1. GLOMUS JUGULARE TUMOR: (Chemodectoma, non-chromaffin paraganglioma, carotid body tumor, tympanic body tumor, glomus tympanicum)[1, 7, 29, 36, 40] Glomus jugulare tumor arises from the glomus bodies located in the adventitia of the dome of the jugular bulb or along branches of the tympanic plexus.

Pathology: Glomus jugulare tumors usually arise in the hypotympanum at the site of the entrance of Jacobson's nerve in the adventitia of the jugular bulb. In many instances they arise on the promontory.

The incidence is five times more often in women than in men. The tumors consist of vascular sinuses supplied by the ascending pharyngeal artery which enters the tympanum along with Jacobson's nerve. These tumors grow slowly but are progressively destructive by invasion into the surrounding structures. Instances of multicentric origin and association with carotid body tumors have been reported. The tumors occasionally metastasize to the lungs and cervical nodes.

Clinical features: The earliest symptom is pulsating tinnitus which is synchronous with the pulse. The hearing loss follows as the tumor enlarges. As it invades the tympanic membrane, spontaneous bleeding and discharge, due to secondary infection, will occur. Isolated facial paralysis is frequently present. Invasion along the course of the jugular wall results in multiple involvement of the 9th, 10th, 11th and 12th cranial nerves. Invasion of the cochlea and petrous tip is a late occurrence resulting in sensorineural hearing loss and (rarely) paralysis of the 5th and 6th cranial nerves.

Diagnosis: Examination in the early stage may reveal a reddish swelling behind the tympanic membrane which with magnification may be seen to pulsate. If the drum head is dull and the tumor small, this appearance may be confused with the Schwartze sign in otosclerosis. As the tumor enlarges, it causes the inferior portion of the tympanic membrane to bulge and finally burst revealing a smooth large red polypoid mass which bleeds very easily (and often massively) on manipulation. Application of pressure with the pneumatic otoscope causes the tumor to increase in pulsation. As the pneumatic pressure is raised to exceed systolic pressure, a sudden blanching occurs(Brown's pulsation sign). Radiographic examination is of little value in early cases but as the tumor advances will reveal the extent of bony destruction. In advanced tumors, external carotid angiography, polytomography and retrograde jugularography are helpful in delineating the extent of tumor. The diagnosis is confirmed by biopsy which must be done carefully in the hospital because of the severe hemorrhage which may occur. With an intact tympanic membrane the biopsy is best done through a tympanotomy approach and combined with total excision.

Classification: Rosenwasser classified glomus tumors into three groups: Group I include those cases in whom the tympanic membrane is intact and the lesion is small and confined to the middle ear; Group II include those cases in whom the middle ear, aditus, antrum and mastoid bone appear to be involved and Group III include those cases in whom there is a wide spread extension, at times with intracranial involvement. (Rosenwasser)[28, 29]

Alford and Gilford classified the tumor into four stages:[1]

Stage O: The earliest manifestation of a glomus tumor. The patient complains of hearing loss and/or pulsating tinnitus. There will be normal hearing or a conductive hearing loss. The drum head is intact but discolored. Radiographs will be normal.

Stage I: Aural discharge due to involvement of the tympanic membrane by the tumor is noted. Radiographs show clouding of the middle ear but no bone erosion. There is no cranial nerve involvement.

Stage II: Facial paralysis now present, and there is sensorineural hearing loss. Radiographs may show enlargement of the jugular forament but no bone erosion.

Stage III: Involvement of the jugular foramen with paralysis of the 9th, 10th, 11th, 12th and/or 7th cranial nerves. Radiographic evidence of erosion of the petrous bone and enlargement of the jugular foramen is noted.

Stage IV: Intracranial extension producing papilledema, extensive involvement of the petrous bone, and paralysis of the 3rd, 4th, 5th, 6th, and 7th cranial nerves.

Treatment: Early cases may be cured by surgical excision but advanced cases should be treated with palliative radiation. The treatment may be summarized as follows:

Group I:	Tumor involving the middle ear only (glomus tympanicum)	Excision via 1. Tympanotomy 2. Endaural hypotympanotomy of Shambaugh[39] 3. Postauricular facial recess approach (House and Glasscock)[17]
Group II:	Tumor extending into the attic or mastoid	Radical mastoidectomy (with ligation of ascending pharyngeal artery or external carotid artery) followed by radiation when removal was incomplete.
Group III:	Tumor involving the jugular foramen with cranial nerve paralysis	1. Partial excision with radiation (in most cases) 2. Temporal bone resection with dissection and ligation of lateral sinus and jugular vein (in some cases) (Hilding)[15] 3. Cryosurgery (palliative)

Radiation is often used especially when complete removal is not possible. Tumor doses of 2400 to 6000 r are given over a period of two to four weeks. Palliative benefit from radiotherapy is probably due to reduction in vascularity as the tumor cells are not considered to be radiosensitive.[1, 29, 48]

INTERNAL EAR:

ACOUSTIC NEUROMA: Acoustic neuroma accounts for 78% of all tumors of the cerebellopontine angle. It is found in about 8% of all intracranial tumors and constitutes even a greater percentage of all posterior fossa lesions. The tumor most often becomes symptomatic between the ages of 30 and 40 years. Routine autopsies have revealed a 2.4% incidence of asymptomatic acoustic neuroma. It is commoner in females in the ratio of 3:2.

Pathology: Acoustic neuroma is a benign encapsulated tumor arising from the sheath of Schwann (neurilemma) of the 8th nerve. The usual site of lesion is the vestibular portion of the nerve in the region of Scarpa's ganglion. The incidence of involvement of vestibular and auditory nerves is a 2:1 ratio. The 8th nerve loses the neurilemmal sheath at the porus acousticus and hence it is unlikely that the tumor would arise proximal to the porus. It usually begins in the internal auditory canal, slowly enlarges within the canal and with some degree of erosion extends toward the cerebellopontine angle. It is usually unilateral, but bilateral lesions may be noted as in the case of von Recklinghausen's disease. The size of the tumor may reach 5.0 cm., although the more common size outside the canal is about 2.5 - 3.0 cm.

Histologically, the tumor is characterized by streams of elongated spindle cells, with the elongated nuclei often arrayed in a palisade pattern. Tumors in which there is a thick concentration of cells are called Antoni, Type A, whereas those in which the cells are loose are called Antoni, Type B.

Clinical features:

1. The earliest symptoms are tinnitus and unilateral progressive hearing impairment. In the early stages of acoustic neuroma, dizziness is also an extremely common complaint, appearing in the form of unsteadiness in about 83% of the patients.
2. Vertigo is not common initially, but may become a more prominent symptom with continued growth of the tumor.
3. Other early complaints are sensation of prickling and itching, and pain in the ear.
4. Late manifestations of the disease develop from great pressure upon the auditory canal and extension of tumor into the posterior cranial fossa. The sensory part of the fifth nerve may become involved first, producing unilateral numbness of the face. The motor part of the 7th nerve may be affected, causing facial weakness. Eventually the cerebellum may be disturbed, producing slurring of the speech, ataxia, and incoordination of one or both upper extremities. With continued growth the tumor can obstruct the flow of cerebrospinal fluid, creating an internal hydrocephalus. Headache, nausea, vomiting and dullness of mental faculties may accompany these complications.

Diagnosis: Any patient suspected of acoustic neuroma should undergo a complete audiologic, vestibular, and neurologic evaluation.

Audiometric examination: [21, 22, 26, 30]

1. All the patients have sensorineural hearing loss. Approximately 64% have a high tone loss, but others can present with a flat-type of curve.
2. Impairment of speech discrimination is much greater than would be expected from pure tone loss. Discrimination scores of 0-30% occur in over half of the patients.
3. The short increments sensitivity index (SISI score) is in the region of 0-35% with retrocochlear lesions.
4. Approximately 50-60% of the patients with acoustic tumors show Type III and Type IV Bekesy tracings.

Vestibular examination: Diminished or absent response to caloric testing is an important and early sign of acoustic tumor. About 96% of patients with acoustic neuroma have an abnormal caloric response. Electronystagmography may show spontaneous nystagmus away from the side of the lesion. In some patients positional nystagmus may be noted. Vertical nystagmus may suggest posterior fossa involvement. [27]

Neurologic evaluation: With an increase in intracranial pressure there may be blurred optic discs, impairment of occular motor function, diminished sensation of the face, and facial weakness. Hitselberger and House noted hypesthesia of the posterior wall of the external auditory canal (Hitselberger's sign). Lacrimation, taste, and blink reflexes should be tested. A complete neurological examination should be a must in all suspected cases of acoustic neuroma.

Radiologic evaluation: The radiologic examination for an acoustic tumor usually includes conventional films, polytomography and posterior fossa myelogram. The x-rays most valuable in evaluation of the internal auditory canal are Stenvers, transorbital, Towne's and submentovertical projections. These views demonstrate enlargement of the canal or erosion of the petrous portion of the temporal bone in about 85% of patients. Polytomography and Pantopaque posterior fossa myelogram may increase the diagnostic accuracy to 90-100%. Vertebral angiography is useful in evaluating atypical cerebellopontine angle tumors.

Laboratory examination:

1. Cerebrospinal fluid examination shows elevated protein more often in acoustic neuroma than in any other intracranial tumor.
2. Radioisotope brain scan may show a high incidence (85%) of positive scan.
3. Diagnostic labyrinthotomy (Silverstein). Small acoustic neuromas produce an elevated protein content of the perilymph of the inner ear in the presence of a normal content of the cerebrospinal fluid. Through a tympanotomy approach, a small hole is made in the footplate and a capillary tube is placed into the vestibule and the perilymph is obtained. A protein content of 1000 mg. % or greater is diagnostic of an acoustic neuroma. (Silverstein). [43]

Differential Diagnosis:

1. Endolymphatic hydrops is the most easily and frequently confused with acoustic neuroma. Clinical history, further radiologic and laboratory tests will help to differentiate these lesions.
2. Cystic arachnoiditis of the cerebellopontine angle from previous acute or chronic otitis media producing otitic hydrocephalus may stimulate an acoustic neuroma. The history of otorrhea is important.
3. Meningioma arising from the posterior surface of the petrous pyramid produces the angle syndrome. Involvement of other cranial nerves generally occur earlier in meningioma and loss of hearing and vestibular response occur later than in acoustic neuroma. The spinal fluid protein is generally not elevated in meningioma. Radiologic studies show hyperostosis, calcification or destruction of the petrous pyramid or an increased vascularity on angiography.
4. Congenital cholesteatoma of the petrous pyramid may produce the angle syndrome. Facial nerve paralysis occurs earlier than in acoustic neuroma and the x-ray changes are characteristic.
5. Multiple sclerosis may stimulate an angle tumor except for its characteristic remissions. Spinal fluid protein is not greatly elevated in multiple sclerosis.

Surgical treatment: A classification of patients and a system of management on the surgery removal of acoustic tumors were suggested by Pulec, et al.[26] and summarized as shown in Table 4-1.

TUMOR-LIKE CONDITIONS OF THE TEMPORAL BONE:[40]

1. HISTIOCYTOSIS X: (Reticuloendotheliosis) The characteristics of the three clinical syndromes or varients of histocytosis X (all involving the skin, skeleton, and reticuloendothelial system) may be summarized as follows:

A. Letterer-Siwe Disease: This is a rare and rapidly fatal form of acute disseminated histiocytosis occurring in children before the age of two years, and characterized by fever, splenomegaly, hepatomegaly, lymphadenopathy, skeletal lesions, purplish skin rash and anemia.

B. Hand-Schuller-Christian Disease: This is a less severe and more chronic form in children and young adults, characterized by exophthalmos and diabetes insipidus from involvement of the sphenoid bone. When the temporal bone is affected, it may involve the mastoid cortex, the external auditory canal, labyrinth, the facial nerve, and the jugular foramen.

The characteristic histologic feature is the presence of lipoid-filled histiocytes (foam cells).

Treatment: Irradiation. The mortality is 30 percent.

SIZE OF TUMOR	ASSOCIATED CONDITIONS	MANAGEMENT
Intracanalicular tumor (up to 8 mm diameter)	Some hearing	Removal via middle cranial fossa approach (Facial nerve preserved and hearing can be saved in 60% of cases
Intracanalicular tumor	No hearing	Translabyrinthine approach
Medium-sized tumor (2.5 - cm. in diameter)	With or without 5th nerve sign but no increased intracranial pressure, no papilledema, no cerebellar or long tract signs	Translabyrinthine approach
Large tumor (2.5 cm. or more in diameter)	Increased intracranial pressure, 5th nerve signs, papilledema, cerebellar and long tract signs, headache, depressed mental ability	Suboccipital decompression with removal of occipital bone from the midline to the sigmoid sinus, removal of arch of the atlas, incision of the atlanto-occipital ligament without opening the dura, followed in 5-7 days by translabyrinthine approach for removal of tumor
Bilateral medium or large tumor	Useful hearing	Retrolabyrinthine approach with preservation of labyrinth and endolymphatic sac, and removal of major portion of tumor leaving only a small part over the 7th and 8th nerves and internal auditory artery. Purpose: 1. preserve hearing, 2. Relieve the life threatening tumor mass. Repeat surgery when and if indicated.
Small, medium or large tumor	High risk case with disabling symptoms of vertigo, nausea, and ataxia.	Translabyrinthine approach. To accomplish labyrinthectomy and brief subtotal removal of tumor

C. Eosinophilic Granuloma: This is a less acute condition occurring in children and young adults, characterized by osteolytic lesions in one or several bone areas and a predilection for the frontal or temporal bone.

Otological manifestations include swelling over the mastoid, granulations in the external auditory canal, otorrhea, deafness and facial paralysis.

Histologically, the lesion presents two types of cells:

a) large, pale mononuclear histiocytes with mitotic figures, and
b) eosinophils

Treatment:

(1) Surgical excision or curettage of individual lesions.
(2) Radiotherapy for recurrences and inaccessible lesions. Useful for relief of pain.

2. FIBROUS DYSPLASIA: (Osteitis fibrosa cystica) Fibrous dysplasia may involve a single bone (monostotic type), or, less often, several bones (polyostotic type). Fibrous dysplasia of bone usually first becomes manifest during childhood or early adult life and the lesions grow slowly. The polyostotic type characteristically involves the long bones and rarely the skull. The monostotic type may occur in the long bones, facial bones, or membranous bones. Occasionally the polyostotic type of fibrous dysplasia occurs in a form known as Albright's syndrome which is characterized by multiple involvement of the long bones, pigmentation of the skin, and precocious puberty in females.

Fibrous dysplasia of the temporal bone manifests itself as a painless swelling in the region of the mastoid and the external auditory canal. Conductive hearing loss due to occlusion of the external auditory canal may be the only symptom.

Histologically, fibrous dysplasia is characterized by replacement of marrow with fibrous tissue containing spicules of bone undergoing resorption and formation. Active osteoblastic and osteoclastic activity is usually present and islands of cartilage may be seen.

Fibrous dysplasia has a female sex preponderance in a ratio of three to one. The onset is usually in childhood, and the lesions, when multiple, are often unilateral.

Differential diagnosis include hyperparathyroidism, Ollier's enchondromatosis, von Recklinghausen's disease, Paget's disease, Hand-Schuller-Christian disease, and other bone tumors. The history of painless swelling associated with the characteristic radiographic appearance (a typical loss of cellular structure and increased radiolucency due to replacement of osseous substance by fibrous tissue) and biopsy are adequate to differentiate fibrous dysplasia from these conditions.

Treatment of fibrous dysplasia is surgical excision. Radiotherapy appears to have a predisposing propensity to malignant degeneration and is considered as contraindicated for treatment of fibrous dysplasia (Schuknecht).[36]

VI. PRESBYCUSIS

This can be classified under the following sub-headings: (Schuknecht).[32]

1. SENSORY:
   a) atrophy of the organ of Corti and the auditory nerve in the basal end of the cochlea. It is characterized by abrupt high frequency loss.
   b) begins at middle age and is slowly progressive.

2. NEURAL:
   a) loss of ganglion cells and degeneration of nerve fibers.
   b) significant disability in discrimination of speech.
   c) occurs late in life.

3. METABOLIC:
   a) stria atrophy
   b) good discrimination
   c) flat audiometric curve

4. MECHANICAL:
   a) descending audiometric curve. The basal turn is most involved.
   b) questionable stiffening of basilar membrane.

MISCELLANEOUS

1. 75% of ganglion cells can be missing and yet pure tone thresholds are maintained.

2. Loss of spiral ganglion cells does not necessarily produce hair cell degeneration.

3. Loss of hair cells with normal supporting cells does not produce spiral ganglion cell degeneration.

4. The stria vascularis is the source of +80 mv DC potential of the scala media.

REFERENCES

1. Alford, B. R. and Gilford, R. R.: A comprehensive study of tumors of the glomus jugulare. Laryngoscope, 72:765-787, 1962.

2. Armstrong, B.W.: Traumatic perforation of the tympanic membrane: observe or repair? Laryngoscope 82:1822-1830, 1972.

3. Brown, J.S.: Meningitis following stapes surgery. Laryngoscope, 77:1295-1303, 1967.

4. Cody, D.T.: Complications of stapedectomy, In M.M. Paparella, et al. (Ed.) Clinical Otology. C.V. Mosby Co., St. Louis, Chapter 7, pp. 53-74, 1970.

5. Feldman, B.A., and Schuknecht, H.F.: Experiences with revision stapedectomy procedures. Laryngoscope, 80: 1281-1291, 1970.

6. Gacek, R.R.: The diagnosis and treatment of poststapedectomy granuloma. Ann. Otol. 79:970-975, 1970.

7. Glasscock, M.E. III, et al.: Glomus tumors: diagnosis and treatment, Laryngoscope 84:2006-2032, 1974.

8. Glasscock, M.E.: The stapes gusher. Arch. Otolaryng. 98: 82-91, Aug. 1973.

9. Goodhill, V.: The conductive loss phenomenon in poststapedectomy perilymphatic fistulas. Laryngoscope, 77:1179-1190, 1967.

10. Goodhill, V.: Posterior arch stapedectomy. Ten commandments for stapedectomy. Arch. Otolaryng. 100:460-464, 1974.

11. Goodhill, V.: Sudden deafness and round window rupture. Laryngoscope, 8:1462-1474, 1971.

12. Goodhill, V., et al.: Sudden deafness and labyrinthine window ruptures: audiovestibular observations. Ann. Otol. Rhin. & Laryng. 82:2-12, 1973.

13. Healy, G.B., et al.: Ataxia, vertigo and hearing loss: result of rupture of inner ear window. Arch. Otolaryng. 100:130-135, 1974.

14. Hemenway, W.G., et al.: Poststapedectomy perilymph fistula in the Rocky Mountain area. Laryngoscope. 78:1687-1715, 1968.

15. Hilding, D.A. and Greenberg, A.: Surgery for large glomus jugulare tumor. Arch. Otolaryng. 93:227-231, 1971.

16. Hildyard, V., et al.: Diagnosis and management of far-advanced otosclerosis. Arch. Otolaryng. 96:530-534, 1972.

17. House, W.F. and Glasscock, M.E. III: Glomus tympanicum tumors. Arch. Otolaryng. 87:550-554, 1968.

18. House, H.P. and Linthicum, F.H.: Sodium fluoride and the otosclerotic lesion. Arch. Otolaryng. 100:427-430, 1974.

19. Jaffe, B.F.: Sudden deafness--an otologic emergency. Arch. Otolaryng. 86:55-60, 1967.

20. Jaffe, B.F.: Sudden sensori-neural deafness. Maico Audiological Library Series, Vol. XI, Report Two.

21. Jerger, J., et al.: Acoustic reflex in eighth nerve disorders. Arch. Otolaryng. 99:409-413, 1974.

22. Jerger, J. and Jerger, S.: Audiologic comparison of cochlear and eighth nerve disorders. Ann. Otol. Rhin. Laryngol. 83: 275-285, 1974.

23. Kaufman, R.S. and Schuknecht, H.F.: Reparative granuloma following stapedectomy--a clinical entity. Ann. Otol. 76:1008-1017, 1967.

24. Morimitsu, T.: New theory and therapy of sudden deafness, paper presented at the Shambaugh 5th International Workshop on middle ear microsurgery and fluctuating hearing loss. March, 1976.

25. National registry for idiopathic sudden deafness.

26. Pulec, J.L., et al.: A system of management of acoustic neuroma based on 364 cases. Trans. Acad. Ophthal. Otolaryng. 75:48-55, 1971.

27. Pulec, J.L., et al.: Vestibular involvement and testing in acoustic neuroma. Arch. Otolaryng. 80:677-681, 1964.

28. Rosenwasser, H.: Tumors of the middle ear and mastoid. (In Paparella, M.A. and Shumrick, D.A. (ed.): Otolaryngology, Vol. 2, Chapter 13, W.B. Saunders Co., Philadelphia, 1973.

29. Rosenwasser, H.: Glomus jugulare tumor, Monograph. Arch. Otolaryng. 88:29-66, 1968.

30. Sanders, J.W., et al.: Audiologic evaluation in cochlear and eighth nerve disorders. Arch. Otolaryng. 100:283-289, 1974.

31. Schiff, M. and Brown, M.: Hormones and sudden deafness. Laryngoscope 84:1959-1981, 1974.

32. Schuknecht, H.F.: Further observations on the pathology of presbycusis. Arch. Otolaryng. 80:369-382, 1964.

33. Schuknecht, H.F.: Cupulolithiasis. Arch. Otolaryng. 90:765-778, 1969.

34. Schuknecht, H.F.: Stapedectomy, Little, Brown Co., Boston, 1971.

35. Schuknecht, H.F. and Gacek, R.R.: Surgery on only-hearing ears. Trans. Am. Acad. Ophth. 77:257-266 (ORL), 1973.

36. Schuknecht, H.F.: Pathology of the ear. Harvard University Press, Cambridge, Mass., 1974.

37. Shaia, F.T. and Sheehy, J.L.: Sudden sensori-neural hearing impairment: A report of 1220 cases. Laryngoscope 86:389-398, 1976.

38. Shambaugh, G.E., et al.: New concept in management of otospongiosis. Arch. Otolaryng. 100:419-426, 1974.

39. Shambaugh, G.E., Jr.: Surgical approaches to glomus jugulare tumors of the middle ear. Laryngoscope, 65:185-198, 1955.

40. Shambaugh, G.E., Jr.: Surgery of the ear, 2nd ed. W.B. Saunders & Co., Philadelphia, 1967.

41. Sheehy, J.L. and Perkins, J.H.: Stapedectomy: gelfoam compared with tissue grafts. Laryngoscope, 86:436-444, 1976.

42. Sheehy, J.L.: Vasodilator therapy in sensorineural hearing loss. Laryngoscope 70:885-914, 1960.

43. Silverstein, H.: Indications for diagnostic labyrinthotomy. Arch. Otolaryng. 94:195-196, 1971.

44. Silverstein, H., Fabian, R.L., Stool, S.E. and Hong, S.W.: Penetrating wounds of tympanic membrane and ossicular chain. Trans. Am. Acad. Ophth. 77:125-135 (ORL), 1973.

45. Simmons, F.B.: Theory of membrane breaks in sudden hearing loss. Arch. Otolaryng. 88:41-48, 1968.

46. Snow, J.B., Jr., and Suga, F.: Labyrinthine vasodilators. Arch. Otolaryng. 97:365-370, 1973.

47. Snow, J.B., Jr.: Sudden deafness. In Paparella, M.M. and Shumrick, D.A. (ed.): Otolaryngology, Vol. 2, Chapter 22, W.B. Saunders Co., Philadelphia, 1973.

48. Spector, G.J., Fierstein, J. and Ogura, J.H.: A comparison of therapeutic modalities of glomus tumors in the temporal bone. Laryngoscope 86:690-696, 1976.

CHAPTER 5

VERTIGO

The term dizziness has often been used imprecisely. It is imperative for an otolaryngologist to be able to differentiate the following terms:

Dizziness: encompasses any discomfort, other than pain, related to the head. The etiology could be visual, cerebral, vestibular or gastrointestinal.

Vertigo: describes a discomfort in a patient experiencing an actual sensation of motion in which either the patient or his environment is moving. The direction of motion is often rotatory.

Unsteadiness: is a loss of equilibrium in relationship to one's environment. It is often described by the patient as "bumping into things" or "almost falling". The etiology could be cerebellar, cerebral, pyramidal tract, posterior column, or vestibular. A pure labyrinthine etiology seldom gives rise to unsteadiness without vertigo.

Lightheadedness: is described by the patient as a feeling of "going to faint". It is also used to describe mild vertigo.

The next step when evaluating a "dizzy" patient is to determine the duration of each attack, the frequency of each episode and whether it is constant, episodic, or related to position. Past medical history of dizziness, no matter how remote, should be taken into consideration when arriving at the diagnosis. It is also imperative to obtain a general medical history to rule in or out diabetes mellitus, hypertension, and other cardiovascular or neurological disease.

A complete ENT and neurological examination which includes observation for spontaneous nystagmus in 3 directions of gaze, either through Frenzel glasses (+20 lenses) or other methods, is a prerequisite to other studies. Audiometric tests, mastoid and internal acoustic meatus view, caloric tests or ENG can be obtained if needed. Positional testing is performed if the symptoms are questionably induced or provoked when the patient assumes a particular position. One should note that a sudden change of position may aggravate the symptoms in any type of dizziness without necessarily implying a disease of labyrinthine origin or positional vertigo. A feeling of lightheadedness upon rapidly assuming an upright position does not indicate a labyrinthine or vestibular disorder.

I. NYSTAGMUS

The slow phase of the nystagmus is the direction of the flow of the endolymph and it is vestibular in origin, whereas the quick phase is most likely initiated by the reticular formation as a compensatory mechanism.

Spontaneous: nystagmus present without positional or other labyrinthine stimulation.
Induced: nystagmus elicited by stimulation, e.g. caloric, rotation, parallel swings, etc.
Positional: nystagmus elicited by assuming a specific position as in positional testing.

SPONTANEOUS NYSTAGMUS: Spontaneous nystagmus can be pendular without a fast or slow phase. Pendular nystagmus usually points to a congenital disorder, ocular disease (Miner's nystagmus) or multiple sclerosis. Labyrinthine nystagmus usually has a fast and a slow phase. By convention, the direction of the nystagmus is determined by the fast component.

Spontaneous dissociated nystagmus is also indicative of central nervous system disease.

Spontaneous rotatory nystagmus is rare although not infrequently observed with a horizontal component during positional testing of patients with positional vertigo of the Benign Paroxysmal Type.

Spontaneous vertical or diagonal nystagmus is very rarely observed. It usually signifies a central nervous system disorder. Vertical or diagonal nystagmus induced by stimulation on positional testing also suggests central disorders.

1st degree Spontaneous Nystagmus:	Nystagmus present only when gazing in the direction of the fast component.
2nd degree Spontaneous Nystagmus:	Nystagmus present when gazing in the direction of the fast component and when on straight gaze.
3rd degree Spontaneous Nystagmus:	Nystagmus present in all 3 directions of gaze.
Clinical Correlation:	1st degree = peripheral lesion 2nd degree = central lesion 3rd degree = central lesion

When testing for spontaneous nystagmus one should not bring the patient to a complete lateral gaze as this will induce fatigue or "end point" nystagmus. The patient should be tested with eyes in straight gaze, 30°-45° to the left and 30°-45° to the right.

Spontaneous nystagmus due to peripheral disease can be inhibited by fixation - its manifestation is made possible by eliminating fixation through eye closure or darkness. Spontaneous nystagmus of the central type is present during eye fixation and may be eliminated during eye closure or darkness. When the lesion is below the level of the vestibular nuclei, spontaneous nystagmus is exaggerated by eye closure or darkness. When above, spontaneous nystagmus is subdued by eye closure or darkness.

POSITIONAL NYSTAGMUS: Positional nystagmus is nystagmus elicited during positional testing.

TECHNIQUE OF POSITIONAL TESTING:

1. Sit the patient on a bench in an upright position with arms folded.
2. Reassure the patient that he is not going to fall regardless of his sense of direction. Insist that it is of utmost importance to keep his eyes open during the test.
3. Bring the patient backward swiftly with head hanging. Watch for nystagmus induced by assuming this position. Notice a) the latency between assuming the position and the onset of nystagmus, b) the character and direction of nystagmus, c) the duration of the nystagmus. (If the nystagmus has a rotatory component it is classified as clockwise or counter-clockwise as illustrated in Figure 5-1.)

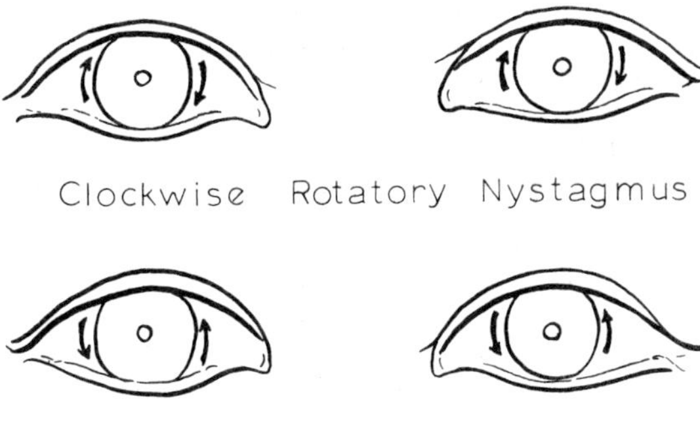

FIGURE 5-1.

4. Bring the patient back to the upright position either after the nystagmus has stopped or after 3 minutes and determine, a) the direction of the nystagmus, b) the duration of the nystagmus.
5. Repeat steps 3 and 4 except that now the head is positioned with the left ear down in step 3.
6. Repeat steps 3 and 4 again except that now the patient's head is positioned with the right ear down in step 3.

The nystagmus elicited can be classified according to Nylen's classification or as modifed by Aschan.

NYLEN'S CLASSIFICATION

Type I: The direction of nystagmus varies with the positions of the head in the positional testing.

Type II: The direction of nystagmus remains fixed regardless of the position of the head during positional testing. When present in different head positions, the nystagmus is stronger in a particular position.

Type III: The nystagmus is irregular, characterized by variations in its behavior. It is thus sometimes direction-changing, sometimes direction-fixed and sometimes changes its direction with the same head position. Type III is used to label all forms of positional nystagmus that cannot be classified under Type I or Type II.

CLINICAL CORRELATION:
Type I: implies central lesion, e.g. multiple sclerosis or cerebellar tumor.
Type II: implies peripheral lesion or acoustic neurinoma.
Type III: ? significance.

ASCHAN'S CLASSIFICATION

Type I: Nystagmus is non-fatigable and persistent; its direction changes with head position.
Type II: Nystagmus is non-fatigable and persistent; its direction remains fixed with change of head position.
Type III: All varieties of transitory positional nystagmus with latency and fatigue.

CLINICAL CORRELATION:
Type I: The majority of these patients have CNS disorder.
Type II: Possible end organ lesion, but mainly CNS
Type III: Peripheral disease; usually indicating positional vertigo of the Benign Paroxysmal Type.

The positional testing has many implications. However, the only practical clinical application to date is to separate positional vertigo of the Benign Paroxysmal Type from positional vertigo secondary to CNS disease. Characteristics of positional vertigo of the Benign Paroxysmal Type are:

a) The nystagmus elicited is rotatory.
b) If the left ear is the pathological ear, the patient will manifest a clockwise rotatory nystagmus when assuming the left ear down position.
c) There will be a latency of 5-15 seconds between assuming that position and the onset of nystagmus.
d) The nystagmus will "fatigue out" (stop after a while).
e) Upon re-assuming the upright position, the patient may manifest a nystagmus in the opposite direction.
f) On repeat testing without rest in between, the positional nystagmus can no more be elicited.

	Peripheral	Central
Latency:	5 - 15 seconds	No latency
Persistence:	Disappears within 50 seconds	Lasts longer than one minute
Fatigability:	Disappears on repetition	Repeatable
Position:	Present in one head position	Present in multiple head positions
Vertigo:	Always present	Occasionally absent

	Peripheral (Cont'd)	Central (Cont'd)
Direction of nystagmus	One direction	Changing with different head positions
Incidence:	85% of all positional vertigo	10-15% of all positional vertigo

II. STIMULATION TESTS

SIMPLE CALORIC TEST: There are many modifications of this test. The important point is that it is a qualitative test measuring the difference in response between the right and left ears. It does not matter which modification of this test is used provided the physician is familiar with the test chosen as well as with its clinical implications and limitations. It is important that the irrigating fluid reaches the tympanic membrane and is not just reflected by the anterior osseous canal or cerumen impaction. This is particularly crucial if small amounts of water are used.

In order to bring the horizontal canal to a vertical plane for the caloric test, it is necessary to tilt the head back 60° when the patient is in an upright position or elevate the head 30° when the patient is supine.

The test as devised by Kobrak (Kobrak Test) used 0.2 cc up to 5 cc of ice water instilled against the tympanic membrane of the patient in a sitting position with head tilted 60° back. The latency and duration of nystagmus are measured. Other tests include Veit's minimal caloric test, Barany Mass Caloric Test and Dundas Grant cold air test for patients with perforated tympanic membranes.

DIRECTIONAL PREPONDERANCE: This is a standardized test to measure canal paresis and directional preponderance. To determine directional preponderance Fitzgerald and Hallpike used the following system:

The patient is placed supine with head elevated 30°. Each ear is douched in turn with water at exactly 30°C (86°F) and with water at 44°C (112°F), each douche consisting of no less than 250 cc. At least 5 minutes should elapse between each douche. Directional preponderance is calculated as follows.

a) Right ear irrigated with cold H_2O = Duration of nystagmus to (L) = (a)
b) Right ear irrigated with warm H_2O = Duration of nystagmus to (R) = (b)
c) Left ear irrigated with cold H_2O = Duration of nystagmus to (R) = (c)
d) Right ear irrigated with warm H_2O = Duration of nystagmus to (L) = (d)

If (a) + (b) is less than (c) + (d), the right ear is hypoactive. If (a) + (d) is less than (b) + (c), there is directional preponderance to the right.

Directional preponderance is believed to be towards the side of central lesion and away from the side of peripheral lesion.

ENG: This test is based on the difference in potential between the cornea (+) and the retina (-). During nystagmus, movements of the eyes cause this corneal-retinal potential to be displaced laterally giving rise to changes in potential that can be recorded by electronic equipment. This electronic recording of the nystagmus is called electronystagmography or ENG.

1. Electrodes are placed as shown: A, B, C, D, E. (See Figure 5-2).

    AC = vertical axis
    BE = horizontal axis
    D = grounding

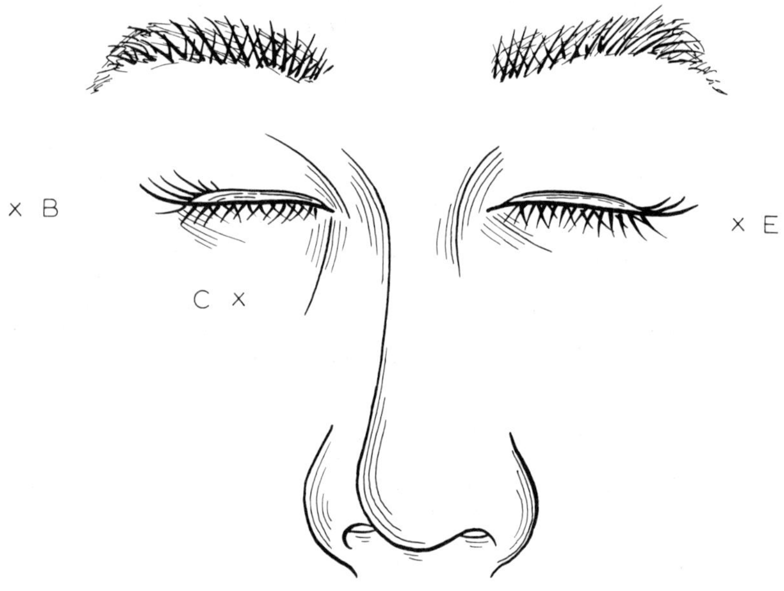

FIGURE 5-2.

2. By convention and calibration, an upward swing of the pen indicates nystagmus to the right while a downward swing indicates nystagmus to the left.
3. The patient lies supine with the head elevated 30°. He is 8-1/2 feet from the wall and gazes at points A, B, C for calibration. (See Figure 5-3).
4. Recordings are then taken with eyes open and eyes closed to check for spontaneous nystagmus.
5. ENG recordings can be obtained from the Rotation Test, Positional Test, etc.

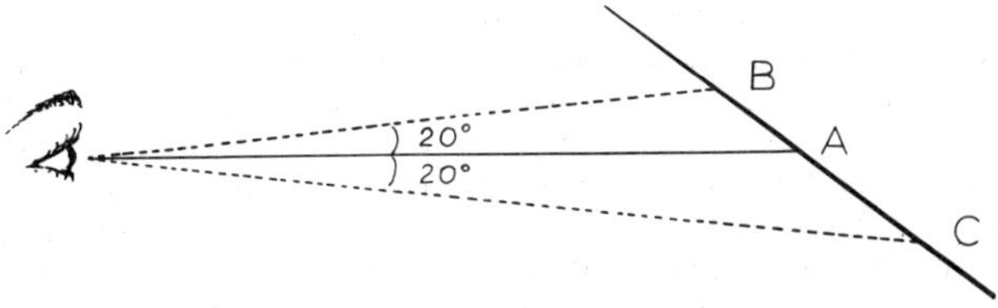

FIGURE 5-3.

6. The patient is then irrigated with 250 cc of 30°C and 250 cc of 44° C water in turn as outlined in the Fitzgerald and Hallpike test.
7. The parameters measured by electronystagmography include Intensity (frequency of beats, amplitude of pen displacement, and velocity of slow component), and Duration.

ROTATION TEST: This test stimulates the labyrinth by the force of rotation. It has little clinical application because it stimulates both ears simultaneously.

TECHNIQUE:
1. Sit patient up with head brought forward 30°.
2. Rotate the chair at the speed of approximately 10 turns per 20 seconds then stop abruptly.
3. If the subject was rotated to his right, the normal response would be nystagmus to the left with past pointing to the right. A patient rotated to his right and brought to an abrupt stop undergoes the same effect as beginning a turn to his left, i.e. the quick phase is to the left, slow phase to the right. The direction of the slow phase is that of the flow of the Endolymph.

Past pointing and falling would also be to the right, in the direction of the slow phase. Past pointing is a compensatory body musculature reflex, its nerve pathways being entirely separate from those of the ocular reflex.

PARALLEL SWING: It tests Utricular function and is still a research tool.

FISTULA TEST: In the presence of a fistula, stimulation of the ear with (+) pressure causes nystagmus to the same side while (-) pressure brings about nystagmus to the opposite side. The presence of nystagmus may be accompanied by vertigo. However, it is the presence of the nystagmus that is significant in this test. If the patient experiences vertigo without nystagmus of the type mentioned, he could be undergoing a cool caloric stimulation without a (+) Fistula Test. Example: when a fistula is present in the right ear, stimulation of this ear with:

(+) pressure gives nystagmus to the (R)
(-) pressure gives nystagmus to the (L)

OPTOKINETIC NYSTAGMUS: Optokinetic Nystagmus can be elicited by various methods. One practical way is to have the patient watch a drum 30 cm. high by 25 cm. in diameter. The surface has 1.5 cm. wide white vertical stripes. The drum is rotated about its vertical axis taking 1 to 2 seconds for a complete revolution. The optokinetic nystagmus is measured while the drum is rotated in one direction. The direction is then reversed and the measurements taken again. When the optokinetic nystagmus is asymmetrical for the two directions of drum rotation, a central lesion is implied. Labyrinthine spontaneous nystagmus can be altered to optokinetic nystagmus by fixation on a rotating drum, whereas spontaneous nystagmus of central origin remains unchanged.

Practical Benefits of ENG:

a) to record spontaneous nystagmus and positional nystagmus with eyes open and eyes closed
b) to record caloric responses
c) to study Optokinetic Nystagmus (eye-tracking is still non-clinical)

III. DIFFERENTIAL DIAGNOSIS

When evaluating a patient with vertigo, one should try to differentiate between vertigo of peripheral origin and that of central origin.

Peripheral	Central
A definite sensation of movement is present in this type of vertigo.	The vertigo is mild and more like a sensation of unsteadiness.
Vertigo is severe and paroxysmal.	Vertigo is vague with no specific onset or termination.
The attacks of vertigo last from minutes to days and are accompanied by spontaneous nystagmus and associated with autonomic nervous system disorders. The patient almost never loses consciousness.	The attacks of vertigo last for weeks, often with no apparent nystagmus.

The following list of differential diagnoses constitutes the more common etiologies of the "dizzy" patient:

1. Ménière's Disease
2. Acoustic neurinoma
3. Vestibular neuronitis
4. Bacterial labyrinthitis
5. Non-bacterial "labyrinthitis"
6. Positional vertigo of the Benign Paroxysmal Type
7. Congenital syphilis
8. Cogan's Syndrome
9. Vertigo due to whiplash injury
10. Temporal bone fracture and labyrinthine concussion
11. Multiple sclerosis
12. Vascular insufficiency
13. Cervical vertigo
14. Vertiginous epilepsy

1. MÉNIÈRE'S DISEASE: The medical history of Ménière's Disease is usually quite typical. The patient suffers episodic vertigo lasting from 30 minutes to 2 hours. The attack is associated with nausea, vomiting, and prostration. The patient may experience fluctuating hearing loss, tinnitus, and a sensation of fullness in the affected ear or ears during an attack of vertigo. After a severe attack, he may feel lightheadedness for half a day or so but is completely well by that evening or the next day. In the early stage of the disease, the episodic vertigo may occur once every year or so but sometimes as far apart as 5 to 10 years. In the majority of the patients the disease affects only one ear (85%). Should the second ear be involved, it usually happens within 36 months.

Diagnostic labyrinthotomy through the oval window may reveal the characteristics of endolymph rather than perilymph. However, the fluid obtained from the round window is perilymph, unchanged from normal conditions.

Audiometric testing will document fluctuating hearing loss usually in the low frequencies with high SISI score, Type II Békésy, and little or no tone decay. Caloric testing or ENG will demonstrate hypofunction of the vestibular labyrinth in the affected ear.

Crisis of Tumarkin: This is a variant of Ménière's Disease in which the patient loses his extensor powers and falls to the ground during a sudden, severe, and short episode of vertigo. He is completely conscious throughout this episode and recovers promptly afterwards.

Lermoyez Syndrome: This is generally agreed to be a rare variant of Ménière's Disease in which there is a dramatic restoration of hearing after an episodic attack of vertigo. Recurrence of this phenomenon can be expected.

Glycerol Test: It has been speculated that administration of glycerol in the dose of 1.2 cc per Kg of body weight with addition of an equal amount of physiological saline, to a patient with Ménière's disease with sensorineural hearing loss, tinnitus and sensation of fullness in the ear, has improved his symptoms within an hour with maximum effects in 2 to 3 hours. After 3 hours, the symptoms return slowly.

2. ACOUSTIC NEURINOMA: (Accounts for 80% of angle tumors) Most patients with acoustic neurinomas complain of unsteadiness rather than episodic vertigo. However, it has been reported that about 10% of acoustic neurinoma patients presented with episodic vertigo of the Ménière's type.

Classically, the caloric reaction is markedly depressed. Audiometric studies reveal a high frequency hearing loss in many of the cases. However, other audiometric patterns are not uncommon. The patients usually have a disproportionately low discrimination score, low SISI score, high tone decay score and Type III or Type IV Békésy. Definitive diagnosis of this disease is made from x-rays of the internal auditory canal.

3. VESTIBULAR NEURONITIS: (50% unilateral, 50% bilateral) This usually follows an upper respiratory tract infection. A patient experiences a sudden onset of vertigo with nausea, vomiting, the sensation of blacking out accompanied by severe unsteadiness. This severe attack can last from days to weeks. Cochlear symptoms are surprisingly absent and without associated neurological deficits. When seen initially, the patient has spontaneous nystagmus to the contralateral side. A caloric test would show marked hypofunction of the labyrinth. Audiometric tests and x-rays of the internal auditory canal are within normal limits.

After the acute episode has subsided, which may take weeks, the patient continues to experience a slight sensation of lightheadedness for some time, particularly in connection with sudden movements. In some patients, there may be an exacerbation of the acute attack within 3 to 6 months. The caloric reaction may remain mildly hypoactive for the duration of the patient's life. The acute episode may also be followed by a period of positional vertigo of the Benign Paroxysmal Type.

4. BACTERIAL LABYRINTHITIS: This is usually a complication of an ear infection which makes the diagnosis obvious.

5. NON-BACTERIAL "LABYRINTHITIS": Some patients have presented with a sudden attack of vertigo associated with nausea, vomiting, and sensori-neural hearing loss without previous history of vertigo. There is no associated neurological deficit. Is this the 1st attack of Ménière's Disease, or does the patient have an Acoustic Neurinoma? Perhaps it is viral labyrinthitis or thrombosis of one of the labyrinthine vessels? Should one consider the possibility of a round or oval window rupture? A careful evaluation and long follow-up may reveal the mystery.

6. CUPULOLITHIASIS: Is a term used by Schuknecht to designate positional vertigo of the Benign Paroxysmal Type. The symptoms include sudden attacks of vertigo precipitated by certain head positions. These attacks have been reported to be prompted by sudden movement of the head to the right or left or by extension of the neck when looking upward. The sensation of vertigo is always of short duration even when the provocative position is maintained. Diagnosis can be confirmed by positional testing which will indicate positional nystagmus with latency and fatigability.

Etiologies include degenerative changes, otitis media, labyrinthine concussion, previous ear surgery, and occlusion of the anterior vestibular artery. Histopathologically, otoconia has been found deposited in the posterior semicircular canal ampulla. It is probable that some of these deposits have resulted from postmortem degeneration of the utricular otolithic membrane. Treatment of this disease is symptomatic and reassurance.

7. CONGENITAL SYPHILIS: The majority of these patients develop hearing loss during young adulthood. This hearing loss is of a flat sensori-neural type. When the onset of hearing loss occurs in adulthood, the loss in both ears is asymmetrical and fluctuates with the

episodic vertigo and tinnitus. However, when the onset occurs in childhood, the hearing loss is abrupt, bilaterally symmetrical, and more severe.

Acquired syphilis seldom gives hearing loss but neurosyphilis and congenital syphilis (38% of congenital syphilis) frequently give rise to hearing loss, with bilateral hearing loss being more prevalent than unilateral hearing loss. Vertigo in congenital syphilis is episodic, similar to Ménière's Disease.

These patients usually have a (+) Hennebert's sign, i.e. (+) fistula test without any demonstrable fistula along with normal external auditory canal and tympanic membrane. The (+) fistula test indicates an abnormally mobile footplate. They may also demonstrate Tullio's phenomenon. (See Chapter 6 or 18).

Histopathologically, mononuclear leukocytic infiltration is evident with obliterative endarteritis. Inflammatory fibrosis and endolymphatic hydrops are present. Osteolytic lesions are often seen in the otic capsule. Interstitial keratitis is another common manifestation of congenital syphilis.

8. COGAN'S SYNDROME: (Refer to Chapter 18: SYNDROMES AND EPONYMS)

9. VERTIGO DUE TO WHIPLASH INJURY: Patients often complain of dizziness following a whiplash injury. In some cases, there was no physiological evidence for this complaint. In others, ENG has documented objective findings such as spontaneous nystagmus. The onset of dizziness often occurs 7 to 10 days following the accident, particularly upon head movements toward the side of the neck most involved in the whiplash. The symptoms may last for months or years after the accident.

Otological examination is usually normal. Audiometric studies are normal unless there is associated labyrinthine concussion. Vestibular examination can reveal spontaneous nystagmus or positional nystagmus with the head turned in the direction of the whiplash. The use of ENG is essential in evaluating these patients.

10. TEMPORAL BONE FRACTURE AND LABYRINTHINE CONCUSSION:

A. <u>Transverse Fracture</u>: Since this fracture destroys the auditory and vestibular function, the patient has no hearing or vestibular response in that ear. When seen initially, he presents with spontaneous nystagmus to the contralateral side and is severely vertiginous very much like a recently post-operative labyrinthectomized patient. The severe vertigo subsides after a week or so and the patient remains mildly unsteady for 3 to 6 months depending on his age and athletic inclination. The patient may also have labyrinthine concussion in the opposite ear. During the acute phase, he usually falls to the involved side.

B. Longitudinal Fracture: (Constitutes 80% of temporal bone fractures) In this type of fracture, there is usually bleeding into the middle ear, with perforation of the tympanic membrane and disruption of the tympanic ring. Hence, the patient has a conductive hearing loss as well as a sensorineural high frequency hearing loss from the concomitant labyrinthine concussion. His dizziness is mild and he may not have vertigo except during positional testing.

C. Labyrinthine Concussion: This is secondary to head injury. The patient complains of mild unsteadiness or lightheadedness particularly with change of head position. Audiometric testing reveals high frequency hearing loss. ENG may show spontaneous or positional nystagmus; occasionally, the caloric response is hypoactive.

11. MULTIPLE SCLEROSIS: This is one of the more common neurological diseases encountered in a clinical practice. Vertigo is the presenting symptom of multiple sclerosis in 7 to 10% of the patients or eventually appears during the course of the disease in up to 1/3 of the cases. The patient usually complains of unsteadiness along with vertigo. Diagnosis of the disease depends on other signs of demyelination. Vertical nystagmus, bilateral internuclear ophthalmoplegia, ataxic eye movements are other clues for this disease. Charcot's triad (nystagmus, scanning speech, intention tremor) may be present.

12. VASCULAR INSUFFICIENCY: Vascular insufficiency can be a very common etiology for vertigo among the over 50-year-olds as well as in patients with diabetes, hypertension or hyperlipidemias. The following syndromes have been recognized among patients with vascular insufficiency:

A. Labyrinthine Apoplexy: This is due to thrombosis of the internal auditory artery or one of its branches. The symptoms include acute vertigo with nausea and vomiting. Hearing loss and tinnitus may or may not occur.

B. Wallenberg Syndrome: (See Chapter 18) This is also known as lateral medullary syndrome secondary to infarction of the lateral portion of the medulla which is supplied by the posterior inferior cerebellar artery. This syndrome is believed to be the most common brain stem vascular disorder. The symptoms include:

1. vertigo, nausea, vomiting, nystagmus.
2. ataxia, falling to the side of the lesion.
3. loss of the sense of pain and temperature sensations on the ipsilateral face and contralateral body.
4. dysphagia with ipsilateral palate and vocal cord paralysis.
5. ipsilateral Horner's syndrome.

C. Subclavian Steal Syndrome: (See Chapter 18) This syndrome is characterized by intermittent vertigo, occipital headache, blurred vision, diplopia, dysarthria, pain in the upper extremity, loud bruit or palpable thrill over the supraclavicular fossa, a difference of at least 20 mm of Hg in systolic blood pressure between the two arms, and a delayed or weakened radial pulse. The blockage can be surgically corrected.

D. <u>Anterior Vestibular Artery Occlusion:</u>

1) sudden onset of vertigo, without deafness.
2) slow recovery followed by months of positional vertigo of the benign paroxysmal type.
3) histologically, utricular macula, the cristae of the lateral and superior semi-circular canals and the superior vestibular nerve show signs of degeneration.
4) this symptom complex was first described by Lindsay and Hemenway in 1956.

E. <u>Basilar-Vertebral Insufficiency:</u> Symptoms include vertigo, hemiparesis, visual disturbances, dysarthria, headache, vomiting. These symptoms are a result of a drop in blood flow to the vestibular nuclei and surrounding structures. The posterior and anterior inferior cerebellar arteries are involved. Tinnitus and deafness are unusual symptoms.

Drop attacks without losing consciousness are characteristic of Basilar-Vertebral Insufficiency. These drop attacks can be precipitated by neck motion.

13. CERVICAL VERTIGO: It can be caused by cervical spondylosis as well as by other etiologies. Cervical spondylosis in turn can be brought about by degeneration of the intervertebral disc. As the disc space narrows, approximation of the vertebral bodies takes place. With mobility, the bulging of the annulus is increased causing increased traction on the periosteum to which the annulus is attached and stimulating proliferation of bone along the margins of the vertebral bodies to produce osteophytes.

Barre believed that the symptoms of cervical spondylosis (including vertigo) are due to irritation of the vertebral sympathetic plexus, which is in close proximity to the vertebral artery. Laskiewicz claims that spondylosis irritates the periarterial neural plexus in the wall of the vertebral and basilar arteries leading to contraction of the vessels. Temporary ischemia then gives rise to vertigo. Another author claimed that the loss of proprioception in the neck can give rise to cervical vertigo. Emotional tension, rotation of the head and extension of the head can cause the neck muscle (including scalenus anticus) to be drawn tightly over the thyrocervical trunk and subclavian artery compressing these vessels against the proximal vertebral artery. In elderly individuals a change from the supine to the upright position may give rise to postural hypotension which in turn may cause vertebral-basilar insufficiency. Aortic Arch Syndrome and Subclavian-Steal Syndrome may also cause cervical vertigo.

<u>Symptoms:</u>

a) headache, vertigo
b) syncope
c) tinnitus and loss of hearing (usually low frequencies)
d) nausea and vomiting (vagal response)

e) visual symptoms such as flashing lights are not uncommon. This is due to ischemia of the occipital lobe which is supplied by the posterior cerebral artery, a branch of the basilar artery.

f) physical examination may reveal a supraclavicular bruit in 1/3 of the patients.

All the above symptoms usually present themselves when the head or neck assumes a certain position or change of position.

Treatment: Proper posture, neck exercises, cervical traction, heat massage, and anesthetic infiltration. Immobilization of the neck with a collar temporarily are all good therapeutic measures. If traction is required it can be given in a few pounds horizontally for several hours at a time. In cervical spondylosis without acute root symptoms, heavy traction (100 lbs.) for 1 to 2 minutes continuously or 5 to 10 minutes intermittently is considered by some as more effective.

14. VERTIGINOUS EPILEPSY: Cortical vertigo can either be severe and episodic like Ménière's Disease, or may manifest as a mild unsteadiness. It is usually associated with hallucination of music or sound. The patient may exhibit "daydreaming", purposeful or purposeless repetitive movements. Motor abnormalities such as chewing, lip smacking, facial grimacing are not uncommon. The patient may experience an unusual sense of familiarity (déja vu) or a sense of strangeness (jamais vu). Should the seizure discharge spread beyond the temporal lobe, grand mal seizures may ensue.

15. VERTIGO IN MIGRAINE: Vertebral-basilar migraine is due to impairment of circulation of the brainstem. The symptoms include vertigo, dysarthria, ataxia, paresthesia, diplopia, diffuse scintillating scotomas or homonymous hemianopsia. The initial vasoconstriction is followed by vasodilatation giving rise to intense throbbing headache, usually unilateral. A positive family history is obtained in over 50 percent of these patients. Treatment of migraine includes fiorinal, ergot derivatives and Sansert. (Sansert has the tendency to cause retroperitoneal fibrosis).

IV. MISCELLANEOUS

1. Streptomycin sulfate is believed to destroy the cristae of the semicircular canals and not the maculae of the utricle and saccule.

2. Ewald's Law:
   A. When a semicircular canal is stimulated, it tends to elicit nystagmus in its own plane.
   B. The horizontal semicircular canal is maximally stimulated by an ampullopetal flow (i.e. endolymph directed towards the ampulla). The superior semicircular canal and posterior semicircular canal are maximally stimulated by ampullofugal flow (i.e. endolymph directed away from the ampulla).
   C. When a semicircular canal is maximally stimulated, it elicits a quick phase of nystagmus to its own side.

3. a. Coriolis Forces: Any body which is set in motion off the surface of the earth towards a distant earth target is deflected from a straight course due to the fact that the earth is revolving. When a subject is on a machine which is rotating at a steady velocity, any movement of the body, head or limbs which are made about an axis different from and at an angle to that of the machine, generates extra forces, some of which are also described as Coriolis forces or acceleration.

b. Coriolis Phenomenon: When the subject's head is tilted about an axis which is perpendicular to the main axis of rotation, he will experience spatial disorientation.

4. Internuclear Ophthalmoplegia is a disturbance of the lateral movements of the eyes which is characterized by a paralysis of the internal rectus on one side and weakness of the external rectus on the other side. In testing, the examiner has the patient follow his finger, first to one side, and then to the other, as in testing for horizontal nystagmus. Internuclear ophthalmoplegia is recognized when the adducting eye (III Nerve) is weak while the abducting eye (VI Nerve) moves normally and displays a coarse nystagmus (? vestibular nuclei involvement). The pathology is in the medial longitudinal fasciculus. When the disorder is bilateral it is pathognomonic of multiple sclerosis, when unilateral, one should consider a tumor or vascular process.

REFERENCES

1. Aschan, G., et al.: Nystagmography, Recording of Nystagmus in Clinical Neuro-Otological Exam., Acta Oto-Laryng. Suppl. 129: 1, 1956.

2. Hallpike, C.: Some Types of Ocular Nystagmus and Their Neurological Mechanisms, Proc. Roy. Soc. Med. 60: 1043, 1967.

3. Igarashi, M., Watanabe, T. and Maxian, P.: Role of the Neck Proprioceptors for Maintenance of Dynamic Bodily Equilibrium in the Squirrel Monkey, Laryngoscope 79: 1713, 1969.

4. Jongkees, L.B.W.: Cervical Vertigo, Laryngoscope 79: 1473, 1969.

5. Lindsay, J. and Hemenway, W.: Postural Vertigo Due to Unilateral Sudden Partial Loss of Vestibular Function, Ann. Otol. Rhin. Laryng. 65: 692, 1956.

6. McCabe, B. and Gillingham, K.: The Mechanism of Vestibular Suppression, Ann. Otol. Rhin. Laryng. 73: 816, 1964.

7. McCabe, B. and Ryu, J.: Experiments on Vestibular Compensation, Laryngoscope 79: 1728, 1969.

8. Nylen, C.: Clinical Study on Positional Nystagmus in Cases of Brain Tumor, Acta Oto-Laryng. Suppl. 15, 1931.

9. Nylen, C.: Positional Nystagmus, J. Laryng. 64: 295, 1950.

10. Schuknecht, H.F.: Cupulolithiasis, Arch. Otolaryng. 90: 113, 1969.

11. Wolfson, R.J.: Vertigo, Otolaryngol. Clin. N. Am., Vol. 6: February, 1973.

CHAPTER 6

CONGENITAL DEAFNESS

GENERAL INFORMATION:

1. One person in 8 carries a recessive gene for deafness; one in 4,000 live births has hereditary deafness.

2. 1% of hereditary hearing loss is sex-linked, 9% are due to an autosomal dominant inheritance and 90% are the results of an autosomal recessive transmission. Hereditary deafness constitutes 15% of all congenital deafness.

3. Dominant hearing loss usually progresses while the recessive type is nonprogressive.

4. Hereditary deafness can be classified as follows:

   a. Hereditary (Congenital) Deafness without associated abnormalities. (Autosomal dominant, autosomal recessive, or sex-linked).
   b. Hereditary Congenital Deafness associated with integumentary system disease. (Autosomal dominant, autosomal recessive or sex-linked).
   c. Hereditary Congenital Deafness associated with skeletal disease. (Autosomal dominant, autosomal recessive, or sex-linked).
   d. Hereditary Congenital Deafness associated with other abnormalities. (Autosomal dominant, autosomal recessive or sex-linked).

Each category can be subdivided along 3 kinds of hearing impairment: sensori-neural, conductive, and mixed.

5. Otologists have attempted to classify inner ear developmental anomalies. One of the classifications is:

Michel: Complete failure of development of the inner ear (bony and membranous aplasia). The middle ear and external auditory canal may be normal.

Mundini-Alexander: Incomplete development of the bony and membranous labyrinth. The cochlea may be represented by a single curved tube. The vestibular labyrinth is not developed either.

Scheibe: Membranous cochlea-saccular aplasia (pars inferior). The bony labyrinth is normal. The utricle and semi-circular canals (pars superior) are normal.

Alexander: Partial aplasia of the cochlear duct giving rise to high frequency hearing loss.

Bing-Siebenmann: The membranous vestibular apparatus is maldeveloped. The membranous cochlea may or may not be normal.

6. The Scheibe type of inner ear anomaly is the most commonly encountered. It is believed to be transmitted autosomal recessively. The next most common is the Mundini-Alexander which is believed to be autosomal dominant.

7. The rubella syndrome includes congenital cataract, cardiovascular anomalies, mental retardation, retinitis and deafness. It has been reported that 5 to 10% of the mothers with rubella in the first trimester gave birth to children with deafness. Alford reported 90 out of 141 rubella syndrome children presented with deafness. The eye is the most commonly involved organ followed by the ears and then by the heart. Histologically, the middle ear as well as inner ear anomalies have been described. Confirmatory tests for rubella syndrome include identification of fluorescent antibody, serum hemagglutination and viral cultures from stool and throat. Deafness of a viral etiology shows: (a) degeneration of the organ of Corti; (b) adhesions between the organ of Corti and Reissner's membrane; (c) rolled up tectorial membrane; (d) partial or complete stria atrophy; (e) scattered degeneration of neural elements (cochlea-saccule degeneration).

8. Twenty percent of the Kernicteric babies will have severe deafness secondary to damage to the dorsal and ventral cochlear nuclei as well as the superior and inferior colliculi nuclei. Clinically, bilateral sensory-neural loss especially in high frequencies is manifested. The most accepted indication for exchange transfusion is a serum bilirubin of greater than 20 mg. per 100 ml.

9. Syphilitic Deafness: Tamari and Itkin estimated that hearing loss occured in:
   17% of early congenital syphilis
   18% of late congenital syphilis
   25% of late latent syphilis
   29% of asymptomatic neurosyphilis
   80% of symptomatic neurosyphilis

Congenital: Contrary to the above, Karmody and Schuknecht reported 25 to 38% of patients with congenital syphilis had hearing loss. There exist two forms of congenital syphilis: early (infantile) and late (tardive). The infantile form is often severe, bilateral. These children usually have multisystem involvement and hence a fatal outcome.

Late congenital syphilis has progressive hearing loss of various severity and time of onset. Those that have the onset in early childhood are usually bilateral, sudden and severe associated with vestibular symptoms. The symptom complex is similar to Ménière's disease. The late onset form (sometimes as late as the fifth decade of life) has mild hearing loss. Karmody and Schuknecht also pointed out that the vestibular disorders of severe episodic vertigo are more common in the late onset group than in the infantile group. Histopathologically, one noticed osteitis with mononuclear leukocytosis, obliterative endoarteritis and endolymphatic hydrops. Serum and CSF serology may or may not be (+). Treatment with steroids and penicillin seems to be of benefit. Other sites of congenital syphilis are:

(1) nasal cartilaginous and bony framework
(2) periostitis of the cranial bones (bossing)
(3) periostitis of the tibia (sabre shin)
(4) injury to the odontogenous tissues (Hutchinson's teeth)
(5) injury to the epiphyseal cartilages (short stature)
(6) commonly interstitial keratitis (cloudy cornea)

Two signs are associated with congenital syphilis:

(1) Hennebert's sign consists of a positive fistula test without clinical evidence of middle ear or mastoid disease or a fistula. Nadol postulated that the vestibular stimulation is mediated by fibrous bands between the footplate and the vestibular membranous labyrinth. He observed that Hennebert's sign may also be present in Ménière's disease. The other explanation was that the vestibular response is due to an excessive mobile footplate. The nystagmus in Hennebert's sign is usually more marked upon application of a negative pressure. (Refer to Chapter on Syndromes and Eponyms on Hennebert's sign)

(2) Tullio's phenomenon consists of vertigo and nystagmus on stimulation with high intensity sound such as the Barany noise box. This phenomenon occurs not only in congenital syphilis patients with a semicircular canal fistula but also in post-fenestration patients if the footplate is mobile and the fenestrum patent. It can also be demonstrated in chronic otitis media should the patient have an intact tympanic membrane, ossicular chain and a fistula...(rare combination).

In order for Tullio's phenomenon to take place, there need to be a fistula of the semicircular canal and intact sound transmission mechanism to the inner ear (i.e., intact tympanic membrane, intact ossicular chain, mobile footplate). The pathophysiology is that the high intensity noise energy transmitted through the footplate finds the course of least resistance and displaces towards the fistula instead of towards the round window membrane.

Acquired: Hearing loss may occur in the secondary or tertiary forms of acquired syphilis. Histopathologically, one noticed osteitis with round cell infiltration. In tertiary syphilis, gummatous lesions may involve the auricle, mastoid, middle ear and petrous pyramid. These lesions can cause a mixed hearing loss. Since penicillin and other antibiotic therapy is quite effective in treating acquired syphilis, this form of deafness is rare nowadays.

10. Cretinism: retarded growth, mental retardation and mixed hearing loss.

I. HEREDITARY DEAFNESS WITHOUT ASSOCIATED ABNORMALITIES

1. STRIA ATROPHY: (Hereditary, not congenital)
   a) Autosomal dominant.
   b) The sensori-neural hearing loss begins at middle age and is progressive.
   c) Good discrimination is maintained.
   d) Flat audiometric curve
   e) (+) SISI Test.
   f) Bilaterally symmetrical hearing loss.
   g) The patient never becomes profoundly deaf.
2. OTOSCLEROSIS (Hereditary, not congenital)
   a) See Chapter 6.

II. HEREDITARY CONGENITAL DEAFNESS ASSOCIATED WITH INTEGUMENTARY SYSTEM DISEASE

1. ALBINISM WITH BLUE IRIDES:
   a) Autosomal dominant or recessive
   b) Sensori-neural hearing loss
2. ECTODERMAL DYSPLASIA, HIDROTIC: (Anhidrotic ectodermal dysplasia is sex-linked recessive. Mixed or conductive hearing loss).
   a) Autosomal dominant
   b) Small dystrophic nails
   c) Coniform teeth
   d) Elevated sweat electrolytes
   e) Sensori-neural hearing loss
3. FORNEY'S SYNDROME:
   a) Autosomal dominant
   b) Lentigines
   c) Mitral insufficiency
   d) Skeletal malformations
   e) Conductive hearing loss
4. LENTIGINES:
   a) Autosomal dominant
   b) Brown spots appear on the skin. These begin to appear at age 2.
   c) Ocular hypertelorism
   d) Pulmonary stenosis
   e) Abnormalities of the genitalia
   f) Retarded growth
   g) Sensori-neural hearing loss
5. LEOPARD SYNDROME:
   a) Autosomal dominant with variable penetrance
   b) Variable sensori-neural hearing loss
   c) Ocular hypertelorism
   d) Pulmonary stenosis
   e) Hypogonadism
   f) EKG changes with widened QRS or bundle branch block
   g) Retardation of growth
   h) Normal vestibular apparatus
   i) Lentigines
   j) Skin changes progressive over the 1st and 2nd decades

6. PIEBALDNESS:
   a) Sex-linked or autosomal recessive
   b) Blue irides
   c) Fine retinal pigmentation
   d) Depigmentation of scalp, hair, and face
   e) Areas of depigmentation on limbs and trunk
   f) Sensori-neural hearing loss
7. TIETZ'S SYNDROME:
   a) Autosomal dominant
   b) Profound deafness
   c) Albinism
   d) Eyebrow absent
   e) Blue irides
   f) No photophobia or nystagmus
8. WAARDENBURG'S DISEASE:
   a) Autosomal dominant with variable penetrance
   b) Contributes 1 to 7% of all hereditary deafness
   c) Widely spaced medial canthi. This is present in all cases.
   d) Flat nasal root in 75% of the cases.
   e) Confluent eyebrow
   f) Sensori-neural hearing loss (unilateral or bilateral). Hearing loss is present in 20% of the cases.
   g) Colored irides
   h) White forelock
   i) 10% of these patients have areas of depigmentation
   j) Abnormal Tyrosine metabolism
   k) 75% of these patients have diminished vestibular function
   l) 10% of these patients are associated with cleft lip and palate

III. HEREDITARY CONGENITAL DEAFNESS ASSOCIATED WITH SKELETAL DISEASE

1. ACHONDROPLASIA:
   a) Autosomal dominant
   b) Large head, short extremities
   c) Dwarfism
   d) Mixed hearing loss (fused ossicles)
   e) Saddle nose, frontal and mandibular prominence
2. APERT'S DISEASE: (Acrocephalosyndactyly)
   a) Autosomal dominant
   b) Syndactylia
   c) Flat conductive hearing loss secondary to stapes fixation
   d) Patent cochlear aqueduct has been noted histologically
   e) Frontal prominence, exophthalmos
   f) Craniofacial dysostosis, hypoplastic maxilla
   g) Proptosis, saddle nose, high arched palate, and occasionally, with spina bifida.
   h) Occurs in about 1:150,000 live births.
3. ATRESIA AURIS CONGENITA:
   a) Autosomal dominant
   b) Unilateral or bilateral involvement are possible
   c) Middle ear abnormalities with VII nerve anomaly
   d) Internal hydrocephalus
   e) Mental retardation
   f) Epilepsy
   g) Choanal atresia and cleft palate

4. CLEIDOCRANIAL DYSOSTOSIS:
   a) Autosomal dominant
   b) Absent or hypoplastic clavicle
   c) Failure of fontanelles to close
   d) Sensori-neural hearing loss
5. CROUZON'S DISEASE:(Craniofacial Dysostosis)
   a) Autosomal dominant
   b) One-third of the cases are associated with hearing loss
   c) Mixed-hearing loss in some cases
   d) Cranial synostosis
   e) Exophthalmos and divergent squint
   f) Parrot-beaked nose
   g) Short upper lip
   h) Mandibular prognathism and small maxilla
   i) Hypertelorism
   j) The external auditory canal may be atretic
   k) Congenital enlargement of the sphenoid bone
   l) Premature closure of the cranial suture lines can lead to mental retardation.
6. ENGELMANN'S SYNDROME:(Diaphyseal Dysplasia)
   a) Autosomal dominant; ? recessive
   b) Progressive mixed hearing loss
   c) Progressive cortical thickening of diaphyseal regions of long bones and skull.
7. HAND-HEARING SYNDROME
   a) Autosomal dominant
   b) Congenital flexion contractures of fingers and toes
   c) Sensori-neural hearing loss
8. KLIPPEL-FEIL (Brevicollis)(Wildervanck's) SYNDROME:
   a) Autosomal recessive or dominant
   b) The incidence in females is greater than in males
   c) Sensori-neural hearing loss along with middle ear anomalies
   d) Short neck due to fused cervical vertebrae
   e) Spina bifida
   f) External auditory canal atresia
9. MADELUNG'S DEFORMITY:(related to Dyschondrosteosis of Leri-Weill)
   a) Autosomal dominant
   b) Short stature
   c) Ulna and elbow dislocation
   d) Conductive hearing loss secondary to ossicular malformation with normal tympanic membrane and external auditory canal.
   e) Spina bifida occulta
   f) The ratio of female to male is 4 to 1
10. MARFAN'S SYNDROME: (Arachnodactyly, Ectopia Lentis, Deafness)
   a) Autosomal dominant
   b) Thin elongated individuals with long spidery fingers
   c) Pigeon breast
   d) Scoliosis
   e) Hammer toes
   f) Mixed hearing loss
11. MOHR SYNDROME: (Oral-Facial-Digital Syndrome II)
   a) Autosomal recessive
   b) Conductive hearing loss

c) Cleft lip, high arched palate
d) Lobulated nodular tongue
e) Broad nasal root, bifid tip of nose
f) Hypoplasia of the body of the mandible
g) Polydactyly and syndactyly

12. OSTEOPETROSIS: (Albers-Schönberg Disease) (Marble Bone Disease)
a) Autosomal recessive (A rare dominant transmission has been reported)
b) Conductive or mixed hearing loss
c) Fluctuating facial nerve paralysis
d) Sclerotic, brittle bone due to failure of resorption of calcified cartilage
e) Cranial nerves, II, V, VII may be involved also
f) Optic atrophy
g) Atresia of paranasal sinuses
h) Choanal atresia
i) Increased incidence of osteomyelitis
j) The widespread form of this disease may lead to obliteration of the bone marrow, severe anemia and rapid demise
k) May have hepatosplenomegaly

13. OTO-FACIAL-CERVICAL SYNDROME:
a) Autosomal dominant
b) Depressed nasal root
c) Protruding narrow nose
d) Narrow elongated face
e) Flattened maxilla and zygoma
f) Prominent ears
g) Pre-auricular fistulas
h) Poorly developed neck muscles
i) Conductive hearing loss

14. OTO-PALATAL-DIGITAL SYNDROME:
a) Autosomal recessive
b) Conductive hearing loss
c) Mild dwarfism
d) Cleft palate
e) Mental retardation
f) Broad nasal root, hypertelorism
g) Frontal and occipital bossing
h) Small mandible
i) Stubby, clubbed digits
j) Low set small ears
k) Winged scapulae
l) Malar flattening
m) Downward obliquity of eye
n) Down-turned mouth

15. PAGET'S DISEASE:(Osteitis Deformans)
a) Autosomal dominant with variable penetrance
b) Mainly sensori-neural hearing loss but mixed hearing loss is seen as well.
c) Occasionally may develop cranial nerve involvement
d) Onset usually at middle age, involving skull and long bones of the legs.
e) The Endochondral bone is somewhat resistant to this disease.

16. PIERRE-ROBIN SYNDROME:(Cleft Palate, micrognathia and glossoptosis)
    a) Autosomal dominant with variable penetrance. Possibly not hereditary but due to intrauterine insult.
    b) It occurs 1:30,000 live births to 1:50,000 live births.
    c) Glossoptosis
    d) Micrognathia
    e) Cleft palate (in 50% of the cases)
    f) Mixed hearing loss
    g) Malformed auricles
    h) Mental retardation
    i) Hypoplastic mandible
    j) Möbius Syndrome
    k) Subglottic stenosis not uncommon
    l) Aspiration is a common cause of death
17. PYLE'S DISEASE:(Craniometaphyseal Dysplasia)
    a) Autosomal dominant (less often autosomal recessive)
    b) Conductive hearing loss can begin at any age. It is progressive and it is secondary to fixation of the stapes or other ossicular abnormalities. Mixed hearing loss is also possible.
    c) Cranial nerve palsy secondary to narrowing of the foramen
    d) Splayed appearance of long bones
    e) Choanal atresia
    f) Prognathism
    g) Optic atrophy
    h) Obstruction of sinuses and nasolacrimal duct
18. ROAF'S SYNDROME:
    a) Not hereditary
    b) Retinal detachment, cataracts, myopia, coxa vara, kyphoscoliosis and retardation.
    c) Progressive sensori-neural hearing loss
19. DOMINANT PROXIMAL SYMPHALANGIA AND HEARING LOSS:
    a) Autosomal dominant
    b) Ankylosis of proximal interphalangeal joint
    c) Conductive hearing loss early in life
20. TREACHER-COLLINS DISEASE:(Mandibulofacial Dysostosis) (Franceschetti-Zwahlen-Klein Syndrome)
    a) Autosomal dominant or intrauterine abuse
    b) Antimongoloid palpebral fissures with notched lower lids
    c) Malformation of ossicles (stapes is usually normal)
    d) Auricular deformity, atresia of external auditory canal
    e) Conductive hearing loss
    f) Preauricular fistulas
    g) Mandibular hypoplasia and malar hypoplasia
    h) "Fish-mouth"
    i) Normal I-Q
    j) Usually bilateral involvement
    k) May have cleft palate and cleft lip
    l) Arrest in embryonic development occurs at 6 to 8 weeks to give the above findings.
21. VAN BUCHEM'S DISEASE:(Hyperostosis Corticalis Generalisata)
    a) Autosomal recessive
    b) Generalized osteosclerotic overgrowth of skeleton including skull, mandible, ribs, long and short bones.
    c) Cranial nerve palsies due to obstruction of the foramina

d) Increased serum alkaline phosphatase
e) Progressive sensori-neural hearing loss

22. VAN DER HOEVE'S SYNDROME: (Osteogenesis Imperfecta)
   a) Autosomal dominant with variable expressivity
   b) Fragile bones, loose ligaments
   c) Blue or clear sclera, triangular facies, dentinogenesis imperfecta
   d) 60% of osteogenesis imperfecta patients have blue sclera and hearing loss which are most frequently noticed after age 20. The hearing loss is conductive and is due to stapes fixation by otosclerosis. Hearing loss can also be due to ossicular fracture. (Some use the term Van der Hoeve's Syndrome to describe osteogenesis imperfecta with otosclerosis. Others use the term interchangeably with osteogenesis imperfecta regardless of whether otosclerosis is present or not).
   e) The basic pathological defect is "abnormal osteoblastic activity".
   f) When operating on such a patient, it is important to avoid fracture of the tympanic ring or the long process of the incus. It is also important to realize that the stapes footplate may be "floating".
   g) The sclera may have increased mucopolysaccharide content.
   h) These patients have normal calcium, phosphorus, and alkaline phosphatase in the serum.
   i) Occasionally capillary fragility is noticed in these patients.

IV. HEREDITARY CONGENITAL DEAFNESS ASSOCIATED WITH OTHER ABNORMALITIES

1. ACOUSTIC NEURINOMAS:(Inherited)
   a) Autosomal dominant
   b) Progressive sensori-neural hearing loss in the 2nd or 3rd decades of life.
   c) Ataxia, visual loss
   d) No café-au-lait spots

2. ALPORT'S DISEASE:
   a) Autosomal dominant
   b) Progressive nephritis and sensori-neural hearing loss
   c) Hematuria, proteinuria beginning the 1st or 2nd decade of life
   d) Males with this disease usually die of uremia by the age of 30. Females are less severely affected.
   e) Kidneys are affected by chronic glomerulonephritis with interstitial lymphocytic infiltrate and foam cells.
   f) Progressive sensori-neural hearing loss begins at age 10. Although it is considered not sex-linked, hearing loss affects almost all males but not all females. Histologically, degeneration of the Organ of Corti and stria vascularis is observed.
   g) Spherophalera cataract
   h) Hypofunction of the vestibular organ
   i) Contributes 1% of hereditary deafness

3. ALSTROM'S DISEASE:
   a) Autosomal recessive
   b) Retinal degeneration giving rise to visual loss
   c) Diabetes, obesity
   d) Progressive sensori-neural hearing loss
4. COCKAYNE'S SYNDROME:
   a) Autosomal recessive
   b) Dwarfism
   c) Mental retardation
   d) Retinal atrophy
   e) Motor disturbances
   f) Progressive sensori-neural hearing loss bilaterally
5. CONGENITAL CRETINISM: (To be distinguished from Pendred's Syndrome)
   a) 35% of the patients with congenital cretinism present with congenital hearing loss of the mixed type (irreversible).
   b) Goiter, hypothyroid
   c) Mental and physical retardation
   d) Abnormal development of the petrous pyramid
   e) This disease is not inherited in a specific Mendelian manner. It is restricted to a certain geographical locale where a dietary deficiency exists.
6. DUANE'S SYNDROME:
   a) Autosomal dominant (some sex-linked recessive)
   b) Inability to abduct eyes, retract globe.
   c) Narrowing of palpebral fissure
   d) Torticollis
   e) Cervical rib
   f) Conductive hearing loss
7. FANCONI ANEMIA SYNDROME:
   a) Autosomal recessive
   b) Absent or deformed thumb
   c) Other skeletal, heart and kidney malformations
   d) Increased skin pigmentation
   e) Mental retardation
   f) Pancytopenia
   g) Conductive hearing loss
8. FEHR'S CORNEAL DYSTROPHY:
   a) Autosomal recessive
   b) Progressive visual and sensori-neural hearing loss
9. FLYNN-AIRD SYNDROME:
   a) Autosomal dominant
   b) Progressive myopia, cataracts, retinitis pigmentosa
   c) Progressive sensori-neural hearing loss
   d) Ataxia
   e) Shooting pains in the joints
10. FRIEDREICH'S ATAXIA:
   a) Autosomal recessive
   b) Childhood onset of nystagmus, ataxia, optic atrophy, hyperreflexia and sensori-neural hearing loss.
11. GOLDENHAR'S SYNDROME:
   a) Autosomal recessive
   b) Epibulbar dermoids
   c) Preauricular appendages

d) Fusion or absence of cervical vertebrae
e) Colobomas of the eye
f) Conductive hearing loss

12. HALLGREN'S SYNDROME:
a) Autosomal recessive
b) Retinitis pigmentosa
c) Progressive ataxia
d) Mental retardation occurs in 25% of these patients
e) Sensori-neural hearing loss
f) This constitutes about 5% of hereditary deafness

13. HERMANN'S SYNDROME:
a) Autosomal dominant
b) Onset of photomyoclonus and sensori-neural hearing loss in late childhood or adolescence.
c) Diabetes mellitus
d) Progressive dementia
e) Pyelonephritis and Glomerulonephritis

14. A. HURLER'S SYNDROME: (Gargoylism)
a) Autosomal recessive
b) Abnormal mucopolysaccharides are deposited in tissues. (When mucopolysaccharide is deposited in the neutrophiles they are called Adler bodies). Middle ear mucosa with large foamy gargoyle cells staining PAS (+).
c) Chondroitin Sulfate B and heparitin are found in urine
d) Forehead prominence with coarsening of the facial features and low set ears.
e) Mental retardation
f) Progressive corneal opacities
g) Hepatosplenomegaly
h) Mixed hearing loss
i) Dwarfism
j) Cerebral storage of 3 gangliosides, $GM_{3,2,1}$
k) Beta-galactosides deficient

B. HUNTER'S SYNDROME:
a) Same as above except that it is sex-linked

15. JERVELL-LANGE-NIELSON SYNDROME:
a) Autosomal recessive
b) Profound bilateral sensori-neural hearing loss. The high frequencies are more severely impaired.
c) Associated with Heart Disease (prolonged QT interval on EKG). Has been associated with Stokes-Adams Disease.
d) Recurrent syncope
e) Usually terminates fatally; death being sudden
f) Histopathologically, PAS (+) nodules can be seen in the cochlea.

16. LAURENCE-MOON-BIEDL-BARDET SYNDROME:
a) Autosomal recessive
b) Dwarfism
c) Obesity
d) Hypogonadism
e) Retinitis pigmentosa
f) Mental retardation
g) Sensori-neural hearing loss

17. (RECESSIVE) MALFORMED LOW-SET EARS AND CONDUCTIVE HEARING LOSS:
    a) Autosomal recessive
    b) 50% of these patients show mental retardation
18. (DOMINANT) MITRAL INSUFFICIENCY, JOINT FUSION AND HEARING LOSS:
    a) Autosomal dominant with variable penetrance
    b) Conductive hearing loss, usually due to fixation of the stapes
    c) Narrow external auditory canal
    d) Fusion of the cervical vertebrae, carpal and tarsal bones
19. MÖBIUS SYNDROME (CONGENITAL FACIAL DIPLEGIA):
    a) Autosomal dominant, ? recessive
    b) Facial diplegia
    c) External ear deformities
    d) Ophthalmoplegia
    e) The hands or feet may be missing
    f) Mental retardation
    g) Paralysis of the tongue
    h) Mixed hearing loss
20. (DOMINANT) SADDLE NOSE, MYOPIA, CATARACT AND HEARING LOSS:
    a) Autosomal dominant
    b) Saddle nose
    c) Severe myopia
    d) Juvenile cataract
    e) Sensori-neural hearing loss which is progressive, moderately severe and of an early onset.
21. NORRIE'S SYNDROME:
    a) Autosomal recessive
    b) Congenital blindness due to pseudotumor retini
    c) Progressive sensori-neural hearing loss in 30% of the patients
22. PENDRED'S DISEASE:
    a) Autosomal recessive
    b) Variable amount of bilateral hearing loss secondary to atrophy of the Organ of Corti. A U-shaped audiogram is often seen.
    c) These patients are euthyroid. They develop diffuse goiter at the time of puberty. It is said that the metabolic defect is faulty iodination of Tyrosine.
    d) (+) Perchlorate Test
    e) The goiter is treated with exogenous hormone to suppress TSH secretion.
    f) Normal I.Q.
    g) Unlike congenital cretinism, the bony petrous pyramid is well developed.
    h) Constitutes 10% of hereditary deafness
23. REFSUM'S DISEASE: (Heredopathia Atactica Polyneuritiformis)
    a) Autosomal recessive
    b) Retinitis pigmentosa
    c) Polyneuropathy
    d) Ataxia
    e) Sensori-neural hearing loss
    f) The visual impairment usually begins in the 2nd decade
    g) Ichthyosis is often present
    h) The patient is noted to have elevated plasma phytanic acid levels.
    i) Etiology: Neuronal lipid storage disease and hypertrophic polyneuropathy.

24. (RECESSIVE) RENAL, GENITAL, MIDDLE EAR ANOMALIES:
   a) Autosomal recessive
   b) Renal hypoplasia
   c) Internal genital malformation
   d) Middle ear malformation
   e) Moderate to severe conductive hearing loss
25. RICHARDS-RUNDEL DISEASE:
   a) Autosomal recessive
   b) Mental deficiency
   c) Hypogonadism (decreased urinary estrogen, pregnanediol and total 17-keto steroids).
   d) Ataxia
   e) Horizontal nystagmus to bilateral gazes
   f) Sensori-neural hearing loss begins at infancy
   g) Muscle wasting in early childhood and absent deep tendon reflexes
26. TAYLOR'S SYNDROME:
   a) Autosomal recessive
   b) Unilateral microtia or anotia
   c) Unilateral facial bone hypoplasia
   d) Conductive hearing loss
27. TRISOMY 13-15 (GROUP D) (PATAU'S SYNDROME):
   a) Low set pinnae
   b) Atresia of external auditory canals
   c) Cleft lip and cleft palate
   d) Colobomas of the eyelids
   e) Micrognathia
   f) Tracheo-esophageal fistula
   g) Hemangiomas
   h) Congenital heart disease
   i) Mental retardation
   j) Mixed hearing loss
   k) Hypertelorism
   l) Incidence of 0.45 per 1000 live births
   m) These patients usually die early in childhood
28. TRISOMY 16, 17, 18 (GROUP E):
   a) Low set pinnae
   b) External canal atresia
   c) Micrognathia, high arched palate
   d) Peculiar finger position
   e) Prominent occiput
   f) Cardiac anomalies
   g) Hernias
   h) Pigeon breast
   i) Mixed hearing loss
   j) Incidence of 0.25 to 2 per 1000 live births
   k) Ptosis
   l) These patients usually die early in life
29. TRISOMY 21 OR 22 (DOWN'S SYNDROME) (G TRISOMY):
   a) Extra chromosome on No. 21 or No. 22
   b) Mental retardation
   c) Short stature
   d) Brachycephaly
   e) Flat occiput
   f) Slanted eyes

g) Epicanthus
h) Strabismus, nystagmus
i) Seen in association with leukemia
j) Subglottic stenosis not uncommon
k) Decreased pneumatized or absent frontal and sphenoid sinuses
l) 1:600 live births

30. TURNER'S SYNDROME:
a) Not inherited; ? due to intra-uterine insult
b) Low hairline
c) Webbing of neck and digits
d) Widely spaced nipples
e) XO; 80% are sex chromatin negative
f) Gonadal aplasia
g) Incidence of 1 in 5000 live births (Klinefelter's Syndrome is XXY)
h) Ossicular deformities
i) Low set ears
j) Mixed hearing loss
k) Large ear lobes
l) Short stature
m) Abnormalities found in the heart and kidney
n) Some with hyposmia

31. (DOMINANT) URTICARIA, AMYLOIDOSIS, NEPHRITIS AND HEARING LOSS:
a) Autosomal dominant
b) Recurrent urticaria
c) Amyloidosis
d) Progressive sensori-neural hearing loss due to degeneration of the Organ of Corti, ossification of the basilar membrane and cochlear nerve degeneration.
e) The patient usually succumbs to uremia

32. USHER'S SYNDROME: (Recessive retinitis pigmentosa with Congenital severe deafness)
a) Autosomal recessive
b) Retinitis Pigmentosa giving rise to progressive visual loss. Usually, the patient is completely blind by the second or third decade.
c) These patients are usually born deaf secondary to atrophy of the Organ of Corti. Hearing for low frequencies may be present in some patients.
d) Ataxia and vestibular dysfunction are very common. Usher's Syndrome, among all congenital deafness, is the one most likely to include vestibular symptoms.
e) It constitutes 10% of hereditary deafness

33. WEIL'S SYNDROME:
a) Nephritis
b) Hearing loss
c) Autosomal dominant

MIDDLE AND EXTERNAL EAR CONGENITAL DEFORMITIES

1. These have been classified into Class I, II, III. However, the classification is less commonly used than that for inner ear developmental anomaly.

Class I:
a) Normal auricle in shape and size
b) Well pneumatized mastoid and middle ear
c) Ossicular problem
d) This type is the most common

Class II:
a) Microtia
b) Atretic canal and abnormal ossicles
c) Normal aeration of mastoid and middle ear

Class III:
a) Microtia
b) Atretic canal and abnormal ossicles
c) Middle ear and mastoid poorly aerated

2. External deformity does not correlate necessarily with the middle ear abnormality.

3. Patients with congenitally fixed footplate have the following points to differentiate them from those patients with otosclerosis.
a) Onset in childhood
b) Non-progressive
c) Negative family history
d) Flat 50 to 60 dB conductive hearing loss
e) Carhart's Notch is not present
f) Schwartze sign is not present

REFERENCES

1. Alford, B.R.: Rubella-La Bête Noire De La Medecine, Laryngoscope 78:1623, October, 1968.

2. Hemenway, W.G. and Bergstrom, L.: Symposium on Congenital Deafness, The Otolaryngologic Clinics of North America, Vol. 4: No. 2, June, 1971, W.B. Saunders Co., Philadelphia.

3. Hemenway, W.G., et al.: Temporal Bone Pathology Following Maternal Rubella, Arch. Ohr. Nas.-Kehlk-Heilk. 193: 287, 1969.

4. Hennebert, C.: Un Syndrome Nouveau Dans La Labyrinthite, Heredo-Syphilitique, Clinique, Brux 25: 545 also Presse Med. 63: 467, 1911.

5. Karmody, C. and Schuknecht, H.F.: Deafness in Congenital Deafness, Arch. Otolaryng. 83: 18, 1966.

6. Lindsay, J., et al.: Inner Ear Pathology Following Maternal Rubella, Ann. Otol. Rhinol. Laryng. 62: 1201, 1953.

7. Perlman, H. and Leek, J.: Late Congenital Syphilis of the Ear, Laryngoscope 62: 1175, 1952.

8. Schuknecht, H.F.: Pathology of the Ear, Harvard University Press, Boston, 1974.

9. Tamari, M. and Itkin, P.: Penicillin and Syphilis of the Ear. Eye, Ear, Nose, Throat Monthly 30:252, 301, 358, 1951.

10. Tietz, W.: A syndrome of Deafmutism Associated with Albinism Showing Dominant Autosomal Inheritance, Am. J. Hum. Genet. 15:259, 1963.

CHAPTER 7

FACIAL NERVE

I. EVALUATION

Evaluation of a patient with peripheral facial nerve paralysis (partial or complete) not associated with any trauma or surgery must include an audiogram and mastoid x-rays to rule out any potentially hazardous and yet treatable condition, e.g. facial nerve or acoustic neurinoma, and primary cholesteatoma. If no etiology can be found after a careful, thorough ENT examination, the diagnosis of Bell's Palsy can be made.

STEPS IN EVALUATING A BELL'S PALSY

Is it partial or total ?

<u>Partial</u>

No treatment
Close follow-up

<u>Total</u>

1. Determine the level of involvement:
   a) Taste impairment?
   b) Presence of Stapedial Reflex?
   c) Schirmer's Test (It is important to note that this is a gross test and it is of no significance unless the normal eye tears at least 30% more than the involved eye).
2. One or more of the following tests can be performed:
   a) Nerve Excitability Test
   b) Conduction Latency Test
   c) Strength - Duration Studies
   d) Electromyography (EMG)
   e) Maximal Stimulation Test
   f) Salivary Flow

When increasing difficulty in eliciting response in these tests is noted, one should consider the fact that the nerve is showing signs of denervation. If one believes in decompression of the nerve, it should be done as soon as it is feasible.

1. NERVE EXCITABILITY TEST: This test uses a once per second square-wave pulse, 1 msec in duration. This test has no clinical usage in a partial paralysis or within 3 days of total paralysis. After the 3rd day of total paralysis, the normal side is first tested to obtain the threshold needed to elicit the slightest flicker of facial muscle movement. The electrode is placed percutaneously along the stylomastoid foramen and then along the main branches of the facial nerve. After recording the thresholds for the normal side, the electrode is placed at the same locations on the diseased side. The respective thresholds are then compared. A greater than 3 to 4 mamps difference is considered significant, suggesting denervation. For those who

believe in decompression of the facial nerve, the Nerve Excitability Test should be performed daily after the 3rd day of total paralysis. As soon as a consistent 3 to 4 mamps difference or more in threshold between the normal and the abnormal sides appears, decompression is performed. In the Nerve Excitability Test, one must avoid stimulating the muscle directly so as not to obtain a false threshold.

2. CONDUCTION LATENCY TEST: This test also uses a once per second square-wave pulse, 1 msec in duration. A 2nd electrode is placed in a distal facial muscle. The time taken by the impulse to reach the distal electrode is recorded as conduction latency. The normal conduction time from the angle of the mandible to the facial muscle in the midline is about 4 msec. Like the Nerve Excitability Test, it does not demonstrate prolonged conduction times till 72 hours after denervation. After 72 hours, a completely transected nerve shows increasing conduction time until no excitability is demonstrable. A lengthening of conduction time may also imply partial denervation.

Unlike the Nerve Excitability Test, the Conduction Latency Test is harder to perform both for the doctor and the patient. Hence it is not used clinically in the office.

3. STRENGTH-DURATION STUDIES: A particular muscle is selected for this test. A square-wave pulse of varying duration and intensity is applied until a just visible twitch is noted. As one goes from a longer pulse duration to a shorter pulse duration, the threshold needed to elicit a just visible twitch is recorded. The intensities for various pulse duration are recorded for the normal side. A denervated nerve will show considerably higher thresholds. The strength-duration curve is not altered in neuropraxia and is not altered till 7 days after denervation.

Rheobase = The strength of current just strong enough to depolarize (mamps).

Chronaxie = The length of duration needed to depolarize using an intensity 2 times the rheobase (msec).

4. ELECTROMYOGRAPHY (EMG): This test determines the activity of the muscle itself. A needle electrode is inserted into the muscle and recordings are made during rest and voluntary contraction (Figure 7-1 illustrates a voluntary unit discharge, fibrillation potential and polyphasic reinnervation potential). Degeneration of a lower motor nerve is followed in 14 to 21 days by spontaneous activity called fibrillation potential. Hence the EMG is not of diagnostic value till 2 weeks after denervation. The practical clinical usage of EMG is in the determination of reinnervation. Polyphasic reinnervation potentials are present 6 to 12 weeks prior to clinical return of facial function.

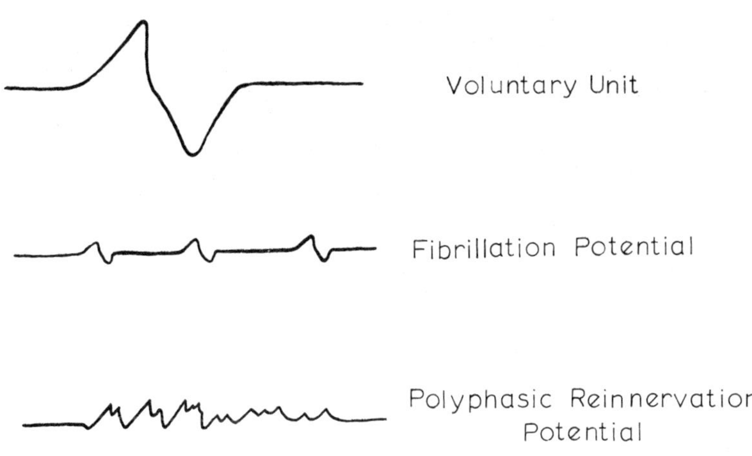

FIGURE 7-1: Schematic Representation of Electromyographic Responses to Facial Paralysis.

5. MAXIMUM STIMULATION TEST: This test is similar to the Nerve Excitability Test except in that it uses maximal rather than minimal stimulation. The main trunk as well as each major portion of the distal branches of the nerve (forehead, eye, nose, mouth, lower lip and neck) on the normal and abnormal sides are stimulated with an intensity that produces discomfort. The results of the test are expressed as a difference in facial muscle movement between the normal and involved side. "The finding of a difference is considered evidence of abnormality".

6. SALIVARY FLOW TEST: This test is based on the fact that the preganglionic parasympathetic nerve fibers are on the outside of the VII nerve bundle and hence it is assumed that these fibers will be injured before the motor fibers. The proponents of this test further reason that the Nerve Excitability Test examines the nerve distal to the injury while the Salivary Flow Test checks the nerve at the site of injury.

After anesthetizing the anterior floor of the mouth, the test is performed by first dilating the Wharton's ducts. A polyethylene tube is then cannulated into each duct. Lemon juice is next used to stimulate salivary flow of which the number of drops secreted per minute is counted for each side. A differencc of 70% or greater is considered significant and warrants surgical decompression of the VII nerve.

II. TREATMENT OF BELL'S PALSY

Before one can specifically advocate one mode of treatment over another, it is imperative to realize that the great majority of Bell's

Palsy are either partial paralysis or total paralysis without degeneration (i.e. maintaining the neuropraxia state). It is also fairly well recognized that, unless denervation has occurred, the patient more than likely will recover spontaneously with little synkinesis. Hence, surgical treatment, if proposed, is reserved for those of total paralysis that have shown signs of denervation. There is no conclusive evidence to date that surgical decompression is of definite benefit. Some protocols treat Bell's Palsy of all severities with steroids, others treat only cases of total facial palsy with steroids. Some believe that if the nerve is allowed to degenerate completely, the prognosis is poor and synkinesis is common.

III. A GUIDELINE FOR THE MANAGEMENT OF FACIAL NERVE PARALYSIS

BELL'S PALSY (complete otological, audiometric and radiographic work-up needed)

Partial: No treatment

Total: Determine level of involvement
Daily Electrical Test until:
(a) threshold of the involved side increases to 4 mamps greater than the normal side.
(b) there is evidence of some return of facial function

If (a) is found, decompression of the facial nerve from the stylomastoid foramen to the level of blockage is performed (should do a "middle fossa" decompression if the greater superficial petrosal nerve is involved).

POST-EAR SURGERY: (Rule out effects of local anesthetics and too tight a mastoid packing).

Delayed onset (partial or complete): Follow like Bell's Palsy

Immediate onset (partial or complete): Explore the nerve before the "sun sets".

TRAUMATIC (Head Injury)

Delayed onset (partial or complete): Follow like Bell's Palsy

Immediate onset (partial or complete): Explore the nerve when patient is stabilized

HERPES ZOSTER OTICUS: (The most common motor nerve involved is the VII nerve, the next are III, IV and VI). Treat like Bell's Palsy.

CHRONIC OTITIS MEDIA:

Partial or Complete: Mastoidectomy and Facial Nerve Decompression ? Tympanoplasty.

ACUTE OTITIS MEDIA:
? Treat like Bell's Palsy
? Simple Mastoidectomy
? Myringotomy

ACUTE MASTOIDITIS WITH FACIAL PARALYSIS: Simple Mastoidectomy and decompression of the Facial Nerve and Myringotomy or Simple Mastoidectomy and Myringotomy.

IV. MISCELLANEOUS

1. Neuropraxia: Blockage due to localized pressure without axonal degeneration or nerve sheath interruption. ? Chemical basis.

2. Axonotmesis: Blockage of replenishment of axoplasm to distal segment. Degeneration of myelin sheath without disruption of neurolemmal sheath.

3. Neurotmesis: Disruption of nerve trunk.

4. Synkinesis: A single axon innervating widely separated facial muscles. (It has also been postulated that unmyelinated nerve regeneration gives rise to more synkinesis and as more myelin is laid down, less synkinesis is noted).

5. Möbius Syndrome: Facial paralysis in the newborn due to central nerve lesion or agenesis of facial muscles.

6. Melkersson-Rosenthal Syndrome: Recurrent unilateral or bilateral facial palsy associated with chronic or recurrent edema of face and with fissured tongue. Unknown etiology. Peak age is 20's; histologically, dilated lymphatic channels, giant cells and inflammatory cells are seen.

7. "Crocodile Tears": Regenerating fibers innervate the lacrimal gland instead of the submaxillary gland.

8. Faradic Current: Is a high frequency interrupted current that stimulates the nerve directly and elicits an all or none response.

9. Galvanic Current: Is a constant direct current that stimulates the muscle directly.

10. Bell's Phenomenon: The orbit turns up and out during an attempt to close the eyes.

11. Facial Paralysis of Central Origin is characterized by:
    a) Intact frontalis and orbicularis oculi.
    b) Intact Mimetic function.
    c) Absence of Bell's Phenomenon.

12. Blood Supply of the facial nerve: (See Figure 7-2)
    a) ECA ⟶ Post Auricular Artery ⟶ Stylomastoid Artery
    b) ECA ⟶ Middle Meningeal Artery ⟶ Greater Superficial Petrosal Artery

13. Pons to IAM = 23 to 24 mm
    IAM = 7 to 8 mm
    Labyrinthine = 3 to 4 mm
    Tympanic = 12 to 13 mm
    Mastoid = 15 to 20 mm
    Parotid before branching = 15 to 20 mm
    75 to 89 mm

14. The Chorda tympani branches off at about 5 to 7 mm before the stylomastoid foramen.

15. Facial nerve paralysis not involving the greater superficial petrosal nerve would give a "tearing" eye because of
    a) Paralysis of Horner's muscle that dilates the nasolacrimal duct orifice.
    b) Ectropia and so produces malposition of the puncta.
    c) Absence of winking, i.e. lack of the pumping action.

16. The most likely areas of compression in Bell's Palsy have been noted to be in the stylomastoid area and around the pyramidal eminence.

17. Korczyn reported that among 130 patients with Bell's Palsy, 66% had either frank diabetes or abnormal Glucose Tolerance Test. It has also been stated that the percentage of denervation in Bell's Palsy is higher in diabetics.

18. In parotid surgery, the facial nerve can be identified at 6 to 8 mm below the inferior "drop off" of the tympanomastoid fissure. This was described by H.G. Tabb in the Laryngoscope 80:559, 1970.

19. 25% of longitudinal fractures involve the facial nerve. 50% of transverse fractures involve the facial nerve.

20. The facial nerve regenerates at 3 mm. per day.

21. Incapacitating facial spasm (particularly of the orbicularis oculi) can be treated by selective avulsion of the facial nerve branches through a parotidectomy approach.

REFERENCES

1. Frey, L.: Le Syndrome du nerf auriculo-temporal, Rev. Neurol. 2: 97, 1923.

2. Korczyn, A.: Bell's Palsy and Diabetes Mellitus, Lancet 1:108, 1971.

3. May, M., et al.: The Prognostic Accuracy of the Maximal Stimulation Test Compared with that of the Nerve Excitability Test in Bell's Palsy, Laryngoscope 81: 931, 1971.

4. May, M. and Harvey, J.E.: Salivary Flow: A Prognostic Test for Facial Paralysis, Laryngoscope 81: 179, 1971.

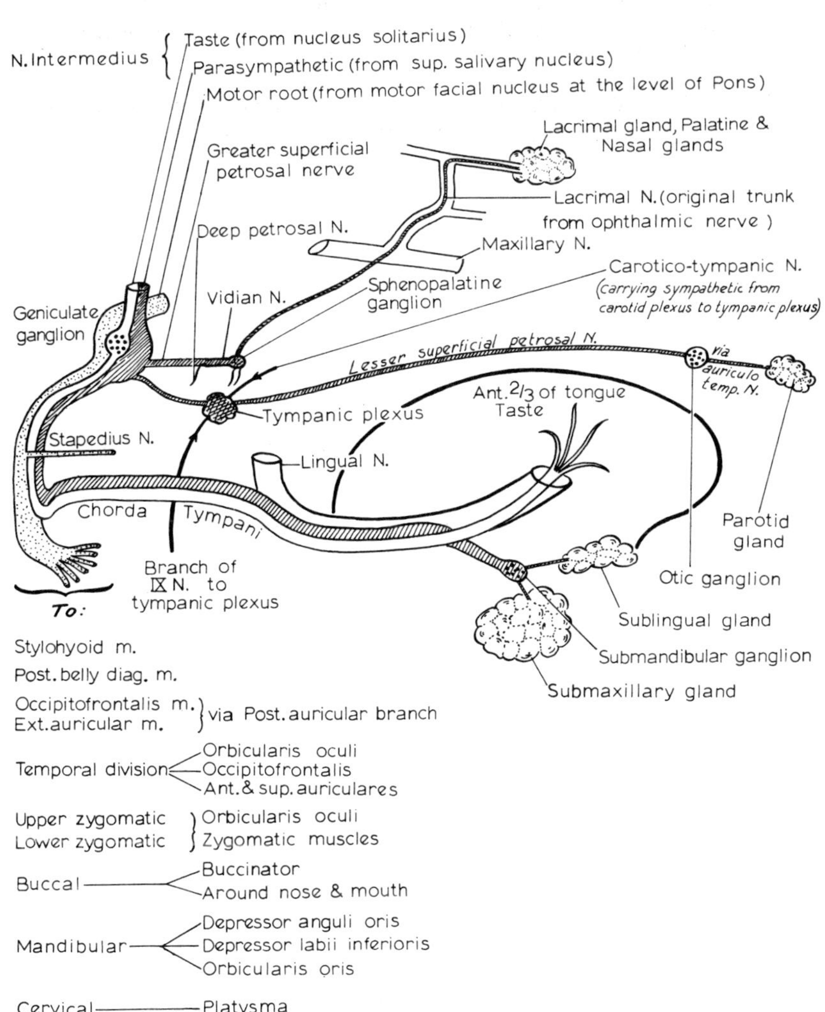

FIGURE 7-2. Course of the Facial Nerve

5. Melkersson, E.: Et fall ay recidiverande facilspares i samband med angioneurotiskt öden, Hygiea 90: 737, 1928.

6. Rosenthal, C.: Klinisch-erbbiologischer Beitrag Zur Konstitutionspathologie. Gemeinsames Auftreten von (rezidivierender familiärer) Facialislähmung, Angioneurotischem Gesichtsödem und Lingua Plicata in Arthritismus-Familien, Z. Neurol. Psychiat. 131: 475, 1931.

7. Tabb, H.G. and Scalco, A.N.: Exposure of the Facial Nerve in Parotid Surgery, Laryngoscope 80: 559, 1970.

CHAPTER 8

EMBRYOLOGY OF THE CLEFTS AND POUCHES

I. CORRELATION BETWEEN AGE AND SIZE OF EMBRYO

Age		Size
2-1/2 weeks	=	1-1/2 mm
3-1/2 weeks	=	2-1/2 mm
4 weeks	=	5 mm
5 weeks	=	8 mm
6 weeks	=	12 mm
7 weeks	=	17 mm
8 weeks	=	23 mm
10 weeks	=	40 mm
12 weeks	=	56 mm
16 weeks	=	112 mm
5 to 10 months	=	160-350 mm

II. 1. The first 8 weeks constitutes the period of greatest embryonic development of the head and neck. There are 5 arches named Pharyngeal or Branchial arches. Between these arches are the grooves or clefts externally and the pouches internally. Each pouch has a ventral or dorsal wing. The derivatives of arches are usually of mesoderm origin. The groove is lined by ectoderm while the pouch is entoderm lined. (See Figure 8-1)

Each arch has an artery, nerve and cartilage bar. These nerves are anterior to their respective arteries except in the 5th arch where the nerve is posterior to the artery. (Embryologically, the arch after the 4th is called the 5th or 6th arch depending on the theory one follows. For simplicity in this synopsis, it will be referred to as the 5th arch). Caudal to all the arches lies the XII nerve. From the cervical somites posterior and inferior to the above arches is derived the sternocleidomastoid muscle.

2. There are 2 ventral and 2 dorsal aortas in early embryonic life. The 2 ventral ones fuse completely while the 2 dorsal ones fuse caudally only. (Figure 8-2A). In the course of embryonic development, the 1st and 2nd arch arteries degenerate. The 2nd arch artery has an upper branch which passes through a mass of mesoderm which later chondrifies and ossifies as the stapes. This stapedial artery degenerates in late fetal life. The 3rd arch artery is the precursor of the carotid artery in both left and right sides. The left 4th arch artery becomes the arch of the aorta. The right 4th arch artery becomes the proximal subclavian. The rest of the right subclavian and the left subclavian are derivatives of the 7th segmental arteries. The left 5th arch artery becomes the pulmonary artery and ductus arteriosus. The right 5th arch artery becomes the pulmonary artery with degeneration of the rest of this arch vessel. (Figure 8-2B).

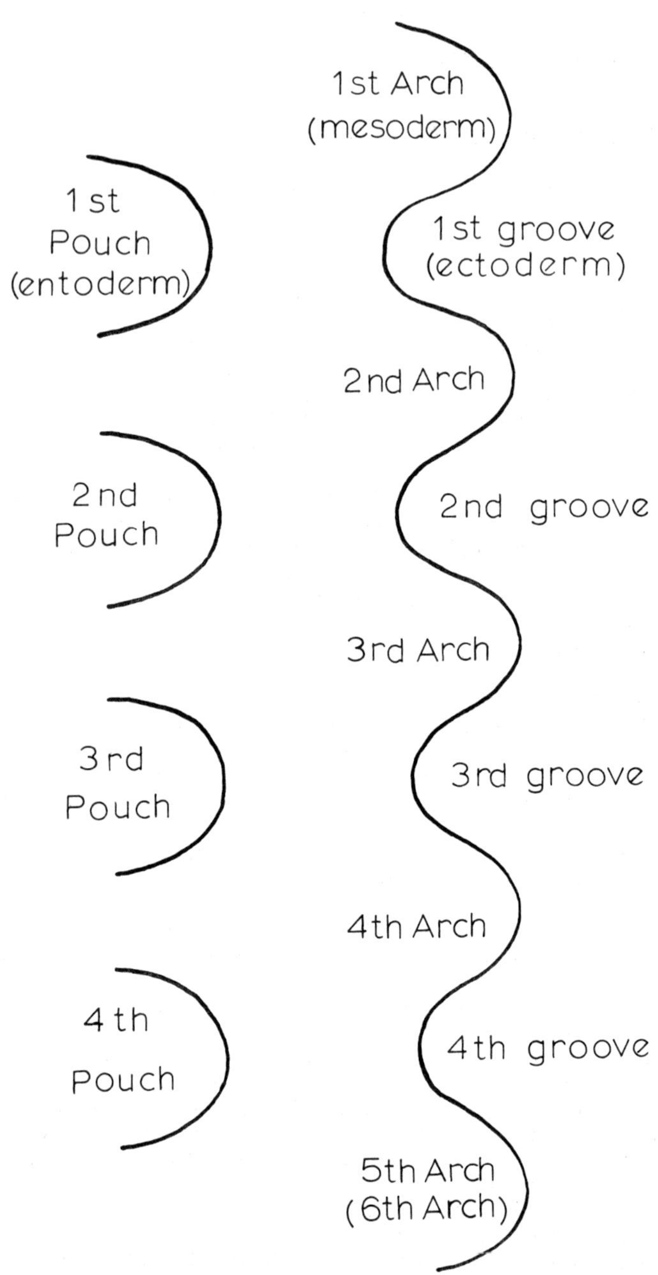

FIG. 8-1. Diagrammatic Illustration of the Pouches and Grooves

Ventral Aorta
1
2
3
4
5
Dorsal Aorta
Carotid Artery
Carotid Artery
1
2
3
4
Arch of the Aorta
Subclavian
Ductus Arteriosus
5
Descending Aorta
1
2
3
4
5
Right Subclavian
Dorsal Aorta

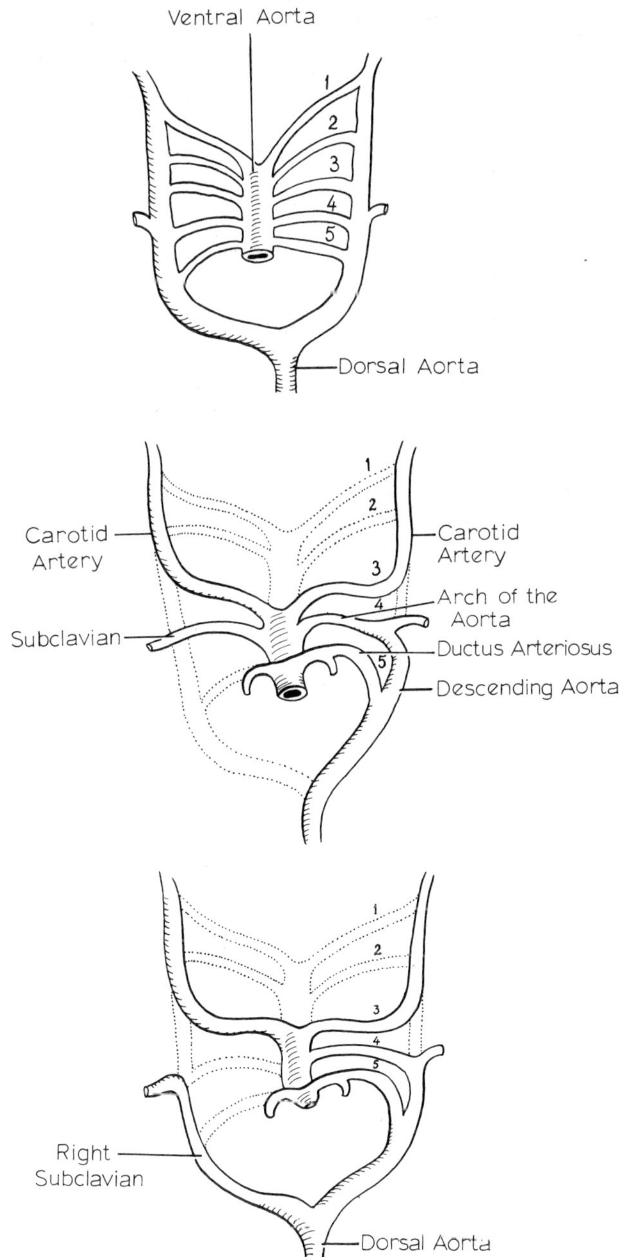

FIG. 8-2

3. a) Should the right 4th arch artery degenerate and the right subclavian arise from the dorsal aorta instead (as shown in Figure 8-2C, the right subclavian would become posterior to the esophagus thus causing a constriction of the esophagus without any effect on the trachea (dysphagia lusoria).

b) The innominate artery arises ventrally. Hence, when it arises too far from the left, an anterior compression of the trachea results.

4. The 5th arch nerve is posterior and caudal to the artery. As the connection on the right side between the 5th arch artery (pulmonary) and the dorsal aorta degenerates, the nerve (recurrent laryngeal nerve) loops around the 4th arch artery which subsequently becomes the subclavian. On the left side, the nerve loops around the ductus arteriosus and the aorta.

III. DERIVATIVES OF THE POUCHES

1. Each pouch has a ventral and a dorsal wing. The 4th pouch has an additional accessory wing. The entodermal lining of the pouches proliferates into glandular organs.

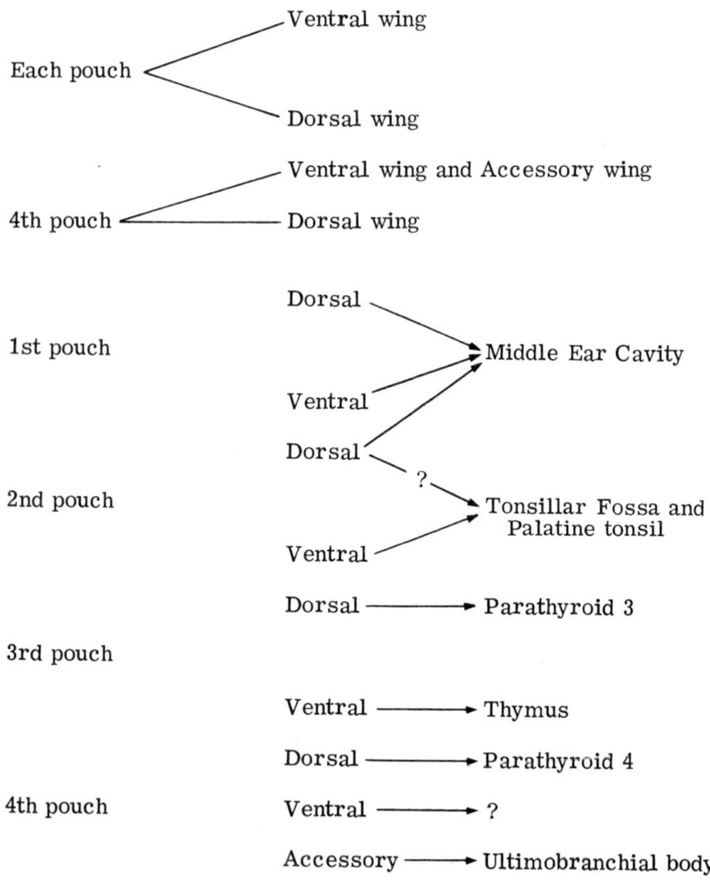

2. During embryonic development, the thymus descends caudally pulling with it Parathyroid 3. Consequently, Parathyroid 3 is inferior to Parathyroid 4 in the adult.

3. The fate of the ultimobranchial body is unknown.

4. As these "out-pocketing" pouches develop into glandular elements, their connections with the pharyngeal lumen referred to as pharyngobranchial ducts become obliterated. Should obliteration fail to occur, branchial sinus (cyst) is said to have resulted.

The 2nd pharyngobranchial duct (between the 2nd and 3rd arches) is believed to open into the tonsillar fossa, while the 3rd pharyngobranchial duct opens into the pyriform sinus and the 4th opens into the lower part of the pyriform sinus or larynx. An alternative school of thought believes that Branchial Sinuses and Cysts are not remnants of patent pharyngobranchial ducts but are rather remnants of the cervical sinus of HIS (Davies, J.: Embryology of the Head and Neck in Relation to the Practice of Otolaryngology, A Manual, AAOO, 1965).

5. The cutaneous openings of branchial sinuses, if present, are always anterior to the anterior border of the sternocleidomastoid muscle. The tract always lies deep to the platysma muscle which is derived from the 2nd arch. (Figure 8-3)

The course of a 3rd arch branchial cyst:

- a) Deep to 2nd arch derivatives and superficial to 3rd arch derivatives.
- b) Superficial to the XII nerve and anterior to the sternocleidomastoid.
- c) In close relationship with carotid sheath but superficial to it.
- d) Superficial to the IX nerve, pierces middle constrictor, deep to stylohyoid ligament, opens into Tonsillar Fossa.

The course of a 2rd arch branchial cyst:

- a) Again, it is subplatysmal and opens externally anterior to the sternocleidomastoid muscle.
- b) Superficial to the XII nerve, deep to the internal carotid artery and the IX nerve.
- c) Pierces the thyrohyoid membrane above the internal branch of the superior laryngeal nerve and opens into the pyriform fossa.

The course of a 4th arch branchial cyst:

Right:

- a) The tract lies low in the neck beneath the platysma and anterior to the sternocleidomastoid muscle.
- b) Loops around the subclavian and deep to it, deep to the carotid, lateral to the XII nerve, inferior to the superior laryngeal nerve, and opens into the lower part of the pyriform sinus or into the larynx.

Left:

- a) Since the 4th arch vessel is the adult aorta, the cyst may be intrathoracic, medial to the ligamentum arteriosus and the arch of aorta.

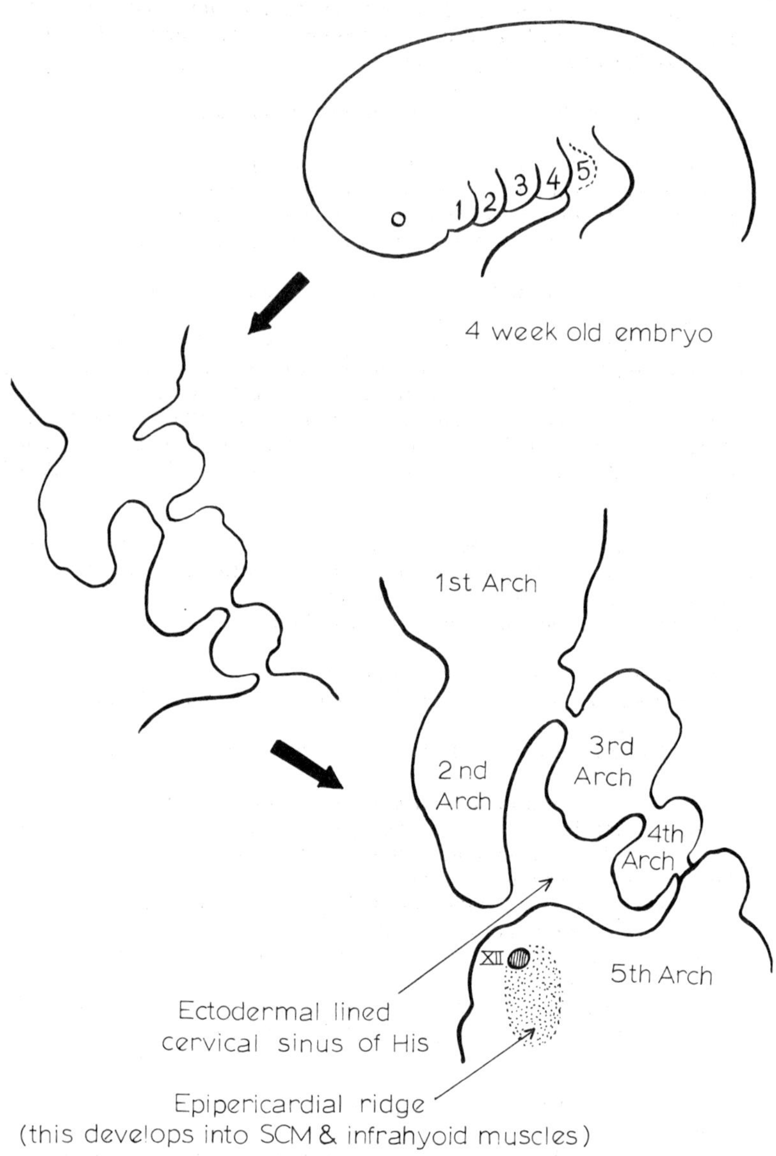

FIG. 8-3. Diagrammatic Representation of the Pharyngobranchial Ducts

b) Lateral to the XII nerve, inferior to the superior laryngeal nerve.
c) Opens into the lower pyriform sinus or into the larynx.

IV. On a 4-week-old embryo, a ventral (thyroid) diverticulum of endodermal origin can be identified between the 1st and 2nd arches on the floor of the pharynx. It is also situated between the tuberculum impar and the copula. (The tuberculum impar together with the lingual swellings becomes the anterior 2/3 of the tongue while the copula is the precursor of the posterior 1/3 of the tongue). The ventral diverticulum develops into the thyroid gland. During development, it descends caudally within the mesodermal tissues. At 4-1/2 weeks, the connection between the thyroid diverticulum and the floor of the pharynx begins to disappear. By the 6th week, it should be obliterated and atrophied. Should it persist through the time of birth or thereafter, a thyroglossal duct cyst is present. This tract travels through the hyoid and reaches the foramen cecum (Figure 8-4).

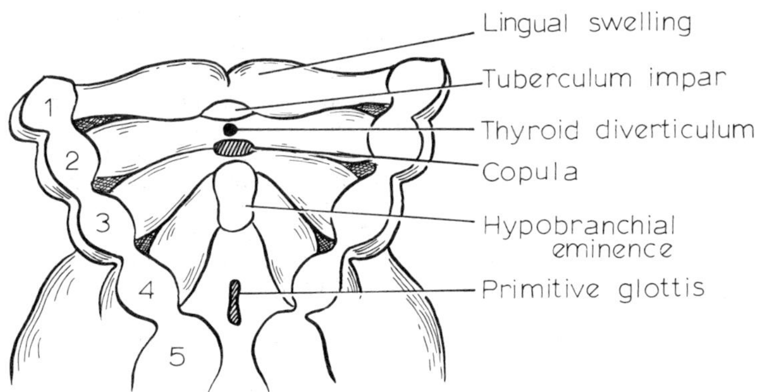

FIG. 8-4. Diagrammatic Representation of a 4-week-old embryo

V. The tongue is derived from ectodermal origin (anterior 2/3) and entodermal origin (posteriorly). At the 4th week, 2 lingual swellings are noted at the 1st arch and a swelling, the tuberculum impar, appears between the 1st and the 2nd arches. These 3 prominences develop into the anterior 2/3 of the tongue. Meanwhile, another swelling is noted between the 2nd and 3rd arches, called the copula. It develops into the posterior 1/3 of the tongue. On the 7th week the somites from the high cervical areas differentiate into voluntary muscle of the tongue. The circumvallate papillae develop between the 8th and 20th week while filiform and fungiform papillae develop at the 11th week.

VI. Palatine Tonsil (8 weeks old)	from	2nd Pouch (Ventral or Dorsal)	
Lingual Tonsil (6-1/2 weeks old)	from	Between 2nd and 3rd Arches ventrally	
Adenoids (16 weeks old)		Develops as a subepithelial infiltration of lymphocytes	
VII. Parotid (5-1/2 weeks old)		Ectodermal origin	1st Pouch
Submaxillary (6 weeks old)		Ectodermal origin	1st Pouch
Sublingual (8 weeks old)		Ectodermal origin	1st Pouch

TABLE 8-1

ARCHES	GANGLION OR NERVE	DERIVATIVES
1st Arch	Semilunar Ganglion $(V)_3$	Mandible Head, neck, manubrium of malleus Body and short process of incus Anterior malleal ligament Sphenomandibular ligament Tensor Tympani Mastication muscles Anterior belly of digastric muscle Tensor Palati muscle
2nd Arch	Geniculate Ganglion VII	Manubrium of malleus Long process of incus All of stapes except vestibular portion of footplate and annular ligament Styloid process Stylohyoid ligament Lesser cornu of hyoid Part of body of hyoid Stapedius muscle Facial muscles Buccinator, posterior belly of digastric muscle Styloid muscle Part of pyramidal eminence Lower part of facial canal
3rd Arch	IX	Greater cornu of hyoid and rest of hyoid Stylopharyngeus muscle

ARCHES	GANGLION OR NERVE	DERIVATIVES
4th Arch	Superior laryngeal nerve	Thyroid cartilage, cuneiform, Inferior pharyngeal constrictor, Cricopharyngeus, crico-thyroid muscles
5th Arch (Often called the 6th arch from the standpoint of evolution and comparative anatomy)	Recurrent laryngeal nerve	Cricoid, arytenoids Corniculate Trachea Intrinsic laryngeal muscles

REFERENCES

1. Davies, J.: Embryology of the Head and Neck in Relation to the Practice of Otolaryngology, American Academy of Ophthalmology and Otolaryngology Manual, 1965.

2. Hough, J.V.D.: Malformations and Anatomical Variations Seen in the Middle Ear During Operations on the Stapes, American Academy of Ophthalmology and Otolaryngology Manual, 1961.

3. Pearson, A.A., et al.: The Development of the Ear, American Academy of Ophthalmology and Otolaryngology Manual, 1967.

4. Simpson, R.A.: Lateral Cervical Cysts and Fistulas, Laryngoscope 79: 30, 1969.

5. Strickland, E.M., et al.: Branchial Sources of Auditory Ossicles in Man, Arch. Otolaryng. 76: 200, 1962.

6. Tucker, J.A. and O'Rahilly, R.: Observations on the Embryology of the Human Larynx, Ann. Otol. Rhinol. Laryng. 81: 520, 1972.

7. Van Alyea, O.E.: The Embryology of the Ear, Nose and Throat. American Academy of Ophthalmology and Otolaryngology Manual, 1965.

CHAPTER 9

CLEFT LIP AND PALATE

ANATOMY OF THE LIP: The lip is composed primarily of muscles, covered by skin on the outer surface and mucosa on the inner surface. The lip edge or vermillion is covered by non-keratinized epithelium made red by numerous highly vascular connective tissue papillae. The junction between the vermillion and skin is called the mucocutaneous ridge or white line. This line forms a gentle arch in the upper lip and is depressed lightly in the middle to form the center of "cupid's bow". Lateral extension of the white line completes "cupid's bow". From the ends of this central depression of the white line, small ridges extend upward to the base of the columella enclosing a small depressed skin area called the philtrum. A slight protrusion of the vermillion below "cupid's bow" is called the tubercle. These anatomical landmarks are used for orientation in repairing clefts of the upper lip. (Figure 9-1)

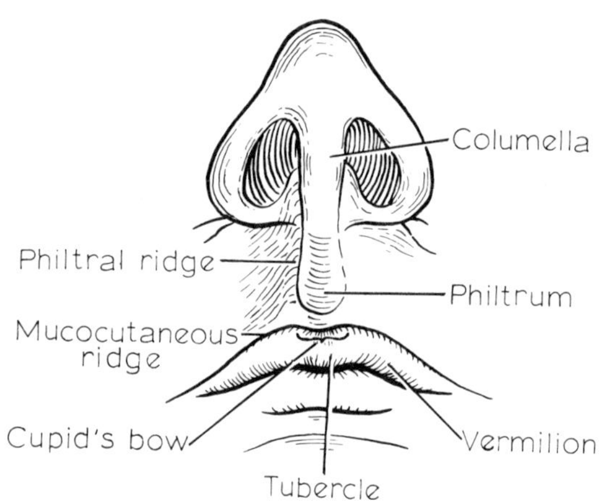

FIG. 9-1. Anatomy of the Lip

The lip is a movable muscular curtain composed primarily of the orbicularis muscle which creates a sphincter and is formed by significant contributions from paired muscles converging on the mouth. (Figure 9-2). The muscle substance arches around the lips and interlaces at the angle of the mouth. The muscle lies between the skin and mucous membrane of the lips being limited superiorly by the nose and inferiorly by the chin.

An almost infinite variety of movements can be obtained by the lips by the individual action, inaction or antagonistic action of these various paired muscles.

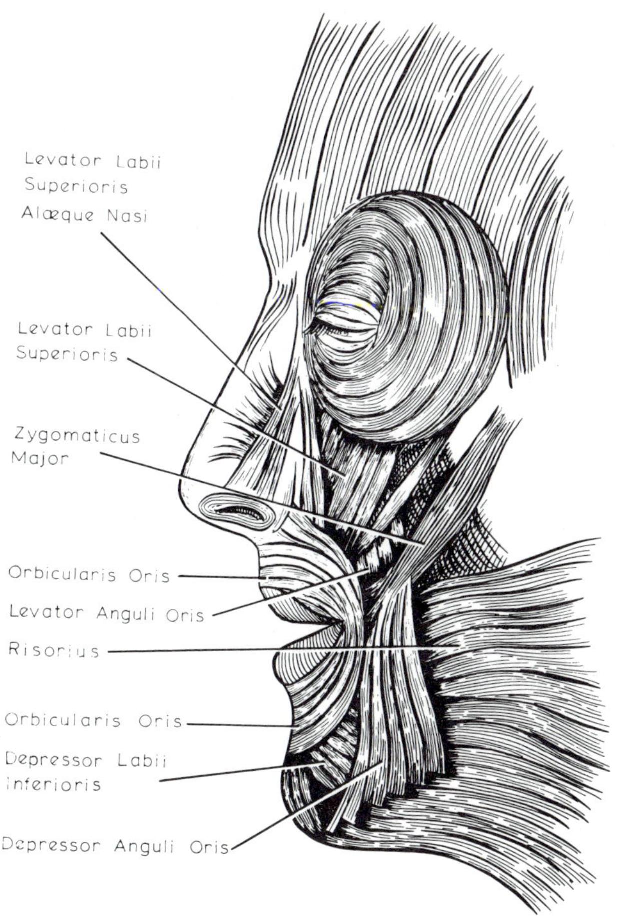

FIG. 9-2. Facial Musculature

The main arterial blood supply to the upper lip is provided by the paired superior labial arteries which are located near the mucous membrane deep to the muscle. Sensation to the upper lip is supplied mainly by fibers from the inferior orbital branches of the Vth cranial nerve. Motor fibers are derived from the labial branches of the VIIth cranial nerve.

ANATOMY OF THE PALATE: The palate is composed of a bony anterior portion and a soft muscular posterior portion. The tooth-bearing alveolar ridges surround the hard palate. An anterior wedge-shaped portion of the alveolar ridge carrying the 4 incisor teeth and a triangular section behind constitute the premaxilla or primary palate. The remaining hard palate is made up of palatine processes of the maxillary bone, and to a lesser degree by the palatine processes of the palatine bone. The maxillary and palatine portion of the hard palate plus the soft palate constitute the secondary palate.

The oral surface of the hard palate is covered by firm mucoperiosteum of variable thickness. Anteriorly this membrane has raised ridges called palatine rugae. The nasal surface of the hard palate is divided into two portions by the nasal septum and is lined by a thin mucoperiosteum surfaced anteriorly by stratified squamous and posteriorly by respiratory epithelium. The blood supply to the hard palate is provided chiefly by the anterior palatine artery which is derived from the internal maxillary via the greater palatine foramen. The nerve supply is chiefly from the anterior palatine and nasopalatine branch from the sphenopalatine ganglion. The nerve supply follows the arterial blood supply in distribution.

The soft palate is a movable muscular curtain covered on its oral surface by stratified squamous epithelium and on its nasal surface by pseudo-stratified columnar epithelium. This structure contains numerous muscles and glands. The palate has five muscles as follows:

	MUSCLE	NERVE SUPPLY	ACTION
1.	Tensor veli palatini	Vth	tense and depress soft palate
2.	Levator veli palatini	pharyngeal plexus	elevate the palate
3.	Musculus uvulae	pharyngeal plexus	draw uvula upward and forward
4.	Glossopalatine	pharyngeal plexus	draw palate down and narrow the pharynx
5.	Palatopharyngeus	pharyngeal plexus	draw palate down and narrow pharynx

The arterial blood supply to the soft palate is the descending palatine branch of the internal maxillary, the ascending palatine branch of the external maxillary, the palatine branch of the ascending pharyngeal and twigs from tonsilar branch of dorsalis linguae. The sensory nerve supply is mainly from the lesser and middle palatine branches from the sphenopalatine ganglion.

EMBRYOLOGY OF THE CLEFT LIP: The central upper lip is formed by growth of the nasomedian process in a downward medial and forward direction. This process provides the central lip consisting of philtrum, labial tubercle, the central alveolar ridge containing the paired central and lateral incisor teeth, the anterior nasal septum and an anterior palatal triangle (primary palate). Paired lateral maxillary processes grow medialward toward the descending nasomedian process. These processes provide the lateral upper lip elements. Failure of the structure to unite on one side or both provides clefts of the lip, extending into the nose and through the alveolus between the lateral incisor and cuspid teeth. Paired processes or shelves arise from the maxillary processes. They converge upon the primary palate, on each other and the septum to fuse from before backward to provide the secondary palate. The lip and hard palate formation is completed by the 8th week of embryonic life and the soft palate and uvula are completed by the 12th week of embryonic life.

(Note: The genesis of harelip has not been agreed upon by various investigators. Some believe it is the result of failure of fusion between the maxillary and frontonasal processes. Others believe that it is the lack of "filling up" between the premaxillary and maxillary centers that result in a furrow and hence a harelip).

TYPES OF CLEFT LIP AND PALATE. (Figure 9-3)

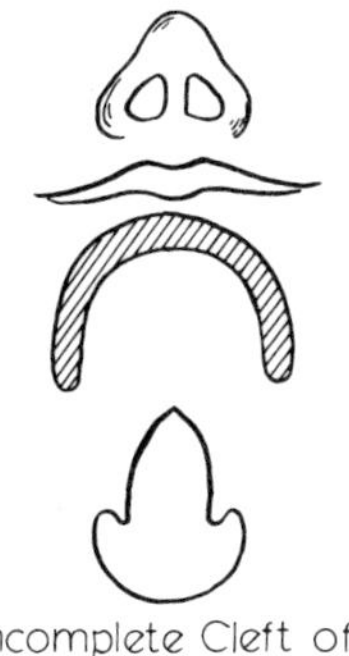

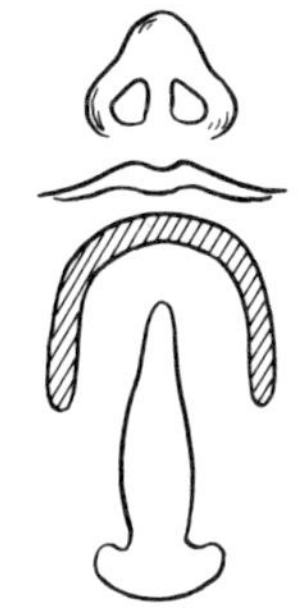

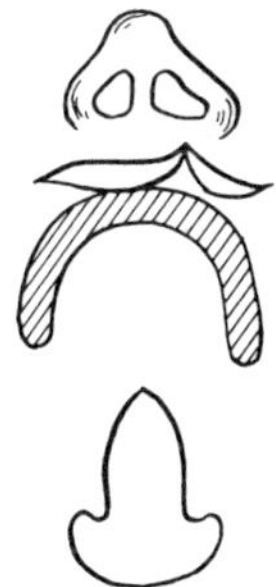

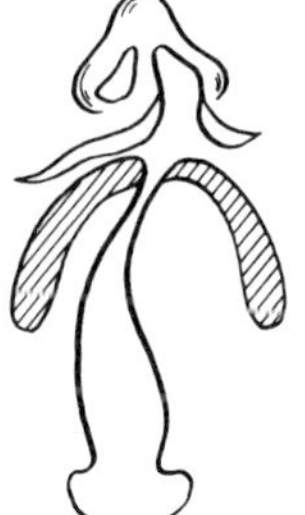

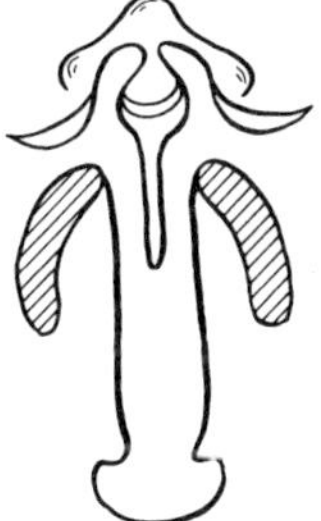

FIG. 9-3. Types of cleft palate

1. Unilateral cleft lip: occurs in varying degrees and may involve the alveolus in varying degrees.
2. Unilateral cleft lip with cleft palate.
3. Bilateral clefts of the lip: usually involve complete clefts of the secondary palate but can (rarely) occur without the presence of a cleft palate.
4. Bilateral clefts of the lip, alveolus and palate: both nasal cavities are exposed to the oral cavity.

5. Clefts of the secondary palate: occur in varying degrees such as bifid uvula, submucous cleft and complete division up to the primary palate.
6. Median cleft of the upper lip: very rare.

INCIDENCE OF CLEFT LIP AND CLEFT PALATE: (Cleft lip with cleft palate is the most common; cleft palate alone is next; cleft lip alone is the least common). The incidence of cleft lip with or without cleft palate varies from 0.8 to 1.6 per 1000 births. The incidence of combined cleft lip and cleft palate is 1.5 to 3 times as frequent as cleft lip alone. The incidence of cleft lip with cleft palate is greater in males. The incidence of cleft palate alone is greater in females. The frequency of single cleft lip is greater on the left than on the right. The incidence of cleft lip is 3 times as great in Caucasians as in the Negro. Genetic factors in cleft lip with or without cleft palate are:

a) Mutant genes
b) Chromosomal aberration
c) Environmental teratogens
d) Multifactorial inheritance

INCIDENCE OF CLEFT PALATE: Cleft palate is embryologically and genetically different from cleft lip alone or combined cleft lip and cleft palate. The rate is 0.45 per 1000 Caucasian births. The cleft palate is more common in females. Genetic factors in cleft palate are:

a) Mutant genes
b) Chromosomal aberration
c) Environmental teratogens
d) Multifactoral inheritance

COUNSELING PARENTS REGARDING LIP AND/OR PALATE CLEFTS:

SITUATION A: Parents normal, first child affected with cleft lip with or without cleft palate.

<u>Question 1:</u> What are the chances for the next child if there are no affected relatives?
<u>Answer:</u> 4%
<u>Question 2:</u> What are the chances for the next child if there is an affected relative?
<u>Answer</u> 4%
<u>Question 3:</u> What is the chance for the next child if the affected child has another malformation?
<u>Answer:</u> 2%
<u>Question 4:</u> What is the chance for the next child if the parents are related?
<u>Answer:</u> 4%

SITUATION B: Both parents are normal and have 2 affected children with cleft lip with or without cleft palate.

<u>Question:</u> What are the chances for the next child to have the same defect?
<u>Answer:</u> 9%

SITUATION C: One affected parent with cleft lip or cleft palate and no affected children.
Question: What is the chance for the next child of having a defect?
Answer: 4%

SITUATION D: One parent affected and have one affected child.
Question: What is the chance that the next child will be affected?
Answer: 17%

COUNSELING FOR CLEFT PALATE ALONE:

SITUATION A: The parents normal - one child affected with cleft palate.
Question 1: What is the chance for the next baby to have cleft palate if there are no affected relatives?
Answer: 2%
Question 2: What is the chance for the next baby to have cleft palate if there is an affected relative?
Answer: 7%
Question 3: What is the chance for the next baby to have cleft palate if the affected child has other malformations?
Answer: 2%

SITUATION B: The parents are normal but have 2 children, both with cleft palate.
Question 1: What is the chance for the next baby to have a cleft palate?
Answer: 1%

SITUATION C: One of the parents has a cleft palate.
Question 1: With no affected children, what is the chance of the next baby to have a cleft palate?
Answer: 6%
Question 2: What is the chance for the next baby with one child having a cleft palate?
Answer: 15%

TIMING AND TECHNIQUES

1. LIPS: There is no set time for repair of cleft lip. Since cleft lip is a congenital deformity, adequate time should be allowed to properly observe and examine the infant to determine the possibility of other associated congenital defects. Closure is usually performed within three months; however, social pressures often dictate that the defect be closed before the infant leaves the hospital. The rule of over 10 is advocated, over 10 weeks in age, over 10 lbs. in weight, and hemoglobin of over 10 gms.

The Millard rotation advancement technique of closure is accepted by many as the standard for repair of unilateral cleft lips. (Figure 9-4). Other techniques include the triangular flaps and the quadralateral flaps. At the time of closing the lip cleft, the floor of the nose is also closed, allowing the alveolus to unite by contact thus leaving the infant in the case of a complete lip and palate cleft with the posterior hard and soft palate defect to be closed at a later date.

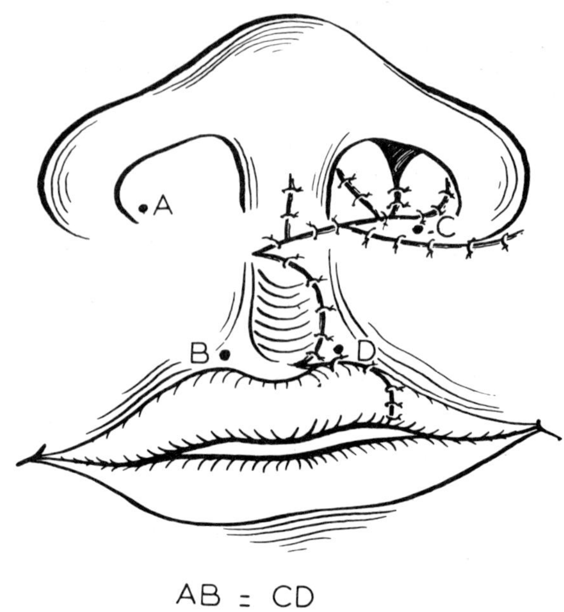

FIG. 9-4. Millard Repair of Unilateral Cleft Lip

The bilateral cleft lip technique may involve simultaneous closure of both sides or staged single procedures, starting with the side with the wider cleft and repairing the remaining cleft two months later. (Figure 9-5). Preoperative maxillary orthopedics has been advocated but is not universally accepted.

Maxillary growth and dental arch malalignment secondary to scar contracture following primary closure are factors which have influenced timing of the procedures. Simple closure of the lip without muscle approximation and closure of the soft palate portion of the complete cleft palate has been advocated. Dental appliances adjusted frequently to accommodate growth, serve to cover the osseous portion of the cleft. The defect of the hard palate is closed after optimum maxillary and alveolar arch growth has occurred. Redirection of the fibers of the orbicularis oris muscle displaced by the cleft is receiving increased attention in the repair of primary clefts.

Techniques for surgical repair of the cleft lip are numerous and are listed according to the names of the surgeons who developed the techniques. The operation provides closure of the floor of the nose back to the beginning of the secondary palate and brings the cleft portion of the lip into alignment with each other. Minor secondary repairs on the cleft lip are usually performed prior to school age.

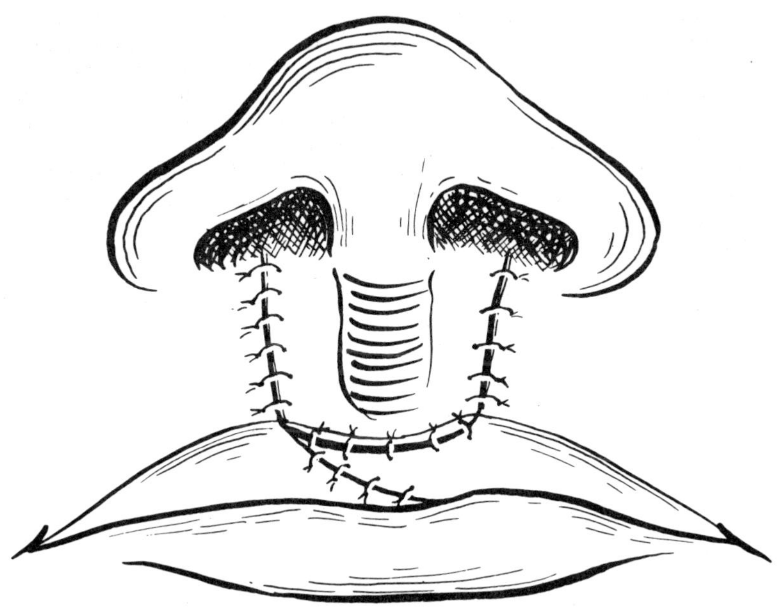

FIG. 9-5. Repair of Bilateral Cleft Lip

2. PALATE: The timing for closure of the palate is less variable than the lips. The most popular is about 18 months. Variations in time of closure are related to such factors as speech, hearing, swallowing, dental occlusion and facial growth.

3. TECHNIQUES BY NAME:

a) Von Langenbeck: Bilateral relaxing incisions with freshening of the cleft margins. The bi-pedicle oral mucoperiosteal flaps are elevated. The nasal layer is elevated and cleft is closed in 2 layers.

b) V-Y Retropositioning: (Wardill-Kilner): Bilateral relaxing incisions are performed. The anterior part of each relaxing incision is angled backward towards the midline to form a "W". The cleft edges are freshened. The oral mucoperiosteal flaps are elevated to the posterior border of the hard palate. The nasal layer is elevated and the cleft is closed in two layers. The oral mucoperiosteum is anchored to the unelevated anterior tip of the oral mucoperiosteum.

c) Dorrance: Bilateral relaxing incisions are performed and continued around behind the anterior teeth to meet each other. The entire oral mucoperiosteum is elevated back to the posterior border of the hard palate. The margins of the cleft are freshened and the nasal layers and the oral mucoperiosteum are returned to the hard palate about 1-2 cm distal to its original position and anchored by passing sutures through holes drilled in the hard palate.

d) Vomer flap: In both single and bilateral clefts of the hard palate, flaps from the vomer may be elevated laterally to be joined with flaps from the lateral (nasal) aspect of the cleft. Closure of the hard palate defect may be performed with the lip surgery. The usual time is 10 - 18 months as a separate procedure and the soft palate is closed shortly thereafter. Great controversy exists regarding timing of closure of the hard palate defect and its relation to maxillary arch growth and development of orthodontic problems. Some surgeons close the soft palate early and delay closure of the hard palate to avoid affecting maxillary bone growth.

VARIOUS FLAPS ASSOCIATED WITH TREATMENT OF CLEFT LIP AND PALATE PROBLEMS.

1. ABBE: is a lip switch flap based on the coronal (labial) artery and used to correct defects up to 50% of either lip. Mostly used for late correction of defects in the upper lip following bilateral cleft lip repair.

2. MILLARD FORKED FLAP: utilizes scars of the upper lip to lengthen the columella and raise the tip of the nose in cases of previously repaired bilateral cleft lip.

3. ECKER BUCCAL FLAPS: used in primary cleft palate repair and in secondary lengthening procedures to reduce the side to side tightness of the soft palate.

4. DORRANCE PALATE FLAP: is incision along palatal border of the maxillary teeth for raising the mucoperiosteum of the entire palate in both primary and secondary palate procedures.

5. WARDILL (V-Y) FLAPS: is incision similar to the Dorrance incision but angles backward to the midline in the cuspid region.

6. LANGENBECK (Bi-PEDICLE FLAP): is similar to the Wardill incision but stops at the cuspid area. Is used as a primary relaxing incision for cleft palate repair.

7. PHARYNGEAL FLAP:

a) Inferiorly based: may be used for additional tissue in closure of primary clefts of the soft palate. May be used to decrease hypernasal speech in short or paralyzed palates.

b) Superiorly based: used in conjunction with palatal lengthening procedures requiring replacement of mucosal lining or nasal resurfacing of a retropositioned palate.

c) Hynes Pharyngeoplasty: are crossed vertical flaps on the posterior pharyngeal wall to build up a contact pad for the soft palate on phonation.

8. CRONIN NASAL FLAP: mucoperiosteum covering the nasal surface of the hard palate posteriorly is carried backward along with the oral mucoperiosteum in palatal lengthening procedures. This tissue provides nasal epithelial covering for the retropositioned soft palate.

9. ISLAND FLAP: (Millard) is a cut section of anterior hard palate mucoperiosteum still attached to the greater palatine artery. This flap is turned over and sutured to the raw area created by the palatal pushback procedure.

10. NASOPHARYNGEAL PUSHBACK: the lateral wall of the nasopharynx directly behind the hard palate and overlying the medial surface of the medial pterygoid plate is elevated widely and incised up to the base of the skull to provide accommodation in the pharynx for retropositioning of the soft palate making repeat palatal pushback procedures possible.

REFERENCES

1. Chase, S.W.: The Early Development of the Human Pre-Maxilla, J. Am. Dental Assoc. 29: 1991, 1942.

2. Fugh-Anderson, P.: Inheritance of Harelip and Cleft Palate, Copenhagen, Nyt. Nordisk Forhag-Arnold Busck, 1942.

3. Fulton, J.T.: Closure of the Human Palate in Embryo, Amer. J. Obst. & Gynec. 74: 179, 1957.

4. Grabb, W.C.: Cleft Lip and Palate; Little, Brown & Co., Boston, 1971.

5. Patten, B.M.: Foundations of Embryology, 2nd ed., McGraw-Hill, New York, 1964.

6. Smith, H.W. and Lee, K.J.: Nasopharyngeal Pushback in Treatment of Velopharyngeal Insufficiency, Arch. Otolaryng. 102: 83, 1976.

7. Woolf, C.M., et al.: Cleft Lip and Heredity, Plastic & Rec. Surg. 34: 11, 1964.

CHAPTER 10

FACIAL TRAUMA

I. NASAL FRACTURES

1. ANATOMY: The nasal skeleton is composed of paired nasal bones which are thick above and thin below. They meet on their long medial side at an angle in the midline of the face, are met from below and joined to the bony portion of the nasal septum. Laterally they are joined to and supported by the maxilla. The paired upper lateral cartilages attach to the lower border of the nasal bones, meet each other in the midline and are met from below and joined to the septal cartilage. The paired lower lateral cartilages are wing-like and provide substance to the nostril framework, overlie the upper lateral cartilages and are situated at the caudal end of the septum. The septum, like the whole nose, is bony in the upper part (ethmoid and vomer) and cartilaginous in the lower part (quadrilateral cartilage).

The internal blood supply to the nose is provided by the anterior ethmoidal artery (from the internal carotid), the nasopalatine branch of the sphenopalatine (from external carotid). Externally the nose is supplied by the lateral nasal and septal branches of the facial artery (external carotid) and the dorsal nasal from the ophthalmic (internal carotid).

The nerve supply to the internal part of the nose is from the internal nasal branches of the anterior ethmoidal and branches from the sphenopalatine ganglion. Externally the upper part of the nose is supplied by the supratrochlear and infratrochlear nerves, the external nasal branch of the anterior ethmoidal and the infraorbital nerve supply the lower part of the nose.

2. DIAGNOSIS: The history of nasal trauma is quite important and should include how the injury occurred, when it occurred and what the nose looked like before and if there was any change after the injury. The question of nasal obstruction should be investigated for any change following injury. The nasal bones are the most frequently fractured bones of the whole facial skeleton. The nose may be pushed to one side or pushed inward. The bony portion of the septum usually is fractured. The cartilaginous portion may only be deflected. A deformity which is obvious to the patient at the time of injury may be obscured when examined at a later time due to a development of edema and ecchymosis. Fractures of the cartilaginous portion of the septum should be searched for. Palpation of the external nose will frequently produce crepitation. X-rays on many occasions will appear normal in the presence of a clinically obvious fracture. Exaggerated Water's lateral and occlusal views are compared in the search for nasal fractures.

3. TREATMENT: Early treatment is usually simple and reliable unless there is severe hemorrhage requiring control prior to undertaking reduction of the nasal bone fracture. The usual treatment is to elevate the depression and depress the elevation. Topical anesthesia, using cotton tipped applicator rods moistened in adrenaline 1:1000 and dipped in cocaine flakes are placed at the internal branch of the nasociliary nerve and at the sphenopalatine ganglion. In more severe cases, where extensive manipulation is anticipated, local anesthesia placed at the infratrochlear area, external nasal area and infraorbital foramen will produce satisfactory anesthesia. Nasal fracture reduction may be postponed up to one week in the presence of severe edema and ecchymosis. If an open reduction method is selected, care must be exercised to avoid separation of the upper lateral cartilages from the nasal bones.

4. COMPLICATIONS:

a) Septal hematoma and subsequent abscess producing dissolution of the nasal cartilages and subsequent deformity of the nose.
b) Failure to recognize pre-existing septal deflection which may produce gradual deflection of the nasal bones during healing of the nasal bone fractures.
c) Impacted fractures, unrecognized and unreduced by simple means and left untreated.
d) Fractures of the cartilaginous septum only recognized by continual growth of nose and developing deformity.
e) Air passage synechia and stenosis.

II. ZYGOMATIC FRACTURES

1. ANATOMY: The zygoma (malar) or cheek bone provides prominence to the lateral side of the face. It provides the lateral inferior rim of the orbit, is supported below by the maxilla and braced behind by an arch extending to the temporal bones. It provides lateral attachment for the suspensory ligament of the eye and partial support for the eye and its musculature. It constitutes a portion of the roof of the maxillary sinus and lends protection via the arch for the temporalis muscle passing to the mandible and also provides attachment for the masseter (jaw) muscle. By virtue of its position, the zygoma serves as a keystone in the reconstruction of severe midfacial fractures.

2. DIAGNOSIS:

a) History of the traumatic incident is helpful since blows producing fracture dislocation in different directions affect the method of treatment.

b) Observation: prior to the development of edema one should look for a depression of the cheek, flatness of the face, lowering of the eyeball, limited eye movements, and restricted mouth opening. The presence of periorbital ecchymosis within two hours of injury usually implies zygomatic fracture. The lateral canthal ligament is attached to the zygomatic bone. In a fracture of the zygoma, slight ptosis may be present.

c) Examination: palpation is essential even after edema develops. Separation (steps) can usually be felt along the inferior orbital rim, occasionally at the upper lateral border of the orbital rim, and usually intraorally high on the lateral maxillary wall above the molar teeth. The presence of anesthetic areas of skin (especially the upper lip) and diplopia should be determined.

d) X-rays show the fracture well in certain views such as Water's and routine submento-vertical. Exaggerated submental vertical view with low exposure will demonstrate fractures of the arch.

3. TREATMENT: There are three basic approaches to surgical treatment of fracture dislocations of the zygoma and arch.

a) Intra-oral (Keen): A small incision is made above the molar teeth and a uterine dilator or a blunt periosteal elevator is inserted above the periosteum into the area below and behind the body of the zygoma. The fracture is elevated up and out and frequently will snap into position requiring no further treatment.

b) Temporal (Gillies): A small incision is made into the hairline in the temporal fossa area. A heavy periosteal elevator is passed beneath the arch below the temporalis fascia and above the temporalis muscle. The arch fracture and occasionally the body are elevated into position through this approach.

c) Open reduction and interosseous wiring of the orbital rim: when simple reduction of the fracture remains unstable and requires immobilization, interosseous wiring of the rim alone or combined with sinus packing if the floor of the orbit is also unstable, is the treatment of choice.

4. PITFALLS AND COMPLICATIONS:

a) Failure to recognize the fracture clinically because of edema and ecchymosis and left untreated.
b) Failure to recognize accompanying blow-out fracture of the orbit.
c) Failure to appreciate that the extent of dislocation is greatly minimized in the Waters x-ray view and that submento-vertical and lateral views must be compared for proper diagnosis.
d) Permanent dislocation of a closed simple reduction.
e) Permanent anesthesia of the infraorbital nerve.
f) Malunion.
g) Traumatic enophthalmus.
h) Hemorrhage into the orbit causing blindness.
i) Fracture of the temporal fossa by improper use of the Gillies approach.

III. MAXILLARY FRACTURES

1. ANATOMY: The paired maxillary bones essentially provide a platform for the middle one-third of the face. They support the nose medially and are reinforced laterally by the zygomas. They each contain a cavity (the maxillary sinus) which provides in its roof the major portion of the floor of the orbit. The inferior border (alveolar ridge) of the maxilla support the maxillary teeth. The weakest part of the maxilla is a horizontal plane at the level of the tooth apices. Terminal branches of the internal maxillary artery enter posteriorly and pass through to facial soft tissue leaving twigs to supply the maxillary bone. The arteries are accompanied by fibers from the maxillary division of the Vth cranial nerve.

2. DIAGNOSIS: History of injury, direction of blow and nature of objects causing injury are helpful factors. Perhaps more helpful is the knowledge that the maxilla is likely to fracture in a certain pattern established experimentally by Doctor Le Fort. These were listed by number and in the order of severity: (Figure 10-1)

Le Fort I (Guerin): Transverse fracture above the level of the apices of the teeth.

Le Fort II (Pyramidal): Triangular fracture line which includes the nasal bones but excludes the zygomas.

Le Fort III (craniofacial disjunction): Includes separation of the maxilla, nasal bones, and zygoma from their cranial attachments.

Knowing these three basic possibilities and that various combinations can occur, aids greatly in the diagnosis which may only be completed at the time of surgery.

a) Observation: Severe fractures of all facial bones may occur without significant soft tissue injury. Edema soon obscures visual landmarks. The face may be elongated and occlusion visibly disturbed. Nasal hemorrhage and edema may obscure the nasal passages. Orbital edema may obscure observation of eye movements and bulbar ecchymosis.

b) Examination: Perhaps most helpful is routine palpation of the orbital rims, nose, zygomatic process of the maxilla plus testing for mobility of the maxillary compound. Nasal drainage and posterior pharyngeal wall leak should be looked for, and if present, tested for cerebral spinal fluid content.

c) X-rays: All views should be obtained. The unconed Water's view is the most helpful and areas to be examined carefully include:

(1) zygomaticofrontal suture.
(2) root of the nose.
(3) zygomatic process of the maxilla.
(4) inferior orbital rim.

The most important areas to look for on the lateral film are:

(1) the relation of the overlapping lateral recesses of the maxillary sinus into the zygoma.
(2) relation of the paired posterior walls of the maxillary sinuses.
(3) continuity of the root of the nose with the frontal bone.

The submentovertical view is helpful for evaluating the arches of the zygoma and the anterior wall of the maxilla. Occasionally x-rays may be poor due to technical difficulties, excessive blood in the sinuses and other air-containing spaces coupled with edema and ecchymosis.

3. TREATMENT: Emergency treatment is the essential first step in establishing and maintaining an airway, control and replacement of blood, evaluation and treatment of more serious other injuries of the cranium, chest or abdomen. Definitive treatment of maxillary

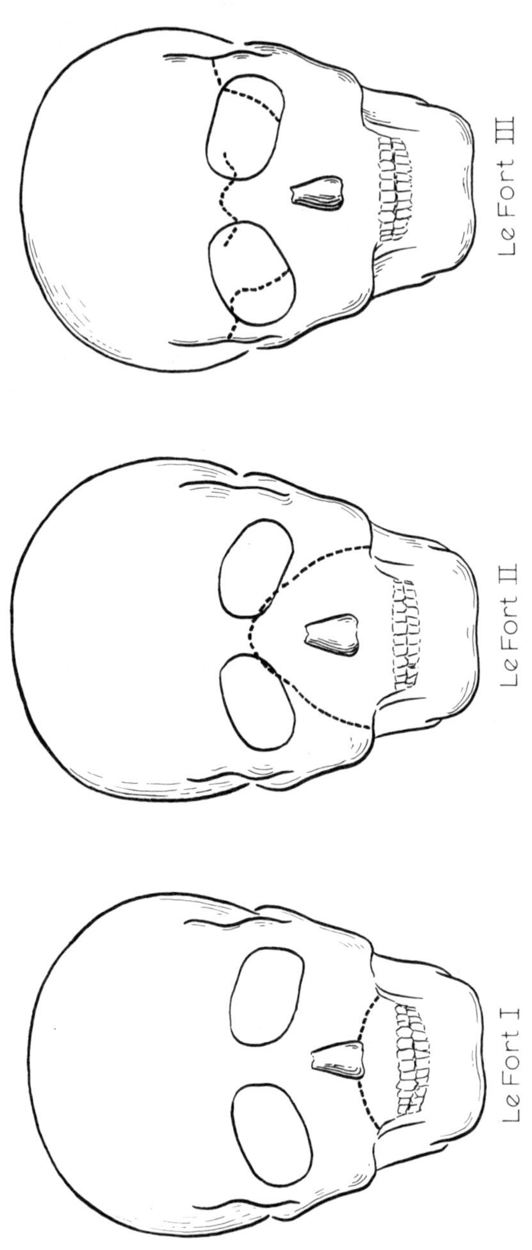

FIG. 10-1. Le Fort Fractures

fractures excluding medical and surgical care of other injuries, can be quite complicated depending on the remaining usable anatomical components.

Le Fort I: In the presence of sufficient mandibular and maxillary teeth the maxilla is reduced onto the mandible and immobilized by intermaxillary wiring aided with a head cap and chin support. In the absence of teeth, the maxilla has to be reduced onto the structures above and immobilized from above down. This may be accomplished by internal wiring, use of wired-in dentures, external traction to orthopedic weights or a variety of head frames.

Le Fort II: In the presence of sufficient mandibular and maxillary teeth, the maxilla is reduced onto the mandible and immobilized by intermaxillary wiring. The inferior orbital rim and nasal frontal areas may be immobilized by interosseous wiring. The accompanying nasal fractures will require reduction, internal and external splinting and possibly transnasal wiring over external splints. In the absence of teeth, the dentures may be wired in prior to performing the above procedures. In the absence of dentures, reduction and immobilization will be accomplished from above down, plus external orthopedic and/or headframe traction.

Le Fort III: The Le Fort III fracture adds the zygomatic compounds to the Le Fort II fracture and treatment represents a combination of these two methods. An added feature is cranial facial wire suspension (from the frontal bone to the maxilla or mandible). This is useful in a limited number of cases where there is a need for upward tractions. Forward traction must be obtained by other methods such as orthopedic weights or from head traction.

4. PITFALLS AND COMPLICATIONS:

a) The magnitude of facial bone injuries is unappreciated by initial observation and review of preliminary x-rays.
b) Poor selection of airway for delivery of general anesthesia.
c) Unnecessary use of wiring suspension for facial fracture immobilization.
d) Failure to establish and maintain centric occlusion.
e) Unrecognized intracanthal trauma.
f) Impacted nasal fracture unreduced by closed reduction efforts and left untreated.
g) Treatment of soft tissue injuries without regard for facial skeletal injuries.
h) Vital structures discarded at the time of initial treatment.
i) Failure to replace missing dental elements early to avoid contracture.
j) "Dropped" canthus, enophthalmos, diplopia, epiphoria, decreased mandibular excursion and permanent paresthesia may occur.

IV. MANDIBULAR FRACTURES

1. ANATOMY: The mandible is a horseshoe-shaped bone forming the bony framework of the lower one-third of the face. It is attached at its end (condyloid processes) to the base of the skull in a sliding-hinge joint (ginglymoarthroidal). The horizontal portion (body)

supports the dentition, is supplied by the inferior alveolar nerve and artery (internal maxillary) which passes out the mental foramen to supply the lower lip. The mental foramen is at about the area of the 2nd premolar. The mandible is weakest at the mental foramen. The ascending portion on its medial surface accepts the inferior alveolar nerve and artery at the mandibular foramen about mid-portion. The anterior superior tip (coronoid process) receives the tendinous attachment of the temporalis muscle. The condyloid process articulates with the temporal bone (glenoid fossa).

Major Muscles of Mastication: (Figure 10-2)

a) Temporalis:
Nerve = mandibular division of Vth cranial nerve.
Arises from the floor of the temporal fossa.
Attachment is to the coronoid process of the mandible.
Action - powerful elevator of mandible.

b) Masseter:
Nerve = mandibular division of Vth cranial nerve.
Arises from the lower and medial border of the zygomatic arch
Attachment to the mandible is the lower one-half of the lateral surface.
Action - powerful elevator of mandible.

c) Internal Pterygoid: (Medial Pterygoid)
Nerve = mandibular division of the Vth cranial nerve.
Arises from the medial surface of the lateral pterygoid plate and tuberosity of the maxilla.
Attachment is to the lower one-half of the mandible on the inner surface.
Action - to pull the mandible upward, inward and forward

d) The External Pterygoid: (Lateral Pterygoid)
Nerve = mandibular division of the Vth cranial nerve.
Arises from the lateral surface of the lateral pterygoid plate and from the greater wing of the sphenoid.
Attachment is to the inner and anterior aspect of the neck of of the condyle.
Action - to pull the mandible forward.

Depressors of the Mandible:

a) Geniohyoid:
Nerve = hypoglossal.
Attachment is to the genial tubercle at the mandibular symphysis.
Action - to open mouth.

b) Digastric: (Anterior Belly)
Nerve = mandibular division of the Vth cranial nerve.
Attachment is to the lower border of the mandible near the midline.
Action - to open mouth.

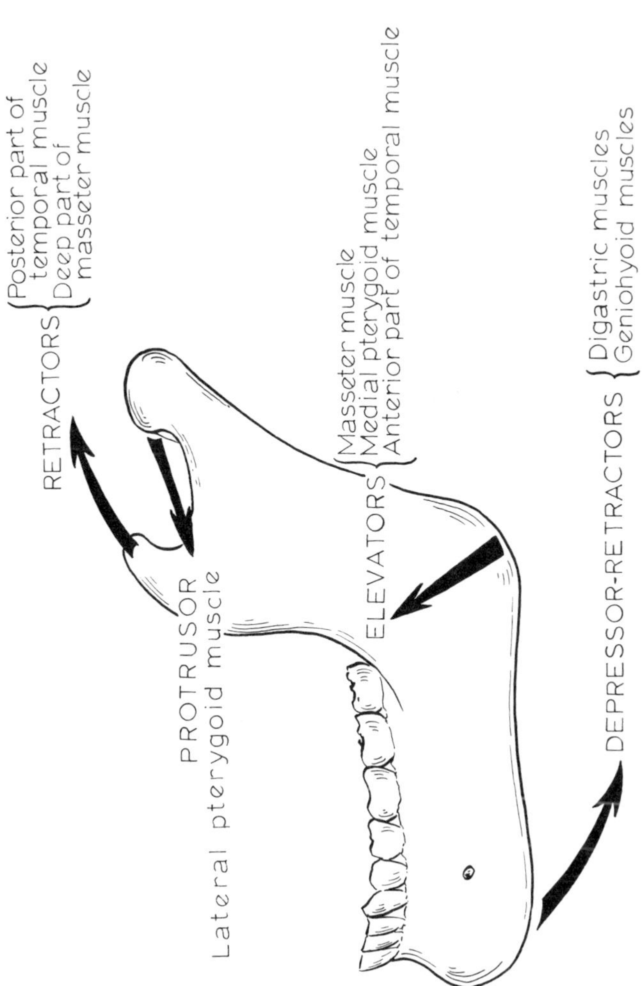

FIG. 10-2. Muscles of the mandible

c) Mylohyoid:
Nerve = mandibular division of Vth cranial nerve.
Attachment is to the mylohyoid ridge of the mandible and to the hyoid bone.
Action - raises the hyoid bone as well as opens the mouth.

To open mouth: Lateral pterygoid pulls the condyle forward while the digastric, mylohyoid and geniohyoid depress the jaw.

MUSCLES ATTACHED TO THE LATERAL SIDE OF THE MANDIBLE: (Figure 10-3) Masseter, part of the temporalis on the coronoid, lateral pterygoid muscle on the condyle.

MUSCLES ATTACHED TO THE MEDIAL SIDE OF THE MANDIBLE: (Figure 10-4) Digastric, mylohyoid, medial pterygoid, temporalis, lateral pterygoid on the neck of the coronoid.

The Temporal-Mandibular Joint: This is a ginglymoarthrodial joint with a hinge and gliding action. It is innervated by the masseter and auriculotemporal nerves. The meniscus that separates the upper cavity from the lower cavity is made of fibrocartilage. The 3 ligaments attached here are (a) temporomandibular ligament, (b) stylomandibular ligament and (c) sphenomandibular ligament.

Teeth: There are 20 deciduous teeth. They start arriving by the sixth month and are all in by the 24th month. Permanent teeth start arriving at 6 years and are all in by the 24th year and are 32 in number. The angle of the mandible is slightly greater than 90° in the young and becomes more obtuse as the patient gets older and becomes edentulous.

2. DIAGNOSIS:

a) History of the direction, severity, and nature of the trauma influences the type of injury. Knowledge of the weak points of the mandible and muscle attachment provide a variety of classifications. Favorable or unfavorable fractures depend upon whether the muscle pull tends to keep the fracture elements apart or together. Classification according to location seems reasonable for both description and treatment planning such as fractures of the symphysis, body, angle, ramus, condyle and coronoid process. (See Figure 10-5)

b) Observation of patients with fractured mandible is very helpful. The face is distorted, the bite may be open or uneven. swallowing is difficult, speech is difficult. It is essential to ask the patient before he is put to sleep whether he has any knowledge of what his normal bite should be.

c) Examination - Bi-manual palpation of the jaw throughout while looking for mobility between teeth, bleeding between the teeth, and eliciting areas of painful response is most helpful. Evaluation of occlusion may be quite easy with a full complement of teeth and in the presence of a previously normal bite. Malocclusion, missing teeth and multiple dental replacements call for careful examination of the teeth for wear and possible positions of the mandible for rendering a satisfactory bite. Crepitation at the fracture site and loss of sensation in the lower lip may be elicited.

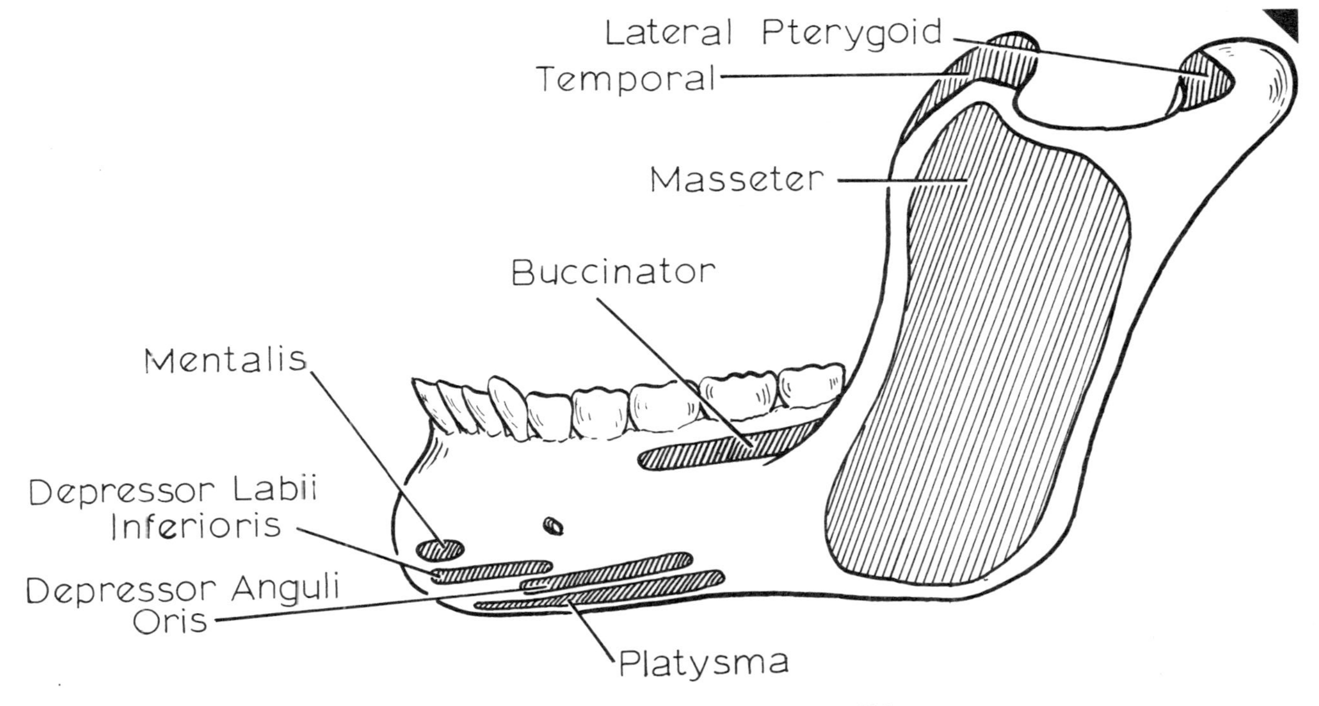

FIG. 10-3. Lateral aspect of the mandible

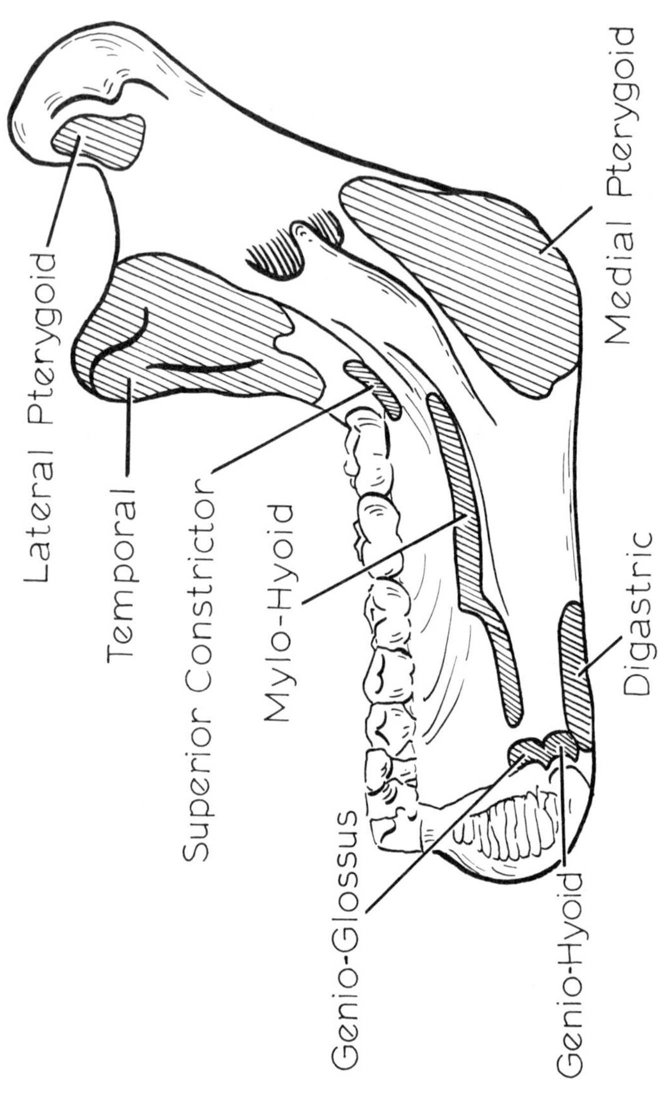

FIG. 10-4. **Medial aspect of the mandible**

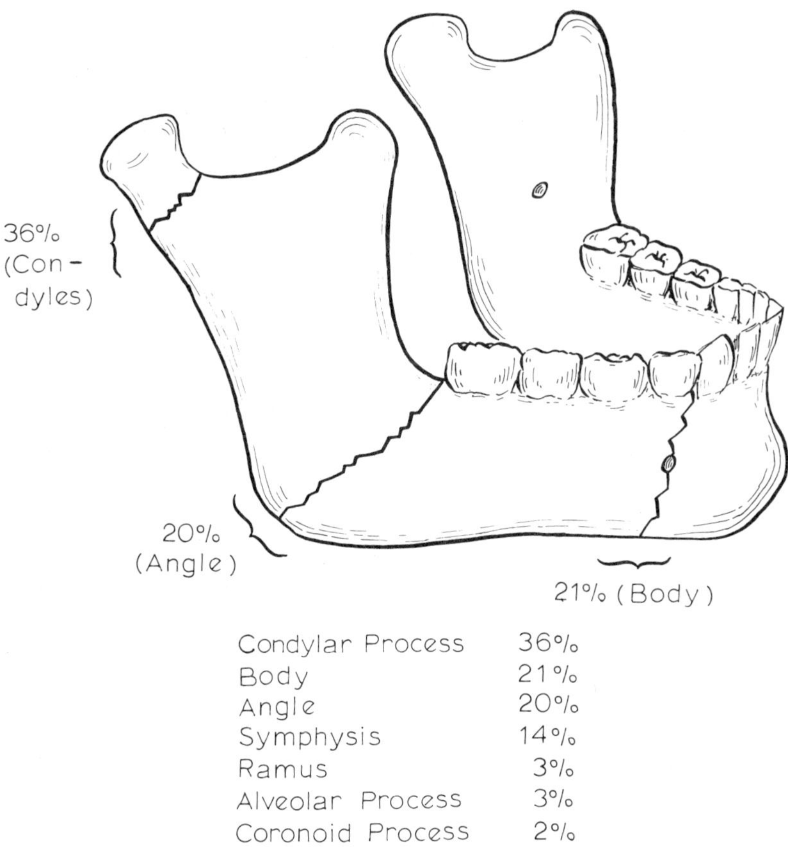

FIG. 10-5. Frequencies of mandibular fracture by site

X-rays may be limited to an AP and lateral of the skull in severely injured patients placing greater reliance on the clinical examination. When possible, the following views are selected:

(1) Right and left lateral jaw - good for fractures of the body especially at the angle and mental foramen.
(2) PA of the mandible - good for angle fractures and occasionally symphysis fractures.
(3) AP mandible - good for ascending ramus, condyle and coronoid processes.
(4) Panorex (orthoplanography) - excellent for condyle, ascending ramus and body including tooth structures.
(5) Occlusal - excellent for symphysis area.

3. TREATMENT: Overall general treatment is aimed toward restoration of occlusion. In the presence of teeth, fractures in the following areas are treated as follows:

a) Symphysis: may require only arch bar immobilization if undisplaced. If severe, with displacement, open reduction and internal wiring plus arch bar would be necessary.

b) Body: intermaxillary wiring alone or with arch bars. (In a body fracture, the anterior segment is pulled down and back by the digastric, mylohyoid and geniohyoid muscles. The posterior segment is pulled up by the masseter, medial pterygoid and temporalis muscles).

c) Angle: if favorable (when the internal pterygoid and temporalis muscles hold the fracture in line) only intermaxillary fixation is required. If unfavorable, open reduction and interosseous wiring plus intermaxillary fixation are applied.

d) Ascending ramus: usually surrounded by muscles which support the fracture once the teeth are immobilized with intermaxillary wiring or splints.

e) Condyle: one or both may be fractured. Treatment is by intermaxillary fixation. If unable to place the teeth in normal occlusion it may be necessary to perform open reduction and interosseous wiring of the fractured neck of the condyle either through a preauricular or submandibular approach. Condylar fractures in children may not require treatment if the mandibular teeth can be placed in centric occlusion. The angulated position of a condyle fracture over a number of years may be observed to right itself and restore the condyle head to the glenoid fossa; occasionally as in adult cases, it is necessary to reduce and immobilize condylar fractures to allow the teeth to meet normally.

f) Coronoid fractures: usually require no treatment.

In the absence of teeth:

a) Symphysis: open reduction and wiring with heavy gauge wire. Possible addition of circumferential wiring of denture or gunning splint.

b) Body: circumferential wiring to denture or gunning splint. Possibly require open reduction either intraorally or externally prior to circumferential wiring.

c) Angle of the mandible: open reduction and wiring plus circumferential wiring to denture or gunning splint.

d) Condyle: circumferential wiring of dentures or gunning splint. May be left alone if unilateral.

e) Coronoid process: usually left alone.

4. COMPLICATIONS:

a) Non union - may result from a number of factors such as infection, non approximation of fractures, excess mobility during healing and tooth in the line of fracture.

b) Loss of bone substance at the time of injury.

c) Ankylosis of the temporomandibular joint.

d) Deformity following removal of fixation, especially in a thin edentulous mandible in older patients.

e) Failure to properly diagnose and leave significant fractures untreated.

f) Permanent anesthesia of the lower lip.

V. BLOW-OUT FRACTURES OF THE ORBITAL FLOOR

1. ANATOMY: The majority of the floor of the orbit is a thin shelf of maxillary bone forming a roof of the maxillary sinus. This shelf of bone is continuous posteromedially as a portion of the palatine bone and anterolaterally as a portion of the zygomatic bone. The inferior orbital fissure separates the floor from the lateral wall of the orbital cavity. The floor of the orbit slopes upward from lateral to medial. It transmits the inferior orbital nerve and vessels from about the midportion of the inferior orbital fissure forward in a canal which exits as a foramen below the inferior orbital rim. Blow-out fractures involve the following structures:

a) Bony orbital floor (posterior medial portion) is most frequent.
b) Orbital periosteum (orbital septum).
c) Suspensory ligament (Lockwood).
d) Inferior rectus muscle (most frequently trapped in blow-out fractures).
e) Inferior oblique muscle (secondarily involved in blow-out fractures).
f) Orbital fat (major cause of enophthalmos).
g) Eye globe.
h) Inferior orbital nerve and vessels.

2. DIAGNOSIS: Direct trauma to the orbit by an object sufficiently large to produce compression of the orbital contents may cause collapse of the orbital floor. In the process, the orbital fascia (orbital septum) is ruptured with herniation of fat and muscle into the maxillary sinus. With release of pressure, after the energy of the traumatic object is spent, the contents of the orbit may return, becoming trapped in the orbital floor or remain in the sinus depending on the severity of the injury. The following signs and symptoms indicate blow-out fracture:

a) Diplopia (chiefly on upward gaze).
b) Altered sensation over the side of the nose, cheek and upper lip.
c) Inability to move the eye ball on upward gaze.
d) Enophthalmos with drooping of the upper lid.
e) Nasal bleeding.
f) X-rays
    (1) Water's view may show herniation of orbital elements into the antrum.
    (2) Actual fracture in the bony orbital floor.
    (3) Orbitogram (contrast media injected into the orbit outlines the defect in the orbital floor).
g) Traction test: The tendon of the inferior rectus muscle is grasped by forceps and traction applied. If the muscle is trapped in the fracture, the eyeglobe will not rotate upward.

3. TREATMENT: Treatment will vary according to the severity of the injury. In general, the objective is to free the trapped muscles and restore the continuity of the orbital floor. The approach through the maxillary sinus may be made for inspection but a direct approach through the lower lid or along the inferior orbital rim offers both an opportunity for inspection and exposure for reduction

of the herniated contents and repair of the floor. A variety of materials have been used, such as silastic sheating, autogenous cartilage and bone.

4. COMPLICATIONS:
  a) Loss of orbital fat either early or delayed, causing enophthalmos.
  b) Extrusion of the foreign implant material used to repair the orbital floor.
  c) Improper placement of the implant causing injury to the optic nerve.
  d) Scar tissue formation producing muscle imbalance.
  e) Permanent anesthesia of the cheek, side of the nose and lip.

VI. FRACTURE OF THE FRONTAL SINUSES

1. ANATOMY: The paired frontal sinuses invade and weaken the osseous structures of the frontal bone. In this location they provide a mechanism for shock absorption in direct trauma to the anterior skull. Their connection inferiorly with the ethmoid sinuses makes it necessary to maintain a passage for secretions from the mucosal lining. This connection also makes fractures of the posterior wall more serious because of the possibility of ascending infection.

Frontal sinus fractures may be simple or complicated, limited to the outer wall or may involve both walls. Displaced fractures of the posterior wall may cause dural tears or penetration of the frontal lobe of the brain. Anatomical structures involved in frontal sinus fractures include:
  a) Outer wall (depressed, simple or comminuted).
  b) Inner wall (depressed, simple or comminuted).
  c) Floor (roof of the orbit).
  d) Superior orbital rim with superior orbital foramen containing supraorbital nerve and vessels.
  e) Frontonasal ducts.
  f) Dura (CSF leaks).

2. DIAGNOSIS: Minor fractures of the outer wall of the frontal sinus may produce only palpable and visual depression without loss of function. Major injuries may produce any or all of the following:
  a) Irritability, restlessness, or loss of consciousness.
  b) Edema and hemorrhage about the orbit.
  c) Supraorbital anesthesia.
  d) Gross destruction and deformity.
  e) Escape of CSF fluid (test should be made to determine escape of fluid in a dependent position of head or on compression of the jugular veins, bilaterally. Also laboratory tests for the presence of sugar but absence of mucin. Tests with fluorescent dye and radioactive material.)
  f) AP and lateral skull films demonstrate defects in outer and inner walls of the sinus.
  g) Laminograms further confirm location and extent of fractures.

3. TREATMENT: Treatment varies according to the extent of injury. Simple depressed fractures may be elevated into position with hooks at the margins or drilling access holes for both elevation and interosseous wiring. Most often soft tissue access to the fracture is through an existing wound. Depressed fractures of the posterior wall are more serious. Reduction must include assurance that mucous membrane has not been left within the cranial cavity and that dural tears have been repaired with fascia or fat. Depressed fragments, cerebral lacerations and extensive dural tears require intracranial operation. Treatment of cosmetic deformities such as contour may be repaired with self-curing silastic. The frontal sinus duct problem may be treated with obliteration of the cavity (abdominal adipose tissue) or reconstruction of the duct with nasal mucosal flaps. Bone grafting may be required to restore the continuity of the orbital rim.

4. COMPLICATIONS: Complications from frontal sinus fractures are relative to the function of the outer and inner walls, the floor and the cavity itself. Those relating to the outer walls are primarily cosmetic in providing contours for the lower forehead with support for the eyebrows, eyes and eyelids. Those relative to the inner wall which protect the brain are CSF leak, aerocele, meningitis and brain abscess. 25% of patients with fractures of the paranasal air sinuses may be expected to develop a CSF leak. The onset in 50% of the cases is within the first 48 hours and another 20% will develop within the four weeks after injury. In those cases not requiring a neurosurgical procedure, a CSF leak usually stops within 10 days. The risk of meningitis is relatively slight if penicillin and sulfonamides are instituted at the onset of the CSF leak.

REFERENCES

1. Archer, W.H.: Oral & Maxillofacial Surgery, W.B. Saunders Co., Philadelphia, 1952.

2. Boies, L.R.: Fundamentals of Otolaryngology, W.B. Saunders Co., Philadelphia, 1954.

3. Converse, J.M.: Reconstructive Plastic Surgery, W.B. Saunders Co., Philadelphia, 1967.

4. Dingman, R.O. and Natvig, P.: Surgery of Facial Fractures, W.B. Saunders Co., Philadelphia, 1964.

5. Rowe, N.L. and Killey, H.C.: Fractures of the Facial Skeleton, Williams & Wilkins Co., London, 1955.

6. Smith, H.W. and Yanagisawa, E.: Fracture-Dislocation of Zygoma and Zygomatic Arch. Arch. Otolaryng. 73: 172, Feb., 1961.

7. Sobotta, J.: Atlas of Human Anatomy, 8th English Edition, Hafner Publishing Co., New York, 1968.

8. Thoma, K.H.: Traumatic Surgery of the Jaws, C.V. Mosby Co., St. Louis, 1942.

9. Yanagisawa, E. and Smith, H.W.: Radiology of the Normal Maxillary Sinus and Related Structures, Otolaryngol. Clin. N. Am. 9: 55, February, 1976.

CHAPTER 11

NOSE AND SINUSES

I. EMBRYOLOGY OF THE NOSE

The nasal placode is of ectodermal origin and appears between the middle of the 3rd and 4th week of gestation. (Figure 11-1A) It is of interest to note that, at this stage, the eyes are laterally placed, the auricular precursors lie below the mandibular process, and the primitive mouth is wide. Hence, abnormal embryonic development at this stage may result in these characteristics in post-natal life.

On the 5th week the placodes become depressed below the surface and appear as invaginated pits. The nasal pit extends backwards into the oral cavity but is separated from it by the bucco-nasal membrane (Figure 11-1B). This membrane ruptures at the 7th to 8th week of gestation to form the posterior nares. Failure in this step of development results in choanal atresia. While the nasal pit extends backward, it also extends upward towards the forebrain area. Epithelium around the forebrain thickens to become specialized olfactory sensory cells. Anteriorly, the maxillary process fuses with the lateral and medial nasal processes to form the anterior nares. The fusion between the maxillary process and the lateral nasal process also creates a groove called the nasolacrimal groove. The epithelium over the groove is subsequently buried, and when the epithelium is resorbed the nasolacrimal duct is formed, opening into the anterior aspect of the inferior meatus. This duct is fully developed at birth.

The frontonasal process (mesoderm) is the precursor of the nasal septum. (Figure 11-2A, B). The primitive palate (premaxilla) located anteriorly is also a derivative of the frontonasal process (mesoderm). Posteriorly (Figure 11-3A, B), the septum lies directly over the oral cavity until the 9th week at which time the palatal shelves of the maxilla grow medially to fuse with each other and with the septum to form the secondary palate. The hard palate is formed by the 8th to 9th week (Figure 11-4) while the soft palate and the uvula are completed by the 11th to 12th week.

From the 8th week to the 24th week of embryonic life, the nostrils are occluded by an epithelial plug. Failure to resorb this epithelium results in atresia or stenosis of the anterior nares.

Along the lateral wall of the nasal precursor, the maxillo-turbinal is the first to appear. This is followed by the development of five ethmod-turbinals and one nasoturbinal. The following gives the derivatives of each embryonic anlage and a time table of their development:

Maxillo-turbinal	Inferior concha
1st ethmo-turbinal	Middle concha
2nd and 3rd ethmo-turbinal	Superior concha
(4th and 5th ethmo-turbinal	Supreme concha)
Naso-turbinal	Agger Nasi Area

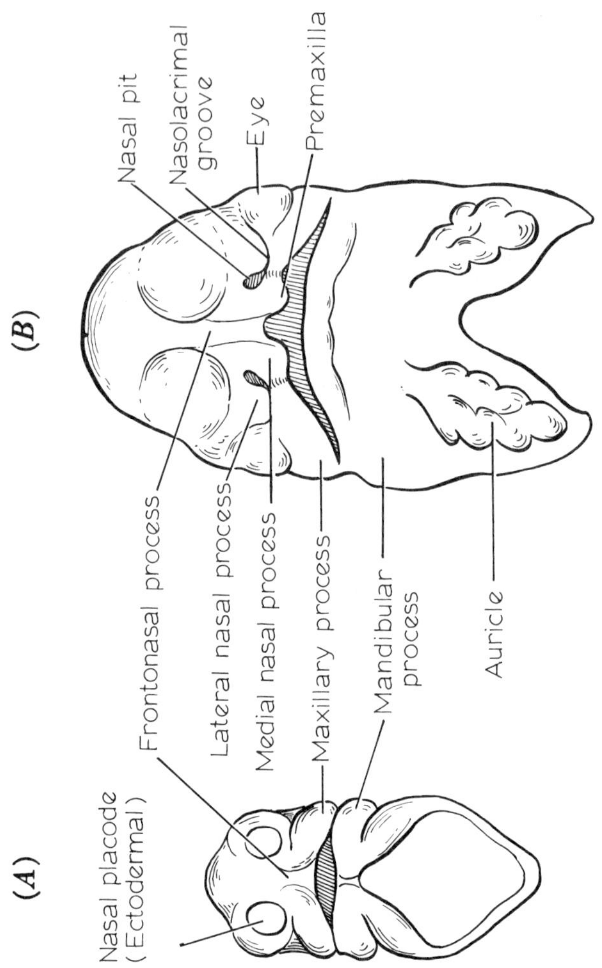

FIG. 11-1. (A) 4-week-old embryo
(B) 5-week-old embryo

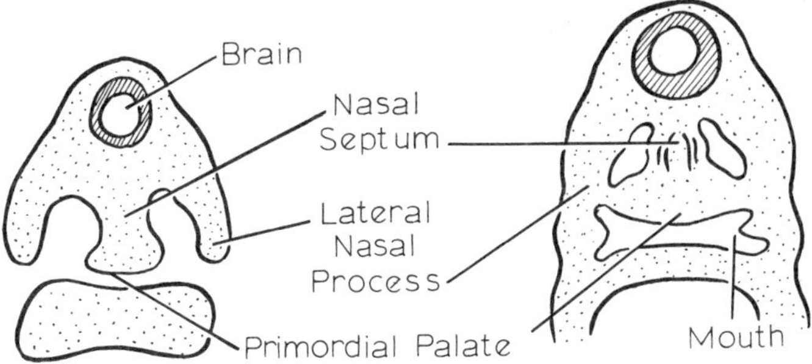

FIG. 11-2. A and B (See Text)

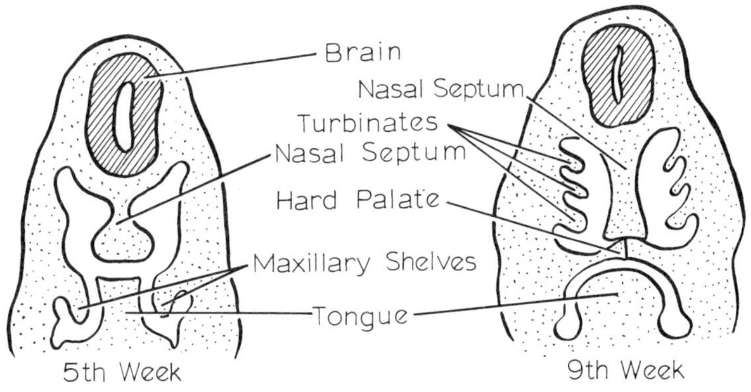

FIG. 11-3. A and B (See Text)

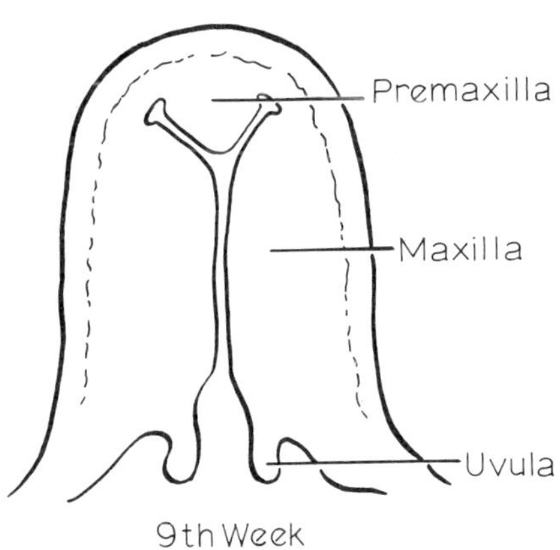

FIG. 11-4. Parts of the palate

Inferior concha formed	7th week
Middle concha formed	7th week
Uncinate process formed	7th week
Superior concha formed	8th week
Cartilage laid down	10th week
Vomer formed and calcified	12th week
Ethmoid bone calcified	20th week
Cribriform plate calcifies	28th week
Perpendicular plate, crista galli calcifies	After birth

Table 11-1 outlines the development of the paranasal sinuses.

TABLE 11-1

Maxillary Sinus:	Arises as a prolongation of the Ethmoid infundibulum--	at 12 weeks
	Pneumatizes----------------	at birth
	Reaches stable size at-------	18 years old
Frontal Sinus:	Arises from the upper anterior area of the middle meatus ---------	Starts at late fetal life or even after birth
	Pneumatizes----------------	After 1 year
	Full Size------------------	20 years old
Sphenoid Sinus:	Arises from the epithelial outgrow of the upper posterior region of the nasal cavity in close relation with the sphenoid bone	starts at 3rd fetal month
	Pneumatization-------------	During childhood
	Full size------------------	15 years old
Ethmoid Sinus:	Arises from the evagination of the nasal mucosa into the lateral ethmoid mass	6th fetal month
	Pneumatization completed----	7 years old
	Full size------------------	12 years old

II. ANATOMY

EXTERNAL NOSE

Bony framework of the external nose consists of:

1. Nasal bone
2. Frontal process of the maxilla
3. Nasal process of the frontal bone

Cartilaginous framework of the external nose consists of:
1. Lower lateral (greater alar), right and left
2. Quadrilateral cartilage of the septum
3. Upper lateral (lateral nasal), right and left
4. Lesser alar, right and left
5. Sesamoid

Muscles of the external nose are:
1. Nasalis (constrictor)
2. Depressor septi (constrictor)
3. Procerus (dilator)
4. Dilator naris (dilator)
5. Angular head of the quadratus labii superior (dilator)
6. Depressor alae nasi (constrictor)

Arterial blood supply is from:
1. External carotid artery:
   Facial artery:
   a) Lateral nasal
   b) Angular
   c) Alar
   d) Septal
   e) External nasal

2. Internal carotid artery:
   Ophthalmic artery:
   a) Dorsal nasal

Lymphatics: Via anterior facial vein to submandibular nodes.

Sensory innervation is the trigeminal nerve through:
1. Ophthalmic division:
   a) Nasociliary
   b) External nasal
   c) Infratrochlear
2. Maxillary division:
   a) Infraorbital

INTERNAL NOSE

1. The roof of the nose is formed by the cribriform plate of ethmoid bone (most of the roof), the frontal bone anteriorly and the sphenoid bone posteriorly.

2. The nasal septum consists of:
   a) Septal cartilage
   b) Vomer
   c) Perpendicular plate of the ethmoid
   d) Maxillary crest
   e) Premaxilla

3. There are three turbinates arising from the lateral wall. The inferior turbinate is the largest. The mucous membrane covering this structure is thick and contains numerous venous plexuses forming a cavernous erectile type of tissue. The bony portion connects

the palatine bone, the ethmoid bone, the maxilla and the lacrimal bone. The middle turbinate is the second largest and lies above the inferior turbinate. The mucous membrane is similar to that found in the inferior turbinate. It is actually a bony projection of the ethmoid bone. The superior turbinate is the smallest of three turbinates having much thinner mucous membrane. This is also a projection of the ethmoid bone. The supreme turbinate is occasionally found and is extremely small.

4. There are three meati in the lateral wall of the nasal cavity:

a) Inferior meatus: Nasolacrimal duct opens here. Damage to the nasolacrimal duct can be minimized by avoiding damage to the attachment of the inferior turbinate. The orifice of the duct is located on the lateral wall from 3 to 3.5 cm. behind the posterior margin of the nostril.

b) Middle meatus: There are two prominent objects in view in the outer wall of the middle meatus, namely the convex surface of the bulla ethmoidalis and immediately beneath it and well defined curved margin of the uncinate process of the ethmoid. Between these two structures there is a narrow interval, the semilunar opening or hiatus semilunaris; this opening serves as a communication between the middle meatus and the small channel or canal named ethmoidal infundibulum.[1]

Anterior ethmoid, maxillary and frontal sinuses drain into the ethmoidal infundibulum. The frontal sinus and anterior ethmoid cells usually drain into the anterior upper portion, and the maxillary sinus drains posteriorly to the frontal sinus.

Accessory ostia of the maxillary sinus are present in 30-40 percent of all sinuses.

c) Superior meatus: Posterior ethmoid sinus opens here.

d) Supreme meatus: Occasionally present.

e) Sphenoethmoidal recess: Sphenoid sinus drains into the sphenoethmoidal recess above and behind the superior turbinate. The ostium is usually in the posterior wall of the recess. The large opening of the sinus in the base of the sphenoid is partially enveloped by a scroll-like bone, the sphenoidal concha or turbinate (bone of Bertin).

5. Arterial supply:

A. Internal carotid artery

Ophthalmic artery:

(1) Anterior ethmoid: (anterosuperior portion of septum and lateral wall). The anterior ethmoidal is the second largest vessel supplying the internal nose.

(2) Posterior ethmoid: (septum and lateral wall superiorly).

B. External carotid artery

Internal maxillary artery:

(1) Sphenopalatine: (most of the posterior part of the nasal septum and most of the lateral wall of the nose, especially posteriorly).

(a) Nasopalatine (posterior septal)
(roof, septum, and floor)
(b) Lateral nasal (lateral wall posteriorly).
(2) Descending palatine (lateral wall posteriorly).
(3) Pharyngeal (roof posteriorly).

(The two terminal branches of the third part of the maxillary artery are the posterior nasal artery and the sphenopalatine artery (Nomina Anatomica, 1966). Others have used the term sphenopalatine to refer to the last centimeter of the maxillary artery and described this as bifurcating into the lateral nasal, and septal branches. (The septal branch has also been called the nasopalatine artery.)[26]

Superior labial artery (from facial artery). (Tip of the septum and ala nasi. Its anastomosis with a branch of sphenopalatine forms Kiesselbach's plexus in Little's area).

6. Venous drainage open into:
   a) Sphenopalatine and anterior facial veins
   b) Ophthalmic veins
   c) Veins of the orbital surface of the frontal lobe of the brain (via foramina in the cribriform plate).
   d) Superior sagittal sinus (via foramen caecum).

7. Innervation:
   a) Anterior ethmoid: (from ophthalmic division of trigeminal)
      (1) Medial
      (2) Lateral
   b) Branches of the sphenopalatine ganglion:
      (1) Lateral posterior superior (short sphenopalatine)
      (2) Medial posterior superior (septal)
      Nasopalatine (long sphenopalatine)
      (3) Greater palatine
   c) Olfactory nerves (roof, upper third of nasal mucous membrane)

8. Lymphatic drainage: Anterior part of cavity to submandibular nodes. Posterior part of cavity to upper deep cervical glands.

9. Mucous membrane:
   a) Pseudostratified ciliated columnar epithelium, except in:
      (1) Vestibule and nares: stratified squamous
      (2) Olfactory-areas: nonciliated pseudostratified columnar epithelium with serous glands of Bowman and bipolar olfactory cells.

PARANASAL SINUSES

1. MAXILLARY SINUS: (ANTRUM OF HIGHMORE)[1,4,14,15,20,23,25]
   a) The largest of the paranasal sinuses located in the body of the maxilla.
   b) A pyramidal cavity with its apex extending laterally and its base directed toward the nasal cavity.

c) The alveolar process forms the floor of the maxilla, which is usually 3 to 5 mm. below the level of the floor of the nasal cavity except in children where the floor is at, or above the level of the floor of the nasal cavity.
d) Its roof is formed by the orbital surface of the maxilla, and the infraorbital nerve is contained in a ridge usually located in the center of this. The roof is also the floor of the orbit.
e) The cheek overlies its anterior wall.
f) The thin medial wall is the lateral wall of the nasal cavity.
g) The posterior wall overlies the pterygoid space.
h) The opening of the sinus is seen as a small slit behind the projection made by the uncinate process of the ethmoid. Often an accessory opening is seen posterior to the primary opening (30-40 percent).
i) The capacity of the maxillary sinus is about 15 ml.

2. ETHMOID SINUSES:
a) The multiple thin-walled cavities located between the middle turbinate and the thin medial wall of the orbit are the ethmoid sinuses. Approximately 7 to 15 in number.
b) The lateral wall of the ethmoid sinuses (the medial wall of the orbit) is known as the lamina papyracea (paper-thin plate). Indeed, so thin is the bone that occasionally natural dehiscences occur in its surface, which permit the development of an orbital cellulitis from an ethmoiditis. At the superior edge of the lamina papyracea at its articulation with the frontal bone, lie the two ethmoidal foramina (anterior and posterior), each containing an arterial and a neural twig. A line connecting these is on a parallel and just inferior to the anterior cranial fossa. The posterior foramen lies 3 to 8 mm anterior and on a parallel to the optic nerve.[28]
c) The anterior ethmoid sinuses (usually small and numerous) are found below the attachment of the middle turbinate and forms the bulla ethmoidalis, while the posterior group (usually larger and few) is superoposterior to the attachment of the middle turbinate. The anterior cells open into the middle meatus while the posterior cells open into the superior meatus.
d) The volume of the ethmoid cells in adults is about 14 ml.
e) The ethmoid cells may invade any of the surrounding bones, including frontal, sphenoid, and maxillary bones. The anterior group of cells will extend into the agger nasi and the uncinate process.
f) The middle turbinate is an osseous shelf approximately 3.5 to 4 cm in length and sometimes pneumatized with an ethmoidal cell (4% to 12%). Its anterior attachment is rooted to the cribriform plate.[28] Length of cribriform plate averages 2 cm, width 0.5 cm, thickness 0.2 cm. These relatively small dimensions leave little room for error.[14] During intranasal surgery, any instrumentation medial to the attachment of the middle turbinate should be done with extreme caution.
g) The relationship of the posterior ethmoidal cells to the optic nerve is variable being dependent on the degree of pneumatization of the sphenoid bone. Occasionally the sphenoidal

sinus may surround the nerve - if the sinus fails to pneumatize, posterior ethmoidal cells may invade the bone and come into intimate relationship with the optic nerve; however, even in a well developed sphenoidal sinus the posterior ethmoidal cells are never far from this nerve. In cases where there is poor access by intranasal or transantral approach, the relative safety and better exposure of an external operation may be a judicious choice if effective surgery is to be combined with maximum safety.[14]

3. FRONTAL SINUSES:[4,15,20,25]
   a) Two frontal sinuses which are usually unequal in size have the shape of an irregular pyramid with their apex directed upward.
   b) About 15% of adult skulls have only one sinus, and about 5% have no frontal sinus.
   c) They are located in the frontal bone above and deep to the superior orbital ridge.
   d) The sinuses are separated by a thin septum of bone which is not always present and only occasionally in the midline.
   e) The opening of the nasofrontal duct is found on the anteromedial aspect of the floor.
   f) The duct then continues through the ethmoidal labyrinth and enters the ethmoidal groove at the anterior end of the middle meatus. Variations in the location of the opening of the frontal sinus are as follows: (1) drainage into the frontal recess anterior to the infundibulum (55%); (2) drainage above but not into the infundibulum (30%); (3) drainage into the infundibulum (15%); and (4) drainage above the bulla (1%).[15]
   g) The capacity is about 6 to 7 ml.

4. SPHENOID SINUS:[4,15,27,28]
   a) The sphenoid sinuses vary greatly in their size and shape, probably because they represent an ingrowth from the nasal cavities. They lie behind the upper part of the nasal cavity. The sinus is commonly very deep in its anteroposterior dimension.
   b) They can spread laterally to invade the greater and lesser wings, pterygoid process and lateral pterygoid plate of the sphenoid.
   c) They are separated by a septum which usually deviates to one side but sometimes is absent.
   d) The openings of the sinuses are medial and superior in the rostrum of the sphenoid. It drains into the superior meatus indirectly through the sphenoethmoidal recess.
   e) The cavernous sinus and its contents as well as the optic nerve are located laterally to the sphenoid sinuses.
   f) The pituitary gland is located posteriorly and superiorly and commonly bulges into the superior wall.
   g) The carotid artery and vidian nerve commonly cause a ridge on the lateral wall if the sinus pneumatically expands laterally for any distance.
   h) The superior and anterior walls of the sphenoidal sinus are its thinnest. The lateral and superior walls are the ones to respect with great care. The inferior wall is the safest.

i) The capacity is about 7.5 ml.
j) Three types of pneumatization are recognized: [4]
   (1) Conchal pneumatization (about 1%). The sinus is rudimentary, having little depth. A contraindication to transphenoidal hypophysectomy.
   (2) Presphenoid pneumatization (about 40%) The sinus is pneumatized as far as the anterior bony wall of the pituitary fossa.
   (3) Postsphenoid pneumatization (about 60%) Pneumatization extends posteriorly below the pituitary fossa so that the sella turcia projects its anterior wall and its floor into the sinuses.

These types of pneumatization are well shown in the lateral x-ray view of the sinuses.

NASAL PHYSIOLOGY

1. Functions of the nose are:
   a) Respiration (warms, humidifies, and filters the inspired air).
   b) Olfaction (site of olfaction. Aid in sense of taste).
   c) Phonation (Amplifies sound. Alters timbre)

2. Functions of the paranasal sinuses are thought to be:
   a) Resonance of voice
   b) Air conditioning
   c) Lightening of the skull

3. Ideal temperature for the nose is 70°F.

4. Ideal humidity is 45-55% at 70°F.

5. Nasal lysozyme is most active in slightly acid medium. (Do not use alkaline or too acid nose drops. They will restrain the lysozyme and ciliary action).

6. pH of nose is 7.3

7. The nose secretes 1000 cc per 24 hours.

III. SELECTED DISORDERS OF THE NOSE AND SINUSES

DISEASES OF THE EXTERNAL NOSE

1. FURUNCULOSIS: An acute circumscribed inflammatory condition ending in suppuration, usually found in or about the vestibule of the nose where the hair follicles and sebaceous glands are located.

Etiology: Staphylococcus aureus.

Symptoms: Redness, swelling and a marked tenderness, may become fluctuant and drain.

Complications: Cavernous sinus thrombosis.

Treatment: Systemic antibiotics are administered because of the extreme danger of intracranial extension of the infection. The infection spreads through the facial vein to the angular and ophthalmic veins up into the cavernous sinus. When there is a sign of upward spread with facial cellulitis, oxacillin is the antibiotic of choice. Incision and drainage should be carried out when the lesion points. Warm saline applications help to localize the furuncle.

2. IMPETIGO CONTAGIOSA: Acute, contagious inflammatory skin disease.

Etiology: Staphylococcus.

Symptoms: Lesion begins as an elevated vesicle that becomes pustular on the external surface of the nose, in the vestibule or in the nares. These rupture rapidly and form yellowish crusts. Removal of the crust shows a reddish moist area.

Treatment: Local and systemic antibiotics.

3. ERYSIPELAS: An acute inflammatory condition of the skin and subcutaneous tissue of the nose.

Etiology: Streptococcus.

Symptoms: Initially there is a localized red, elevated area that is hot and tender to touch. Vesicle formation may result. The patient usually has fever, chills, and a generalized headache with associated malaise. The skin condition usually lasts from three to six days.

Treatment: Systemic penicillin is the drug of choice. Local treatment consists of cold, wet compresses of a saturated solution of magnesium sulfate.

4. LUPUS VULGARIS: Is a tuberculous process characterized by reddish patches composed of papules, nodules and flat infiltration. The terminal stage is ulceration, with resulting scarring.

Etiology: Tubercle bacillus is the causative agent.

Treatment: Systemic chemotherapy of tuberculosis with isoniazid, PAS and dehydrostreptomycin. Curettage followed by cauterization is helpful.

5. LUPUS ERYTHEMATOSUS: A systemic autoimmune disease which frequently involves the skin of the nose. There is usually a fatal outcome if the disorder becomes disseminated. In the early stages reddish spots appear on the lesions. These are elevated, rounded, and have a sharp margin. From the nose these spots extend into the cheeks and give the appearance of a butterfly. This has given the condition the name of "butterfly fever". Atrophic scarring with adherent whitish scales.

6. SYPHILIS: Is a specific chronic infectious disease that can infect the nose as well as any other area of the body.

Etiology: Treponema pallidum - The disease may be either congenital or acquired.

Symptoms: The primary lesion (chancre) appears three to four weeks after contact and is hard and papular, slightly painful, red and tender. The secondary lesions occur about six weeks following the primary lesion and cover every area of the body. They may be papular, macular or pustular. The nose may be thus involved with the secondary lesions. A persistent rhinitis results at this stage, along with generalized lymphadenitis. Deep fissures form in the vestibule.

Tertiary syphilis develops slowly, and the nose may show nodular gummatous formation, which may be ulcerative. These are painless and firm. Nasal obstruction, crusting, and a foul smelling discharge from the nose are present. Septal perforation may develop. In congenital syphilis the nares are usually involved and bony destruction takes place resulting in a "saddle nose" deformity.

Treatment: Penicillin.

7. SENILE KERATOSIS: Is a benign, slightly elevated brown-pigmented or black pigmented lesion covered with crusts or scales. May become malignant. The surface under the crusts and scales is vascular, and bleeding may occur if the crusts and scales are removed.

Treatment: By electrodesiccation and curettage.

8. RHINOPHYMA: Rhinophyma is a chronic inflammatory hypertrophy of the skin of the nose, primarily involving the area covering the cartilaginous portion. This actually resembles a benign tumor. This condition is caused by fibrosis and hyperplasia of the sebaceous glands of the nose, usually as a result of acne rosacea. It is most commonly seen in men past 40 or 50 years of age, and, associated with heavy drinking of alcoholic beverages.

Treatment: Shaving off excessive tissues. Skin grafting may be necessary. Radiation is of no benefit.

DISEASES OF THE INTERNAL NOSE

1. PERFORATION OF SEPTUM:
   Etiology:
   (1) Trauma (septal surgery, constant picking)
   (2) Hematoma or abscess
   (3) Wegener's granulomatosis
   (4) Rhinitis sicca
   (5) Foreign body. Rhinoliths
   (6) Syphilis. Tuberculosis (rare)
   (7) Tuberculosis (rare)

(8) Lupus erythematosus
(9) Carcinoma (rare)
(10) Acute infections (typhoid fever, scarlet fever, diphtheria) rare.
(11) Acid fumes

Symptoms:
(1) Crusting and epistaxis are common
(2) Whistling sound on inspiration
(3) Foul crusts and discharge with pain if syphilitic
(4) Obstruction if crusts become large
(5) The perforation is usually in the bony part of the septum in syphilis and in the cartilaginous part in all other cases.

Treatment:
(1) Alkaline douche
(2) Ointment to reduce crusting
(3) Silver nitrate
(4) Surgical closure

2. SEPTAL HEMATOMA: A collection of blood beneath the mucoperichondrium and mucoperiosteum of the septum.

Etiology:
(1) Usually trauma. Diagnosis often missed.
(2) Septal surgery.
(3) Blood dyscrasias. Rare.

Symptoms:
(1) Nasal obstruction. Often complete.
(2) Fever and headache
(3) Septal abscess and cartilage necrosis if not recognized and treated early. The result is saddle nose.

Treatment:
(1) Incision and drainage
(2) Nasal packing to prevent reaccumulation of blood or pus.
(3) Systemic antibiotic

3. CHOANAL ATRESIA:[13,20,35] Choanal atresia is due to the failure of the bucconasal membrane to rupture at the 7th-8th week of embryonic life. It shows a familial tendency. It may be bilateral or unilateral, complete or incomplete. 75% of choanal atresia cases are unilateral. The incidence of bony atresia is 9 in 10, while that of membranous atresia is 1 in 10.

Symptoms: If the condition is unilateral, nasal obstruction and characteristic tenacious nasal discharge on the affected side are noted. If the condition is bilateral, the symptoms become evident immediately after birth and present a characteristic picture: cyclic dyspnea and cyanosis, which disappear on crying; discharge from the nares and difficulty in feeding. This may be fatal if the condition is not diagnosed and treated early. If the condition is unilateral, it does not require emergency measures. Excoriation of the nasal vestibule is frequently present.

Treatment: Surgical. The most successful operative technique is by the transpalatal approach.

4. FOREIGN BODIES: In children, a history of the introduction of a foreign body may not be obtained. Unilateral persistent purulent discharge (often in spite of antibiotic therapy) is characteristic. Epistaxis, pain, sneezing and obstruction are associated symptoms. A radiograph will confirm if the foreign body is radiopaque.

Treatment: Removal. General anesthesia may be necessary.

5. RHINOLITHS: A calcareous mass formed in the nasal passage by the deposit of salts from the nasal secretions. This is a condition produced by an endogenous foreign body composed of mineral salts, chiefly calcium and magnesium, encrusted upon an organic or inorganic nucleus of foreign body nature, or blood clot or secretion in the nasal passage.

Symptoms:
- (1) Unilateral nasal obstruction.
- (2) Progressive increase in severity.
- (3) Nasal discharge - watery, turning purulent and bloody if ulceration occurs.
- (4) Epistaxis if ulceration occurs.
- (5) Headache.

Treatment: Removal

6. CEREBROSPINAL RHINORRHEA:[19,20] A flow of cerebrospinal fluid from the nose. It may originate in the frontal sinus, sphenoid sinus, ethmoid sinus or cribriform plate. It may even originate in the mastoid or middle ear and reach the nasal space by way of the eustachian tube.

Etiology:
- (1) Traumatic:
  - a) Fracture of the anterior fossa of the skull involving the cribriform plate.
  - b) Penetrating wound
  - c) Postoperative intranasal and sinus surgery, transphenoidal hypophysectomy, etc.)
- (2) Nontraumatic:
  - a) Extracranial tumor (Osteomas of the ethmoid and frontal sinus are the most common)
  - b) Intracranial tumor (tumor of olfactory bulb and pituitary gland)
  - c) Congenital defects (encephalocele)

Symptoms:
- (1) Clear, watery, odorless and tasteless nasal discharge.
- (2) It is odorless, tasteless and free from albumin, mucin and sediment and contains glucose.
- (3) May be intermittent or constant and most often unilateral.
- (4) Has a specific gravity of 1.006.

(5) Flow of rhinorrhea may be characteristically accelerated with change in position.
(6) Discharge may be tested with paper strips for glucose.
(7) X-rays of the skull may show a fracture or air in the cranial cavity. The usual site of fracture is in the area of the frontal sinus or the cribriform plate.
(8) A most important method of identification and location of the source is by intrathecal injection of either indigo carmine or fluorescein.

Treatment:
(1) Conservative initially
(2) Avoid nose-blowing, sneezing and straining
(3) Surgical closure is indicated:
  a) When the leakage lasts more than six weeks.
  b) When the leakage is intermittent
  c) When pneumoencephalocele is present.
  d) When there is a history of meningitis and cerebrospinal otorrhea.
(4) Close the tear by fascia graft or mucoperiosteum of the nasal septum (Montgomery).

7. RHINOSCLEROMA: Rhinoscleroma is a chronic, specific, infectious type of disease, usually affecting the nose and the upper respiratory tract, with or without concomitant involvement of the skin around the nose and the mouth. The most frequent primary site is the anterior nare.

Etiology: Scleroma bacillus is rare on the North American continent and is usually found in the Orient, Russia and Central and South America. Living conditions and climate seem to be important predisposing factors.

Pathology:
(1) The blood vessels become thick-walled, and scattered hyaline bodies are noticed.
(2) Foam cells of Mikulicz containing the scleroma bacillus are seen in the dense fibrotic mucosa and submucosa. This fibrotic tissue compresses the blood vessels and causes the characteristic nasal stenosis.

Symptoms:
(1) Foul smelling secretions
(2) Crust formation
(3) Tumor formation
(4) Painless
(5) Nasal obstruction
(6) Nasal stenosis

Treatment:
(1) Deep x-ray and radium
(2) Streptomycin or tetracycline
(3) Surgical excision
(4) Potassium iodide or saline for foul smell

8. RELAPSING POLYCHONDRITIS: This is a disease of unknown etiology characterized by recurrent fever and inflammation of the nasal, vesicular and joint cartilages. 87% of this entity involves the auricle. It affects mainly the Caucasian race. The symptoms could include:

(1) Chondritis of the nasal cartilages, auricle, larynx, trachea and joints
(2) episcleritis and conjunctivitis
(3) anemia, elevated ESR

Pathologically there is a loss of basophilia with invasion of cartilage by histiocytes and plasma cells. Definitive diagnosis is made by the clinical course and a biopsy specimen.

Treatment: Steroids may help. The urine of the patients may contain acid mucopolysaccharides.

9. LETHAL MIDLINE GRANULOMA:[25] Lethal midline granuloma affects the male twice as often as the female. The age of predilection is in the 40's. It will ultimately involve all the midline structures about the head and neck but sparing the tongue. Pathologically, a broad zone of necrosis with lymphocytes, plasma cells, neutrophils is noted. Treatment consists of cortisone and supportive measures. Lethal midline granuloma is a localized disease while Wegener's Granulomatosis is a generalized disorder with three distinct pathological findings:

(1) Necrotizing granulomatous lesions in the upper respiratory tract.
(2) Glomerulitis, characterized by necrosis and thrombosis of loops of capillary tufts.
(3) Generalized focal necrotizing vasculitis involving both the arteries and the veins.

10. RHINOSPORIDOSIS:
Etiology: Rhinosporidium kinealyi or seeberi. Seen in India and Africa.

Symptoms:
(1) Bleeding, polyps in the nose

Treatment:
(1) Local excision
(2) Amphotericin B

11. GLANDERS: A contagious disease caused by Bacillus mallei, characterized by a purulent inflammation of nasal mucosa and nodules on the skin.

12. MUCORMYCOSIS: (Phycomycosis)[17,25,34,37] A malignant fungal infection of cranial (most often) pulmonary and, occasionally gastrointestinal blood vessels due to the class Phycomycetes. Mucor and Rhizopus are representative genera of the family Mocoraceae. Rhizopus is the most common cause of rhinomucormycosis, which

starts in the nose and rapidly spreads into the sinuses, orbit and cranial structures through the walls of vessels. Thrombosis of vessels is the main feature of this disease.

Symptoms:

(1) The patient is most often an uncontrolled diabetic. Also seen in patients with leukemia, burns, chronic renal disease, and on steroid therapy.
(2) A most characteristic sign is the thrombosed black nasal turbinate.[34] Bloody discharge may be present.
(3) Diagnosis is best made by culture and biopsy of the involved tissues. Broad non-septate hyphae are readily demonstrated.
(4) The most frequent manifestations are complete ophthalmoplegia (both internal and external), signs of acute diffuse cerebrovascular disease, and uncontrolled diabetic acidosis.
(5) X-rays show diffuse cloudiness of the involved sinuses without fluid level.
(6) Usually fatal within a few days after onset of the disease if unrecognized and untreated.

Treatment:

(1) Amphotericin B
(2) Local drainage and resection of the infected tissues in the nose and sinuses.
(3) Control of systemic disease.

13. EPISTAXIS:

Etiology: The local and systemic causes are summarized as follows:

	LOCAL	GENERAL CAUSES
CONGENITAL:	Telangiectasis (See Chapter 18, Osler-Rendu-Weber Disease)	Haemophilia or other coagulation defect
ACQUIRED:	Septal deformity	
TRAUMATIC:	Fractured nose, Foreign body, Nose picking	Crush injury Fractured skull and/or Middle one-third of face
INFLAMMATORY:		
acute:	Acute rhinitis Sinusitis	Hay fever, Exanthemata, glandular fever
chronic:	Chronic rhinitis, sinusitis, Syphilis, tuberculosis Actinomycosis	Pyacemia and septicemia

NEOPLASTIC:	Benign hemangioma, Carcinoma	Lymphosarcoma Leukemias
CIRCULATORY:	Back pressure from enlarged adenoids	Hypertension
BLOOD:		Purpuras
DYSCRASIAS:		Agranulocytosis
OTHERS:		Vicarious menstruation

The most common cause (90%) of this condition is a rupture of the veins or arteries in Kiesselbach's plexus on the nasal septum. Of the remaining cases (10%) most originate in the back of the nose, from the sphenopalatine vessels or from the nasopalatine plexus (of Woodruff), (from external carotid artery). If the bleeding occurs superiorly on the septum, it is usually from the anterior or posterior ethmoid vessels which are branches of the ophthalmic artery (from internal carotid artery).

Symptoms:

(1) Nasal hemorrhage
(2) If severe and uncontrolled, syncope anemia and death.

Treatment:

(1) Find bleeding point (seat the patient in a chair unless he is weak or in shock):
  a) Suction of clots and blood from the nose.
  b) Shrinkage (ephedrine, cocaine)
(2) Stop bleeding:
  a) Epinephrine or ephedrine packs. Apply pressure.
  b) Petrolatum gauze packs
  c) Premarin
  d) Thrombin packs
(3) Cauterize:
  a) Chemocautery (silver nitrate)
  b) Electrocautery: (5% cocaine or 2% pontocaine provides sufficient anesthesia.)
(4) Ensure rest-Hospitalization:
  a) Sedatives
  b) Morphine
(5) Avoid trauma of all types to nose
(6) Treat cause of bleeding
(7) May require transfusion
(8) Severe forms may require:

a) Postnasal packing: (for severe epistaxis from vessels in the posterior part of the nose, most commonly from the sphenopalatine vessels) -- Conventional posterior pack, Steven's balloon, etc.

b) Ligation of anterior ethmoid artery: (Kirchner 1961)[16] (for severe epistaxis from vessels high in the nose posteriorly) -- This procedure done via an external ethmoidectomy approach is sometimes combined with ligation of the maxillary artery when bleeding site of severe posterior epistaxis cannot be identified.[29] In such event, anterior ethmoid artery ligation should precede transantral maxillary artery ligation to avoid oral contamination of the orbital contents.

c) Transantral ligation of internal maxillary artery: (Chandler 1965)[4,7,18,20,28] (for uncontrolled posterior epistaxis) --

(1) When packing is ineffective in controlling the epistaxis from vessels below the level of the middle turbinate, maxillary artery ligation via the Caldwell-Luc approach is indicated.

(2) Maxillary artery ligation is indicated in recurrent, severe posterior epistaxis when the risk of continued medical treatment with packing, sedation, and blood transfusions outweighs the risks of operation. After this procedure the nasal mucosa does not become necrotic from ischemia, and some blood supply continues to perfuse the nose. For this reason maxillary artery ligation should be thought of as an adjunctive procedure in the overall management plan. (Pearson)[23]

(3) Study x-rays of the sinuses preoperatively to determine the size and configuration of the antrum. A small undeveloped or one severely sclerosed from infection or prior surgery contraindicates this procedure.[28]

(4) Branches of the third division of the maxillary artery seen in the pterygopalatine fossa are:
   (1) posterior superior alveolar artery
   (2) infraorbital artery
   (3) vidian artery
   (4) descending palatine artery
   (5) pharyngeal artery
   (6) sphenopalatine artery

(5) According to Pearson[26], three clips are essential to sequester the arterial segment that can supply the nasal cavity. These are;
   (1) on maxillary artery just proximal to the origin of the descending palatine artery
   (2) on maxillary artery as high and medially as possible behind orbital process of palatine bone
   (3) on descending palatine artery as distally as possible

(6) The periosteum outside the posterior wall of the antrum is thin. Do not incise it deeply or the maxillary artery lying behind it may be transected.

(7) Selective external and internal carotid angiography may define the site of bleeding in patients with uncontrolled epistaxis.[10]

Recent elucidation of normal angiography anatomy has made this technique increasingly useful.[3]

Intractable epistaxis may be controlled by percutaneous transcatheter Gelfoam embolization.[36]

d) Ligation of external carotid artery

e) Ligation of superior labial artery: (for recurrent anterior septal bleeder) (Saunders)
f) Submucous resection
g) Septodermoplasty: (Saunders)[12,30] Indicated for hemorrhagic hereditary telangiectasia (Rendu-Osler-Weber disease), an unusual cause of recurrent and severe nosebleeds. The disorder affects most organs and epithelial surfaces, but usually the patient bleeds only from the nose or gastrointestinal tract. Saunders' septal dermoplasty is an effective operation to control bleeding in these patients. It uses as its principle the fact that although these patients have telangiectases on the skin and oral mucosa, lesions covered by squamous epithelium are tough and resist trauma. Nasal mucosa, on the other hand, is exceptionally fragile.

   A graft of split-thickness skin from the thigh is placed in the nose to cover the anterior parts of the septum and the floor and lateral walls of the nose anteriorly. A raw surface for grafting is created by scraping off the mucous membrane, but not the perichondrium. The grafts are held in place five days by appropriate nasal packing. Usually there is great reduction in the severity and frequency of epistaxis after septal dermoplasty. Some patients never bleed again.
h) Cryotherapy[15,24]
i) Injection of pterygopalatine fossa with glycerin.[39]

14. ANOSMIA:

Etiology:

(1) Intranasal:
   a) polyps
   b) infection
   c) tumor
   d) atrophic rhinitis
   e) allergy
   f) deviated septum, marked
(2) Intracranial:
   a) meningioma
   b) frontal lobe tumor (Foster Kennedy syndrome, see Chapter 18)
(3) Trauma
(4) Infection:
   a) meningitis
   b) brain abscess
   c) osteomyelitis
(5) Congenital
(6) Hysterical
(7) Idiopathic

For the idiopathic group, Vitamin A at a dosage of 100,000 units per cc. given intramuscularly once a week for six weeks followed by 50,000 units once a day orally for 12 weeks has been advocated as a treatment.

Parosmia: perverted sense of smell
Hyperosmia: over-sensitive sense of smell
Hyposmia: impaired sense of smell
Anosmia: total loss of smell
Cocosmia: a sense of foul smell when none is present

COMPLICATIONS OF SINUS DISEASE:[5,12,20,25]

ORBITAL MANIFESTATIONS OF SINUS DISEASE:

1) Orbital pain
2) Exophthalmos
3) Lid swelling
4) Epiphora
5) Mass in the orbit
6) Orbital cellulitis
7) Cavernous sinus thrombosis
8) Retrobulbar neuritis
9) Superior orbital fissure syndrome

ORBITAL CELLULITIS:

Symptoms:

1) Lid edema
2) Exophthalmos
3) Chemosis of conjunctiva
4) Progressive immobility of the eye
5) Very ill with high fever
6) Severe pain
7) X-rays show the origin of infection
8) The ethmoid sinus is the most common site of origin

Treatment:

1) Intensive antibiotic therapy
2) Exploration of orbit with I&D. A point of breakthrough may be seen.
3) External ethmoidectomy

RETROBULBAR NEURITIS:

1) Approximately 15% of retrobulbar neuritis are caused by sinus disease.
2) Spread of infection directly through the sinus wall or by phlebitis.
3) Loss of vision may be sudden or gradual.
4) Remember that benign and malignant tumors of the sinuses and the pituitary gland can also cause blindness.

Treatment:

1) Antibiotics
2) Specific surgery of involved sinus

SUPERIOR ORBITAL FISSURE SYNDROME:

1) Superior orbital fissure contains
   a) third CN
   b) fourth CN
   c) sixth CN

d) first division of the fifth CN
e) ophthalmic vein
f) sympathetic nerve from the cavernous plexus

2) The lateral wall of the sphenoid sinus, when well pneumatized, is in close proximity to the superior orbital fissure.
3) This syndrome involves the above mentioned structures and may be caused by:
   a) Acute and chronic sphenoiditis
   b) Cystic lesions (mucocele, craniopharyngioma)
   c) Benign and malignant neoplasm
4) The 6th nerve is the first to be affected, followed by the 3rd, 4th and 5th nerves, exophthalmos and, finally, total ophthalmoplegia.

Treatment: Immediate exploration via the transethmoidal approach.

CAVERNOUS SINUS THROMBOSIS: [20,25]

Etiology:
1) Sphenoid sinusitis (directly)
2) Frontal sinusitis (via frontal diploic, supraorbital and ophthalmic veins)
3) Infection of upper face (via facial and ophthalmic veins).
4) Infection of the ear (via superior and inferior petrosal sinus).
5) Infection of the pharynx and maxilla (via the veins of the pterygoid plexus).

Clinical features:
1) May be unilateral or bilateral. Symptoms develop abruptly
2) Sudden periorbital edema and orbital cellulitis
3) Exophthalmos
4) Orbital pain
5) Papilledema
6) Complete external and internal ophthalmoplegia
7) Very ill with chills, fever, nausea and vomiting, mental dullness
8) Terminal symptoms are similar to those of meningitis. May be fatal.

Treatment:
1) Conservative sinus surgery
2) Intensive antibiotics
3) Anticoagulation

OSTEOMYELITIS OF THE FRONTAL BONE: [20]

Osteomyelitis is most commonly seen in the frontal sinus and rarely in the others. This results from thrombophlebitis of the dural vessels. In the adults, the frontal bone derives all its nourishment from these vessels. It is more common in females.

Organism:
1) Staphylococcus (most common), Streptococcus, pneumococcus

Etiology:
1) In children the origin is hematogenous
2) In adults from trauma during acute frontal sinusitis. Often follows swimming.
3) Frontal sinus surgery

Symptoms:
1) In fulminating acute types:
   a) Edema of upper eye lid
   b) Fever and headache
   c) Soft, doughy swelling (Pott's puffy tumor) or pericranial abscess is pathognomonic
2) In chronic localized type:
   a) Insidious onset
   b) Low grade fever
   c) Local pain and tenderness
   d) Doughy swelling of forehead
   e) Fistula may form

Diagnosis: X-rays show localized discalcification of the bone or actual destruction.

Treatment:
1) Antibiotics (Penicillin is the choice)
2) I&D
3) Trephine operation of frontal sinus (es)
4) Osteoplastic adipose obliteration operation (later)

OSTEOMYELITIS OF THE SUPERIOR MAXILLA:[20]
Etiology:
1) Usually secondary to dental infection
2) Occasionally, in infants, due to buccal infection
3) May produce periosteitis and osteitis with fistula tract formation extending to:
   a) facial surface of cheek breaking down of Bichat's pad
   b) to the palatine and alveolar process with fistula into the roof of the mouth
   c) to the zygomatic process with necrosis of zygomatic arch and extension into pterygoid fossa.

Symptoms:
1) Swelling and chemosis of the cheek
2) Exophthalmos
3) Limitation of eye movement

Treatment:
1) Antibiotics
2) Surgical drainage
3) Heat

4. OSTEOMYELITIS OF THE SPHENOID BONE:[20]
Quite rare.

Etiology: Usually hemolytic streptococcus and beta hemolytic staphylococcus aureus.

Symptoms:
1) Profound postnasal discharge
2) Deep seated headache "behind the eyes"
3) May develop "superior orbital fissure syndrome"
4) Sepsis
5) Increase in retroorbital and temporal pain
6) Cavernous sinus thrombosis, brain abscess, encephalitis and intracranial hemorrhage
7) Usually not diagnosed till late

Treatment:
1) Antibiotic therapy
2) Surgical drainage

FRONTAL SINUS PNEUMATOCELE: (Pneumocele)[20, 23]

1. A collection of air, under pressure, in the tissues. The air escapes from a defect in the bony wall of the frontal sinus and collects adjacent to the sinus.
2. If the defect is on the forehead, an external pneumocele results.
3. If the defect is in the posterior wall of the sinus, an internal or intracranial pneumocele develops.
4. An excessive dilation of the sinus (pneumosinus dilations) may also occur, often associated with acromegaly or localized osteitis.
5. Pneumocele may follow trauma, operation, congenital cleft, dehiscence or necrosis of the bone.

INTRACRANIAL COMPLICATIONS OF SINUS DISEASE:[20,25]

1. Possible intracranial complications from nasal and sinus diseases include:
   a) Meningitis
   b) Extradural and subdural abscess
   c) Dural fistula
   d) Brain abscesses
   e) Thrombosis of the cavernous sinus or superior longitudinal sinus.

2. Intracranial complications are more apt to result from acute infections of the sinuses then from chronic infections.

3. More common in males than in females (4 to 1).

4. Pathways of infection from the nose and sinuses to the intracranial structures are:
   a) Through traumatic defects
   b) Through congenital dehiscences or nonclosure of fetal defects.
   c) Directly through the sinus wall.
   d) Along the sheath of the olfactory nerve.
   e) Via communicating veins
   f) Via diploic veins with a retrograde thrombophlebitis to the cavernous sinus

g) Via the angular or ethmoid veins to the cavernous sinus
h) Via the orbit

5. Temporal lobe abscess most commonly originates from infection in the temporal bone and lateral sinus.

6. Temporal lobe abscess can originate from the sphenoid sinus or indirectly from the other sinuses by way of the cavernous sinus.

7. Frontal lobe abscess may result from acute and chronic frontal sinusitis or tumors of the frontal sinus (such as osteoma) following surgical treatment of frontal and ethmoidal sinus or trauma to the forehead.

Symptoms: Chills, fever, severe headache, nausea, vomiting, and mental dullness. Increasing intracranial pressure will bring on ophthalmic symptoms such as pupil changes, optic nerve changes, visual disturbances, muscle paralysis and papilledema. Mental symptoms include mental dullness, convulsions, personality changes, aphasia, and twitching. The terminal symptoms are coma, rapid pulse, stiff neck, high fever, delirium, twitching, hyperesthesia, paralysis, and death.

Treatment: Surgical drainage and antibiotics.

8. Meningitis is seen in infections of the frontal, sphenoid, or ethmoid sinuses.

Symptoms: Consist of severe headache, fever, nausea, vomiting, anorexia, neck rigidity, increased reflexes, slow pulse, prostration, Cheyne-Stokes respiration, cranial nerve involvement, papilledema, and positive spinal taps. The terminal stages are coma and death.

Spinal fluid examination and culture of the fluid help identify the causative organism. This helps in the selection of the antibiotic.

Treatment:
1. High doses of the antibiotics
2. Surgical intervention to establish drainage is often necessary.

BENIGN TUMORS OF THE NOSE AND SINUSES: [8,23,25]

PAPILLOMA:

1. Usually found in the area of the alae or the nasal vestibule. No malignant degeneration.
2. These are hard, dry, wartlike tumors of various sizes.
3. If this type of tumor is found more posteriorly in the nasal passage, it has a tendency to be more mucoid, softer, varying in size, and rather vascular.
4. The tumor may extend into the sinuses and, if so, is of the cauliflower type. These may be single or multiple, unilateral or bilateral. There is an excessive proliferation of the lining epithelium and connective tissue, and less proliferation of the underlying stroma.

5. These tumors may be asymptomatic, or they may produce nasal obstruction.
6. Occasionally nasal hemorrhage occurs.

Treatment:
1. Surgical removal followed by cautery.
2. Simple electrocautery is sufficient for the lesion in the area of the vestibule.

INVERTING PAPILLOMA: [8,11,25]
1. Usually arises from the lateral wall rather than from the septum.
2. About 13% become malignant.
3. Characterized by microscopic invagination of surface epithelium into the stroma of the polyp. Histological section shows a papilloma covered by epithelium with islands of epithelium within and completely surrounded by a fibrous stroma.
4. May present as a fleshy polyp.

Treatment: Complete wide excision via lateral rhinotomy. Inadequate excision is followed by local recurrences, each progressively more destructive. Although histologically benign, this tumor acts clinically in a malignant fashion.

LIPOMA: The lipoma is an extremely rare type of tumor in the nasal cavity. If found there, these tumors are usually pendulous and smooth or lobulated. They are composed of fatty cells covered with mucous membrane. Usually they are found near the alae of the nose.

Treatment: Surgical excision.

POLYPS: [21, 31, 38] Polyps are probably the most common form of tumor to be found in the nose.

ADENOMA: An epithelial tumor of glandular structure surrounded by a fibrous capsule. Such tumors are usually very vascular and when found are located in the nasal cavity, on the septum, or in the ethmoid area.

Symptoms: Nasal obstruction and possibly a bloody nasal discharge.

Treatment: Complete surgical excision followed by electrocautery of an extensive nature.

LYMPHANGIOMA: The lymphangioma is a rare type of benign tumor, so far as the nose is concerned. These grossly appear as a smooth type of growth, having a bright red color and varying in size. They may be single or multiple. Treatment should consist of excision followed by electrodesiccation.

HEMANGIOMA: Hemangioma may be of either the capillary or the cavernous type.
1. Capillary hemangiomas consist of loosely arranged tissue containing thin-walled blood vessels. They are covered with stratified or pedunculated, dark red-colored tumor occurring most frequently on the nasal septum. It is very vascular.

Treatment: Excision and electrocautery.

2. The cavernous type of hemangioma consists of thin-walled growth with an afferent and an efferent vein that do not communicate with the neighboring capillaries. These tumors usually are seen in the lateral wall of the nose, and they grow by infiltration. Thus they can destroy the surrounding tissue and cause severe epistaxis. This type of hemangioma may become so large that it can fill the entire nasal cavity.

Treatment:
1. Surgical removal and electrocautery
2. Ligation of the external carotid artery may be necessary in some cases.

Hemangiomatous polyps of the nasal septum are found, but they are not a common type of nasal tumor. They are chiefly found in the Kiesselbach's area. Found more in adults.

Treatment: Removal by snare followed by cautery of the base.

OSTEOMA:[2] The osteoma is a true bone tumor. The most common site is the frontal sinus, and then the ethmoid, the maxillary, and the sphenoid, in that order.

Osteomas can produce obstruction if their size is sufficiently large. These tumors are composed of dense, compact cancellous bone. They are slow-growing, but they may be dangerous because they may extend into the orbital or nasal cavities or even into the cranial fossa. Headache is common. Massive necrosis of the brain tissue may prove to be fatal. The formation of osteomas may be related to the development of the paranasal sinuses.

Diagnosis: By radiologic examination.

Treatment: Surgical removal. Incomplete removal will result in recurrence: Osteoplastic obliteration may be indicated for larger osteomas.[2,33]

ANGIOFIBROMA: (Juvenile Nasopharyngeal Angiofibroma)[5,6,8,9] Relatively rare tumor composed of vascular and fibrous tissue. Predominantly found in adolescent males. Derived from the perichondrium of the embryonal cartilage that joins the basiocciput to the body of the sphenoid. They may also arise from the internal ptorygoid plate, the pterygoid maxillary fossa, the nasal choanae, the first two cervical vertebrae, or the eustachian tube orifice.

Symptoms:
1. Nasal obstruction and epistaxis (recurrent and severe).
2. Biopsy, rarely necessary, is best done under general anesthesia in the operating room prepared for severe hemorrhage.
3. The tumor may be pedunculated or sessile.
4. Classic radiographic picture is a soft tissue mass in the nasopharynx associated with an anterior bulge of the posterior wall of the maxillary sinus.

5. Carotid angiography coupled with subtraction technique further support the diagnosis and aid in the selection of surgical approach. Polytomography is also very useful.

Treatment:
1. Transpalatal excision
2. Lateral rhinotomy and antrostomy may be necessary. Recurrence of the lesion is commonly 50%.
3. Hormonal therapy may be helpful.
4. Cryotherapy
5. Radiation is of minor adjunctive use.

Prognosis: The tumor may involute with increasing age.

NASAL GLIOMA:
1. This is not a neoplasm, but rather a congenital abnormality consisting of herniation of brain tissue through a dehiscence in the floor of the anterior cranial fossa.
2. It may present as rounded, firm swellings either on the bridge or the nose or intranasally.
3. Intranasally it is firmly fixed to the turbinate and vault of the nasal cavity.
4. There may be a bone defect in the frontal bone through which a stalk connects the tumor with the brain.

Treatment:
1. Intracranial repair of an encephalocele first, followed by intranasal removal of the tumor. Otherwise, cerebrospinal rhinorrhea may result.
2. Recurrence is rare.

MENINGOCELE:[25, 32] A meningocele is actually a herniated protrusion of the meninges, which may extend intranasally, but it is rare. The mucous membrane may be pushed forward and there may be brain tissue within the meningocele. It is then called meningo-encephalocele. The tumor appears to be continuous with the mucous membrane of the septum. These tumors are elastic, and frequently pulsations are visible.

CHONDROMA: Is a rare type of tumor found on the cartilaginous portion of the nasal septum. Grossly it resembles an osteoma. These tumors develop very slowly and have a great tendency toward recurrence.

Treatment: Excision and cautery.

CYST:
Radicular cyst develops from an apical abscess of an erupted tooth.

Globulomaxillary cyst is a fissural cyst in the bone at the junction of the premaxilla and maxillary process. No relation to teeth.

Nasoalveolar cyst is a developmental cyst located in the soft tissue at the junction of the premaxilla and the alveolar process of the maxilla. The etiology is believed to be incomplete degeneration of trapped respiratory epithelium from the floor of the nose during fusion between the premaxillary and maxillary processes.

Rathke's pouch tumor. These are microscopic cysts lined with squamous cells and filled with keratin. Embryologically, the anterior lobe of the pituitary gland is formed by a fusion between the infundibulum and an invagination of oral ectoderm. The pouch formed by this invagination is called Rathke's pouch. Normally it is obliterated. Squamous inclusion cysts may develop in the pouch.

Dermoid cysts are seen most frequently in children. They are painless swellings in the midline of the nose, often associated with indentation of the adjacent skin. The embryologic features of these cysts are not clear, but dermoid elements may persist as deeply as the cribriform plate. Some dermoid cysts originate from remnants of dura mater situated between the nasal septal cartilages.

Nasopharyngeal cyst (Tornwaldt's cyst). A cyst which develops in the nasopharyngeal sac situated just beneath the adenoid and its remnants. This sac, which derives from the pharyngeal segment of the notochord, extends backward and upward to the periosteum of the occipital bone.

MUCOCELE:[5,12,22,25] Mucocele is defined as the accumulation and retention of mucoid material within a sinus as a result of continuous or periodic obstruction of the osteum of the sinus. When infected, it is called a pyocele.

Mucoceles are most frequently found in the frontal sinus. Mucoceles erode and expand the sinus walls as the intraluminal pressure increases. They may erode either the anterior or posterior wall of the frontal sinus. A tender fluctuant mass may be present in the supraorbital region. It may displace the globe. If the posterior wall is eroded, epidural or subdural abscess, meningitis or brain abscess may develop. Treatment is surgical removal. Osteoplastic obliteration procedure is recommended.[2,20,33]

Mucocele of the ethmoid sinus may displace the orbital contents resulting in exophthalmos and diplopia or orbital apex syndrome. Treatment is surgical.

Mucoceles of the sphenoid sinus are rare. Recurrent headache and visual disturbances are characteristic symptoms. Exophthalmos and cerebrospinal rhinorrhea may be present. Radiographic examination shows cloudiness of the sphenoid sinus with erosion of the interseptum, ballooning and rarefaction of the sinus wall. Tomography and angiography are essential. The mucocele of the sphenoid sinus should not be mistaken for a malignant lesion because of destruction of the bony structures.

It is essential that the correct diagnosis be made before planning treatment (radiotherapy). Transethmoidal sphenoidotomy will confirm the diagnosis and adequate drainage and exenteration of the sinus may dramatically cure this condition.[22]

REFERENCES

1. Alberti, P.W.: Applied surgical anatomy of the maxillary sinus. Otolaryngol. Clin. N. Am. 9:3-20, 1976.

2. Alford, B.R., Gorman, G.N. and Mersol, V.F.: Osteoplastic surgery of frontal sinus. Laryngoscope 75:1139-1150, 1965.

3. Allen, W.E., Kier, E.L. and Rothman, S.L.G.: The maxillary artery: normal arteriographic anatomy. Am. J. Roentgenol. 118:517-527, 1973.

4. Bernstein, L. (ed.): Symposium on surgery of the nasal sinuses. Otolaryng. Clin. N. Am. Vol. 4, No. 1, 1971.

5. Ballenger, J.J. (ed.): Diseases of the nose, throat and ear. 11th ed. Lea and Febiger, Philadelphia, 1969.

6. Biller, H.F., Sessions, D.G. and Ogura, J.H.: Angiofibroma: treatment approach. Laryngoscope 84:695-706, 1974.

7. Chandler, J.R. and Serrins, A.J.: Transantral ligation of internal maxillary artery for epistaxis. Laryngoscope 75:1151-1159, 1965.

8. Chandler, J.R., de laCruz, A. and Pickard, R.E.: Tumors of the nose and sinuses and their surgical treatment, in Maloney, W.H. (ed.): Otolaryngology, Harper & Row, Hagerstown, Md., Chapter 22, 1973.

9. Christiansen, T.A., et al.: Juvenile nasopharyngeal angiofibroma. Trans. Am. Acad. Ophthalmol. Otolaryng. 78:140-147, 1974.

10. Coel, M.N. and Janon, E.A.: Angiography in patients with intractable epistaxis. Am. J. Roentgenol. 116:37-40, 1972.

11. Cummings, C. and Goodman, M.L.: Inverted papillomas of the nose and paranasal sinuses. Arch. Otolaryng. 92:445-449, 1970.

12. DeWeese, D.D. and Saunders, W.H.: Textbook of otolaryngology. 3rd ed. St. Louis, C.V. Mosby Co., 1968.

13. Fearon, B. and Dickson, J.: Bilateral choanal atresia in the newborn: plan of action. Laryngoscope 78:1487-1499, 1968.

14. Harrison, D.F.N.: Surgical anatomy of maxillary and ethmoidal sinuses - a reappraisal. Laryngoscope 81:1658-1664, 1971.

15. Hollingshead, W.H.: Anatomy for surgeons: Vol. 1 - the head and neck, ed. 2. Hoeber Medical Division, Harper & Row Publishers, New York, 1968.

16. Kirchner, J.A.: Surgical treatment of nasal hemorrhage. Surgery. 50:899-904, 1961.

17. Lowe, J. T. and Hudson, W. R.: Rhinocerebral phycomycosis and internal carotid artery thrombosis. Arch. Otolaryng. 101: 100-103, 1975.

18. Montgomery, W.W., Katz, R. and Gamble, J.F.: Anatomy and surgery of the pterygomaxillary fossa. Ann. Otol. Rhin. & Laryng. 79:606-618, 1970.

19. Montgomery, W.W.: Surgery for cerebrospinal fluid, rhinorrhea and otorrhea. Arch. Otolaryng. 84:538-550, 1966.

20. Montgomery, W.W.: Surgery of the upper respiratory system. Vol. 1, Lea and Febiger, Philadelphia, 1973.

21. Myers, D. and Myers, E.N.: Medical and surgical treatment of nasal polyps. Laryngoscope 84:833-847, 1974.

22. Norman, P.S. and Yanagisawa, E.: Mucocele of sphenoid sinus: report of a case. Arch. Otolaryng. 79:646-652, 1964.

23. Noyek, A.M. and Zizmor, J. (ed.): Symposium on the maxillary sinus. Otolaryng. Clin. N. Am., Vol. 9, No. 1, 1976.

24. Ozenberger, J.M.: Cyrosurgery in chronic rhinitis. Laryngoscope 80:723-734, 1970.

25. Paparella, M.M. and Shumrick, D.A.: Otolaryngology, Vol. 3: head and neck. W.B. Saunders Co., Philadelphia, 1973.

26. Pearson, B.W., MacKenzie, R.G. and Goodman, W.S.: Anatomic basis of transantral ligation of maxillary artery in severe epistaxis. Laryngoscope 79:969-984, 1969.

27. Peele, J.C.: Unusual anatomical variations of the sphenoid sinuses. Laryngoscope 67:208-237, 1957.

28. Ritter, F.N.: The paranasal sinuses: anatomy and surgical technique. C.V. Mosby Co., St. Louis, 1973.

29. Rosnagle, R.S., Yanagisawa, E. and Smith, H.W.: Specific vessel ligation for epistaxis: survery of 60 cases. Laryngoscope 83:517-525, 1973.

30. Saunders, W.H.: Septal dermoplasty - ten years' experience. Trans. Am. Acad. Ophthal. Otol. 72:153-160, 1968.

31. Schenck, N.L.: Nasal polypectomy in the aspirin - sensitive asthmatic. Trans. Am. Acad. Ophthal. Otol. 78:109-119, 1974.

32. Schmidt, P.H. and Luyendijk, W.: Intranasal meningoencephalocele. Arch. Otolaryng. 99:402-405, 1974.

33. Sessions, R.B., Alford, B.R., Stratton, C., Ainsworth, J.Z. and Shill, O.: Current concepts of frontal sinus surgery: appraisal of osteoplastic flap fat obliteration operation. Laryngoscope 82:918-930, 1972.

34. Smith, H.W. and Kirchner, J.A.: Cerebral mucormycosis: a report of three cases. Arch. Otolaryng. 68:715-726, 1958.

35. Smith, H.W. and Holmes, R.: Congenital choanal atresia - a technique for surgical correction. Trans. Am. Acad. Ophthal. Otolaryng. 80: (ORL) 527-535, 1975.

36. Sokoloff, J., et al.: Therapeutic percutaneous embolization in intractable epistaxis. Radiology 111:285-287, 1974.

37. Stephan, T., et al.: Rhinocerebral phycomycosis (mucormycosis). Laryngoscope 83:173-178, 1973.

38. Taylor, B., Evans, J.N.G. and Hope, G.A.: Upper respiratory tract in cystic fibrosis: ear - nose - throat survey of 50 children. Arch. Dis. Child. 49:133-136, 1974.

39. Weingarten, C.A.: Injection of pterygopalatine fossa with glycerin for posterior epistaxis. Trans. Am. Acad. Ophthal. 76:932-937, 1972.

CHAPTER 12

THE LARYNX

I. EMBRYOLOGY OF THE LARYNX

Figure 12-1.A, B, C, D [3, 17, 47]

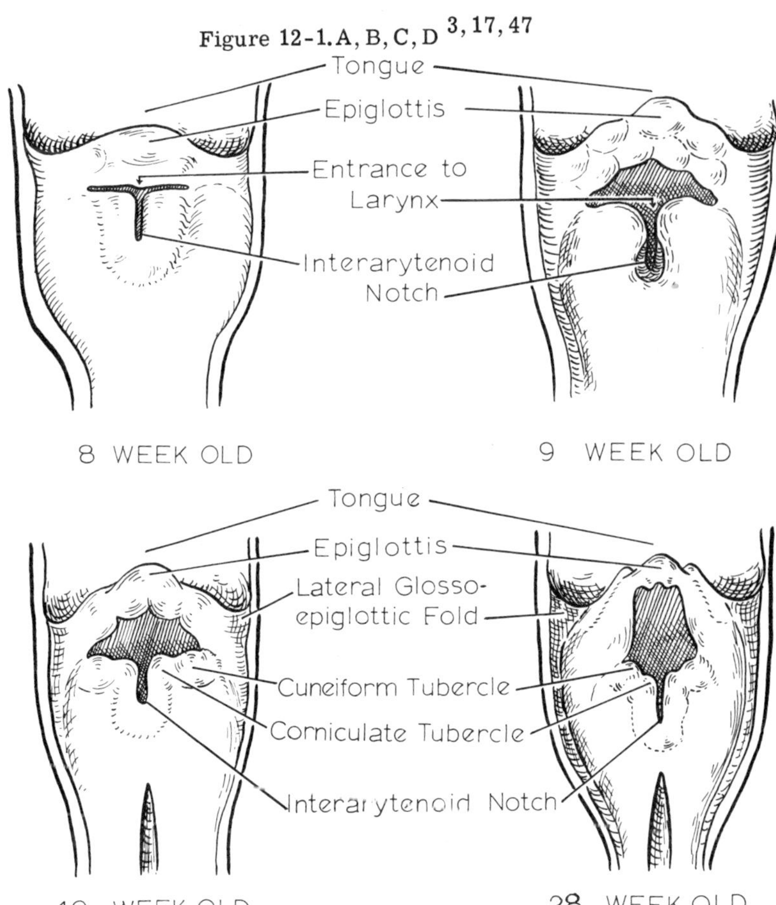

FIGURE 12-1.A, B, C, D

The entire respiratory system is an outgrowth of the primitive pharynx. At $3\frac{1}{2}$ weeks, a groove called the Laryngotracheal groove develops in the embryo at the ventral aspect of the foregut. This groove is just posterior to the hypobranchial eminence and is located closer to the 4th Arch than to the 3rd Arch. In embryonic development, when a single tubal structure is to later become two tubal structures the original tube is first obliterated by a proliferation of lining epithelium, then, as resorption of the epithelium takes place, the 2nd tube is formed and the 1st tube is recannulized. Hence, any malformation will involve both tubes. This process of growth accounts for the fact that more than 90% of tracheal-esophageal fistulae are associated with esophageal atresia. During development, the mesenchyme of the foregut grows medially from the sides, "pinching off" this groove to create a separate opening. With further maturation, two separate tubes are formed: the esophagus and the laryngotracheal apparatus.

This laryngotracheal opening is the primitive laryngeal aditus and lies between the 4th and 5th Arches. The sagittal slit opening is altered to become a T-shaped opening by the growth of three tissue masses:

1. The hypobranchial eminence which first appears on the 3rd week. This mesodermal structure gives rise to the <u>furcula</u> which later develops into the epiglottis.
2. The two arytenoid masses which appear on the 5th week. Later, each arytenoid swelling shows two additional swellings which eventually mature into the cuneiform and corniculate cartilages.

As these masses grow between the 5th and 7th week, the laryngeal lumen is obliterated. On the 9th week the oval shape lumen is reestablished. Failure to recannulize may result in atresia or stenosis of the larynx. The true and false cords are formed between the 8th and 10th week. The ventricles are formed at the 12th week.

The two arytenoid masses are separated by an "interarytenoid notch" which later becomes obliterated. Failure of this obliteration to occur would result in a posterior cleft up to the cricoid cartilage and opening into the esophagus, the culprit of severe aspiration in the newborn.

The following tables illustrate the muscular and cartilaginous development of the larynx.

<u>Muscular Development of the Larynx</u>

4 weeks old: Inferior pharyngeal constrictor and cricothyroid muscles are formed

$5\frac{1}{2}$ weeks old: Interarytenoid and post cricoarytenoid muscles are formed

6 weeks old: Lateral cricoarytenoid muscle is formed

<u>Cartilage Development</u>

3 weeks old: Development of epiglottis takes place (Hypobranchial eminence)
5 weeks old: Thyroid cartilage (IV Arch) and cricoid cartilage (V Arch) appear
7 weeks old: Chondrification of these two cartilages begins
12 weeks old: Development and chondrification of arytenoid (V Arch) and corniculate (V Arch) takes place. (Vocal process is the last to develop)

20 weeks old: Chondrification of the epiglottis occurs
28 weeks old: Development of the cuneiform cartilage (IV Arch) occurs

The laryngeal muscles are derivatives from the mesoderm of the 4th and 5th Arches and hence are innervated by the X nerve.

The infant larynx is situated at a level between the 2nd and 3rd cervical vertebrae. In the adult, it lies opposite the body of the fifth cervical vertebrae.

II. ANATOMY [3, 10, 32]

The larynx consists of a framework of cartilages, held in position by an intrinsic and extrinsic musculature, and lined by mucous membrane which is arranged in characteristic folds.

The larynx is situated in front of the fourth, fifth, and sixth cervical vertebrae. The upper portion of the larynx, which is continuous with the pharynx above, is almost triangular in shape; the lower portion leading into the trachea presents a circular appearance.

LARYNGEAL CARTILAGES:

1. Laryngeal cartilages form the main framework of the larynx and consist of:
   a) Thyroid cartilage (unpaired)
   b) Cricoid cartilage (unpaired)
   c) Epiglottis (unpaired)
   d) Arytenoid cartilage (paired)
   e) Corniculate cartilage (paired)
   f) Cuneiform cartilage (paired)

2. Thyroid cartilage (hyaline cartilage) is the largest and encloses the larynx anteriorly and laterally, thus shielding it from all but the most forceful blows. This cartilage is composed of two alae which meet anteriorly, dipping down from above to form the thyroid notch before meeting at the protuberance of the Adam's apple. Posteriorly, each wing has a superior cornu, extending upward about 2 cm. and a much shorter inferior cornu, which articulates with the cricoid cartilage below. This is the only direct articulation of the thyroid cartilage, all other relationships with contiguous structures being maintained by muscles or ligaments.

3. Cricoid cartilage (hyaline cartilage) lies directly below the thyroid cartilage. It is the strongest of the laryngeal cartilages, and is shaped like a signet ring. The flat portion of the ring or lamina is located posteriorly and extends upward to form the posterior border of the larynx. Since the cricoid cartilage forms the only complete annular support of the laryngeal skeleton, its preservation is essential for the maintenance of the enclosed airway. In the adult, the cricoid cartilage is at the level of C6-C7 and in the child at the level of C3-C4.

Posterolaterally, the cricoid articulates with the inferior cornua of the thyroid cartilage with which it shares true synovial joints. These joints permit a rocking action of the cricoid cartilage on the thyroid cartilage and also a slight anteroposterior sliding motion. Also through synovial joints, the cricoid cartilage on its posterosuperior aspect supports the two arytenoid cartilages.

4. Epiglottis (fibroelastic cartilage) is a leaf-shaped structure attached to the inside of the thyroid cartilage anteriorly and projecting upward and backward above the laryngeal opening. The petiole is the small, narrow portion of the epiglottis that is attached to the thyroid cartilage.

5. Arytenoid cartilages (mostly hyaline cartilages) are much smaller in size, yet they are primarily responsible for the opening and closing of the larynx. Roughly pyramidal in shape, they rest on the upper edge of the cricoid lamina at the posterior border of the larynx. The anterior projection of each arytenoid, or vocal process, receives the attachment of the posterior or mobile end of each vocal cord. The lateral prominence of each arytenoid cartilage is known as the muscular process because of the insertion of numerous muscles. The arytenoids articulate with the cricoid cartilage at the cricoarytenoid joint, which permits a wide range of motion in three directions.

6. Corniculate cartilages (fibroelastic cartilage), also called cartilages of Santorini, are small cartilages above the arytenoid and in the aryepiglottic folds.

7. Cuneiform cartilages (fibroelastic cartilages) also called cartilages of Wrisberg, are elongated pieces of small yellow elastic cartilages in the aryepiglottic folds.

8. Triticeous cartilage (Cartilago triticea) is a small elastic cartilage in the lateral thyrohyoid ligament. When calcified, it could be mistaken for a foreign body on the soft tissue x-ray film.

9. Ossification:

a) Thyroid cartilage ossifies at 20-30 years of age. Ossification begins in the inferior margin, and progresses cranially.

b) Cricoid cartilage ossifies after the thyroid cartilage. The first part to be calcified is the superior portion and could be mistaken for a foreign body. Calcification progresses caudally.

c) Arytenoid cartilages calcify at the third decade.

d) The hyoid ossifies from six centers shortly after birth and is completed by two years of age.

LARYNGEAL LIGAMENTS AND MEMBRANE:

1. Extrinsic: The extrinsic ligaments of the larynx bind the cartilages to the adjoining structures and to one another, and round out the laryngeal framework.

a) Thyrohyoid membrane and ligaments attach the thyroid cartilage to the hyoid bone. The thyrohyoid membrane is pierced on each side by: (1) Superior laryngeal vessels; (2) Internal branch of superior laryngeal nerve. Median thyrohyoid ligament is the thickened median portion of the thyrohyoid membrane. Lateral thyrohyoid ligament forms the thickened posterior border of the thyrohyoid membrane on each side, and the cartilago triticea is often found in this ligament.

b) Cricothyroid membrane and ligaments connect the thyroid and cricoid cartilages. This ligament may be pierced for emergency tracheotomy (cricothyrotomy) with little fear of bleeding. However, because of the proximity of the vocal cords, this space should not be utilized for prolonged tracheal intubation since scar tissue may be produced to interfere with the mobility of the cords.

c) The cricotracheal ligament attaches the cricoid cartilage to the first tracheal ring.

d) The epiglottis is suspended in position by membranous connections to the hyoid bone, the thyroid cartilage, and the base of the tongue.

2. Intrinsic: The intrinsic ligaments unite the cartilages of the larynx and perform an important role in the closure of this organ.

a) Elastic membrane of larynx is the fibrous framework of the larynx. It lies beneath the laryngeal mucosa and is divided into upper and lower parts by the ventricle of the larynx.

b) Quadrangular membrane is the upper part of the elastic membrane of the larynx, extending from the lateral margin of the epiglottis to the arytenoid and corniculate cartilages, and inferiorly to the false cord. It forms part of the wall between the upper pyriform sinus and the laryngeal vestibule. The quadrangular membrane and the conus elasticus are separated by the ventricle of Morgagni.

c) Conus elasticus (cricovocal membrane) is the name given to the lower part of the elastic membrane of the larynx. It is composed mainly of yellow elastic tissue. It is attached to:

Inferiorly: Superior border of the cricoid cartilage.
Superoanteriorly: Deep surface of angle of the thyroid cartilage.
Superoposteriorly: Vocal process of the arytenoid cartilage.

d) Median cricothyroid ligament is formed by the thickened anterior part of the conus elasticus.

e) Vocal ligament which forms the framework of the vocal cord is the free upper edge (the strongest part) of the conus elasticus.

f) Thyro-epiglottic ligament attaches the epiglottis to the thyroid cartilage.

CAVITY OF THE LARYNX:

1. The cavity of the larynx is divided into three parts:
   a) Vestibule
   b) Ventricle
   c) Subglottic space

   by two folds of mucous membrane:
   a) false cords
   b) true cords

2. The vestibule lies between the inlet and the edges of the false cords and is bordered by:

Anteriorly: Posterior surface of the epiglottis
Posteriorly: Interval between the arytenoid cartilages
Laterally: Inner surface of the aryepiglottic folds and upper surfaces of the false cord

3. The ventricle of the larynx (Ventricle of Morgani) is a deep, spindle-shape recess between the false and true cords, and lined by a mucous membrane which is covered externally by the thyroarytenoid muscle.

4. The saccule is a conical pouch which ascends from the anterior part of the ventricle. It lies between the inner surface of the thyroid cartilage and the false cord. Numerous mucous glands open on to the surface of its lining mucosa for lubricating the vocal cords.

5. The glottis (rima glottidis) is the space between the free margin of the true vocal cords. This space is wide and triangular in shape when the vocal cords are abducted (as in respiration), but assumes a slitlike appearance during adduction of the cords (in phonation). The posterior glottic chink in the adult is 18-19 mm. In the newborn it is 4 mm. The total glottic chink in a newborn is 14 sq. mm.

6. The subglottic space lies between the true vocal cords and the lower border of the cricoid cartilage.

7. The pre-epiglottic space is a wedge-shaped space lying in front of the epiglottis and bounded by:

Anteriorly:	Thyrohyoid membrane
Anterosuperiorly:	Hyoid
Superiorly:	Vallecula
Posteriorly:	Part of the epiglottis
Laterally:	Hyoepiglottic ligament

8. The false cords (ventricular bands) are the upper set of two horizontal folds on each side of the laryngeal cavity and extend from the angle of the thyroid cartilage anteriorly to the bodies of the arytenoid cartilages posteriorly, and have a primitive constricting function.

9. The true cords (the lower set) are directly concerned with the production of voice and with the protection of the lower respiratory passages. These folds stretch from the angle of the thyroid cartilage anteriorly to the vocal processes of the arytenoid cartilages posteriorly; they enclose the vocal ligament and a major portion of the vocalis muscle. The covering epithelium is closely bound down to the underlying vocal ligament and the blood supply is poor; hence the pearly white appearance of the vocal cords in life.

LARYNGEAL JOINTS:

1. Cricothyroid joint: A synovial joint with a capsular ligament between the inferior cornu of the thyroid cartilage and the facet on the cricoid cartilage at the junction of arch and lamina. Two movements occur:
   a) Rotation-through a transverse axis
   b) Gliding-slightly

2. Cricoarytenoid joint: A synovial joint with a capsular ligament between the base of the arytenoid cartilage and the facet on the upper border of the lamina of the cricoid cartilage. Two movements occur:
   a) Rotation-Of the arytenoid, on a vertical axis. The vocal process moves medially or laterally.
   b) Gliding-The arytenoids move towards or away from each other. A strong posterior crico-arytenoid ligament prevents excessive movements of the arytenoid on the cricoid.

LARYNGEAL MUSCLES:

1. Extrinsic muscles of the larynx are concerned with the movement and fixation of the larynx as a whole and consist of levator and depressor groups.

2. Depressor group consists of:
   a) Sternohyoid (C2, C3)
   b) Thyrohyoid (C1)
   c) Omohyoid (C2, C3)

3. Elevator group consists of:
   a) Geniohyoid (C1)
   b) Digastrics (Anterior, V and posterior, VII)
   c) Mylohyoid (V)
   d) Stylohyoid (VII)

4. The middle constrictor muscle is attached to the greater cornua of the hyoid bone. The inferior constrictor muscle is attached to the oblique lines of the thyroid cartilage and to the cricoid cartilage. These muscles influence the position of the larynx during phonation.

5. Intrinsic muscles of the larynx are directly concerned with its protective and phonatory functions, and consist of one unpaired muscle, the transverse arytenoid, and four paired muscles which act on the cricoarytenoid and cricothyroid joints, respectively.
   a) Interarytenoid muscle (unpaired)
      (1) transverse
      (2) oblique
   b) Posterior cricoarytenoid muscle (paired)
   c) Lateral cricoarytenoid muscle (paired)
   d) Thyroarytenoid muscle (paired)
   e) Cricothyroid muscle (paired)

6. Interarytenoid muscle is unpaired and consists of transverse and oblique fibers connecting the bodies of two arytenoid cartilages. This muscle is innervated bilaterally by the recurrent laryngeal nerve and therefore is not paralyzed by unilateral recurrent nerve disease. Action: Approximation of arytenoids and closure of glottis.

7. Posterior cricoarytenoid muscle passes from the posterior surface of the cricoid lamina to the muscular process of the arytenoid cartilage. Action: Lateral rotation of arytenoids and abduction of vocal cords (main abductor).

8. Lateral cricoarytenoid muscle passes from the cricoid arch to the muscular process of the arytenoid cartilage. Action: Medial rotation of arytenoids and adduction of vocal cords.

9. Thyroarytenoid or vocalis muscle arises from the inner aspect of the thyroid angle anteriorly and inserts into the vocal ligament and into the arytenoid cartilage. Action: Fine control of the vocal cords--relaxation of cord, firming of edge, changing of mass, etc.

10. Cricothyroid muscle arises from the arch of the cricoid anteriorly, and inserts into the inferior horn and body of the thyroid cartilage above. It elevates the arch of the cricoid cartilage as a level, and thus tilts the lamina with the attached arytenoid cartilages posteriorly. Action: Elongation and tension of the cords. (chief tensor)

11. Laryngeal movements:

Abduction:	Posterior cricoarytenoid
Adduction:	a) Lateral cricoarytenoid
	b) Transverse portion of interarytenoid
	c) Thyroarytenoid
Tension:	a) Cricothyroid (chief tensor)
	b) Thyroarytenoid or vocalis (internal tensor)

MUCOUS MEMBRANE OF THE LARYNX:

1. Stratified squamous epithelium is found over:
   a) Vocal cords
   b) Upper part of vestibule of larynx

2. Ciliated columnar epithelium lines the remainder of the cavity.

3. Mucous glands are found in:
   a) Ventricles and saccules.
   b) Posterior surface of epiglottis.
   c) Margins of aryepiglottic folds. There are none on the free edges of the vocal cords.

4. Reinke's layer of connective tissue lies immediately under the epithelium of the larynx and superficial to the elastic layer. There are no glands beneath it and no lymph vessels in it.

NERVE SUPPLY:

1. The larynx is supplied by two branches of vagus nerve: superior laryngeal and inferior (recurrent) laryngeal nerves.

2. The superior laryngeal nerve divides extralaryngeal into:
   a) Internal branch (sensory)
   b) External branch (motor)

The larger internal branch supplies sensory innervation to those areas of the larynx above the glottis. The smaller external branch gives motor innervation to the cricothyroid muscle and sensory supply to the infraglottic larynx at the level of the cricothyroid membrane.

3. The recurrent or inferior laryngeal nerve supplies motor innervation to all the intrinsic laryngeal muscles of the same side except for the cricothyroid and to the interarytenoid muscle of both sides. It also supplies sensory innervation to those portions of the larynx below the glottis.

4. Recurrent laryngeal nerve has a much longer course on the left side than on the right. On the left side it turns round the arch of the aorta. On the right side it turns round the subclavian artery. In the neck it lies between the trachea and esophagus as it approaches the larynx. Its terminal part passes upwards, under cover of the ala of the thyroid cartilage, immediately behind the inferior cricothyroid joint.

5. Each nucleus ambiguus is the somatic motor nucleus of the 9th, 10th, and 11th nerves.

6. Nucleus ambiguus is supplied by posterior inferior cerebellar artery (branch of vertebral) and anterior inferior cerebellar artery (branch of basilar).

BLOOD SUPPLY

1. Upper larynx:
   External carotid artery; Superior thyroid artery; Superior laryngeal artery
2. Lower larynx:
   Subclavian artery; Thyrocervical artery; Inferior thyroid artery; Inferior laryngeal artery

VENOUS DRAINAGE

1. Upper larynx:
   Superior laryngeal vein; Superior thyroid vein; Internal jugular vein
2. Lower larynx:
   Inferior laryngeal vein; Inferior thyroid vein; Innominate vein

LYMPHATIC DRAINAGE:

1. The lymphatics arising from the larynx drain mainly into the deep cervical group of lymph nodes. It is of great clinical importance that the vocal cords themselves contain scarcely any lymphatic channels.

2. The lymphatic network of the supraglottic structures is extensive. The channels collect in a pedicle at the anterior end of the aryepiglottic fold and pass laterally, anterior to the anterior wall of the pyriform fossa and leave the larynx with the neurovascular bundle through the thyrohyoid membrane. Almost all (98%) of the channels end in the upper deep cervical nodes between the digastric tendon and the omohyoid muscle. The remainder pass to the lower cervical chain or the spinal accessory chain.

3. The lymphatics of the infraglottic area have a more variable drainage pattern than those of the supraglottic network. The channels leave the area in three pedicles. The anterior pedicle passes through the cricothyroid membrane and many vessels end in the prelaryngeal (Delphian) nodes in the region of the thyroid isthmus. Channels then leave these nodes with the remaining anterior channels to travel to the deep inferior cervical nodes. The two posterolateral pedicles leave the larynx through the cricotracheal membrane with some channels going to leave the larynx through the cricotracheal membrane with some channels going to the paratracheal chain of nodes, while others pass to the inferior jugular chain.

4. Generally, lymphatic drainage from each half of the larynx is quite separate and little cross-over or mixing occurs.

5. There is evidence that lymphatic channels do cross the midline in the supra-and infraglottic areas. Contralateral drainage is more likely to occur spontaneously from the infraglottic areas, thus lesions of this area may be associated with less consistent patterns of metastases.

III. FUNCTIONS OF THE LARYNX[3, 10, 32]

1. Functions of the larynx include:
   a) Phonation: Voice produced by vibration of vocal cords
   b) Respiration: Reflex adjustment of glottic aperture assists in the regulation of gaseous exchange with the lung and in the maintenance of acid-base balance.
   c) Protection:
      (1) Closure of the laryngeal inlet
      (2) Closure of the glottis
      (3) Cessation of respiration
      (4) Cough reflex, expulsion of secretions and foreign bodies
   d) Fixation of the chest: Closure of glottis to fix intrathoracic and intra-abdominal pressure and aid in lifting, defecation, vomiting, urination or childbirth.
   e) Swallowing:
      (1) The epiglottis acts as a protective factor by shielding the central opening and by directing the stream of food laterally.

(2) The larynx is drawn upward by the inferior pharyngeal constrictors, for its own protection and to permit passage of the food bolus into the esophagus.

(3) The larynx is closed to prevent the aspiration of food.

2. There are two major theories of voice production:

a) The traditional or myoelastic theory, maintains that the mechanism of voice production is primarily an aerodynamic process controlled by the air pressure in the trachea and by the elasticity of the vocal cords. According to this interpretation, the lungs, acting as bellows, drive air under pressure against the lower surfaces of the closed vocal cords. The vocal cords are pushed apart, and some of the air escapes through this opening. Meanwhile the innate elasticity of the cords and the reduced lateral pressure cause reapproximation of the cords, which in turn blocks any further escape of air. This same cycle is repeated again and again as soon as the subglottic pressure rises sufficiently to overcome the resistance of the vocal cords.

b) The neuromuscular theory, now disproven, suggests that laryngeal vibrations are under the direct control of the central nervous system, and that each vibratory cycle is initiated by a separate nerve impulse to the appropriate muscles in the larynx. Under this theory the vocal cords are pulled apart actively by the vocalis muscle at the beginning of each vibration, while the process of reapproximation is the result of muscular relaxation.

3. Arrhythmia, bradycardia, and occasionally cardiac arrest may result from stimulating the larynx. The mechanism appears to be related to stimulation of nerve fibers which arise in aortic baroreceptors, and in some individuals, travel to the central nervous system by way of the recurrent laryngeal nerve, ramus communicans, and superior laryngeal nerve. These can result from light anesthesia, prolonged laryngoscopy, repeated attempts at intubation, respiratory obstruction and tracheal irritation. The reflex cardiac effects can be controlled by atropine and enhanced by morphine.[40]

IV. SELECTED DISORDERS OF THE LARYNX

INFLAMMATORY DISEASES:

ACUTE EPIGLOTTITIS:[4,15,22,25] A special form of rapidly progressive acute laryngitis in which the inflammatory changes mainly involve the epiglottis. It occurs mainly in children age 2 to 7 years,[32] although infants, older children, and even adults may be affected.[15]

Etiology: Hemophilus influenzae

Symptoms:

1. Rapidly progressive dyspnea, especially in children. May be fatal within a few hours of onset unless immediately diagnosed and treated. This is a surgical emergency!

2. Dysphagia. Starts with sore throat, difficulty in swallowing, then refusal of oral feedings.

3. Dehydration, fever, tachycardia, restlessness, exhaustion with respiratory and circulatory collapse.

4. The voice is usually not hoarse but may present with a "hot potato voice".

5. Patient prefers upright position and leaning slightly forward. Do not place the patient in a recumbent position.

6. The most important clinical feature is the swollen, bright-red epiglottis obstructing the pharynx at the base of the tongue.

7. Blood culture usually shows H. influenzae.

Treatment:

1. Immediate hospitalization and constant observation.

2. All upper airway emergency instruments including bronchoscope, laryngoscope, endotracheal tubes and tracheotomy set should be at the bedside.

3. Tracheotomy as soon as the diagnosis of acute epiglottitis is made.[4,25]

4. Tracheotomy should be done after the airway is established with a bronchoscope or an endotracheal tube.

5. Antibiotic treatment. Ampicillin is the drug of choice; Chloramphenicol and Streptomycin are also effective to a lesser degree.

6. Steroids may be of value in limiting the progression of inflammation and edema.

7. Nasotracheal intubation is suggested[45], but it is safer to rely on time-tested tracheotomy.

ACUTE LARYNGOTRACHEOBRONCHITIS: Laryngotracheobronchitis is an acute infection of the lower respiratory passages, extending from the larynx down into the smaller subdivisions of the bronchial tree. It is endemic throughout the year, but may react in epidemic proportions in any locality during the winter season.

Etiology: Probably a virus. Para Influenza Types 1 to 4 have been isolated frequently. Haemophilus influenzae, streptococcus, staphylococcus, pneumococcus are commonly cultured. The disease occurs in children, especially between the ages of one and three years.

Pathology: A descending inflammation of the mucous membrane lining the lower respiratory tract, followed by congestion, edema and exudation of a thick tenacious secretion. Anatomically, the conus elasticus is the most involved site.

Symptoms:

1. At the onset, the disease is not unlike an ordinary cold except for the early presence of a croupy cough.

2. Hoarseness is noted shortly thereafter.

3. As the swelling increases, inspiratory stridor develops.

4. Retractions then occur.

5. Circumoral pallor and cyanosis usually precede a decrease in breath sounds that, in turn, is an indication that death may be imminent.

6. In addition to these symptoms of respiratory embarrassment, anorexia, and fever are common in the early stages while restlessness, dehydration, and exhaustion may be noted later.

Prognosis: Entirely depends on early recognition of the disease and upon timely hospitalization and treatment.

Treatment:

A. Medical:
   1. Cold humidification (a most important treatment)
   2. Corticosteroids
   3. Rest
   4. Antibiotics
   5. Fluids
   6. Oxygen
   7. Racemic epinephrine via IPPB[13]

B. Surgical:
   1. Timely tracheotomy. When in doubt, do it.

TUBERCULOUS LARYNGITIS:[46]

Etiology: Almost always secondary to active pulmonary tuberculosis.

Pathology:

1. Cellular infiltrator
2. Proliferation and nodular function
3. Granulation tissue in the interarytenoid fold
4. Perichondritis, cartilage necrosis
   a) Multiple small superficial ulcers in the interarytenoid fold, false and true cords, and the epiglottis.
   b) Perichondritis and cartilage necrosis

Symptoms:

1. Hoarseness
2. Cough, late, with production of blood streaked sputum
3. Pain, and referred earache are fairly common
4. In advanced cases, dyspnea from edema of the larynx and scar contraction or destruction of underlying cartilages.
5. Biopsy is essential for diagnosis to rule out malignancy. The tuberculous granuloma similar to that of pemphigoid is subepithelial. The pemphigus involvement is intraepithelial.
6. The most common site of tuberculosis of the larynx is the posterior larynx (interarytenoid fold). The next common site is the laryngeal surface of the epiglottis.

Prognosis: If diagnosed and treated early, prognosis is good. If the local manifestations include cartilaginous involvement, the prognosis is more serious, since irreparable harm may have been inflicted upon the framework or soft tissues of the larynx.

Treatment:

1. Streptomycin and para-aminosalicylic acid
2. Treatment of pulmonary lesion
3. Voice rest
4. Narcotics for pain

5. Inspection of superior laryngeal nerve (Novocaine or alcohol for relief of pain).
6. Tracheotomy for obstruction
7. Surgery for secondary stenosis, if indicated

SYPHILITIC LARYNGITIS:
Etiology: Treponema pallidum. Extremely rare in the congenital form and now very rare also in the acquired form of the disease.

Pathology: The larynx is never affected in the primary stage of the disease. During the secondary stage, infection and mild edema of the larynx are common and mucous patches may be observed; these lesions are temporary and disappear with the resolution of this phase. The gummata are characteristic of laryngeal involvement in the tertiary stage. Ultimate breakdown of these lesions results in the development of ulcerations, perichondritis and fibrosis.

Symptoms:
1. A mild hoarseness is often the only symptom. Gummata and ulcerations may lead to varying degrees of hoarseness.
2. There is no pain.
3. As the swelling increases or fibrosis develops, symptoms of respiratory embarrassment may occur.
4. The diagnosis is confirmed by serologic tests and biopsy.

Prognosis: In early lesions, the prognosis is quite favorable, but destruction of cartilages cause permanent changes.

Treatment:
1. Penicillin
2. Supportive measures
3. Tracheotomy for respiratory obstruction
4. Reconstructive operation for severe laryngeal stenosis

SARCOIDOSIS: A systemic granulomatous disease of unknown etiology. It affects primarily the lung and mediastinal nodes but laryngeal involvement may occur.

Pathology: The lesion is characterized by noncaseating granuloma. The lack of caseation distinguishes sarcoid from tuberculosis, pathologically.

Symptoms:
1. Hoarseness is the prominent feature
2. Pain is not usually present
3. If the lesion is large, dyspnea may be present.
4. Usually involves the epiglottis and false cords. Marked edema may be present.
5. Biopsy is essential for diagnosis.

Prognosis: Permanent clinical remission usually occurs.

Treatment:
1. Steroids
2. Tracheotomy for laryngeal obstruction

SCLEROMA OF THE LARYNX:
Etiology: Klebsiella rhinoscleromatis (von Frisch bacillus). Rare in the United States.

Symptoms:
1. Hoarseness, cough and increasing dyspnea
2. The most common site of scleroma of the larynx is the subglottic region. Pale pinkish swelling may be seen below the vocal cords.

Treatment:
1. Streptomycin
2. Steroids
3. Tracheotomy (often needed)

PERICHONDRITIS OF THE LARYNX:
Etiology:
1. Infection (tuberculosis, syphilis, septic laryngitis, etc.)
2. Trauma
3. High tracheotomy
4. Radiotherapy
5. Neoplasm with secondary infection

Pathology:

1. Perichondritis leads to subperichondrial abscess, necrosis of cartilage and, later, stenosis.

2. Perichondritis of the thyroid cartilage is more common than perichondritis of the epiglottis. This is because the epiglottis is fibroelastic cartilage where the perichondrium is adhered to the cartilage.

Symptoms:
1. May be insidious or of sudden onset
2. Fever and malaise (acute form)
3. Local pain and tenderness
4. Enlargement of laryngeal framework; swelling of the neck
5. Abscess and fistula
6. Hoarseness, cough, dysphagia and dyspnea

Diagnosis:
1. Syphilis and malignant disease should be ruled out
2. Rule out unsuspected foreign body

Treatment:
1. Hospitalization
2. Systemic antibiotics
3. Tracheotomy
4. I&D if indicated
5. Dilation for stenosis
6. Laryngofissure
7. Laryngectomy for extensive necrosis of a cartilage

GLANDERS: Glanders is a serious infectious disease marked by the occurrence of multiple granulomatous abscesses throughout the body, caused by Actinobacillus mallei. Perichondritis, and cartilage destruction may complicate the laryngeal disease.

LEPROSY OF THE LARYNX: Leprosy of the larynx is rare. It affects the larynx in 10% of cases. It is caused by Mycobacterium leprae or Hansen's bacillus.

Treatment:
1. DDS (Diaminophenylsulfone) (for 1-4 years)
2. Steroids
3. Tracheotomy

DIPHTHERITIC LARYNGITIS: Rare
Etiology: Corynebacterium diphtheriae

Symptoms:
1. Onset insidious
2. Hoarse, croupy cough is the first symptom
3. Grayish-white membrane on the larynx. Its removal is followed by bleeding.

Treatment:
1. Antitoxin
2. Penicillin
3. Tracheotomy

MYCOTIC INFECTION OF THE LARYNX: Fungus infections of the larynx are rare. Blastomycosis, histoplasmosis, and candidiasis are the ones most commonly encountered.

1. Blastomycosis: Seen in endemic proportions in North America and mainly a disease of the skin and lungs. However, primary involvement of the larynx does occur. It is caused by Blastomyces dermatiditis and characterized by diffuse nodular infiltration of the larynx, vocal cord fixation, ulcer and stenosis.

The epithelium undergoes marked hyperplasia of the pseudoepithelial type and may be mistaken for carcinoma. Microabscesses containing the organisms, giant cells and mononuclears occur in the epidermis and dermis and are characteristic of this disease.

Symptoms:
- a. Hoarseness and cough occur early.
- b. Dyspnea and dysphagia are late symptoms.
- c. In the early stage, laryngeal mucosa is diffusely inflamed and granular.
- d. Tiny miliary nodules may be seen on the vocal cords.
- e. In advanced stage, mucosal ulceration, covered with foul smelling, greenish exudate, under which a bright red granula bed.
- f. Later, fibrosis, fixation of arytenoids or stenosis develops.

Treatment: Amphotericin B

2. Histoplasmosis is caused by Histoplasma capsulatum and usually associated with pulmonary histoplasmosis.

Treatment:
   a. Amphotericin B.
   b. Sulfonamide

3. Candidiasis (Moniliasis) is caused by Candida albicans, almost always the result of chemotherapeutic suppression of normal bacterial flora, and characterized by white patches on mucosa of a bright red color.

Treatment: Nystatin (Mycostatin)

4. Actinomycosis is caused by Actinomyces bovis characterized by yellowish granulomatous infiltration which suppurates. It involves the neck and perilaryngeal structures.

Treatment: Penicillin or tetracycline

5. Coccidioidomycosis caused by Coccidioides immitus is endemic in the San Joaquin Valley area of California. More often seen in colored races. The lesion consists of nodular masses of granulomatous tissue.

BENIGN TUMORS AND CYSTS OF THE LARYNX:

BENIGN TUMORS: [3, 10, 32, 39] Benign tumors of the larynx are relatively uncommon. They occur in order of the following frequency: papilloma, chondroma, neurofibroma, leiomyoma, angiofibroma, myoma, hemangioma and chemodectoma.

PAPILLOMA: Papilloma is the most common benign tumor of the larynx, and occurs in patients of all ages.

Etiology:
1. The causative agent is thought to be a virus.
2. Seems to be related to hormonal changes. Papillomas usually regress during puberty.

Pathology:
1. Papillary epithelial tumor usually involving the true cords but may affect supraglottic and subglottic regions.
2. May also involve the trachea and bronchus.
3. Papilloma in juveniles is more often multiple, and recurs more frequently than those in adults.
4. Papillomas in adults are usually single, but may undergo malignant change.

Symptoms:
1. Aphonia or weak cry is usually the first sign in infants.
2. Dyspnea
3. Patients with papilloma have low serum magnesium

Treatment:

1. Repeated laryngoscopic removal to maintain an adequate airway is currently the standard treatment.
2. Tracheotomy is occasionally necessary.
3. Cryosurgery [38]
4. Autogenous vaccine
5. Ultrasound therapy
6. In view of high incidence of recurrence, thyrotomy and pharyngotomy are not indicated.
7. Irradiation is contraindicated because of its carcinogenic effects.
8. Laser surgery. [1,41]

CHONDROMA: [21,32,42] Slow growing lesion. Composed of mainly hyaline cartilage. Affects males more often than females (10-1).

The most frequent site of origin is the internal aspect of the posterior plate of the cricoid, followed by thyroid, arytenoid and epiglottis.

Symptoms:

1. Hoarseness, dyspnea and dysphagia (in that order) are the presenting symptoms.
2. Full sensation within the throat may be present.
3. Symptoms are insidious.
4. Dyspnea and hoarseness prominent with a subglottic mass arising from the internal aspect of the cricoid.
5. Dysphagia more common in lesions arising from the posterior aspect of the cricoid.
6. Hoarseness is due to restriction of cord mobility by the mass.
7. Mirror examination shows a smooth, firm, round or modular, fixed tumor covered by normal mucosa.
8. Chondroma of the thyroid, cricoid or tracheal cartilages may present as a hard neck mass.
9. Soft tissue film, laminogram, and laryngogram will delineate the extent and site of lesion.
10. Calcification is commonly seen on x-ray.

Treatment:

1. Excision. The site of origin determines the approach.
2. Thyrotomy for tumors of anterior aspect of cricoid.
3. Lateral external approach with or without pharyngotomy for chondromas of the thyroid, posterior aspect of cricoid, or arytenoid.
4. Recurrence common if not removed completely. Peroral removal is not advised.
5. Total laryngectomy may be necessary for treatment of recurrences.

NEUROFIBROMA:

1. This is a rare tumor arising from Schwann cells.
2. The tumor most commonly arises from the aryepiglottic fold.
3. The incidence favors females 2:1.

GRANULAR CELL MYOBLASTOMA: [7, 32, 43]

1. These tumors are thought to be of neurogenic origin.
2. They occur in any age group and affect males predominantly.
3. The lesion usually occurs at the posterior aspect of the true cords or arytenoids. The lesion is small, sessile, and gray.
4. Hoarseness is often the only symptom.
5. The mucosa may show pseudoepitheliomatous hyperplasia.

Treatment: Excision by direct laryngoscopy.

ADENOMA:

1. Rare. Arises from the mucous glands.
2. The most common site is the false cord or ventricle.

Treatment: Excision perorally or by thyrotomy.

CHEMODECTOMA:

1. Arises from paraganglion tissue.
2. Usually seen in the false cord and aryepiglottic fold.
3. Smooth, cystic and red.
4. Biopsy may be associated with bleeding.

Treatment: Lateral pharyngotomy.

LIPOMA:

1. Rare. Pedunculated or submucosal.
2. Usually arises from the aryepiglottic fold, epiglottis, true cord and pharyngeal wall.

Treatment:

1. Excision via laryngoscope for pedunculated lesion.
2. Lateral pharyngotomy for submucous tumor.

HEMANGIOMA: (adult)

1. Hemangiomas in adults are more common.
2. Occur on vocal cords, subglottic regions, and pyriform sinus.
3. Hemangioma in children (See Congenital Anomalies)

Treatment: Excision is best handled by suspension laryngoscopy (for a small angioma) or by lateral pharyngotomy (for a large angioma).

PSEUDOEPITHELIAL HYPERPLASIA: This is a benign epithelial change that may resemble carcinoma. It can be caused by:

1. Tuberculosis
2. Syphilis
3. Granular cell myoblastoma
4. Blastomycosis
5. Pachyderma laryngis
6. Radiation
7. Papillary keratosis (premalignant)

When a diagnosis of pseudoepithelial hyperplasia is made further biopsy or studies may be necessary to rule out blastomycosis, granuloma cell myoblastoma, etc.

CYSTS AND TUMOR-LIKE LESIONS OF THE LARYNX:

RETENTION CYST:

1. Occur most often where mucous glands are abundant.
2. False cord, ventricle, epiglottis, aryepiglottic fold may be the sites.

Treatment:
1. Laryngoscopic removal
2. Marsupialization

PROLAPSE OF VENTRICLE:

1. Ventricular prolapse is protrusion of ventricular mucosa between the true and false cords.
2. Frequently associated with chronic bronchitis.
3. Presenting symptom is hoarseness.
4. A sessile pink mass arising between the false and true cord is seen.

Treatment: Laryngoscopic removal with a forceps.

LARYNGOCELE:

1. This is an air-filled dilation of the appendix of the ventricle.

2. There are two types:
   a) External laryngocele, the commoner form, in which the sac protrudes above the thyroid cartilage and the thyrohyoid membrane and presents as a mass in the neck.
   b) Internal laryngocele, less common, in which the sac remains within the thyroid cartilage.
   c) The combined type may be present.

Etiology: Unknown

Symptoms:
1. External laryngocele presents as a swelling in the neck which increases in size with increased intralaryngeal pressure.
2. Internal laryngocele presents with hoarseness and dyspnea.
3. Indirect laryngoscopy may show a smooth dilation at false cord level involving the false cord and aryepiglottic fold.
4. Diagnosis may be confirmed by tomogram of the neck showing air within the sac.

Treatment:
1. Laryngoscopic decompression for small lesions.
2. Lateral external approach for larger lesions.

CONTACT ULCER OF THE LARYNX:
Etiology: Unknown

Pathology: The most common site is vocal process of the arytenoid.

Symptoms:

1. Hoarseness
2. Pain on exertion
3. Typical ulceration

Treatment:

1. Absolute voice rest
2. Vocal reeducation
3. Avoidance of irritants

VOCAL NODULE:

1. The most common site is at the junction of the anterior and middle thirds, usually bilateral. (The middle part of the membranous vocal cord has the greatest amplitude of vibration and hence most likely to develop singer's nodule).

2. Vocal nodule arises from the subepithelial layer of the vocal cord called the Rienke's layer.

THE MOST COMMON SITE OF BENIGN LARYNGEAL LESIONS:		
	The most common site	Side
Contact ulcer:	Vocal process of arytenoid	Unilateral or bilateral
Laryngeal polyp:	Junction of anterior and middle thirds	Usually unilateral
Vocal cord nodule:	Junction of anterior and middle third	Bilateral
Post intubation:	Vocal process of the arytenoid	About 50% bilateral

INTUBATION GRANULOMA: [11]

Etiology: Endotracheal intubation.

Age and Sex: All adults. The incidence is higher in females (4 to 1) because the tube falls to the posterior commissure more and because the mucosa is thinner.

Site: Invariably on the vocal process of the arytenoid.

Treatment:

1. Excision when pedunculated.
2. Attempts of removal during the sessile stage should be avoided as recurrence is likely.

CHRONIC NON-SPECIFIC DISEASE OF THE LARYNX:

PACHYDERMA LARYNGIS: Pachyderma laryngis is a specific entity in which the posterior commissure and the posterior third of the true cords are the site of a localized hyperplastic and keratinized process. Histologically, acanthosis, parakeratosis, keratosis and hyperkeratotic papilloma are noticed. There is no dyskeratosis. It is not premalignant. Diagnosis is made by biopsy.

Treatment: Non-specific

KERATOSIS OF THE LARYNX: This is a term used to denote a group of premalignant epithelial lesions in which an abnormality of growth and/or maturation has occurred.

Etiology:
1. Smoking, vocal abuse, chronic laryngitis vitamin deficiences.
2. Exact cause unknown.

Symptoms:
1. Hoarseness is the only symptom.
2. A raised reddish area of mucosal irregularity overlying a portion of one or both cords with chronic inflammation.

Treatment:
1. Cessation of smoking and other causative agents.
2. Direct laryngoscopy with excision.
3. Periodical examination.

LEUKOPLAKIA OF THE LARYNX: This is a pathologic premalignant process characterized by a thick whitish layer of hyperkeratotic epithelial cells.

Etiology: Vocal abuse, excessive smoking and intake of alcohol, irritative environment.

Symptoms:
1. Hoarseness
2. White patches on vocal cords

Treatment:
1. Laryngoscopic excision
2. Removal of causative factors
3. Periodical examination

CHRONIC CICATRICIAL STENOSIS OF THE LARYNX:

Etiology:
1. Trauma to the larynx (Automobile accident most common).
2. High tracheotomy
3. Endoscopic procedures
4. Radiation injuries
5. Prolonged nasogastric intubation
6. Syphilis, tuberculosis, diphtheria, (typhoid fever rare today).

LARYNGEAL STENOSIS CAN BE DIVIDED INTO THREE GROUPS:

	Most common cause	Treatment
Supraglottic stenosis:	1. Lye burn	1. Excision of scarred epiglottis and false cord.
	2. External trauma	2. Pharyngotomy
Glottic stenosis:	1. Most often due to indiscriminate removal of mucosa from both cords at the anterior commissure (web formation) 2. Rarely external trauma	McKnaught keel through thyrotomy
Infraglottic stenosis: (commonest site of stenosis)*	1. External trauma	1. Correction of high tracheotomy
	2. High tracheotomy	2. Excision of stenotic area with anastomosis between the thyroid cartilage and trachea
	3. Endotracheal intubation	3. Arytenoidopexy

* This is the narrowest part of the laryngeal airway and the cricoid cartilage is susceptible to development of perichondritis.

ARTHRITIS OF THE CRICOARYTENOID JOINT:

Etiology:

1. Rheumatoid arthritis is by far the most common cause (about 25% of cases of rheumatoid arthritis).
2. Gout, collagen diseases (lupus erythematosus)
3. Gonorrhea, Tuberculosis, Syphilis, rare.
4. Trauma

Symptoms:

1. Lump in throat
2. Throat pain aggravated by swallowing or speaking
3. Referred ear pain
4. Hoarseness, stridor and dyspnea
5. Striking, bright red swelling over the arytenoid
6. Palpation of the arytenoid produces severe pain
7. Vocal cord may be fixed in the paramedian or intermediate position. Direct laryngoscopy and palpation of the arytenoids is necessary to differentiate fixation from paralysis.
8. Other signs of rheumatoid arthritis (Sedimentation rate, C-reactive protein, gamma globulin, abnormal; positive test for rheumatoid factor.)

Treatment:

1. Control systemic rheumatoid arthritis
2. Salicylates

3. Steroids
4. Tracheotomy
5. Arytenoidectomy or arytenoidopexy for midline fixation of both vocal cords. Unilateral fixation rarely requires therapy.
6. Teflon injection

CONGENITAL ANOMALIES OF THE LARYNX:

CONGENITAL WEB: Develops as a band which extends over part (web) or all (atresia) of the glottis. Anterior two thirds of the glottis is the site of predilection.

Symptoms:
1. Depend on degree of glottic closure.
2. Atresia present as severe dyspnea at birth. Death may follow if unrecognized and untreated promptly.
3. Small web may be asymptomatic.
4. Mainly weak or hoarse cry and cough.

Treatment:
1. Immediate insertion of a bronchoscope or tracheotomy for atresia.
2. Thyrotomy and insertion of McKnaught tantalum plate be-ween the vocal cords.

CONGENITAL LARYNGEAL CYST: Occurs most commonly in the supraglottic area (lateral wall of supraglottis or on epiglottis) or associated with laryngocele producing inspiratory stridor and weak cry. Diagnosis is made by direct laryngoscopy.

Treatment:
1. Emergency treatment by aspiration.
2. Endoscopic excision later.

CONGENITAL SUBGLOTTIC STENOSIS: The subglottic region 2-3 mm. below the true cord is the site of predilection.

Symptoms:
1. Severe barking stridor.
2. Expiratory stridor if subglottic.

Treatment:
1. 40 to 50% need tracheotomy.
2. Dilation.

VOCAL CORD PARALYSIS:

Etiology:
1. Trauma at birth (unilateral)
2. Platybasia (bilateral)
3. Arnold-Chiari syndrome (bilateral)
4. Left vocal cord paralysis may result from stretching of the left recurrent nerve due to a congenital cardiovascular lesion.

Symptoms:

Unilateral-weak cry.
Bilateral-crowing inspiration, severe stridor

Treatment:

Unilateral-no treatment
Bilateral-(1) Tracheotomy; (2) Arytenoidectomy or Arytenoidopexy best delayed until age 5 or 6.

SUBGLOTTIC HEMANGIOMA:[12, 32, 39] A rare anomaly of early infancy which may be associated with a skin hemangioma (50% of cases). Anterior subglottic area is the site of predilection.

Symptoms:

1. Inspiratory stridor is noted at birth or soon thereafter.
2. There may be a history of repeated episodes of croup.
3. Hoarseness is not a common symptom.
4. Direct laryngoscopy reveals a pink to blue, easily compressible, subglottic tumor.
5. Biopsy is never done, since the ensuing hemorrhage may be fatal.
6. The tumor can be seen on a lateral neck x-ray.

Treatment:

1. Tracheotomy is carried out to relieve the airway obstruction which already exists or which may occur during the initial stages of irradiation.
2. Irradiation is the treatment of choice.
3. Occasionally surgery is required.

LARYNGOMALACIA: This is the most common laryngeal abnormality of the newborn and is due to unusual flaccidity of the laryngeal tissues, especially the epiglottis.

Symptoms:

1. Inspiratory stridor and noisy respiration noted soon after birth, usually worse with the infant on his back as compared with the infant on his stomach.
2. Diagnosis requires direct laryngoscopy which reveals a flaccid, curled epiglottis which is drawn over the glottis on inspiration.
3. The vocal cords are normal in appearance and motility.
4. Rule out lower respiratory tract anomalies by bronchoscopy.

Treatment:

1. Observation (Stridor usually disappears by 12-16 months of age).
2. Tracheotomy in rare cases.

LARYNGEAL CLEFTS: Very rare. Irregular and incomplete fusion of the laryngotracheal septum results in a tracheosophageal fistula or cleft of the larynx. These anomalies are manifest very soon after birth.

Symptoms:

1. Cyanosis with feeding
2. Stridor
3. Abnormal cry
4. Pneumonia
5. Usually fatal unless diagnosed early and corrected early.
6. Diagnosis made by direct laryngoscopy.

LARYNGEAL TRAUMA: [3, 9, 28, 39] Blunt trauma to the neck is being seen with increasing frequency. Severe laryngeal injury may occur without open neck injuries. The undiagnosed laryngeal trauma case may succumb early from laryngeal obstruction or develop late laryngeal stenosis that requires the permanent wearing of a tracheotomy tube.

Clinical Manifestations: In any patient who has sustained a possible laryngeal injury, the following symptoms are indicative of some derangement of laryngeal structure:

1. Increasing airway obstruction with dyspnea and stridor
2. Dysphonia or aphonia
3. Cough
4. Hemoptysis
5. Neck pain
6. Dysphagia and odynophagia

Distinctive clinical signs indicative of laryngeal injuries are:

1. Deformities of the neck including alteration in contour and swelling.
2. Subcutaneous emphysema
3. Laryngeal tenderness
4. Crepitus over the laryngeal framework.

Diagnosis:

1. Indirect and direct laryngoscopy.
2. Roentgenograms of the neck and chest must be taken to detect laryngeal fractures, tracheal injuries and pneumothorax.

Treatment: [9, 28, 31]

1. Establishment of an adequate airway which may necessitate tracheotomy. (Avoid high tracheotomy).
2. Cricothyrotomy may be indicated. In such cases, remove the tracheotomy as soon as the patient's condition permits to prevent laryngeal stenosis.
3. Many of these patients have multiple injuries; yet suspicion and recognition of the acute laryngeal injury is imperative.
4. Surgical exploration is indicated in any neck injury with symptoms of stridor, voice change, cartilage disruption and cervical emphysema.
5. Exploration of laryngeal structure is best performed through a horizontal incision at the level of the previous tracheotomy incision to minimize scarring of the anterior neck.
6. Some injuries may be compound with an external opening. If so, debride the wound, splint the fracture, and leave the wound open before closing it later.

7. Laryngeal cartilage fractures, like any other fractures, must be reduced and immobilized. Repair should be done within 7-10 days of the time of injury.
8. Splint a laryngeal fracture by means of a mold or stent in the laryngeal lumen. A rubber finger-cot, filled with Ivalon sponge may be used.
9. The stent is usually inserted through a thyrotomy or infrahyoid laryngotomy and is fixed above and below by stainless steel sutures passed through the skin.
10. The stent is fixed in a position so that the upper end is at the level of the aryepiglottic folds and the lower end is just above the tracheotomy site. It should be left for 4-8 weeks.

PARALYSIS OF THE LARYNX: [3,28,31,36,37]

1. The larynx is supplied by two branches of vagus nerve: superior laryngeal and inferior (recurrent) laryngeal nerves.

The superior laryngeal nerve divides extralaryngeally into: A) Internal branch which supplies sensory innervation to the laryngeal cavity above the glottis, and B) External branch (motor) which supplies the cricothyroid muscle.

The recurrent or inferior laryngeal nerve supplies motor innervation to all the intrinsic laryngeal muscles of the same side except for the cricothyroid and to the interarytenoid muscle of both bodies. It also supplies sensory innervation to those portions of the larynx below the glottis.

2. Paralysis of the laryngeal muscles originates in one of two areas; the central nervous system or the peripheral motor nerves. In most cases (90%) laryngeal paralysis is the result of peripheral nerve involvement. Arising from the ambiguous nucleus in the mid-brain, motor impulses to the intrinsic laryngeal muscles travel via the vagus nerve into the chest, where they enter the recurrent laryngeal nerve. On its passage back to the larynx the right recurrent laryngeal nerve crosses the right subclavian artery, while the left recurrent laryngeal nerve winds around the arch of the aorta in close relation to the heart. The ascent of the recurrent laryngeal nerve occurs in a groove between the trachea and the esophagus in close relation to the mediastinal lymph nodes, thyroid gland, and esophagus. Thus a swelling of any of these structures may cause pressure on one of the recurrent laryngeal nerves and obstruct muscles on the involved side. Depending upon the nerve fibers involved and the muscles they supply, many different types of paralysis may occur.

3. Paralyzed vocal cords are best described by their position--median, paramedian, intermediate, extreme abduction (lateral). In median position, the paralyzed cord remains in the midline. This is a frequent position of a paralyzed vocal cord since the abductor muscles are weaker and more vulnerable than the adductor fibers. The intermediate position, often called cadaveric, is midway between the midline and position of complete abduction. Paramedian is between median and intermediate.

4. Regardless of what type of paralysis it is hard to predict the permanent position of the vocal cord because of:
   a) Continued function of remaining muscles
   b) Muscle fibrosis
   c) Tone of the autonomic system
   d) Cricoarytenoid joint fibrosis
   e) Tension of conus elasticus

5. Unilateral midline paralysis is the most frequent; the left more than the right. The paralyzed vocal cord usually lies lower than the normal cord.

6. Suggested workup for acute laryngeal paralysis after history and physical includes:
   a) CBC, ESR, Urinalysis
   b) Chest x-ray, PA and lateral
   c) Skull series
   d) Cervical spine films
   e) Ba swallow
   f) Glucose tolerance test
   g) L. P.

UNILATERAL PARALYSIS:

Etiology: Unilateral paralysis of the vagus or recurrent laryngeal nerve can be the result of one of the following:
1. Tumor in the thyroid gland, mediastinum or esophagus
2. Surgical trauma. (The most common etiology is thyroidectomy).
3. Pressure on the left recurrent laryngeal nerve by a hypertrophied heart or an aortic aneurysm.
4. Toxic neuritis following influenza or alcohol, lead, or arsenic poisoning.
5. Rarely by a central lesion
6. Unknown cause. About 20%.

Finding:
1. Involvement of the nerve may be partial, with weakness and decreased motility of the ipsilateral cord or total with a resulting unilateral paralysis.
2. The paralyzed vocal cord is usually fixed in the paramedian position (incomplete paralysis).
3. Involvement of the vagus nerve may lead to fixation in an intermediate or lateral position (complete paralysis). Depending on the etiology, the paralysis may be either temporary or permanent.

Symptoms: Hoarseness is usually the only symptom of unilateral laryngeal paralysis. Even this symptom often gradually disappears as the healthy cord increases its excursion beyond the median line and functional apposition of the voice may persist of a somewhat longer period of time. Feebleness of the cough mechanism parallels the degree of hoarseness.

Treatment:
1. Removal of causative agent
2. Voice therapy
3. Surgery (Teflon injection) after six months

BILATERAL ABDUCTOR PARALYSIS: Bilateral abductor paralysis is the most common form of bilateral motor paralysis, and is of great clinical importance.

Etiology: In almost all instances it is by extensive thyroid surgery, with injury of both recurrent laryngeal nerves.

Finding: Bilateral abductor paralysis of the vocal cords is manifested by a paralysis of both vocal cords near the median line.

Symptoms:
1. Destruction of both recurrent laryngeal nerves or injury of these nerves is usually followed by a history of transient hoarseness.
2. Weakness of voice is usually prolonged.
3. Cough mechanism is less forceful.
4. As the vocal cords approach the median line, respiratory embarrassment may become increasingly severe and call for immediate establishment of adequate airway.

Treatment:
1. Tracheotomy for respiratory difficulty.
2. Extralaryngeal arytenoidectomy with cord lateralization with a suture (the procedure of choice).
3. Endoscopic arytenoidectomy.

Several secondary operations have been devised to restore normal respiration. All procedures aim at lateralizing one vocal cord. A 5 mm. posterior glottic chink is needed for an adequate airway in an adult but with a 5 mm. chink the voice is poor. Therefore, it is suggested that the glottic chink be made 4 mm. but to place one vocal cord lower than the other.

SUPERIOR LARYNGEAL NERVE PARALYSIS:

Etiology: Usually secondary to thyroidectomy or supraglottic laryngectomy.

Symptoms:
1. Lowered voice
2. Posterior commissure deviates to the paralyzed side
3. Paralyzed side has a vocal cord that is bowed, flabby and lower. Guttman's Test: Frontal pressure on the thyroid cartilage in the normal subject lowers the voice while lateral pressures raises his voice. In paralysis of the cricothyroid muscle, the opposite is true.

Treatment:
1. As a rule no therapy is necessary
2. Vocal therapy

A surgical procedure to narrow the cricothyroid space may be of benefit if symptoms are severe. Arnold described suturing the thyroid muscle to the cricoid cartilage to elevate the cartilage during phonation.

TRACHEOTOMY:

1. GENERAL CONSIDERATIONS:

A. Tracheotomy is done to form a temporary opening in the trachea. Tracheostomy, in which the trachea is brought to the skin and sewed in place, provides a permanent opening. Tracheostomy is usually done in connection with laryngectomy.

B. Tracheotomy is indicated for two groups of patients.
(1) Those who have an obstruction at or above the level of the larynx (mechanical obstruction).
(2) Those who have no actual obstruction to the airway but cannot raise secretions (secretional obstruction).

Tracheotomy in the second group is becoming increasingly common.

C. Elective tracheotomy may be necessary when respiratory problems are anticipated in the postoperative period in patients being subjected to major head and neck thoracic operations or in patients with chronic pulmonary insufficiency.

Therapeutic tracheotomy is indicated in any case of respiratory insufficiency due to alveolar hypoventilation in order to by-pass obstruction, to remove secretions or to provide for the use of mechanical artificial respiration.

D. Clinical signs of upper airway obstruction: include:
(1) Retraction (suprasternal, supraclavicular, intercostal).
(2) Inspiratory stridor
(3) Restlessness, apprehension, disorientation, leading to coma
(4) Rising pulse and respiratory rates
(5) Pallor (earlier sign) and cyanosis (late danger sign).
(6) Fatigue and exhaustion due to excessive efforts to breathe through an obstructed airway.

The patient's exhaustion must not be regarded as a sign of improvement, but rather a dangerous sign. It is a mistake to wait for late clinical signs of obstruction to appear before performing tracheotomy. The time to proceed with the operation is whenever the possible need was first considered. Surgical manipulation in hypoxemic patients is often associated with cardiac arrest.

E. Function of a Tracheotomy: In addition to the by-pass of an upper airway obstruction, tracheostomy has several other physiologic functions which include:
(1) Decreasing the amount of dead space in the tracheobronchial tree, usually 70 to 100 ml. The decrease in dead space may vary from 10 to 50 percent, depending on the individual's physiologic dead space.

(2) Reduction of resistance to airflow which, in turn, reduces the force required to move air. This will result in increased total compliance and more effective alveolar ventilation, provided the tracheostomy opening is large enough.
(3) Protection against aspiration.
(4) Enables swallowing without reflex apnea which is important in respiratory patients.
(5) Access to the trachea for cleaning.
(6) Pathway to deliver medication and humidification to the tracheobronchial tree, with or without intermittent positive pressure breathing.
(7) Decreasing the power of the cough and thereby preventing peripheral displacement of secretions by the high negative intrathoracic pressure associated with the inspiratory phase normal cough.

F. Tracheotomy in infants and children[18, 48] should always be done after a bronchoscope, endotracheal tube or catheter has been inserted to provide an airway and some rigidity to the trachea. This will convert an emergency tracheotomy to an orderly one. It is easy, in these small patients to carry dissection too deeply and laterally to the trachea with resulting damage to the recurrent laryngeal nerve, the common carotid artery, apex of the pleua, or the cervical esophagus. Caution must be used when incising the tracheal wall not to insert the knife too deeply and lacerate the posterior wall. When the head of a child is turned or keeps moving, a trachea may be entered too laterally. A bronchoscope or endotracheal tube in the trachea will help these complications.[18]

2. INDICATIONS: Indications of tracheotomy may be summarized as below:

A. Mechanical Obstruction:
(1) Obstructive tumors involving the larynx, pharynx, upper trachea, and esophagus, thyroid gland.
  a) When in advanced stage
  b) Edema from radiotherapy
  c) As adjunct to surgery
(2) Inflammation of larynx, trachea, tongue and pharynx.
  a) Acute epiglottis
  b) Viral croup
  c) Ludwig's angina, etc.
(3) Congenital anomalies obstructing larynx or trachea.
  a) Laryngeal web or atresia
  b) Tracheosophageal anomalies, etc.
(4) Trauma of larynx and trachea.
  a) Cartilaginous framework and soft tissues.
  b) Inhalation of steam or fumes (burn)
(5) Maxillofacial trauma with extensive bony and soft tissue damage.
  a) LeFort II, III, multiple fractures of mandible and maxilla, etc.
  b) Hemorrhage
  c) As adjunct to surgery

(6) Bilateral vocal cord paralysis
(7) Foreign bodies

B. Secretional Obstruction:
(1) Retained secretions and inadequate cough.
a) Thoracic and abdominal surgery
b) Bronchopneumonia
c) Burns about face, neck and respiratory tree
d) Conditions producing coma, i.e., diabetes mellitus, uremia, septicemia and liver failure.
(2) Alveolar hypoventilation.
a) Drug intoxication and poisoning
b) Flail chest, fractured ribs and surgical emphysema
c) Paralysis of chest wall
d) Chronic obstructive pulmonary disease, i.e., emphysema, chronic bronchitis, atelectasis, bronchiectasis and asthma.
(3) Both retained secretions and alveolar hypoventilation.
a) Central nervous system disease, i.e., stroke, encephalitis, Guillain-Barré syndrome, poliomyelitis and tetanus.
b) Eclampsia
c) Massive head and chest injuries
d) Neurosurgical postoperative coma
e) Air and fat embolism
f) Several of the conditions noted in (1) and (2) may include both alveolar hypoventilation and retained secretions.

3. TECHNIQUE: Refer to standard textbooks.

4. POSTOPERATIVE CONSIDERATIONS:

A. Immediate postoperative chest x-rays (AP and lateral) are important to ascertain the length and position of the tracheotomy tube and to rule out complications of tracheotomy such as pneumomediastinum or pneumothorax.

B. The inner cannula of the tracheotomy tube should be removed and cleaned every one to two hours for the first two or three days to prevent obstruction by dried mucous. This is especially important in infants.

C. A tracheotomy tube in a fresh tracheotomy should be left in place two to three days before it is changed. By this time a permanent tract exists and there is little danger of being unable to reinsert the tube. Changing a tube before this time may result in loss of the tracheal opening into the neck wound with possible fatality.

D. A string around the neck should never be loosened "for comfort". The tube may slip out of the fresh tracheotomy wound.

E. Suctioning must be done often, especially during the first few days after tracheotomy because of the increase in tracheobronchial secretions secondary to tracheal irritation.

F. A tracheotomy should be left in place no longer than necessary, especially in children. Removal as soon as it is expedient will help reduce the incidence of tracheobronchitis, tracheal ulceration, tracheal stenosis, tracheomalacia and persistent tracheocutaneous fistula.

COMPLICATIONS:[2,5,8,14,16,18,20,24,26,27,29,30,34,35,44,49]
Complications of tracheotomy may be summarized as follows:

A. Immediate:
- (1) Apnea
- (2) Hemorrhage
- (3) Pneumothorax and pneumomediastinum
- (4) Subcutaneous emphysema
- (5) Malpositioned tube
- (6) Tracheoesophageal fistula
- (7) Recurrent laryngeal nerve paralysis
- (8) High tracheotomy (injury to the cricoid cartilage)
- (9) Aerophagia
- (10) Aspiration of gastric contents

B. Delayed:
- (1) Delayed hemorrhage
- (2) Tracheoesophageal fistula
- (3) Tracheocutaneous fistula
- (4) Displacement or obstruction of a tube and a cuff
- (5) Atelectasis and pulmonary infection
- (6) Tracheomalacia
- (7) Dysphagia
- (8) Difficult decannulation
- (9) Problems with neck scar
- (10) Tracheal stenosis

a) Apnea: When tracheotomy is performed on a patient with a history of chronic hypoxia, the patient may take one or two breaths right after the procedure and then suddenly become apneic. This is due to physiologic denervation of the peripheral chemoreceptors by the sudden increase of pO_2 and because hypoxia may be largely responsible for respiratory drive in these patients, apnea results. Some form of respiratory assistance is necessary until enough CO_2 is removed to allow a return of sensitivity of central chemoreceptors. The patient should never be left unattended after an emergency tracheotomy.

b) Hemorrhage: This may occur if hemostasis is not secured at operation.

c) Pneumothorax and pneumomediastinum: Pneumothorax may be caused by injury to the cupula of the pleura which rises into the neck in infants and young children and is subject to injury during the operative procedure. This usually occurs when the tracheotomy is done without prior establishment of an airway by a bronchoscope or an endotracheal tube.

Pneumomediastinum may result from air being sucked through the wound in a child severely obstructed and having violent respiratory movements, or it may result from excessive coughing which forces air into the deep tissue planes of the neck, which then dissects into the mediastinum. Should the parietal pleura rupture, pneumothorax will result. Pneumomediastinum may require no surgical therapy, but pneumothorax often requires the placement of chest tubes with an underwater seal.

d) Malpositioned tube: This is a frequent complication. Careful preoperative selection of a tube followed by postoperative roentgenographic evaluation will prevent this complication. Tubes of excessive length may impinge on the anterior wall of the trachea or the carina producing partial tracheal obstruction as well as ulceration and possible rupture of the innominate artery. The tube may extend down one bronchus with resultant atelectasis of the opposite lung. Too short a tube may predispose to displacement of the tube out of the trachea, especially when the neck is flexed in obese individuals or small children.

e) Tracheoesophageal fistula: This results from penetration through the muscular posterior tracheal wall into the esophagus, or approaching the trachea from the side. Recurrent laryngeal nerve injury rarely occurs. These complications can be avoided by dissecting the midline of the neck and by inserting a rigid endotracheal airway.

f) Aerophagia:[35] Aerophagia is most often seen in infants and young children and should be recognized as a cause of persistent dyspnea; it is treated with nasogastric tube decompression of the swallowed air. Death of an infant secondary to aerophagia with respiratory compromise has been reported.

g) Delayed hemorrhage:[2,5,25,49] This is most often due to erosion of a major vessel by pressure necrosis from the cuff, or occasionally, the tip of the tracheostomy tube. Any bleeding occurring four to five days postoperatively should be given careful and immediate attention because of the threat that it may represent erosion into a major vessel. The innominate artery is the vessel most commonly involved[5] with the common carotid, inferior and superior thyroid arteries aortic arch or, occasionally, the innominate vein.

Mathog et al.[26] proposed possible preventive measures, which include the following: (1) Adequate skin incision to allow visualization or palpation of abnormal vessels. (2) Avoidance of a "low" tracheostomy, i.e., minimal extension of the head, gentle traction with a tracheal hook, and the stoma placed in the second and third tracheal rings. (3) Elimination of metal tubes, with the use of plastic or silicone rubber tubes without a cuff and roentgenographic guidance to be certain the position and length of tubes are appropriate. (4) High humidity and aseptic care of the tracheostomy.

h) Delayed Tracheosophageal fistula: This is usually fatal and results from severe pressure necrosis from an overinflated cuff or from the tip of a malpositioned tube, the erosion occurring through the posterior tracheal wall and the anterior wall of the esophagus. Typically, the aspiration through the fistula results in severe pneumonitis.

i) Difficult decannulation: This is a frequent complication in children. A tracheotomy tube should be decannulated within 8-10 days (or sooner) whenever possible. If not, decannulation becomes difficult because (a) the child gets used to less resistance and less effort (tracheotomy decreases the dead space), (b) the child forgets the apneic reflex during deglutition, and (c) tracheal collapse develops.

j) Neck scar:[24] The use of a vertical skin incision is the most frequent cause of unsightly scar formation. The duration of tracheostomy is also important in scarring which is lessened by early removal of the tube. Vertical contracture and widening of a hypertrophic scar will require a Z-plasty for repair.

k) Tracheal stenosis:[20,22] Stenosis of the larynx follows injury and perichondritis of the cricoid cartilage which is the only circular tracheal support. Tracheal stenosis is most common in children and thought to result from excision of cartilage from the anterior tracheal wall. Exuberant granulations may develop on the anterior tracheal wall due to delayed epithelialization when there is a large defect in the anterior tracheal wall and may cause obstruction and bleeding.

6. ENDOTRACHEAL INTUBATION:

A. Nasotracheal intubation in acute epiglottitis has been recommended. Smooth polyvinylchloride tubes of somewhat smaller caliber than that corresponding to the patient's age are used. After intubation, children are placed in a cool mist-oxygen tent. The tube is tolerated well. Duration of intubation is usually 25-48 hours. Because most children with acute epiglottitis must be intubated to be tracheotomized, and because the critical period for airway obstruction is at most 48 hours, nasotracheal intubation may be preferable to acute tracheotomy in a severely ill child.[45] However, for those who are responsible for the occasional case, it is safer to rely on time-tested tracheostomy. Endotracheal intubation should be done only by an experienced anesthesiologist or otolaryngologist.

B. There has been renewed interest in prolonged endotracheal intubation. Autopsy study showed:[11]

(1) Total damage and laryngeal ulceration in the intubated larynx and trachea were statistically related to duration of intubation but not to age or sex of the patient.

(2) Significant ulcerations were confined to the posterior half of the larynx and the anterior and lateral aspects of the trachea between the 3rd and 10th rings.

(3) Intubation beyond 48 hours was associated with significant laryngeal ulceration, increasingly severe vocal process perichondritis and frequent infestation by microorganisms.

(4) Intubation beyond 96 hours was associated with severe damage to the vocal processes and the subglottis and a higher incidence of inferior vocal fold ulceration.

(5) Tracheal damage in patients with multiple intubations or extubation before death was similar to that in the continuously intubated patients, but inflammation was more widespread and deeper.

(6) Orotracheal intubation of adults for more than 96 hours may cause permanent damage.

C. Causes of inadequate ventilation with intubation include:
(1) Mucous or clot obstruction.
(2) Herniation of the cuff down over the end of the tube.
(3) Collapse of the beveled end of the tube so as to block the lumen.
(4) Lodging of the open portion of the beveled tube against the tracheal wall so as to occlude its lumen.
(5) Kinking of the proximal unarmored end of the tube at its attachement to the adaptor.
(6) Collapse of the endotracheal tube lumen by the inflated cuff.[33]

REFERENCES

1. Andrews, A.H., Jr. and Moss, H.W.: Experiences with carbon dioxide laser in the larynx. Ann. Otol. Rhinol. Laryngol. 83:462-470, 1974.

2. Aubry, M., et al.: Vascular dangers during tracheotomy. Ann. Otolaryng. 87:5-12, 1970.

3. Ballenger, J.J. (Ed.): Diseases of the nose, throat and ear. 11th ed. Philadelphia, Lea and Febiger, 1969.

4. Bass, J.M., et al.: Acute epiglottitis: surgical emergency. JAMA 229:671-675, 1974.

5. Biller, H.F. and Ebert, P.A.: Innominate artery hemorrhage complicating tracheotomy. Ann. Otol. Rhin Laryng. 79:301-306, 1970.

6. Bone, R.C., et al.: Evaluation and correction of dysphagia - producing cervical osteophytosis. Laryngoscope 84:2045-2050, 1974.

7. Canalis, R.F., et al.: Granular cell myoblastoma of the cervical trachea. Arch. Otolaryng. 102:176-179, 1976.

8. Chew, J.Y. and Cantrell, R.W.: Tracheostomy: complications and their management. Arch Otolaryng. 96:538-545, 1972.

9. Cohn, A.M. and Larson, D.L.: Laryngeal injury, a critical review. Arch. Otolaryng. 102:166-170, 1976.

10. DeWeese, D.D. and Saunders, W.H.: Textbook of otolaryngology. 3rd ed. St. Louis, C.V. Mosby Co., 1968.

11. Donnelly, W.H.: Histopathology of endotracheal intubation: autopsy study of 99 cases. Arch. Path. 88:511-520, 1969.

12. Feuerstein, S.S.: Subglottic hemangioma in infants. Laryngoscope 83:466-475, 1973.

13. Gardner, H.G., et al.: Evaluation of racemic epinephrine in treatment of infectious croup. Pediatrics 52:68-71, 1973.

14. Glas, W.W., et al.: Complications of tracheotomy. Arch. Surg. 85:56-63, 1962.

15. Gorkinkel, H.J., et al.: Acute infectious epiglottitis in adults. Ann. Int. Med. 70:289-294, 1969.

16. Grillo, H.C.: Tracheal reconstruction: indications and technics. Arch. Otolaryng. 96:31-39, 1972.

17. Hast, M.H.: Early development of the human laryngeal muscles. Ann. Otol. 81:524-531, 1972.

18. Hawkins, D.B. and Williams, E.H.: Tracheostomy in infants and young children. Laryngoscope 86:331-340, 1976.

19. Hilding, A.C.: Laryngotracheal damage during intratracheal anesthesia: demonstration by staining unfixed specimen with methylene blue. Ann. Otol. Rhin. Laryng. 80:565-581, 1971.

20. Hughes, M., et al.: Skin-lined tube as a complication of tracheostomy. Arch. Otolaryng. 94:568-570, 1971.

21. Hyams, V.J. and Rabuzzi, D.D.: Cartilaginous tumors of larynx. Laryngoscope 80:755-767, 1970.

22. Johnson, G.K., et al.: Acute epiglottitis: review of 55 cases and suggested protocol. Arch. Otolaryngol. 100:333-337, 1974.

23. Krizek, T.J. and Kirchner, J.A.: Tracheal reconstruction with autogenous mucochondrial graft. Plast. & Reconstruction Surg. 50:123-130, 1972.

24. Kulber, H. and Passy, V.: Tracheostomy closure and scar revisions. Arch. Otolaryng. 96:22-26, 1972.

25. Margolis, C.Z., et al.: Routine tracheotomy for hemophilus influenzae type B epiglottitis. J. Pediat. 81:1150, 1971.

26. Mathog, R.H., et al.: Delayed massive hemorrhage following tracheostomy. Laryngoscope 81:107-119, 1971.

27. Meade, J.W.: Tracheotomy - its complications and their management: study of 212 cases. NEJM 265:519-

28. Montgomery, W.W.: Surgery of the upper respiratory system. Vol. 2. Philadelphia, Lea and Febiger, 1973.

29. Nelson, T.G.: Tracheotomy: a clinical and experimental study. Baltimore, Williams & Wilkins, 1958.

30. Ogura, J.H. and Mallen, R.W.: Respiratory insufficiency and tracheostomy, in Ballenger, J.J. (ed.): Diseases of the nose, throat and ear. Philadelphia, Lea & Febiger, 1969, Chap. 26.

31. Ogura, J.H. and Mallen, R.W.: Trauma of the larynx, in Ballenger, J.J. (ed.): Diseases of the nose, throat and ear. Philadelphia, Lea and Febiger, 1969, Chap. 28.

32. Paparella, M.M. and Shumrick, D.A.: Otolaryngology Vol. 3: Head and neck. Philadelphia, W.B. Saunders Co., 1973.

33. Pearson, K.D.: Defective endotracheal tube demonstrated on chest roentgenogram. A case report. Radiology 95:304, 1970.

34. Rabuzzi, D.D. and Reed, G.F.: Intrathoracic complications following tracheotomy in children. Laryngoscope 81:939-946, 1971.

35. Rosnagle, R.S. and Yanagisawa, E.: Aerophagia: unrecognized complication of tracheotomy. Arch. Otolaryng. 89:537-539, 1969.

36. Schechter, G.L. and Kostianovsky, M.: Vocal cord paralysis in diabetes mellitus. Tr. Am. Acad. Ophth. 76:729-740, 1972.

37. Sessions, D.G., et al.: Surgical management of bilateral vocal cord paralysis. Laryngoscope 86:559-566, 1976.

38. Singleton, G.T. and Adkins, W.Y.: Cryosurgical treatment of juvenile laryngeal papillomatosis: eight-year experience. Ann. Otol., Rhin. Laryng. 81:784-790, 1972.

39. Sisson, G.A. (ed.): Symposium on problems of the larynx. Otolaryng. Clin. N. Am., Vol. 3, No. 3, 1970.

40. Strong, M.S., et al.: Cardiac complications of microsurgery of the larynx: etiology, incidence and prevention. Laryngoscope 84:908-920, 1974.

41. Strong, M.S. and Jako, G.J.: Laser surgery in the larynx: early clinical experience with continuous CO_2 laser. Ann. Orol. Rhin. Laryng. 81:791-798, 1972.

42. Swerdlow, R.S., et al.: Cartilaginous tumors of the larynx. Arch. Otolaryng. 100:269-

43. Thawley, S.E. and Ogura, J.H.: Granular cell myoblastoma of the trachea. Arch. Otolaryng. 100:393-394, 1974.

44. Thomas, G.G.: Tracheostomy, in Paparella, M.M. and Shumrick, D.A. (ed.): Otolaryngology. Philadelphia, W.B. Saunders Co., 1973, Chap. 50.

45. Tos, M.: Nasotracheal intubation in acute epiglottis. Arch. Otolaryng. 97:373-375, 1973.

46. Travis, L.W., et al.: Tuberculosis of the larynx. Laryngoscope 86:549-558, 1976.

47. Tucker, J.A. and O'Rahilly, R.: Observations on the embryology of the human larynx. Ann. Otol. 81:520-523, 1972.

48. Tucker, J.A. and Silberman, H.D.: Tracheotomy in pediatrics. Ann. Otol. 81:818-824, 1972.

49. Utley, J.R., et al.: Definitive management of innominate artery hemorrhage complicating tracheostomy. JAMA 220: 577-579, 1972.

CHAPTER 13

ORAL CAVITY AND ESOPHAGUS

The oral cavity is bounded by the lips anteriorly and the cheeks laterally. It extends posteriorly to arches formed by the palatoglossus muscles.

The vestibule is that space lying between the lips and teeth.

The mouth contains: the teeth; the mandible; the maxilla; and the anterior two-thirds of the tongue.

The roof of the mouth consists of the hard palate and soft palate.

The floor of the mouth consists of the anterior two-thirds of the tongue plus the mucosa running from the tongue to the mandible. This area is underlaid by the mylohyoid muscle.

The gums consist of heavy fibrous tissue united with the mucous membrane and covered by stratified squamous epithelium. They attach to the alveolar ridges and surround the bases of the teeth.

The teeth fit into the alveolar ridges of the mandible and maxilla.

Twenty teeth exist in a deciduous set; thirty two teeth replace the deciduous teeth. Both sets are arranged symmetrically bilaterally and are identical above and below. The permanent set consists of two incisors, one canine, two premolars and three molars in each quadrant. Innervation and blood supply arrive within the teeth through the tooth root.

THE TONGUE: This mobile structure occupies much of the space in the oral cavity when the mouth is closed. It acts as the propelling mechanism to move food from the teeth to the pharynx and is vital in producing intelligible speech. The anterior and lateral margins are free.

The frenulum in the midline anteriorly connects with the median raphe of the mandible. Wharton's ducts open on either side of the frenulum.

The inferior surface of the tongue is covered by a thin, smooth mucous membrane with prominent blood vessels underlying it.

The dorsum of the tongue. The anterior two-thirds (palatine segment) is covered with filiform papillae of mucous membrane.

The vallate papillae are a V-shaped group of large papillae marking the junction of the anterior two-thirds of the tongue with the posterior one-third. The apex of the "V" marks the site of the primitive foramen caecum.

The posterior one-third (pharyngeal portion) has no papillae. It does have numerous glands as well as varying amounts of lymphoid follicles (lingual tonsils).

The muscles of the tongue consist of 2 sets - intrinsic and extrinsic.

The intrinsic muscles of the tongue control its shape. They are named according to the location and direction of the fibers: superior longitudinal; inferior longitudinal; transverse; and vertical.

The extrinsic muscles are paired and act to move the tongue:
Styloglossus: retracts tongue and elevates it.
Hyoglossus: depresses tongue.
Genioglossus: protrudes the tip and depresses the tongue as a whole.

Innervation of the tongue comes from the following cranial nerves:

Sensation:
Lingual branch of V: sensation to anterior two-thirds of the tongue.

Chorda tympani branch of VII: taste to the anterior two-thirds of tongue.

Lingual branch of IX: taste and sensation to the posterior third of the tongue.

Superior laryngeal branch of X: sensory branches to the area near the epiglottis.

All motor activity is mediated by the hypoglossal nerve.

The arterial blood supply to the tongue is primarily from the lingual artery although a small contribution is made by the external maxillary and ascending pharyngeal branches. Venous drainage is into the internal jugular.

The lymphatic vessels of the tongue drain chiefly into the deep cervical nodes, lying between the posterior belly of the digastric and the omohyoid muscle. Drainage from the tip area appears to go to the submental and/or omohyoid nodes. Drainage from the lateral area may go to the submaxillary nodes or to the deep cervical region. Central areas drain to both sides.

ISTHMUS OF THE OROPHARYNX:
Boundaries: Tonsillar fauces laterally
The inferior surface of the soft palate
The dorsum of the tongue

The isthmus contains the tonsils.

THE PALATE: The palate marks the superior limit of the oral cavity.

Hard Palate: This is formed from the palatine process of the maxilla and the horizontal plates of the palatine bone. It is covered with the same mucosa which lines the other areas of the mouth. The blood supply arises from the palatine artery. The nerve supply is from the sphenopalatine ganglion.

Torus palatinus is a bony ridge found along the medial suture. It is often protuberant and is mistaken for a tumor. It arises from continued growth of the palatal bones and the horizontal process of the maxilla. Growth proceeds past puberty. The mass may be smooth and symmetrical or irregular and lobulated. Tori are occasionally a problem to denture wearers but rarely require treatment.

The soft palate is continuous with the posterior margin of the hard palate. It is the posterior limit of the oral cavity. The anterior part is free of muscle and contains fibrous connective tissue. Posteriorly, five pairs of muscles can be identified:

The palatoglossus The palatopharyngeus	contracts the lateral dimension
The musculus uvulae	alters the uvula
The levator palati	raises soft palate to contact with posterior pharyngeal wall
The tensor palati	pulls laterally to give firmness and rigidity to the palate

Innervation: The vagus supplies motor function to all except tensor palati which is supplied through the sphenopalatine ganglion.

THE PHARYNX: This tube-like structure extends from the base of the skull to the cricopharyngeus. Its dorsal and lateral walls are complete. The ventral wall has openings for the nasal cavity, the mouth and larynx. It is most commonly divided into: nasopharynx, oropharynx, and laryngopharynx (hypopharynx).

Structures related to the nasopharynx:

- Base of skull
- Adenoids
- Posterior choanae of nose
- Nasal septum
- Torus tubari with eustachian tube orifices
- Pharyngeal recess

Structures related to oropharynx: Tonsils and oral cavity.

Structures related to laryngopharynx:

- Larynx and associated structures
- Epiglottis, valleculae
- Esophagus

Muscles of the pharynx:

- Salpingopharyngeus
- Stylopharyngeus
- Palatopharyngeus

The nerve supply to these muscles comes from branches of the pharyngeal plexus and the glossopharyngeal nerve. They act to elevate and dilate the pharynx during the swallowing mechanism (q. v.).

The external muscles run in an oblique direction and act as constrictors.

The superior constrictor arises from the medial pterygoid plate, the base of the tongue and mandible. It inserts, as do all constrictors, in the median raphe and interdigitates with its corresponding muscle on the opposite side.

The middle constrictor arises from the hyoid bone and stylohyoid ligament.

The inferior constrictor arises from the cricoid and thyroid cartilages. The constrictor muscles have innervation primarily from the pharyngeal plexus although the inferior constrictor may have some additional innervation from the external branch of the superior laryngeal nerve.

Passavant's ridge represents the superior interdigitation of the superior constrictor.

Killian's dehiscence lies at the junction between the upper oblique (thyropharyngeus) and lower transverse (cricopharyngeus) segments of the inferior constrictor. It is through this point of muscular dehiscence that the pulsion diverticulum (Zenker's diverticulum) is thought to arise.

Fascia is not prominent in the pharynx except in areas where muscle is absent. Two major fasciae are recognized:

1. Pharyngobasilar fascia: Hangs the pharynx from the skull and the superior vertebrae.
2. Buccopharyngeal fascia: Attaches posteriorly to the median raphe and to the prevertebral fascia. This fascia prevents retropharyngeal abscesses from crossing the midline. Abscess formation deep to the prevertebral fascia may present as a midline mass because this level lacks the midline fascial insertion.

Blood Supply of the Pharynx: Multiple vessels supply the different levels of the pharynx as it extends from the base of the skull to the cricopharyngeus. These include:

a. The ascending pharyngeal artery: from the external carotid
b. The ascending palatine: from facial artery
c. The tonsillar: from fascial artery
d. Pharyngeal branches of the maxillary artery
e. Greater palatine artery from the maxillary artery
f. Venous drainage from all areas of the pharynx is into the internal jugular vein.

Innervation of the pharynx is supplied through the pharyngeal plexus. This lies on the posterior surface of the middle constrictor and is formed from branches of:

1. Vagus
2. Glossopharyngeus
3. The cranial roots of the spinal accessory nerve
4. The cranial sympathetic trunk

THE PHYSIOLOGY OF MASTICATION: Chewing involves movements of the mandible, lips, tongue, cheeks and teeth. Jaw movements utilizing the teeth convert solid foods to a divided state and mix saliva with bits of food, initiating the digestive process. The tongue and cheeks pass food back and forth between the teeth to facilitate the grinding and dividing action. They then assemble the bolus, ready for swallowing. Swallowing consists of 3 stages:
1. Voluntary collection of food onto the tongue and propulsion back to the isthmus of the pharynx. The mylohyoid, with the assistance of other extrinsic tongue muscles (hyoglossus, palatoglossus and styloglossus), draws the tongue upward and backward, forcing the bolus into the pharynx. At this point protective mechanisms come into play:

(a) The tongue remains elevated while the palatopharyngeus and glossopharyngeus reduce the lumen of the pharyngeal isthmus. This also creates a negative pressure (35 cm. water ±) in the pharynx and nasopharynx.

(b) The nasopharynx is closed off by elevation of the soft palate to appose the tightened superior and middle constrictor muscles. This maneuver utilizes the levator palati, the tensor veli palatini and uvulae muscles.

(c) The pharynx is elevated by contraction of the thyrohyoid muscles. The epiglottis falls over the open glottis to help protect the larynx. Simultaneous closure of the glottis also acts to protect the airway. At the same time the cervical esophagus opens, by virtue of the thyrohyoid contraction. Breathing stops in inspiration at this point. The negative intrathoracic pressure created by this act also helps to distend the esophagus.

2. Reflex movement of the bolus through the pharynx is then carried out utilizing the previously described protective mechanisms. The food is forced downward and the hypopharynx is elevated up around the bolus by the palatopharyngeus and stylopharyngeus muscles.

3. The cricopharyngeus opens. The bolus of food passes and is then propelled by peristaltic waves through the esophagus.

SUMMARY OF THE NEUROLOGIC MECHANISM OF DEGLUTITION: The initial movement of food is voluntary and sets in action a chain of reflex activity encompassing the second and third phases of the swallowing act.

Efferent fibers are furnished by the hypoglossal nerve to the lingual muscles; the third division of the trigeminal nerve to the mylohyoid muscle; and the pharyngeal branches of the glossopharyngeal nerve in conjunction with the pharyngeal and the esophageal plexuses.

Afferent fibers of the swallowing reflex are furnished by branches of the trigeminal, glossopharyngeal and vagus nerves innervating the mucosa at various levels. Blockade by topical anesthesia, particularly the area of the base of the tongue and the pharyngeal wall, inhibits or eliminates the swallowing mechanism in man. Initiation of the entire swallowing mechanism in man depends on stimulation in the mouth. It cannot be initiated in the esophagus. Central control for this activity is mediated through a diffuse mechanism extending through the pons and medulla with a more circumscribed center of control lying in the neighborhood of the vagus nucleus.

LYMPHOID TISSUE QF THE PHARYNX (Waldeyer's ring):

FUNCTION OF WALDEYER'S RING: No clear-cut function for the pharyngeal lymphoid tissue is known. The structures of Waldeyer's ring are well situated to ward off bacteria which might enter through the nose and mouth. Additional protection may be afforded by external secretory antibodies produced in lymphoid tissue and acting directly on these external antigens. This type of system has been shown to exist in tissues adjacent to the nasopharyngeal membranes. In spite of this hypothesis, no evidence yet exists that loss of the lymphoid tissue in Waldeyer's ring lessens human resistance to disease or increases the risk of contracting new disease. In fact, there is strong clinical evidence that repeated infection, with enlargement and scarring of the pre-existing lymphoid architecture, may eliminate any protective function of the system. The controversy surrounding these structures, plus their frequent involvement in otolaryngologic procedures, make the area of special interest to otolaryngologists.

The adenoid (pharyngeal tonsil) lies on the posterior and superior walls of the nasopharynx. It is composed of a lobulated mass of lymphoid tissue enmeshed in fibrous connective tissue. Follicular centers and lymphoid cells are called the follicles of Goodsir. Lymphatic drainage of these structures is to the retropharyngeal and pharyngomaxillary spaces and thence to the neck.

The faucial tonsil is a paired structure, one lying on each side of the pharynx between the palatoglossus (anterior pillar) and palatopharyngeus muscles (posterior pillar). Its development begins in the fourth month of gestation as a simple invagination of mucous membrane at the second branchial pouch, midway between the second and third branchial arches. Crypt formation becomes complex due to the continued epithelial ingrowth of the tissue.

The tonsils vary greatly in size and depth of retraction between the fauces. They are covered over their surface by stratified squamous epithelium which extends into the multiple crypts. Within the structure of the tonsils are three elements:

1. Connective tissue framework along which lie the blood vessels, nerves and lymphatics.
2. Germination follicles where young lymphoid cells are formed.
3. Interfollicular tissue containing lymphoid cells of varying maturity.

Although not a true capsule, the pharyngeal fascia surrounds 4/5 of the tonsil and separates it from its surrounding structures.

The crypts are among the most outstanding anatomical components of the tonsils. They vary in number from 8 to 30 and usually extend the entire depth of the tonsil. Although compound, they are relatively straight. Within the crypts the overlying epithelium lies closely against the lymphatic structure providing little or no obstruction to elements from the outside.

Lymphatic drainage in these structures is all efferent. The lymphatics drain through the buccopharyngeal fascia to the deep cervical nodes, usually ending in one large node near the internal jugular vein, and lying at the side of the posterior belly of the digastric muscle.

Arterial supply is from the lingual, ascending palatine, and tonsillar arteries. The ascending pharyngeal and descending palatine branches also contribute to the arterial supply. The veins begin in the tonsillar plexus, finally draining into the jugular. The nerve supply is derived from branches of the maxillary and glossopharyngeal nerves.

The plica triangularis is a triangular mucosal fold overlying the lower pole of the tonsil and coursing between the anterior and posterior pillars. It often contains small amounts of lymphoid tissue and is the usual source of "regrowth" of the tonsils if not completely excised at the time of tonsillectomy. In some lower animals it actually becomes the faucial tonsil. The plica semilunaris is a thin fold of mucous membrane connecting the palatoglossal and palatopharyngeal folds above the tonsil.

The lingual tonsil lies on the base of the tongue. Anteroposteriorly, it lies between the circumvallate papillae and the epiglottis. Laterally, it is bounded by the faucial tonsils. It is separated from the tongue musculature by a layer of fibrous tissue. It consists of many circular elevations resembling craters. Mucous glands drain into the center of these craters. The surrounding lymphoid tissue drains into the suprahyoid, submaxillary and deep cervical lymph nodes. It is the constituent of Waldeyer's ring most likely to hypertrophy after puberty.

NON-NEOPLASTIC DISEASES OF THE PHARYNX: (Exclusive of the tonsils)

1. SIMPLE PHARYNGITIS:
Etiology: Any of many respiratory pathogens.

Treatment: Specific identification of etiologic agents determines therapy.

Certain patients have chronic pharyngeal irritation based not on infection but allergy, chronic postnasal drainage, smoking, air pollution or other irritating factors. Relief will be obtained only when these irritants are eliminated.

2. MONILIASIS: (Thrush)
Etiology: Long-term antibiotic therapy is probably the most common cause today. Other sources: diabetes, chronic debilitation, failure of newborn to develop normal bacterial responses.

Signs and Symptoms: Sore tongue and mouth with pearly white lesions scattered over the membranes.

Treatment: Reduction of the fungus growth by the use of appropriate medication (Nystatin), discontinuance of antibiotic therapy.

3. RANULA:
Etiology: Apparently represents cyst formation within an area containing lesser salivary glands.

Treatment: Removal is often difficult and recurrence is frequent. Careful dissection should result in elimination of the lesion. Sometimes marsupialization is the most effective means of control.

4. HAIRY TONGUE:
Etiology: Unknown - often seen with respiratory infections and in patients who have not been masticating food. Occasionally seen after penicillin therapy.

Pathology: Elongated filiform papillae with cornified cell material. Usually located in the posterior one-third of the tongue.

Treatment: Careful dietary management. Vitamin supplements, occasionally clipping of the papillae.

5. GEOGRAPHIC TONGUE:
Etiology: Unknown. Seen often in allergic patients, particularly at times of marked allergy manifestation. More often seen in children and young adults.

Finding: Irregular depapillated areas surrounded by a reddish margin combined with a yellow rim. Occasionally painful. Variation in size and position.

Treatment: Characterized by spontaneous remission. No specific treatment known.

6. MEDIAN RHOMBOID GLOSSITIS:
Etiology: Interposition of a portion of base of tongue between the lateral halves of the tongue before fusion in embryonic life.

Finding: Depapillated diamond-shaped area with grooves often present. Almost exclusively seen in men.

Treatment: Unless chronically irritated, no treatment is necessary. The area can be removed if symptoms indicate.

7. EDEMA OF THE UVULA:
Etiology: Often occurs with acute infections. Sometimes seen when the uvula is excessively long and is unconsciously swallowed.

Treatment: Scarification may be necessary to relieve acute edema. Uvulectomy can be employed if recurrent episodes are due to swallowing the uvula.

8. LEUKOPLAKIA:
Etiology: Undetermined. Appears to be related to irritation of the mucosa either by mechanical or chemical factors including smoking, chewing tobacco, and other ingested materials.

Pathology: Increased keratinization of the superficial layers of the mucosa with loss of transparency and flexibility of the tissues. Continued progression may be a precursor of malignant change.

Treatment: Elimination of irritant. Vitamin A supplements, treatment of concurrent diseases (especially syphilis).

9. Many dermatologic diseases have well recognized oral manifestations. Among these are:
  a. Lichen planus
  b. Erythema multiforme (Stevens-Johnson)
  c. Behcet's syndrome
  d. Pemphigus

10. Syphilis produces specific oral changes in each of its stages:
  Congenital - Hutchinson's teeth
  Acute - Primary chancre
  Chronic - Gumma

11. Nutritional deficiencies.

DISEASES OF THE TONSIL:

1. Acute Follicular Tonsillitis:
Infectious agent: Streptococcus, pneumococcus, occasional viruses.

Pathology: Swollen inflamed tonsils, crypts saturated with pus and epithelial debris.

Symptoms: Fever and chills, increasing pain on swallowing, referred ear pain, speech alteration.

Course:
Acute phase: 5-7 days
Rapid loss of symptoms after the fever diminishes
General debilitation following infection

Differential Diagnosis:
a) Diphtheria
b) Infectious mononucleosis
c) Non-bacterial pharyngitis

Treatment: Penicillin is the drug of choice.

2. PERITONSILLAR ABSCESS: Probably develops in a crypt close to the outer aspect of the tonsil. This breaks through either to the supratonsillar area or inferiorly and posteriorly.

Symptoms: Increasing sore throat with dysphagia, trismus, drooling, pain on head movement, "hot potato voice".

Physical findings:
a) Examination is difficult because of trismus.
b) Unilateral swelling and fluctulance of one tonsillar area.
c) Uvula displaced to opposite side.

Differential Diagnosis:
a) Submaxillary space infection
b) Dental infection
c) Infectious mononucleosis

3. INFECTIOUS MONONUCLEOSIS:

Etiology: Probably of viral origin. The disease is characterized by atypical lymphocytes and increasing heterophile titer (Paul-Bunnel Test).

Symptoms: Oral manifestations are often confused with acute follicular tonsillitis.

Physical findings:
a) Marked hyperplasia of the tonsils may take place.
b) Thick white membrane may cover the tonsil.
c) Poor response to antibiotic may be the first hint that infectious mononucleosis is the agent.
d) Throat culture fails to reveal a predominant streptococcal organism.
e) Generalized adenopathy including splenomegaly is present in greater than 50% of cases.

Treatment: Supportive measures including fluids, rest, and analgesics. Steroid therapy may be helpful for extreme cases of pharyngeal infection.

4. BENIGN HYPERPLASIA OF THE TONSILS: This is often associated with recurrent non-specific infections although some persons may have massive lymphoid hypertrophy without any symptoms of infection.

Symptoms: Obstructive breathing. Lymphoid hyperplasia of other structures within Waldeyer's ring.

Treatment: Symptomatic treatment at the time of infection. Superficial scarification with cautery or cryotherapy has produced symptomatic relief.

5. DIPHTHERIA: Although rare now, this is the most serious disease to differentiate from tonsillitis. Diagnosis is based on culture or fluorescent antibody studies.

Physical findings: Exudate extends beyond the tonsils to involve papillae, soft palate and uvula.

Treatment: Antitoxin must be employed before fixation of the endotoxin takes place in the tissue.

6. VINCENT'S ANGINA: This infection takes place when a mixture of fusiform baccilli plus Borrelia Vincentii gain access to the mucosa of the pharynx. This usually a unilateral infection producing ulceration and destruction of the tonsil.

Treatment: Appropriate antibiotics, usually penicillin.

7. LUDWIG'S ANGINA: Often of dental origin, following extraction. Involves submental and submaxillary triangles.

Symptoms: Increasing swelling and pain in floor of the mouth. Tongue is progressively elevated and pushed posteriorly.

Treatment: Involvement of space above geniohyoid muscle allows incision and drainage from within mouth. Penetration of geniohyoid leads to involvement of planes of neck, requring drainage externally. Massive antibiotic therapy is essential. Tracheotomy may be necessary.

8. RETROPHARYNGEAL ABSCESS: Usually due to ear infections in younger children and almost always unilateral. It does not cross the midline because the insertion of the buccopharyngeal fascia prevents progression beyond this point. This disease is usually due to suppurative adenitis of the small nodes between the buccopharyngeal and prevertebral fascia. These nodes are called glands of Henle. They usually regress after age 5. The abscess is characterized by a large mass in the posterior pharyngeal wall which produces dysphagia because of obstruction and pain on swallowing. Dyspnea may occur because of impingement on the arytenoid area.

Treatment: Consists of incision and drainage. Protection of the airway should be exercised to prevent aspiration of pus.

9. PARAPHARYNGEAL INFECTION: Characterized by tenderness and swelling at the angle of the mandible, usually with involvement of the pterygoid muscle area. This infection can travel in the carotid sheath both superiorly and inferiorly. These infections usually respond well to antibiotic therapy and rarely require drainage.

10. TONSILLOLITHS: Arise from retained material in the tonsillar crypts. Usually a cheesy consistency but may become quite hard. Produce discomfort, irritation and foul taste or odor in the mouth.

Treatment: Consists of expression of the tonsilloliths from the crypts. Persistent problems and pain may require tonsillectomy to relieve the symptoms.

Macroglossia (etiologies)
Hemangioma
Myxedema
Acromegaly
Amyloidosis
Cysts
Actinomycosis
Pierre-Robin Syndrome (relative macroglossia)
Tertiary syphilis
von Gierke's disease

ANATOMY OF THE ESOPHAGUS: The esophagus is a mucosal-lined muscular tube which extends from the hypopharynx to the stomach. It differs from the remainder of the gastrointestinal tract in having no serosa. In its average length it extends about 25 cm from the cricopharyngeus to the cardioesophageal junction. Its width varies from 13 mm when relaxed to 30 mm or greater when distended. The cricopharyngeal sphincter is the superior margin in the neck, lying at the level of the cricoid cartilage and the C7 vertebra. The esophagus describes a C-shaped anteroposterior course while descending through the mediastinum anterior to the vertebrae. It begins in the midline of the neck, deviates slightly laterally to the left at the thoracic inlet, returns to the midline and then again deviates to the left near the hiatus of the diaphragm (T_{10}). A small portion (1-2 cm) lies within the abdominal cavity. Three constrictions are recognized:

1. The cricopharyngeus (narrowest area).
2. The broncho-aortic constriction at the arch of the aorta (level of T_4).
3. The cardioesophageal hiatus.

The esophagus has three distinct layers:

1. The inner mucosal layer of stratified squamous epithelium combined with a layer of longitudinally arranged nonstriated muscle.
2. The submucosa contains fibrous connective tissue, vessels, nerves, and mucous glands.
3. The muscularis consists of an inner layer of circularly arranged fibers and an outer layer of longitudinal fibers. The muscle fibers in this layer show gradual transition from striated to smooth muscle as the esophagus descends from the neck to the cardioesophageal junction.

Arterial supply is derived from various vessels as the esophagus passes distally:

1. In the neck: esophageal branches from the inferior thyroid artery.
2. In the chest: esophageal branches from the descending aorta, right intercostal and branchial arteries.
3. In the abdomen: left gastric and inferior celiac arteries.

Venous drainage begins in the plexus on the external surface of the esophagus. Superiorly it drains into the thyroid vein, then into the innominate and on to the superior vena cava. In mid-esophagus, it drains into the azygos and hemiazygos veins.

At the inferior end it drains into the coronary and short gastric veins, thence to the portal vein.

With reduction of flow into the portal vein (as in cirrhosis) the coronary vein shunts blood via the esophageal plexus to the superior vena cava. The massive increase in venous flow through these small vessels produces varices.

Lymphatic drainage also has three major segments:

1. Superior: into the tracheal and inferior deep cervical nodes.
2. Mid-thoracic: into the bronchial nodes.
3. Esophagogastric: into celiac and suprapancreatic nodes.

Innervation is largely autonomic.

Sympathetic: In the neck, a combination of fibers from the superior and inferior cervical ganglia. In the thorax, a combination of upper thoracic ganglia plus the greater and lesser splanchnic nerves. In the abdomen, the celiac plexus.

Parasympathetic: all innervation is supplied via the vagus nerve. The vagus probably supplies all striated muscles in the upper portion of the esophagus via the recurrent laryngeal nerve.

PHYSIOLOGY OF ESOPHAGEAL MOTILITY: The function of the esophagus is to transport food from the hypopharynx to the stomach. This is done primarily as a reflex act, stimulated by the voluntary act of deglutition (q.v.).

Coordination between the hypopharynx and esophagus may be blocked by topical anesthesia or CNS disorders, as in cerebrovascular accidents. Peristalsis in the lower portion of the esophagus is not lost but no mechanical stimulation occurs to produce further activity in the amount.

Esophageal transit begins when a bolus of food is forced to the level of the cricopharyngeus by the superior and middle constrictors. The inferior constrictor and cricopharyngeus relax in response to this mechanical stimulation. The entire esophagus also relaxes at the same time. Liquids entering at this point drop by gravity to the cardioesophageal junction. Solids begin progress when peristaltic waves begin at the level of the cricopharyngeus. These waves require a passage time of about 6 seconds through the esophagus. The cardioesophageal junction, which is tonically closed, relaxes upon the stimulation of the transmitted peristaltic activity. This transmission pattern in the lower portion of the esophagus seems to be an intrinsic mechanism and is probably mediated by the plexus of Auerbach. More proximally, where striated muscle is present, the mechanism is dependent on extrinsic nerve activity. All levels can be influenced by extrinsic stimuli such as central or hormonal mechanisms.

DISEASES OF THE ESOPHAGUS: Multiple disease entities involve the esophagus. Only a few of the major ones, those which may involve the otolaryngologist, will be reviewed here.

1. CORROSIVE ESOPHAGITIS: Found in children predominantly - usually due to ingestion of caustics (lye, acids, oxidizing agents).

Characterized by loss of mucosal surface and scarring of muscle. Tends to progress slowly to obstruction as fibrosis takes place. The natural sequence of lye burns is that of liquefaction necrosis.

- 0 - 24 hours: Dusky, cyanotic edematous mucosa
- 2 - 5 days: Grey-white cast of coagulated protein. Fibroblasts first appear.
- 4 - 7 days: Slough with demarcation of depth of burn (esophagus is probably weakest from day 5 to day 8).
- 8 - 12 days: Collagen first noted
- 6 weeks: Collagen shrinks, stricture becomes evident.

Treatment: (after Kaplan)[1]

a) Careful evaluation of the burn by esophagoscopy should be done at some point early in the course. Time may vary from 24 hours to 5 days. This is the only way of confirming the presence of a burn.
b) Insertion of lumen marker - String on Levin tube.
c) Antibiotics are probably of value if begun early.
d) Corticosteroid use is controversial. It must be started early (within the first 48 hours) to be of any value. It may reduce stricture formation. However, it may only delay repair and also may precipitate perforations of the esophagus or stomach. If used, it is usually employed in tapering amounts over a 3 week period.
e) Dilatation of the stricture, using mercury-filled bougies or string-guided dilators may be started immediately or as soon as burns in the esophagus are identified. Used daily for 10 days, gradually reducing the frequency over the next 3-6 weeks. Careful follow-up, with esophagoscopy for at least 6 months after regular bouginage has been discontinued, is necessary.
f) Uncontrollable stricture formation may require excision and interposition of a colon segment.

2. PEPTIC ESOPHAGITIS: Esophageal mucosa can become irritated by endogenous secretions arising from islands of gastric secretory cells within the esophageal walls or from reflux of gastric juice from the stomach itself.

Cause of reflux:

a) Loss of cardioesophageal spincter tone
b) Hiatus hernia
c) Congenitally short esophagus

Symptoms:

Pain (heart burn)
Bleeding
Dysphagia

Diagnosis: Barium swallow shows spasm, ulceration and stenosis without proximal dilatation. Esophagoscopy confirms position of gastric junction and state of esophageal mucosa. Also useful in ruling out cancer.

3. ACHALASIA: (cardiospasm) (Scleroderma and Dermatomyositis - see Chapter 31: II - 86, 87).

Etiology: No clear-cut cause for this disease has yet been found. The normal peristaltic wave fails to initiate relaxation of the cardio-esophageal sphincter. This results in gradual enlargement of the esophagus. In most cases, degeneration of the nerve cells forming Auerbach's plexus in the wall of the esophagus is found.

Symptoms: Most common in 30's and 40's.

Diagnosis: Usually symptoms of acute and chronic esophageal obstruction with dysphagia:
a) Patient regurgitates food and liquid.
b) Sometimes accompanied by psychiatric disturbances.
c) X-ray shows tight esophageal sphincter with enlarged esophagus. Ulceration is not common.

Treatment: Esophagoscopy should be done before any treatment to rule out ulceration or tumor.

Dilatation of sphincter using mercury bougie or pneumatic dilator under fluoroscopic control is helpful. Cardioplasty with division of the cardioesophageal sphincter musculature has gained increasing popularity. It is essential to perform a complete myotomy.

4. LOWER ESOPHAGEAL RING: (Schatzke's Ring) A radiologic finding of a persistent ring-like constriction in the distal esophagus. Often associated with intermittent dysphagia. Treatment for this is usually by dilatation with mercury dilators.

5. ESOPHAGEAL VARICES: Review of the esophageal anatomy (q.v.) re-emphasizes the critical part which the coronary veins and the esophageal plexus play in diverting blood from the portal system to the superior vena cava. Increasing pressure from the portal system causes enlargement of the esophageal veins in the lower third of the esophagus. Ulceration of the esophageal surface by passing foods or reflux esophagitis may produce massive hemorrhage. Diagnosis is easily made in the known cirrhotic who develops hematemesis and/or melena. The varices are often easily seen on barium swallow. Esophagoscopy, while hazardous, can also define the lesion.

Treatment: Is most effective when portal hypertension can be lowered by a shunt procedure. Specific injection of varices with sclerosing solution is of varying effectiveness.

6. CARCINOMA OF THE ESOPHAGUS: An aggressive malignant disease with high early mortality. Found most often at the natural points of constriction.

Incidence:

Upper one-third - 20%
Middle one-third - 37%
Lower one-third - 43%

Lesions of the upper one-third are found most commonly in women and are often associated with the Plummer-Vincent syndrome - an unusual situation inasmuch as 85% of all esophageal carcinomas are found in men.

7. CONGENITAL ESOPHAGEAL ABNORMALITIES:

Atresia: (tracheal esophageal fistula) - the most common congenital abnormality of the esophagus.

Four major types:

a) Blind upper segment, lower segment connected to trachea. This is the most common form (90%).
b) Upper and lower segments blind.
c) Upper segment attached to trachea, lower segment blind.
d) "H" type - extremely rare.

8. SHORT ESOPHAGUS: Displacement of a portion of the stomach into the thoracic cavity. Usually associated with esophagitis and may be complicated by stricture formation. Easily identified on x-ray by the presence of rugal folds above the level of the diaphragm.

9. VASCULAR RING: Produced by failure of embryonic aortic arch formation to resolve. Compression of esophagus and trachea. Characterized by dysphagia and increasing dyspnea at the time of feeding.

10. ESOPHAGEAL DIVERTICULUM: Three types of diverticulum exist:

Pharyngoesophageal	-	80%
Traction	-	7%
Epiphrenic	-	13%

a) Pharyngoesophageal (Zenker's): Arises from dehiscence between the body of the inferior constrictor and the cricopharyngeus. While thought by some to be congenital, it has not been described in individuals less than 15 years old. Seen most commonly lying to the left of the midline. Progressive enlargement is the general clinical course. Occasionally, carcinoma arises in the pouch, probably due to chronic irritation.

Clinical manifestations:

1) Usually seen in patients over age 50.
2) Increasing dysphagia is most common complaint.
3) Delayed regurgitation of undigested food is common complaint.
4) Often complicated by aspiration pneumonia.

Treatment: Surgical removal, usually through left neck incision. Common wall between the esophagus and diverticulum can be divided by electrodesiccation (Dohlman procedure). Cricopharyngeal myotomy has been advocated for moderate-sized diverticulae.

b) Traction Diverticula: Seen most often at mid 1/3 of esophagus, close to carina. Arise from fixation of esophagus to organizing mediastinal lymph nodes, usually secondary to tuberculosis.

The fundus of the diverticulum is usually above the mouth, preventing accumulation of secretions. Excision is rarely necessary.

c) Epiphrenic Diverticula:
1) Lie just above the diaphragm.
2) Usually associated with achalasia.
3) Occasionally produce ulceration and pain.
4) Symptomatic diverticula can be removed transpleurally.

REFERENCES

1. Kaplan, J., Gandhi, K., Elsen, J., and Oppenheimer, P. "Early Esophagoscopy for Diagnosis of Esophageal Burns", Arch. Otol., 73: 52 (1961).

2. Lindskog, G.E., Liebow, A.A., and Glenn, W.W.L., "Thoracic and Cardiovascular Surgery with Related Pathology", New York, Appleton-Century Crofts, 1962.

3. Mountcastle, V.B., "Medical Physiology", St. Louis, The C.V. Mosby Co., 1974.

CHAPTER 14

SALIVARY GLANDS

ANATOMY OF THE SALIVARY GLANDS: Salivary glands arise early in embryonic life. Solid masses of stratified epithelium within the stomadeum extend into the subjacent mesenchyme. The primordium of the parotid appears at approximately the 4th week. By the 5th week the bud of the parotid is visible at the ectodermal margin of the junction between ectoderm and endoderm.

The submandibular and sublingual glands arise somewhat later from endoderm, close to the parotid bud. All lie in close relationship to the 1st and 2nd branchial arches.

1. THE PAROTID GLAND: This is the largest of the three sets of major salivary glands. It lies in the side of the face, anterior to the external ear. The border of the ascending ramus of the mandible marks the anterior border of the gland. Superiorly, it rises to the level of the zygoma. Inferiorly, it reaches the level of the angle of the mandible. Posteriorly, it follows the margin of the external ear canal and inferiorly sends a tail posteriorly toward the mastoid tip. A smaller medial portion lies deep to the mandible, extending often to the pharyngeal wall.

The gland has a capsule of variable definition. Superficially, it is densely adherent to the gland. Elsewhere it is much less well defined. The surgeon divides the gland into a deep and superficial portion using the facial nerve, which runs directly through the gland, as a dividing line. This definition is not accepted by anatomists who recognize no true isthmus between the two lobes.

STRUCTURES ASSOCIATED WITH THE PAROTID GLAND:

Posteriorly: external auditory meatus, mastoid process and anterior border of the sternocleidomastoid muscle.

Superficial: skin, fascia, lymph nodes, branches of great auricular nerve.

Deep: digastric muscle, styloid process, carotid vessels, jugular vein, cranial nerves X and XI.

Anterior: internal pterygoid and masseter muscles.

Stensen's duct begins in the anterior portion of the gland, crosses anterior to the masseter muscle, pierces the buccinator muscle, and opens into the cheek at the level of the second upper molar. The duct is narrow at its orifice. Proximal to that point its lumen is wider.

The arterial supply is from various branches of the external carotid. The venous drainage is through the internal jugular vein.

Nerves: The auriculotemporal branch of cranial nerve V carries the postganglionic parasympathetic fibers from the otic ganglion to the parotid gland. The preganglionic fibers originate in the inferior salivatory nucleus. They follow the glossopharyngeal nerve to the region of the jugular foramen. Here they join the lesser superficial petrosal nerve and travel to the otic ganglion. This nerve controls secretion by the gland.

Sympathetic innervation comes from the external carotid plexus in a poorly defined manner. The sympathetic nerves act only as vasoconstrictors in the region of the glands and have no control over secretion.

2. THE SUBMANDIBULAR GLAND: This gland lies partly under cover of the mandible with a projection forward under the mylohyoid muscle. Inferiorly it overlaps the digastric muscle. It is separated from the parotid posteriorly by the stylomandibular ligament. The lingual nerve lies medial to the gland and is often tented into the field when the gland is retracted laterally.

Wharton's duct runs forward on the medial surface of the gland, deep to the mylohyoid and superficial to the hyoglossus. It opens through an orifice in the papilla on the frenulum of the tongue. It is accompanied distally by terminal branches of the lingual nerve.

Arterial supply comes from branches of the external maxillary and lingual arteries. Venous drainage follows the course of the arteries.

Preganglionic parasympathetic stimulatory fibers arise from the superior salivatory nucleus and travel along the path of the facial nerve. They separate from the main body of the nerve and pass to the gland via the chorda tympani and submandibular ganglion. Sympathetic innervation to the vessels within the gland arises from the carotid plexus.

3. THE SUBLINGUAL GLAND: This gland is located within the floor of the mouth underlying the mucosa. It runs from the lingual frenulum posteriorly along a depression on the inner surface of the mandible. It lies above the mylohyoid muscle and lateral to the genioglossus muscle and submandibular duct. Multiple orifices may be present.

Arterial supply comes from the sublingual and submental arteries. Innervation is similar to that of the submaxillary gland.

Lesser salivary glands within the oral cavity include: the gland of Blandin situated in the anterior portion of the tongue and the gustatory glands of Ebner connected with the circumvallate papillae.

Numerous small glands are situated throughout the oral cavity, nasopharynx, trachea and bronchi. These secrete continuously and are not under specific autonomic control. It is probably their loss which produces the xerostomia in patients following radiation therapy.

HISTOLOGIC DESCRIPTION OF THE SALIVARY GLANDS: All salivary glands have a racemose pattern. Within this structure two cell types are found. One type usually predominates.

Columnar cells: produce mucin
Cuboid cells: produce serous fluid containing zymogen

The sublingual gland is composed primarily of columnar cells while the parotid gland is composed primarily of cuboidal cells. The submandibular gland is a mixture of the two although the serous type of cell predominates. Accessory salivary glands are mixed but primarily of the mucinous type.

Actions of Saliva:

1. Dissolves materials to facilitate the sense of taste.
2. Alters the consistency of ingested material.
3. Acts to cleanse the mouth of unwanted material.
4. Moistens dry material presented to the mouth.
5. Digestion through the action of ptyalin initiates the breakdown of starches to maltose.
6. Excretes a volume of liquid from the body, dependent on the general hydration of the individual.
7. Lysozyme within the saliva acts as a bacteriocidal agent against many of the common pathogens entering by way of the mouth and respiratory tract.

THE NERVOUS CONTROL OF SALIVARY SECRETIONS: Saliva is needed immediately upon the ingestion of food. Therefore, the salivary glands are primarily under autonomic control via the parasympathetic system. This allows rapid response to various stimuli.

Central control is mediated by the superior and inferior salivatory nuclei. The submaxillary and sublingual glands receive stimulation from the superior salivatory nucleus over the nervus intermedius of Wrisberg. Nerve impulses are then carried via the chorda tympani of the lingual nerve which sends branches into the glands.

The parotid gland obtains its parasympathetic fibers from the inferior salivatory nucleus over the glossopharyngeal nerve via Jacobson's nerve and the lesser superficial petrosal nerve. The synapses take place at the otic ganglion. Postganglionic fibers pass to the gland along the auriculotemporal nerve.

Sympathetic nerves to all salivary glands arise from the superior cervical ganglion and carry only vasoconstrictor fibers to the glands. They do not control salivary secretions.

The secretion of saliva can be stimulated in several ways. Introduction of any material into the mouth will produce salivation. Generally the more palatable the material the more saliva is produced. However, inedible substances with unpleasant taste will also produce great volumes of saliva. The nature of saliva is modified greatly by the material presented. The saliva may act as a lubricant or diluent or it may contain large quantities of organic material including enzymes to promote digestion of starches.

Certain conditioned reflexes produce salivation when no oral stimulation is involved. Saliva production may occur when an individual perceives an odor or when other uses of the special senses produce stimulation.

The amount of saliva secreted varies from 1000 to 1500 cc per 24 hours. The contents of the saliva are 99.5% water, 0.5% solids. Saliva is always acidic in nature and cannot be neutralized or alkalinized for any long period of time.

PATHOLOGY OF THE SALIVARY GLANDS:

1. MUMPS: By far the most common disease related to the salivary glands is a viral infection, affecting primarily the parotid, known as mumps. This disease affects other salivary glands as well but it is best known for its effect on the parotid glands.

Other secreting organs of the body are also affected, especially the pancreas and testicles. Histologically, a lymphocyte infiltrate is seen diffusely throughout the gland coupled with diffuse edema. The disease is self-limiting and is usually without complications.

2. SUPPURATIVE PAROTITIS: (Surgical parotitis) This is usually a staphylococcal infection found in dehydrated debilitated patients. Marked swelling of the gland occurs. A typical acute inflammatory response is seen histologically. The greatest hazard lies in abscess formation. If the abscess breaks spontaneously, it can drain within the cheek area, externally, internally or inferiorly. Treatment usually consists of hydration, antibiotics and, occasionally, small doses of radiation therapy.

3. SALIVARY CALCULI: Calculi are found distributed throughout the salivary glands. They are most commonly found in the submaxillary gland (70-80%). About 20-30% are found in the parotid and sublingual glands. Calculi arise from precipitation of foreign material within the ducts secondary to inflammation or other irritation. Calculi are composed of calcium phosphate or carbonate. In about 75-80% of cases sufficient mineral content is present to make the stones radiopaque. Their presence may obstruct the normal flow of saliva and if chronic obstruction and infection occur, sialectasis and chronic suppurative sialadenitis may result. Not all salivary stones are radiopaque and diagnosis may depend heavily on the history. Sialography is useful in demonstrating obstruction due to a salivary stone. Single acute attacks can often be aborted by removal of the stone, particularly from the submaxillary and sublingual system. Chronic sialolithiasis is a strong indication for removal of the affected gland.

Other sources of non-neoplastic salivary gland enlargement include many of the nutritional diseases such as pellegra, beriberi, kwashiorkor and certain malabsorption syndromes. Diabetes mellitus and hypogonadism are other rare causes of salivary gland enlargement.

Mikulicz' disease is a sequential enlargement of the lacrimal, submaxillary and parotid glands. Histologically a massive small cell infiltration of the interstitial tissue has been described. In recent years, the further understanding of Sjögren's disease has allied this disease to Mikulicz' disease and it is probably more accurate at the present time to speak of Mikulicz-Sjögren's disease. This synrome consists of clinical findings of xerostomia, xerophthalmia, and rheumatoid arthritis. It is primarily found in women (90%). Since rheumatoid arthritis is a major component of the syndrome, it may most easily be found in clinics where a large number of patients with rheumatoid arthritis are present. In some studies as many as 10% of such patients are found to have associated findings of Mikulicz-Sjögren's syndrome.

The primary finding in the salivary glands is atrophy of the secreting tissue associated with infiltration by lymphocytes. A strong argument has been raised that this may be one of the auto-immune diseases. It is almost certain that some abnormality of immunologic response is involved in its pathogenesis.

Some investigators have described marked lymphoid infiltration of a single salivary gland, unaccompanied by other symptoms of Mikulicz-Sjögren's disease. This has been described by Godwin as "benign lymphoepithelial lesion"[2]. It probably represents only a variation of Sjögren's disease and has been described as such by Morgan and Castleman[3]. In these cases lymphoid elements predominate to such a degree that epithelial elements may be obscured.

The presence of Sjögren's disease may predipose the patient to reticulum cell sarcoma or macroglobulinemia[5]. However, this phenomenon seems to be rare. In general, the "lymphoepithelial lesion" may be considered to be benign.

REPRESENTATIVE NEOPLASMS IN THE SALIVARY GLANDS: A wide variety of lesions arise in the salivary glands. Approximately 75% of these are benign. Within that group, 80% are of one type-the mixed tumor. Although site distribution varies in different parts of the world, a general pattern for this country would follow thus: For every 100 parotid tumors, 10 will be found in the submandibular and lesser salivary glands, while 1 will be found in the sublingual gland. Those lesser salivary glands located in the palate are the most likely to develop neoplasia. Neoplasms arising from these glands also have a greater likelihood to be malignant-around 40%. Only about 20% of parotid tumors are malignant, but because of the great total number of parotid tumors they represent about 75% of all malignant growths. Malignant tumors of the other salivary glands account for greater than 50% of total incidence in those areas.

Recently it has been reported that patients with malignant salivary gland tumors are predisposed to carcinoma of the breast. The incidence of breast carcinoma found by Berg et al[1], was greater in patients who had experienced removal of a malignant salivary tumor than that expected for patients who had already had a breast removed for cancer.

1. MIXED TUMOR: (complex adenoma, pleomorphic adenoma) Originally called "mixed tumor" to denote dual origin of the tumor from mixed epithelial and mesenchymal elements, this theory has been almost universally discredited. It is generally agreed that these tumors are of epithelial origin, arising from fully developed salivary gland tissue. The tumors remain a puzzle for classification inasmuch as many different cell forms and proliferation may be found in any single tumor.

Grossly these tumors vary in size. They are usually globular, but may grow irregularly with a fibrous capsule of varying density. Satellite nodules may be found connected only by thin strands of tumor cells. Independent foci have also been found. This multicentricity emphasizes the need for wide lobectomy if the tumor is to be removed completely. In spite of extreme enlargement with compression of surrounding tissue, facial nerve involvement is rare and removal should be possible without sacrifice of nerve function.

Histologically, the tumor must contain both epithelial and mesenchyme-like elements. Beyond this requirement, further classification has proved unsatisfactory due to the extreme morphological complexity demonstrated by these tumors. The tumor should consist of a capsule of varying thickness and completeness; epithelial and myoepithelial elements; and a scanty or abundant stroma having varying composition throughout various parts of the tumor.

2. PAPILLARY CYSTADENOMA LYMPHOMATOSUM: (Warthin's tumor) This tumor is most commonly seen as a swelling beneath the lower pole of the parotid gland, posterior to the angle of the mandible. It is usually seen in white males beyond the age of 40 and may be of multicentric origin. Surgical removal usually results in a cure of the specific tumor although its multicentric origin makes recurrence a possibility. Ten percent have bilateral involvement.

3. ONCOCYTOMA: (Oxyphil Adenoma) These arise in all salivary glands. The exact origin is in dispute. It is characterized by cells with a generous acidophilic cytoplasm, pyknotic nuclei, and the presence of abundant mitochondria. The tumors are round, well encapsulated, and relatively easily removed. Complete removal should result in no recurrence.

4. ACINIC CELL TUMOR: These arise primarily in the parotid gland, particularly in the superficial lobe or tail. They are characterized by cells lying in an acinar pattern. Their general characteristics are so vague as to prevent histologic differentiation between benign and malignant varieties. All should be treated as potentially malignant and widely excised. Fifty percent of patients complain of pain without any evidence of inflammation. It is one of the few salivary tumors which is more common in women than in men.

5. LYMPHANGIOMA: In children this tumor is the most commonly found salivary gland lesion. It appears to represent an error in lymphatic development rather than a true tumor. Complete removal is usually difficult or impossible because of the diffuse nature of the lesion. However, the major portion can be resected with benefit to the patient.

6. HEMANGIOMA: Three types are generally recognized--capillary, cavernous and mixed. The tumor is usually a worm-like mass with fluctuance which can be drained by prolonged pressure. Excision is not always necessary, particularly in young children. The tumor can regress spontaneously in this age group.

7. LIPOMAS: These fatty tumors occur occasionally and are similar to lipomas elsewhere in the body. They are encapsulated and are easily removed.

MALIGNANT SALIVARY GLAND TUMORS: These tumors comprise about 25% of all salivary gland neoplasms. Most malignant tumors are easily recognized by their clinical characteristics. These are (1) rapid growth, (2) pain and (3) in the case of the parotid gland, involvement of the facial nerve.

Seventy-five percent of all malignant salivary gland tumors appear in the parotid, although these comprise only 20-30% of all parotid tumors. A far greater relative incidence of malignant tumors is found in the minor salivary glands (40-50%). In the parotid gland, malignant tumors are more likely to lie in the deep lobe. (Exception: acinic cell carcinoma is usually situated in the superficial lobe). About 30% will present with facial nerve weakness or paralysis.

Spiro et al[4], have developed a staging system for parotid tumors which allows for consistent grading of the tumor:

	T_1	T_2	T_3
	0-3 cm	3.1-6 cm	>6 cm or
	Solitary	Solitary	Multiple nodules or
	Mobile	Decreased mobility or Skin fixation	Deep fixation or Ulceration or
	VII nerve intact	VII nerve intact	VII dysfunction
N_0	Stage I	Stage II	Stage III
N_1			

In a large series reported by Spiro et al, 5 year survival after primary treatment for parotid tumors was:

Stage I: 85%
Stage II: 67%
Stage III: 19%

These figures are in agreement with a report from the Mayo Clinic[6]. That clinic's report also showed that cure rates could be improved by radical surgery. Cell type, age of patient and presence or absence of pain also contributed to altering the prognosis for any of the malignant salivary lesions.

1. MUCOEPIDERMOID TUMOR: These compromise 3 to 9% of all major salivary gland tumors. Histologically, the main components consist of mucous cells and epidermal elements. Varying degrees of differentiation can be found. Capsule formation varies and grossly infiltrating lesions are not uncommon. Because of the wide histologic variation, assessment of malignancy cannot easily be made.

Metastasis seems to be uncommon, unless the tumor is widely anaplastic. For this reason, wide resection of the tumor without neck dissection probably represents adequate treatment in the majority of the tumors. Five year cure rates of 85% have been routinely reported. Incomplete removal leads to recurrence in up to 40% of cases.

2. SQUAMOUS CELL CARCINOMA: These tumors are usually highly malignant although some less malignant varieties do occur. Control of the disease is usually difficult and prognosis is poor, no matter what treatment is employed. Histologically, the tumors consist of islands, nests, and cords of cells showing various degrees of squamous differentiation and infiltration. For the most part, squamous cell carcinomas in the salivary glands are poorly differentiated.

Facial nerve paralysis is seen in about 50% of patients at the time of initial examination. Five year survival is no more than 25% in spite of wide initial removal, with or without neck dissection.

3. ADENOCYSTIC CARCINOMA: (CYLINDROMA) These slow growing lesions have an extremely poor prognosis. Even the most complete initial excision often results in failure because of the tendency for these tumors to grow along perineural lymphatics with extensions beyond the ordinary limits of excision. It is the most common malignant tumor of the submaxillary gland area. However, there is a greater incidence in the minor salivary glands. The inexorable course described above usually results in a 5 year survival rate of 50% or less. Radiation therapy is not of great help in treating this lesion.

Many other malignant tumors are found in the salivary glands, including carcinoid type lesions, intraductal carcinomas, varying types of undifferentiated carcinomas, fibrosarcomas and chondrosarcomas. All of these are extremely infrequent and will not be described here.

General principles for treatment of malignant salivary gland tumors:

1) Many tumors are of low malignancy. Adequate conservative removal is probably sufficient treatment[4, 6].
2) Frankly malignant lesions present with unmistakable signs - facial nerve involvement, pain, rapid growth. These lesions demand radical surgery including en bloc neck dissection if any hope of cure can be expected.
3) A few tumors will lie between these two extremes. However, most of these will also point toward malignancy. A high index of suspicion plus careful consultation with the pathologist should make it possible to treat these lesions adequately.

Incidence of Salivary Gland Tumors:

Benign: (75%)	
Mixed tumor	85%
Warthin's tumor	10%
Adenoma Lymphoepithelial hyperplasia Hemangioma All others	5%

Malignant: (25%)	
Mucoepidermoid	33%
Adenocystic carcinoma	25%
All other malignant lesions	42%

REFERENCES

1. Berg, J.W., et al.: "The Unique Association Between Salivary Gland Cancer and Breast Cancer", JAMA, 204:771 (1968).

2. Godwin, J.I., "Benign Lymphoepithelial Lesion of the Parotid Gland", Cancer, 5:1089 (1952).

3. Morgan, W.S. and Castleman, B., "A Clinicopathological Study of "Mikulicz' Disease", Am. J. Path. 29:471 (1953).

4. Spiro, R.H., et al.: "Cancer of the Parotid Gland", Am. J. Surg., 130:452 (1975).

5. Talal, N., Soholoff, L., and Barth, W.F., "Extrasalivary Lymphoid Abnormalities in Sjögren's Syndrome (reticular cell sarcoma "pseudolymphoma" macroglobulinemia)", Am. J. Med., 43: 50 (1967).

6. Woods, J.E., et al.: "Experience with 1360 Primary Parotid Tumors", Am. J. Surg., 130:460 (1975).

CHAPTER 15

CARCINOMA OF THE ORAL CAVITY AND PHARYNX

INTRODUCTION: Review of therapy for any malignant tumor of the head and neck brings the reader to a firm conclusion that no unanimous opinion exists as to the proper treatment. It is not the aim of this chapter to propose specific modes of therapy for lesions of the oral cavity or pharynx, but rather to present those arguments which are put forth by advocates of surgery, radiotherapy, chemotherapy and combined therapy where appropriate. The reader is expected to have some prior familiarity with the subject and this review is designed to refresh his already established concepts in regard to the treatment of these diseases.

Classification for Carcinoma in the Oral Cavity: The American Joint Committee[1] has developed a method of cancer staging for the oral cavity based on clinical inspection of the oral cavity and neck. The oral cavity is considered as one anatomic region extending from the lips anteriorly, to and including the soft palate, uvula and base of the tongue posteriorly. It is divided into specific sites, including buccal mucosa, lower alveolar ridge, upper alveolar ridge, floor of the mouth, hard palate, anterior 2/3 of the tongue, posterior 1/3 of the tongue (base of tongue) and lip.

DEFINITION OF T N M CATEGORIES IN THE ORAL CAVITY:

T - Primary tumor:

T_{1S}	Carcinoma *in situ*
T_1	Tumor 2 cm or less in diameter
T_2	Tumor greater than 2 cm but less than 4 cm in diameter.
T_3	Tumor greater than 4 cm

N - Regional lymph nodes:

N_0	No clinically palpable cervical lymph node (s): palpable node (s) not suspicious for carcinoma.
N_1	Clinically palpable homolateral cervical lymph node (s). Node not fixed, but metastasis is suspected.
N_2	Clinically palpable contralateral or bilateral cervical lymph node (s) without fixation, metastasis suspected.
N_3	Clinically palpable lymph node (s) that are fixed; metastasis is suspected.

M - Distant metastasis:

M_0	No distant metastasis
M_1	Clinical and/or radiographic evidence of metastasis other than to cervical lymph nodes.

STAGING OF CARCINOMA OF THE ORAL CAVITY:

Staging	T N M Classification
I	T_1 N_0 M_0
II	T_2 N_0 M_0
III	T_3 N_0 M_0
	T_1 N_1 M_0
	T_2 N_1 M_0
	T_3 N_1 M_0
IV	Any primary lesion with N_2 or N_3 with or without distant metastases.

It can be seen from the classification that this system encompasses all of the lesions of the oral cavity, many of which must be dealt with separately when discussing treatment or reviewing the modes of therapy. Certain basic facts are generally true of all lesions in this area, and will be set forth here.

General principles regarding carcinoma of the oral cavity: As with most areas in the upper aero-digestive system, the majority of malignant lesions in the oral cavity are epidermoid carcinoma (85-95%). Behavior of these tumors is similar to that of other epidermoid tumors in that recurrence rarely takes the form of distant metastasis but is more likely to manifest itself as a cervical lymph node or regrowth in the primary area. Concern for the lymphatic drainage of these regions is, therefore, an item of high importance. At the present time there is a great diversity of opinion regarding the proper means of treatment. Jesse[8] has pointed out the value of radiotherapy in treatment of these lesions. He reports that, depending on the anatomic site, metastatic nodes developed in less than 10% of patients where the primary lesion was believed to have been controlled, and who thus might have benefited from elective neck dissection. Furthermore, he suggests that radiation therapy may be of help in preventing contralateral metastases in patients without clinical evidence of nodes at the time of the original treatment.

Southwick[15], on the other hand, favors surgical therapy for the primary lesion with the decision for radical neck dissection dependent on the location, size and cell type of the lesion. He does not advocate radical neck dissection if the primary tumor is small and well differentiated. Neither would he do massive extirpative surgery in the face of grossly disseminated disease. He, as well as others, has pointed out that non-palpable positive nodes found in radical neck dissection are common. Incidence in the literature has been described as being from 25-60%.

Combined therapy may be of value in improving the cure rate of large lesions or in patients with obvious metastasis at the time of initial treatment.

Fletcher and Evans [6] advocate prophylactic radiation as another method of controlling possible metastasis. They reason that early recurrence in almost all tumors is synonymous with poor prognosis for a long-term cure. Early radiation for patients who have high risks of recurrence may reduce the likelihood of this manifestation. They emphasize that even massive recurrences deserve comprehensive radiation therapy to control the further spread of the disease.

Chemotherapy and cryotherapy appear to have only limited application to the treatment of massive tumors in this area at the present time.

Carcinoma of the Floor of the Mouth: Like most cancers of the head and neck, carcinoma of the oral cavity shows a consistent predilection for males. In most series the ratio of men to women is at least 4 : 1. This ratio has diminished over the years. Oral cancer was responsible for 71,000 deaths in the United States in 1969. This accounts for approximately 2% of all cancer mortality.

Many patients developing carcinoma in the floor of the mouth or along the alveolar borders demonstrate preliminary changes that can be recognized. The most important lesion is leukoplakia: This is the most common dyskeratotic lesion of the mouth. It is a grayish adherent patch on the mucosa. It is seen most often on the lower lip, buccal mucosa and pharynx. Histologically, acanthosis and dyskeratosis are seen. Leukoplakia may be reversible if the irritating factors causing it are eliminated. Among these factors are tobacco, alcohol, infection, thermal injury and chemical irritation. Mechanical irritations also contribute to this lesion. It must be differentiated from lichen planus which is grossly similar in appearance. That lesion occurs most commonly on buccal mucosa and is usually seen as white, smooth, slightly elevated patches. Histologically, acanthosis and hyperkeratosis are present in this lesion.

Squamous cell carcinoma found in the floor of the mouth behaves according to the general principles described above. Lesions less than 2 cm in size (Stage I) can probably be treated equally effectively by surgery or radiation. Spiro and Strong [16] have quoted 80% likelihood for control if the primary tumor is 4 cm or less in diameter. Lesions greater than 4 cm uniformly present a poor prognosis, particularly if neck nodes are present. Radical surgery, usually combined with preoperative radiation appears to increase the salvage rate of this group.

While squamous cell carcinoma of the mouth is the most common lesion, a variation is seen in certain individuals who chew tobacco. This consists of a verrucous lesion which is usually noted on the lower buccogingival sulcus. It appears to grow more slowly than the common floor of the mouth carcinoma and it metastasizes less readily. Local resection of this lesion usually produces a satisfactory result unless the lesion has already spread to lymph nodes. In that instance, the tumor must be treated as any other disseminated carcinoma of the floor of the mouth.

Carcinoma of the Tongue: The tongue, while an integral part of the oral cavity, may be considered somewhat separately from lesions of the floor and gingiva.

Tumors of the tongue fall into two categories. Those found in the anterior 2/3 of the tongue are usually of small size and consequently present a better prognosis. Tumors of the posterior third of the tongue are usually initially seen at a later stage (T_3 and T_4 lesions) and as a result have a much poorer prognosis. Treatment of the anterior 2/3 of the tongue can often be done successfully with partial glossectomy and reconstruction in those areas where only a small superficial lesion is present. Radiation therapy may be equally effective for lesions in this area. Radical neck dissection is not advocated unless the primary lesion is advanced (T_3 or T_4) or nodes are palpable.

In lesions involving the posterior third of the tongue, radiation therapy is the treatment of choice, largely because of the advanced stage in which most of these lesions are found. The value of radical neck dissection in such lesions lies primarily in the elimination of disease and reduction of discomfort to the patient. Jesse[8] states that the incidence of metastases is unrelated to the stage of the lesion. This conclusion is somewhat at odds with most observers who report a direct correlation between state of lesion and increasing likelihood of metastasis. All observers of this disease, however, point out the extreme difficulty of evaluating metastases at the time of initial examination. The presence of occult metastasis from tongue cancer has been reported in anywhere from 25-65% of patients undergoing elective neck dissection with removal of the primary tumor. It is this disturbing finding which leads to the advocacy of extensive surgery in the face of these lesions. Elective neck dissection should probably be carried out under the following circumstances:

1. Any tumor present in the posterior third of the tongue.
2. Primary tumor larger than 3 cm.
3. Aggressive nature of the tumor histologically (infiltrating tumor vs. exophytic).

Some centers with strong departments of radiotherapy have increasingly advocated control of possible metastasis by the use of radiation therapy to clinically negative necks. Jesse[8] has described this at length. He has postulated that in lesions where the primary tumor is controlled by radiation only about 5% would have received any possible benefit by subsequent neck dissection. This question requires further evaluation before firm rules can be made for all lesions in this area.

Carcinoma of the Lip: This lesion is seen most frequently on the lower lip of male smokers. The multiple etiologic factors of solar rays, tobacco, skin pigmentation, as well as other less well recognized agents have been incriminated in the production of these lesions. A general 5 year cure rate of 75% probably reflects the ease of diagnosis and resectability for these tumors as well as the fact that they are usually well differentiated. Resection of carcinoma of the lip without palpable cervical nodes should produce a 5 year survival of 85-90%.

In early, well differentiated lesions, wide excision of a V-shaped wedge, usually with primary closure,is sufficient. Occasionally, an Abbe flap, or alternative advancement flap, may be necessary for cosmetic closure. More advanced lesions require a more complex resection including neck dissection. Closure of such a defect may require pedicle flaps from the forehead, chest, etc. Cure of these lesions averages only about 35% for 5 year survival.

Carcinoma of Buccal Mucosa: Malignant lesions of the buccal mucosa present a therapeutic challenge to the physician. They are generally aggressive, although metastasis to lymph nodes is often late. Local recurrence may be due more to inadequate surgery than to the true aggressiveness of the tumor. In general, lesions tend to occur in the posterior one third of the buccal cavity. Curability of this group has been stated by Conley [5] and by others to be considerably lower than tumors located more anteriorly. This may be partly due to the many structures which can be involved in the posterior area, as well as to the extensive lymphatic network involved here. (For a somewhat different experience in this area, the reader should refer to reference 9).

Carcinoma of the Gum: (Alveolar Ridge) This area, like all others in the mouth, is the site of cancer more often in men than women (3:1). The tumor occurs primarily in patients in the sixth through the ninth decades. The usual preponderance of smokers and the heavy user of alcohol are uniform findings [4]. Cure of the lesion is often followed by another lesion elsewhere in the oral cavity. This likelihood can probably be modified if the patient will discontinue smoking and give up the excessive use of alcohol. Most studies document a higher incidence in the lower gum and posterior to the bicuspids. However, cure rates do not vary significantly with location [4,10]. Survival seems to be highly dependent on the presence and/or location of nodes. Cure rates of 60-70% may be expected if localized disease is encountered, whereas the presence of lymph nodes in the region of the sternocleidomastoid muscle or jugular vein reduces the survival prospect to only 30%.

Surgical treatment is adequate for lesions less than 3 cm in diameter. Lesions greater than this present continuing problems. Combined surgery plus radiation seem to provide the greatest likelihood for control in these extensive tumors. Chemotherapy on a long-term basis may also be of value.

Carcinoma of the Pharynx: The Joint Committee for Cancer Staging and End Results Reporting has developed a clinical classification and staging for cancer of the pharynx similar to that for the oral cavity [2].

Familiarity with this classification will help to develop basic concepts relative to cancer in this area.

Initially the cancer is localized in one of 3 regions (nasopharynx, oropharynx, hypopharynx):

1. Nasopharynx: Anterior limit is the choana. The floor is the superior aspect of the soft palate. Its roof is attached to the base of the skull and is continuous with the posterior pharyngeal wall. The inferior limit is level with the free border of the soft palate.

2. Oropharynx: Extends from the free border of the soft palate to the tip of epiglottis. Lateral walls are largely occupied by the palatine tonsils. Mucosa of the anterior wall covers the lingual surface of epiglottis and the pharyngoepiglottic and glossoepiglottic folds bounding the vallecula.

3. Hypopharynx: Extends from the level of tip of epiglottis to level of cervical cartilage. It contains: pyriform sinus, posterior surface of larynx (post-cricoid area) and the lower posterior pharyngeal wall.

The sites within each region are as follows:

1. Nasopharynx:
   a) Posterior superior wall
   b) Lateral wall

2. Oropharynx:
   a) Posterior wall
   b) Lateral wall
   c) Anterior wall (lingual surface of epiglottis and pharyngo-epiglottic and glossoepiglottic folds).

3. Hypopharynx:
   a) Pyriform sinus
   b) Post-cricoid area
   c) Posterior pharyngeal wall

Definition of "T" Categories:

Nasopharynx:

T_1 Tumor limited to one site of the nasopharynx

T_2 Tumor extending to two sites of the nasopharynx

T_3 Tumor extending beyond the nasopharynx

Oropharynx:

T_1 Tumor limited to one site of the oropharynx

T_2 Tumor extending to two sites of the oropharynx

T_3 Tumor extending beyond the oropharynx

Hypopharynx:

T_1	Tumor confined to one site of the hypopharynx
T_2	Tumor extending into two sites of the hypopharynx
T_3	Tumor extending beyond the hypopharynx

Definition of "N" Categories: (Lymph node metastasis)

N_0	No clinically palpable node (s); metastasis not suspected.
N_1	Clinically palpable node (s) that are not fixed; metastasis suspected.
N_2	Clinically palpable node (s) that are fixed; metastasis suspected.

Distant Metastasis: (M)

M_0	No distant metastasis
M_1	Clinical and/or radiographic evidence of metastasis other than to cervical nodes. Radiographic evidence of erosion at the base of the skull or clinical signs of intracranial extension of nasopharyngeal cancer are considered evidence of distant metastasis.

STAGING OF PHARYNGEAL LESIONS:

Stage I	T_1 N_0 M_0
Stage II	T_2 N_0 M_0
Stage II	T_1 T_2 T_3 with N_1 M_0
Stage IV	Any T with N_2 M_0
	Any T with any N M_2

Malignant tumors are more frequent in the pharynx (hypopharynx and tonsils) than elsewhere in the head and neck. In addition, they tend to be more aggressive, with lower overall cure rates. Within each site, however, certain areas prove more amenable to therapy than others. For this reason each area will be dealt with individually.

Carcinoma of the Tonsil: Carcinoma of the tonsil is included with the lesions comprising tumors of the pharynx and has been described in the T N M classification (q.v.). Lesions in this area demonstrate more aggressiveness than tumors in the adjoining buccal mucosa or alveolar ridge.

The following chart illustrates the advanced state of these tumors at initial evaluation[3].

Stage	%
I	15
II	20
III	42
IV	15

In addition, a high incidence of metastatic disease is present on initial examination (more than 50%)[13]. Cancer of the tonsil is the second most common form of cancer in the upper air passages (only carcinoma of the hypopharynx exceeds it). Most of the lesions (90%) are epidermoid carcinoma. The remainder are either sarcomas or lymphomas, or are so grossly undifferentiated as to defy ready classification.

Treatment for these lesions is primarily by radiation therapy. Combined treatment with radiation to the primary followed by composite resection and/or by radical neck dissection seems to improve survival rate slightly. The complication rate from surgery after radiation is generally higher than in other head and neck areas. Survival statistics reported for this lesion are strikingly similar, hovering around 30-35%.

Carcinoma of the Nasopharynx: Lesions of this area are usually recognized late. Often the first indication of such a tumor is a fixed neck node.

The position of this tumor at the base of the skull, surrounded by a rich lymphatic plexus allows multiple paths for metastasis. Direct extension through the foramen lacerum gives access to the middle cranial fossa and cavernous sinus. As a result, cranial nerve involvement is common, especially nerves III, IV, V and VI. Lymphatic spread to the lateral pharyngeal nodes along the carotid sheath involves cranial nerves IX, X, XI, XII. Serous otitis media resulting from eustachian tube obstruction is not uncommon. Any adult patient presenting with unexplained serous otitis media should have a careful nasopharyngeal examination to rule out such a lesion.

This is a unique lesion because of its marked predominance in Chinese. In Singapore it ranks first in incidence of malignant tumors in males, while in the United States it ranks 33rd[11]. Prevailing treatment for this disease is almost universally by radiotherapy. The anatomical inaccessibility of the region makes surgical approach impractical. Million[7] has reported that failure to control neck nodes, rather than failure to control the primary is the only cause of failure in his series of patients. He reports that on primary examination as high as 90% of patients will have clinically positive nodes.

The role of radical neck dissection in control of neck nodes is questionable. Surgery may eliminate gross adenopathy in the neck but it cannot reach the retropharyngeal nodes and does not effectively remove nodes along the base of the skull. It may be of limited benefit as part of planned combined therapy or after radiation where a single local neck recurrence appears.

Carcinoma of the Pyriform Sinus and Post-Cricoid Carcinoma: Carcinoma of the pyriform sinus and hypopharynx has often been included with laryngeal tumors because of their close anatomical relationship. Those lesions lying outside the region of the glottis exhibit a much more aggressive course and must be evaluated independently as pharyngeal neoplasms.

The most common symptom of these lesions is pain. Unfortunately, the source of this often ill-defined discomfort is only recognized late in the course of the disease when lymphatic spread has already occurred. More than 50% of patients have cervical metastases when initially examined. Since diffuse lymphatic spread seems to be an early event with these tumors, control of the disease is predictably low.

Treatment for the majority of these tumors consists of laryngectomy and radical neck dissection, with or without combined radiation therapy. There is some evidence to show that combined therapy may improve the overall cure rate from an average of 20% to as much as 30-35%.

Ogura[12] has pioneered in the application of conservation laryngectomy procedures for these lesions. He has been able to preserve laryngeal function without jeopardizing survival rates. Three year survival rates of 55% have been reported. It must be emphasized that this is done only in properly selected patients. Radical neck dissection should be an integral part of this technique because of the high incidence of cervical metastases.

Radiotherapy is also effective in early lesions. Its effectiveness diminishes rapidly as the lesion increases in size. Overall cure rates using radiation are about the same as for surgery when used alone (20% five-year overall survival)[17].

Post-cricoid carcinoma may be considered almost a combination of lesions with tumor often present in the cervical esophagus as well as in the hypopharynx. Experience by Som[14] and others indicates that this lesion can best be treated by surgical removal. However, overall cure rate has been low (25-30%). Results of radiation therapy seem to be worse (10%). Combined therapy has not produced an improved survival rate and has been accompanied by increased complications.

This lesion is almost exclusively found in women. The most common associated finding is the history of prior hypopharyngeal stricture in 40% of the patients. Post-cricoid carcinoma should be strongly considered in any female who has a history of hypopharyngeal stricture, either present or remote.

REFERENCES

1. American Joint Committee for Cancer Staging and End Results Reporting. "Clinical Staging System for Carcinoma of the Oral Cavity", Chicago, 1968.

2. American Joint Committee for Cancer Staging and End Results Reporting. "Clinical Staging System for Carcinoma of the Pharynx", Chicago, 1965.

3. Barber, R. R. and Weiner, S., "Clinical Management of Tonsil Carcinoma", Surg. Gynec., and Obstet., 119:1035 (1965).

4. Cady, B. and Catlin, D., "Epidermoid Cancer of the Gum", Cancer, 23:551 (March, 1969).

5. Conley, J. and Sadoyama, J., "Squamous Cell Cancer of the Buccal Mucosa", Arch. Otolaryng. 97:330 (April, 1973).

6. Fletcher, G.H. and Evans, W.T., "Radiotherapeutic Management of Surgical Recurrences and Postoperative Residuals in Tumor of the Head and Neck". Radiology, 95:185 (1970).

7. Fletcher, G.H. and Million, R.R., "Malignant Tumors of the Nasopharynx", Am. J. Roentgen, 93:44 (1965).

8. Jesse, R.H. and Lindberg, R.D., "Evaluation of Clinically Negative Neck", JAMA, 217:453 (1971).

9. Krause, C.J., Lee, J.G. and McCabe, B.F., "Carcinoma of the Oral Cavity", Arch. Otolaryng. 97:354 (April 1973).

10. Moore, C. and Catlin, D., "Anatomic Origin and Location of Oral Cancer", Am. J. Surg. 114:510 (1967).

11. Muir, C.S., "Current Concepts in Cancer", JAMA, 220:393 (1972).

12. Ogura, J.H. and Biller, H.F., "Conservation Surgery in Cancer of the Head and Neck", Otolaryng. Clin. N.A., pg. 641-665 (1969).

13. Rubin, P., "Current Concepts in Cancer", JAMA, 217:940 (1971).

14. Som, M. and Nussbaum, M., "Surgical Therapy of Carcinoma of the Hypopharynx and Cervical Esophagus", Otolaryng. Clin. N.A., pg. 631-639 (1969).

15. Southwick, H.W., "Elective Neck Dissection for Intraoral Cancer", Arch. Surg., 80:905 (1960).

16. Spiro, R.H. and Strong, E.W., "Epidermoid Carcinoma of the Mobile Tongue", Am. J. Surg., 122:707 (1971).

17. Wang, C.C., "Radiotherapeutic Approach to Carcinoma of the Hypopharynx", JAMA, 221:79 (1972).

CHAPTER 16

CANCER OF THE LARYNX, EAR AND PARANASAL SINUSES

I CARCINOMA OF THE LARYNX

INCIDENCE: Cancer of the larynx represents less than 2% of all carcinoma. In this regard the American Cancer Society estimates approximately 7000 new patients with laryngeal cancer annually. There appears to be no racial predilection although the incidence is considerably higher in smokers than nonsmokers. In this regard it is of interest that epidermoid carcinoma of the larynx may be experimentally produced in hamsters exposed to chronic cigarette smoke inhalation.[16]

DIAGNOSIS: Clinical diagnosis is usually made by mirror examination. Laryngeal tomography may be helpful in assessing limited portions of the larynx such as the true cords and immediate subglottic space. Xeroradiography may provide similar limited information. When airway obstruction is threatened by tumor size contrast laryngography, which provides more comprehensive examination, may be hazardous and therefore contraindicated. Nevertheless, when possible, laryngography may provide excellent demonstration of difficult-to-examine areas such as the laryngeal surface of the epiglottis at the anterior commissure. During laryngography the modified valsalva maneuver will facilitate examination of the pyriform sinuses, whereas the Mueller maneuver (reverse EE) will aid in evaluating the ventricles of Morgagni by drawing the true cords subglottically, thus dilating the ventricular mucosa. The subglottic arches may also be evaluated by this technique which provides additional opportunity to assess vocal cord mobility on deep inspiration and phonation. Laryngography should generally precede direct laryngoscopy and biopsy since surgical defects or reactive edema produced by the latter render radiologic interpretation difficult if not impossible.

THE BIOPSY: A cc of tissue contains 10^9 cells. In general a carcinoma is detectable palpably when it attains a diameter of 1 cm. Therefore 10^9 cells per cc must be malignant to allow gross detection. Histopathologic detection is possible when 10^6 cells per cc (1 in 1000) are malignant. A lesser ratio of malignant to normal cells per cc of tissue may go entirely unnoticed histopathologically, emphasizing the occasional difficulty in obtaining histologic confirmation of cancer.

TREATMENT MODALITIES: Before deciding on the mode of treatment, it is well to note that, in good hands, the mortality rate of laryngectomy with radical neck dissection varies from 2 to 5%.[9, 11, 13] The risk is higher after the patient has received radiotherapy. MacComb[8] reported that the mortality rate of all composite resections about the head and neck is 4.4% without preoperative irradiation and 8.5% after preoperative irradiation.

This chapter hopes to review established methods of treating laryngeal cancer. It is not intended to promote any specific mode of therapy. To date, surgery, radiotherapy or combined modalities are currently acceptable.

In arriving at a rational treatment plan the theoretical advantages of each require brief review for comparison against large clinical experiences.

The theoretical advantages of radiotherapy:

1. Improved preservation of laryngeal function when tumor extension is limited
2. Control of subclinical disease

The theoretical advantages of surgery:

1. Improved wound healing allowing greater latitude in utilizing conservation and reconstructive techniques
2. Improved detection of tumor recurrence allowing earlier salvage opportunities not often possible after radiation in high doses

In recent years survival rates for each modality have assumed gradual plateaus suggesting each has achieved its maximum effectiveness. With better knowledge of tumor biology and patterns of spread, surgeons have sought alternate means of controlling tumor behavior. In this regard combined radiation and surgical techniques have sought to achieve this goal, radiation theoretically sterilizing the subclinical margins of tumor and surgery removing the center of tumor bulk where radiation is less effective. While this has been clinically successful in treatment of various head and neck cancers, its effectiveness has been most apparent in larger tumors of the oral and pharyngeal cavities. In general, carcinoma of the intrinsic larynx produces symptoms early and is therefore usually detectable when tumor bulk is small, its margins generally precisely defined if not confined by the skeletal framework of the larynx. Combined therapy has therefore enjoyed less popularity in treatment of intrinsic laryngeal carcinoma, but may be indicated when cancer extends beyond the confines of the larynx.

ANATOMIC CLASSIFICATION: The larynx is divided into three regions[2] and these may be subdivided into a number of sites as shown in Fig. 16.1.

Supraglottic: Tip of epiglottis including its free borders to and including false-cords.

Glottic: Floor of ventricle including true cord to 1 cm. infraglottic from the edge of true cord.

Infraglottic: Free edge of cord to lower border of cricoid cartilage.

Transglottic: Lesions that cross the ventricle or involve the larynx above and below true cords.

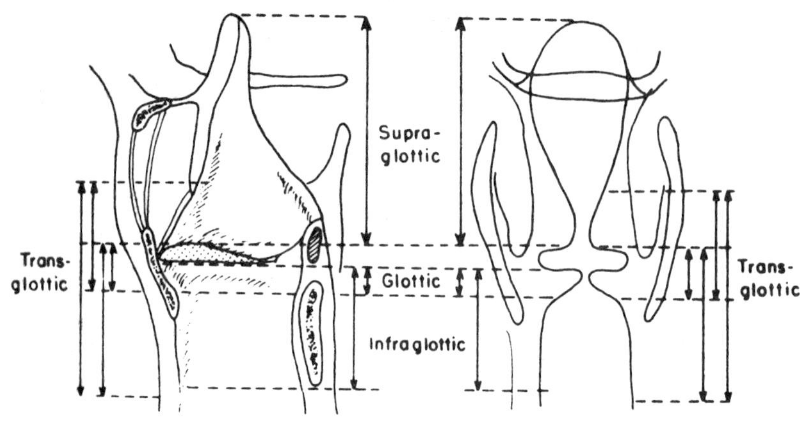

FIGURE 16-1.

TNM CLASSIFICATION AND STAGING: (American Joint Committee on Cancer Staging and End Results Reporting, Geneva, 1972)

T - Primary Tumour:

1. Supraglottis:

T1S Pre-invasive carcinomas (carcinoma in situ).

T1 Tumour limited to the region with normal mobility.

- T1a - Tumour confined to the laryngeal surface of the epiglottis or to an aryepiglottic fold or to a ventricular cavity or to a ventricular band.
- T1b - Tumour involving the epiglottis and extending to the ventricular cavities or bands.

T2 Tumour of the epiglottis and/or ventricles or ventricular bands, and extending to the vocal cords, without fixation.

T3 Tumour limited to the larynx with fixation and/or destruction or other evidence of deep invasion.

T4 Tumour with direct extension beyond the larynx, i.e. to the pyriform sinus, or the postcricoid region or the vallecula or the base of tongue.

2. Glottis:

T1S Pre-invasive carcinoma (carcinoma in situ).

T1 Tumour limited to the region with normal mobility.

- T1a - Tumour confined to one cord.
- T1b - Tumour involving both cords.

T2 Tumour extending to either the subglottic or the supraglottic regions (i.e., to the ventricular bands or the ventricles), with normal or impaired mobility.

T3 Tumour limited to the larynx with fixation of one or both cords.

T4 Tumour extending beyond the larynx i.e., into cartilage or the pyriform sinus or the postcricoid region or the skin.

3. Subglottis:

T1S Pre-invasive carcinoma (carcinoma in situ).

T1 Tumour limited to the region with normal mobility.
- T1a - Tumour limited to one side of the subglottic region and not involving the under surface of the cord.
- T1b - Tumour extending to both sides of the subglottic region and not involving the under surface of the cords.

T2 Tumour involving the subglottic region and extending to one or both cords.

T3 Tumour limited to the larynx with fixation of one or both cords.

T4 Tumour extending beyond the larynx i.e., to the postcricoid region or the trachea or the skin.

N - Regional Lymph Nodes:

N0 Regional lymph nodes not palpable.

N1 Movable homolateral nodes
- N1a Nodes not considered to contain growth.
- N1b Nodes considered to contain growth.

N2 Movable contralateral or bilateral nodes.
- N2a Nodes not considered to contain growth.
- N2b Nodes considered to contain growth.

N3 Fixed nodes.

M - Distant Metastases:

M0 No evidence of distant metastases.

M1 Distant metastases present.

Stage-Grouping:

Stage I	T1	N0 or N1a or N2a	M0
Stage II	T2	N0 or N1a or N2a	M0
Stage III	T3	N0 or N1a or N2a	
	T4	N0 or N1a or N2a	M0
	Any T	N1b or N2b	
Stage IV	Any T	with N3	
	Any T	Any N with	M1

FIVE-YEAR SURVIVAL BY 1972 TNM CLASSIFICATION: The American Joint Committee for Cancer Staging published in July, 1972 the following five-year survival rates on 1632 laryngeal carcinoma, 1061 of which were of glottic origin, 552 supraglottic, 19 subglottic, and one of unknown site or origin (Table I).

Treatment: (Radiation versus Surgery) The recent world literature is deluged with numerous isolated statistics from which comparative analysis appears impossible because of inherent taxonomic ambiguities and varying therapeutic modalities employed. To complicate matters NED (no evidence of disease) statistics are often confused for patient survival rates, which may or may not be clearly defined. Vermund's[21] 1969 series still appears to be the only recent attempt to combine large clinical experiences in a meaningful way. Corrected for the 1972 TNM reclassification his five-year survival statistics appear in Table 2.

TABLE 1

	N0	N1a	N1b	N2b	N3		M	
	Glottic	Supra	Glottic	Supra	Glottic	Supra	Glottic	Supra
T1a	94%	86%	61%	65%	100% (only 1 case)	45%	no cases	
T1b	93%	94%						
T2	85%	82%	62%	45%	(no case)	20%	(no case)	0% (1 case)
T3	65%	76%	53%	36%	0% (4 cases)	20%	no cases	
T4	40%	55%	37%	40%	10%	8%	0% (2 cases)	no cases

TABLE 2

Tumor	Radiation and Surgical Salvage	Surgery
	GLOTTIC	
T1	86%	65%
T2	55%	69%
T3	29%	55%
T4	14%	35%
	SUPRAGLOTTIC	
T1	73%	71%
T2	44%	62%
T3	29%	55%
T4	10%	56%
	SUBGLOTTIC	
T1-4	36%	42%

It would appear that in large series, radiation produces comparable results to surgery when the tumor is small but appears at a decided disadvantage as tumor size increases. The pool of radiation successes in this combined series is even smaller than indicated when survival rates are corrected for surgical salvage following radiation failure.

CONSERVATION SURGERY:

1. According to Som[19] the indication for Horizontal supraglottic laryngectomy is tumor limited to the supraglottic region 3-5 mm. from the anterior commissure with normal vocal cord mobility. Contra-indications are involvement of the vallecula, arytenoid, or pyriform fossa. On the other hand, the criteria proposed by Sisson[18] include:
   a. A margin of 5 mm. must exist between the inferior border of the tumor and the anterior commissure.
   b. The true vocal cords must be mobile.
   c. Only one arytenoid will be removed.

d. There is no clinical or x-ray evidence of extension into the thyroid cartilage. (Theoretically, supraglottic lesions should not involve the thyroid cartilage).
e. There is no evidence of anterior neck invasion. Induration and the presence of enlarged nodes in the suprahyoid space or the thyrohyoid membrane are contraindications to conservation surgery.
f. In case of tongue lesions there must not be fixation of the tongue or extension on the lingual surface to within 5 mm. of the circumvallate papillae or foramen caecum.
g. There must be no extension to either the postcricoid or the interarytenoid space. Prevertebral fascia fixation is a contraindication.
h. Laryngograms and direct endoscopy must prove the apex of the pyriform sinus to be free of disease.
i. Generally, a lesion over 3 cm. in diameter or fixed cervical nodes are contraindications to partial resection.
j. Relatively normal pulmonary function.
k. Under age 60-65.

2. Indications for <u>Vertical hemilaryngectomy</u>[4,5] in nonradiated tumors of the true cord are a) normal mobility, b) less than 30% involvement of the anterior contralateral cord. Contraindications are a) superior involvement of the ventricle or false cord, b) subglottic extension greater than 10 mm. anteriorly. Vertical hemilaryngectomy may be used successfully in salvage of radiation failures of tumors involving the membranous true cord providing strict criteria are met. Contraindications to this procedure in radiated tumors of the true cord are therefore: a) any contralateral cord involvement, b) greater than 5 mm. anterior subglottic extension, c) cord fixation.

3. Indications for <u>Anterior commissure technique</u>[20] are: a) Horseshoe lesions of the membranous vocal cords crossing the anterior commissure, b) less than 10 mm. anterior subglottic extension, c) no arytenoid involvement, d) normal vocal mobility.

DISCUSSION OF SPECIALIZED AREAS:

1. Anterior commissure lesions per se are rare and should not be categorized with cordal tumors that cross the midline anterior commissure. Radiation therapy provides 80% survival rates[15] or 40% five year cure rates according to Kirchner[7] who therefore concludes radiation to be a relatively ineffective treatment modality in this situation. Som[20] provides a 68% surgical cure rate by anterior commissure technique and 81% overall cure rate produced by further salvage surgery.

2. Transglottic carcinoma according to Wang[22] carries a 24% five year survival by radiation therapy alone and 53% five year survival rate when treated by total laryngectomy.

3. Carcinoma in situ of the membranous true cord according to A. Miller[10] carries a 15% probability of invasive change within 3 - 8 months. Vocal cord stripping, the initial treatment of choice,

provides 75% cure rate. Cordectomy is recommended for recurrent carcinoma in situ. Irradiation as the initial treatment is relatively contraindicated because it carries the highest rate of recurrence and invasion.

4. Verrucous carcinoma is characterized by an exophytic warty appearance, slow growth, local invasion, scarcity of metastases and a benign histology. Biller, et al.[3] reported 15 cases of this variant of squamous cell carcinoma. They advocated adequate but conservative surgical excision as opposed to radical radiation therapy.

5. Pyriform sinus carcinoma is rightfully a hypopharyngeal lesion but so often invades the laryngeal framework that its respiratory symptoms, hoarseness, aspiration and pain, justify its brief discussion in this chapter. From a retrospective analysis of 292 patients Ogura[14] concluded that cancer of the laryngopharynx, given low dose preoperative radiation, reduces the incidence of local recurrence from 24% to 9.7%. Preoperative irradiation of 1500-3000 R over a two to three week period, however, did not seem to affect 3 year survival significantly. Using this treatment regimen 3 year survival rates approached 50%.

TREATMENT OF NODAL METASTASIS: There is little disagreement that radical neck dissection is of value in the treatment of the clinically palpable node . However, elective neck dissection remains a controversial issue. The procedure is generally justified when the incidence of occult metastasis for any given tumor approaches 30%. The kind of data that may be helpful in the preoperative decision making process is therefore based on histologic examination of neck specimens in large series.

INCIDENCE OF NODAL METASTASIS:

I.	Norris:[12]	
	Epiglottic	42%
	False cord	29%
	True cord	6%
	Subglottic	16%
II.	McGavran:[9]	
	Supraglottic region	33%
	Transglottic region	52%
	Subglottic region	19%

On the other hand, others might argue that there is in fact no statistical evidence for improved survival rates by elective neck dissection over that performed subsequent to the emergence of a palpable node. Furthermore, there is growing evidence that radiotherapy alone may be effective in controlling occult regional metastases. Bagshaw[1] suggests a 27% five year control rate for N2, N3 adenopathy and in this regard a 95% five year control rate for occult metastasis.

Node fixation is universally an ominous sign. Here radical neck dissection according to Santos[17] provides no substantial role in improving survival in such patients. The effectiveness of standard radical neck dissection is equally questionable when node involvement occurs in the posterior cervical triangle or along the paratracheal chain, the latter notably resulting from a subglottic primary. In this instance Harrison[6] recommends thyroid lobectomy and superior mediastinal dissection of the paratracheal lymphatics.

REFERENCES

1. Bagshaw, M.A., Thompson, R.W.: Elective Irradiation of the Neck in Patients with Primary Carcinoma of the Head and Neck. JAMA 217:456, 1971.

2. Ballenger, J.J.: Diseases of the Nose, Throat and Ear, ed. 11, Philadelphia, Lea & Febiger, 1969. pp. 428.

3. Biller, H.F., Ogura, J.H., Bauer, W.C.: Verrucous Cancer of the Larynx. Laryngoscope 81:1323, 1971.

4. Biller, H.F., Ogura, J.H., Pratt, L.L.: Hemilaryngectomy for T2 Glottic Cancers. Arch. Otolaryng. 93:238, 1971.

5. Biller, H.F., Barnhill, F.R., Ogura, J.H., et al: Hemilaryngectomy following Radiation Failure for Carcinoma of the Vocal Cords, Laryngoscope 80:249, 1970.

6. Harrison, D.F.N.: The Pathology and Management of Subglottic Cancer. Ann. Otol. Rhinol. Laryngol. 80:6, 1971.

7. Kirchner, J.A.: Cancer of the Anterior Commissure of the Larynx, Arch. Otolaryng. 91:524, 1970.

8. MacComb, W.S.: Mortality from Radical Neck Dissection. Amer. J. Surg. 115:352, 1968.

9. McGavran, M.H., Bauer, W.C., Ogura, J.H.: The Incidence of Cervical Lymph Node Metastasis from Epidermoid Carcinoma of the Larynx and their Relationship to Certain Characteristics of the Primary Tumor. Cancer 14:55, 1961.

10. Miller, A.H., Fisher, H.R.: Clues to the Life History of Carcinoma in Situ of the Larynx, Laryngoscope 81:1475, 1971.

11. Nichols, R.R. and Greenfield, D.J.: Experience with Radical Neck Dissection in the Management of 426 Patients with Malignant Tumors of the Head and Neck. Ann. Surg. 167:23, 1968.

12. Norris, O.M.: Laryngectomy and Neck Dissection. Otol. Clin. of N. Amer. October, 1969, pp. 667.

13. Ogura, J.H.: Cancer of the Larynx, Pharynx and Upper Cervical Esophagus, Arch. Otolaryng. 72:66, 1960.

14. Ogura, J.H. and Biller, H.F.: Preoperative Irradiation for Laryngeal and Laryngopharyngeal Cancers. Laryngoscope 80: 802-810, 1970.

15. Olofsson, J., Williams, G.T., Rider, W.D., et al: Anterior Commissure Carcinoma, Arch. Otolaryng. 95:230, 1972.

16. Saffiotti, U., Kaufman, D.G.: Carcinogenesis of Laryngeal Carcinoma, Laryngoscope 85:454, 1975.

17. Santos, V.B., Strong, M.S., Vaughan, C.W., Jr., et al: Role of Surgery in Head and Neck Cancer with Fixed Nodes, Arch. Otolaryng. 101:645, 1975.

18. Sisson, G.A., Goldstein, J.C. and Becker, G.D.: Surgery of Limited Lesions of the Larynx (Past and Present). Otol. Clin. of N. Amer. 3:534, October 1970.

19. Som, M.L.: Conservation Surgery for Carcinoma of the Supraglottis, J. Laryngol. & Otol., 84:655, 1970.

20. Som, M.L., Silver, C.E.: The Anterior Commissure Technique of Partial Laryngectomy, Arch. Otolaryng. 87:138, 1968.

21. Vermund, H.: Role of Radiotherapy in Cancer of the Larynx as Related to the TNM System of Staging. Cancer, 25:485, 1970.

22. Wang, C.C., O'Donnell, A.R.: Cancer of the Larynx. Five Year Results with Emphasis on Radiotherapy. NEJM 252:743, 1955.

II NEOPLASMS OF THE EAR

The majority of ear malignancies involve the auricle (85%)[1] while 10% of such malignancies involve the external auditory canal and only 5% involve the middle ear and mastoid.

EXTERNAL EAR: The majority of tumors of the external ear are squamous cell carcinoma. In Conley's series[1] 62% were squamous and 31% were basal cell epitheliomas. The treatment for basal cell carcinoma of the auricle is wide excision. Miller[5] advocates en bloc resection of most of the auricle with the underlying mastoid cortex when cancer (basal cell or squamous cell) lies within 1 cm. of the external meatus. Squamous cell carcinoma of the helix can be resected widely and primarily reconstructed. Within the canal, the posterior canal wall near the annulus is a common site of malignancy. The lymphatics of this area drain in the direction of the preauricular, mastoid, subparotid, and subdigastric nodes. Lesions of the external auditory canal, particularly of the bony canal, should be treated with "superficial" temporal bone resection leaving intact the facial nerve and the labyrinth. The prognosis for helical and anti-helical lesions (squamous cell as well as basal cell) is 90-95% five year survival. Lesions near the concha and those of the external auditory canal have a five year survival rate of about 30-40%. Lesions of the anterior canal may metastasize to the pre-tragal or parotid nodes through the fissures of Santorini. In general, surgical resection provides a better prognosis than radiotherapy. En-bloc radical neck dissection is not necessary in the absence of clinically palpable nodes. If the parotid region is involved, en-bloc parotidectomy is to be performed.

MIDDLE EAR AND MASTOID: The most common tumor of the middle ear is squamous cell carcinoma while glomus jugulare tumor ranks second in incidence. The most common sarcoma of the middle ear is embryonal rhabdomyosarcoma. Adenoidcystic carcinoma is rare. It is derived from the ceruminous gland duct epithelium of the posterior meatus.[2]

SYMPTOMS OF MALIGNANCY:

1. Deep, unremitting pain due to invasion of bone by tumor.

2. Bleeding from the external auditory canal may be the first and only symptom of disease.

3. Hearing loss may be of the conductive type if tumor obstructs the external auditory canal or destroys the middle ear transformer mechanism. Perceptive hearing loss may result if the inner ear is progressively involved.

4. Vertigo may indicate inner ear destruction.

5. Facial nerve paralysis may occur when disease extends medially to involve the middle and inner ear.

6. Therefore the only symptom that differentiates carcinoma from chronic otitis media or cholesteatoma is pain and its presence should therefore alert the physician to possible malignancy.

DIAGNOSIS: Routine mastoid and skull films show bone destruction in 40% of cases. AP and lateral polytomography are helpful in delineating the extent of bone erosion. Carotid angiography is essential when dural involvement is suspected.

TREATMENT: Early attempts to treat cancer of the temporal bone consisted of radical mastoidectomy followed by radiation therapy which resulted in a five year cure rate of 10%.[5] Osteoradionecrosis and radiation injury to the brain stem often brought devastating sequelae.[7] Temporal bone resection has increased the five year cure rate to 30%.[4] Preoperative radiation should be used cautiously especially when dural involvement is present since the incidence of CSF leaks and meningitis greatly increases when dural grafting follows radiation therapy. In this regard when the dura is involved with carcinoma, radiation used postoperatively avoids life-threatening complications of the dural graft repair.

Lesions involving the middle ear therefore call for subtotal temporal bone resection, a method which Montgomery[6] beautifully describes. Hilding[3] in 1967 described an approach for total resection of the temporal bone. In this regard the facial nerve is sacrificed, a total parotidectomy is performed, and a facial to hypoglossal anastomosis is recommended. Radical neck dissection is recommended when clinical adenopathy is present.

REFERENCES

1. Conley, J.J. and Novack, A.J.: The Surgical Treatment of Malignant Tumors of the Ear and Temporal Bone. Arch. Otolaryng. 71:635, 1960.

2. Goodman, M.L.: Middle Ear and Mastoid Neoplasms. Annals. of Otol., Rhino. and Laryngol. 80:419, 1971.

3. Hilding, D.A. and Selker, R.: Total Resection of the Temporal Bone for Carcinoma. Arch. Otolaryng. 89:636, 1967.

4. Lewis, J.S. and Page, R.: Radical Surgery for Malignant Tumors of the Ear. Arch. Otolaryng. 83:114, 1966.

5. Miller, D.: Cancer of the External Auditory Meatus. Laryngoscope, 65:448, 1955.

6. Montgomery, W.W.: Surgery of the Upper Respiratory Tract, Philadelphia, Lea & Febiger, Vol. 1, pp. 465-481, 1971.

7. Schuknecht, H.R. and Karmody, C.S.: Radionecrosis of the Temporal Bone. Laryngoscope 76:1416, 1966.

III CARCINOMA OF THE PARANASAL SINUSES

Cancer of the paranasal sinuses is relatively rare. According to Martin [3] malignancies here represent 0.2% of all cancer and 3% of cancer of the upper respiratory tract. Carcinoma of the maxillary sinus constitutes 80% of sinus malignancies [1] and has been linked to previous diagnostic introduction of Thorotrast contrast medium into the sinus cavities. [4]

MAXILLARY SINUS:
This is the largest paranasal sinus. Its boundaries are:

Medial Wall	-	Nose
Apex	-	Zygoma
Anterior	-	Face
Posterolateral	-	Infratemporal fossa
Posteromedial	-	Pterygopalatine fossa
Roof	-	Orbit
Floor	-	Alveolar process of the maxilla which holds the three molars and the 2nd premolar. In the adult, the floor of the maxillary sinus is lower than that of the nose, whereas in a child the reverse is true.

Tabb and Barranco [6] reported a male to female ratio of 2:1 with an age distribution greatest in the 6th and 7th decades of life. No racial predilection is reported.

The earliest sign of cancer involving the antrum of Highmore is unilateral nasal obstruction. The next most common symptom is cheek or palate swelling. Nasal bleeding is less commonly encountered. Hypesthesia in the distribution of the infraorbital nerve is an ominous sign which indicates a high and often posterior lesion. Trismus is a sign of pterygoid involvement and ophthalmoplegia points to orbital or intracranial extension.

Most topographical classifications of tumors of the maxillary sinus are based on Ohngren's line, an imaginary line drawn diagonally through the maxillary sinus seen on lateral projection from inner canthus to mandibular angle. Tumors anterior to this line share a better prognosis (71% three year survival) as opposed to tumor posterior to this line (28% three year survival).[2] It is an established fact that tumors lying posteriorly are much more lethal by virtue of their ability to gain access to the anterior cranial fossa through the cribriform plate and into middle cranial fossa via foramen rotundum. Although a TNM classification has not been universally adopted Sisson[5] attempted a classification based on Ohngren's line which may be helpful.

$T_1N_0M_0$ = 1. Invasion of the anterior wall or
2. Inferior naso-antral wall
3. Anterior medial palate

$T_2N_0M_0$ = 1. Invasion of the lateral wall without muscle involvement
2. Invasion of the superior wall without orbital involvement

$T_3N_0M_0$ = 1. Pterygoid muscle invasion
2. Orbital invasion
3. Invasion of anterior ethmoid cells without involvement of cribriform plate
4. Invasion of anterior wall of antrum with skin involvement

$T_4N_0M_0$ = 1. Invasion of cribriform
2. Invasion of pterygomaxillary fossa
3. Extension to nasal fossa or contralateral antrum
4. Invasion of pterygoid plate
5. Invasion of posterior ethmoid cells
6. Extension to ethmo-sphenoid recess or sphenoid sinus

N_0 = No clinically palpable cervical nodes

N_1 = Palpable, non-fixed cervical nodes

N_2 = Palpable, fixed cervical nodes

Stage I	=	$T_1N_0M_0$
Stage II	=	$T_2N_0M_0$, $T_3N_0M_0$
Stage III	=	$T_1N_1M_0$, $T_2N_1M_0$
		$T_3N_1M_0$, $T_4N_0M_0$
		$T_4N_1M_0$, $T_4N_2M_0$

The treatment of choice for maxillary sinus malignancy is en bloc resection of the maxilla including the ethmoid sinus and lateral nasal wall.[6] If indicated, the orbital contents, frontal sinus and cribriform plate are also removed en bloc. Preoperative radiation theoretically improves the ability to encompass the tumor by sterilizing its margins and reducing mechanical spillage at the time of surgery. The average five year survival rate for maxillary carcinoma treated by radical surgery alone is therefore 62%.

The maxillary sinus drains into the retropharyngeal and parapharyngeal nodes. Hence, a routine elective neck dissection is of little benefit. However, if a patient presents with a palpable neck node, neck dissection should be performed although an en bloc dissection is not possible.

The following factors should be considered contraindications to radical surgery of the maxillary sinus:[2]

1. destruction of the base of skull
2. extension of cancer into the nasopharynx
3. inoperable regional metastasis
4. generalized metastasis
5. patient refusal to accept treatment

REFERENCES

1. Ashley, F. L. and Schwartz, A. N.: "Malignant Tumors of the Maxilla." In Converse, J. M. & Littler, J. W., Eds.: Reconstructive Plastic Surgery. Philadelphia, W. B. Saunders Co., 1964, Vol. III. pp. 1038-1052.

2. Jesse, R. H., Butler, J. J., Healey, J. E., Jr., et al: "Paranasal Sinuses and Nasal Cavity" in MacComb, W. S. and Fletcher, G. H.: Cancer of the Head and Neck, Baltimore, Williams and Wilkins Co., 1967, Chap. 10, pp. 329-356.

3. Martin, H.: Cancer of the Head and Neck. JAMA 137:1366, 1948.

4. Schmitz, G. L., Peters, R., and Lehman, R. H.: Thorium Induced Carcinoma of the Maxillary Sinus. Laryngoscope 80: 1722, 1970.

5. Sisson, G., Johnson, E. N., and Amiti, C. S.: Cancer of the Maxillary Sinus. Ann. Otol. Rhinol. Laryngol. 72:1050, 1963.

6. Tabb, H. G. and Barranco, S. J.: Cancer of the Maxillary Sinus. Laryngoscope 81:818, 1971.

FRONTAL, ETHMOID, AND SPHENOID SINUSES

Primary carcinoma of these sinuses is extremely rare. Brownson and Ogura[1] reported five cases of malignancy of the frontal sinus and reviewed the literature for another 28 cases. They concluded that epidermoid carcinoma is the most common form of malignancy in the frontal sinus. The most frequent presenting symptoms are swelling, pain and proptosis. Prognosis is extremely poor. The surgical approach described in their paper recommended that the dura should be sacrificed when the posterior wall is eroded. The ethmoid sinuses should be resected en bloc. The orbit and the contralateral frontal sinus are to be sacrificed when in doubt as to the margin of invasion.

Carcinoma of the ethmoid has a similarly discouraging prognosis. It is interesting to note that ethmoidal carcinoma is unusually common among wood workers. Ketcham[2] has recently reported a series of 48 patients who underwent surgical removal of ethmoid sinuses by a combined intracranial transfacial approach resulting in a 53% five year survival rate. Advantages of this combined approach were: (1) intracranial tumor extension could be established with certainty (2) the brain could be adequately protected during tumor mobilization (3) en bloc removal was possible (4) CSF fistula could be avoided. Preoperative radiation was not used as an adjuvant to surgical resection because of greatly increased morbidity associated with failures of dural grafts and subsequent cerebrospinal fluid leaks and meningitis.

Carcinoma of the sphenoid sinus is very rare with unfavorable prognosis. Because of its inaccessible anatomical location, complete resection is impossible. Consequently, the treatment of choice is radiotherapy. Clinically palpable nodes can be treated with radiation or radical neck dissection.

REFERENCES

1. Brownson, R.J., and Ogura, J.H.: Primary Carcinoma of the Frontal Sinus. Laryngoscope 81:71, 1971.

2. Ketcham, A.S., Chretien, P.B., Schour, L., et al.: "Surgical Treatment of Patients with Advanced Cancer of the Paranasal Sinuses", in Neoplasia of the Head and Neck, Chicago, Year Book Medical Publishers, Inc., pp. 187-202, 1974.

CHAPTER 17

CAROTID BODY TUMOR, HEMANGIOMA, LYMPHANGIOMA, MELANOMA, CYSTS AND TUMORS OF THE JAWS

CAROTID BODY TUMORS: The normal carotid body, situated at the carotid bifurcation, is a chemoreceptor similar to the aortic body. It responds to arterial changes in pH, temperature, oxygen and carbone dioxide tension. The carotid body is different from the carotid sinus, which is a pressoreceptor.

The carotid body tumor is a nonchromaffin paraganglioma associated with a network of chemoreceptors. It is believed to arise from neurocrest cells. Other than at the bifurcation of the carotid, such tumors can be found in other chemoreceptors of the head and neck, middle ear, jugular bulb, carotid bulb, base of skull, lateral pterygoid, vagal and aortic regions. Unlike the carotid body, the tumor has no demonstrable chemoreceptive or hormonal function. These tumors occur generally in equal frequency in men and women, most common in the 3rd and 4th decades of life. The carotid body tumor usually presents as a firm, rubbery, painless, slow-growing mass. When the tumor is large, it may cause a mild pain. Syncopal episodes may occur when the tumor compromises the cerebral blood flow. A bruit is often heard over the tumor. Carotid angiography that shows an "egg shell-like" mass displacing the internal carotid artery laterally and widening the crotch is pathognomonic of this tumor.

Tumors of the carotid body are considered radio-resistant and therefore a symptomatic tumor should be resected. However, an asymptomatic tumor in an elderly patient is best left alone. Carotid body tumor is said to originate from the adventitia of the artery. Consequently, one should be able to free this tumor from the carotid artery. Conley [1] described this tumor as a mass developing in the adventitia of the bifurcation, pushing the internal and external carotid arteries apart. It may eventually encircle both arteries. The weakest point of this encirclement has been determined to be in the posterolateral aspect of the internal carotid artery. Consequently, it is the safest place to begin resection of the tumor. When the internal carotid artery needs to be sacrified, it would be wise to apply a vascular graft. Sacrificing the internal carotid artery without applying a graft carries a 30 to 50% mortality [2] with another 40% incidence of neurological deficits. Nelson [3] in 1962 stated that 5 to 10% of these tumors are malignant. Regional lymph nodes and distant metastases have been reported. However, Conley [1] indicated that multicentricity of paraganglionic foci in the head and neck area is not uncommon. It is, therefore, difficult to differentiate metastases from de novo foci.

REFERENCES

1. Conley, J.J.: The Carotid Body Tumor. Arch. Otolaryng. 81:187, 1965.

2. Lahey, F.H. and Warren, K.W.: A Long Term Appraisal of Carotid Body Tumors with Remarks on Their Removal. Surg. Gynec. Obstet. 92:481, 1951.

3. Nelson, W.R.: Carotid Body Tumors. Surgery 51:326, 1962.

HEMANGIOMAS AND HEMANGIOPERICYTOMA: Hemangiomas are congenital vascular abnormalities rather than true neoplasms. The most common sites are the face and neck. Approximately 63% of hemangiomas are cutaneous, 15% subcutaneous, and 22% mixed. The most common site of deep hemangioma in the head and neck is within the masseter muscles. Females predominate generally in a frequency of 3:1 except for subglottic hemangiomas where the sex ratio is about equal. They may be classified pathologically into 3 types: capillary, cavernous, and mixed. Pathologic classification is probably of little value, compared to clinical classification. Approximately 75% of hemangiomas are present at birth, while 85% will have manifested themselves by the first year of life. Approximately 3% of the patients have a positive family history.

A. Hemangiomas of the Skin and Subcutaneous Tissue:
1. Port-wine hemangioma: This reddish-blue lesion is composed of capillaries with adult endothelium and persists with little change in life. The important features clinically are: (1) the lesion grows only in proportion to body growth and will always cover the same percentage of body surface area; and (2) the lesion is not raised above the surrounding skin. This lesion does not respond to radiation and should be treated with surgical excision, tatooing, or cosmetic coverage. Unless absolutely necessary, treatment is not recommended before the age of two. Hemangiomas that grow rapidly during the first few months of life are also the ones that involute subsequently.

2. Strawberry Hemangioma: This lesion is raised above the surrounding skin, blanches somewhat on pressure, and has a strawberry red color. It is the most common type, accounting for 90% of all infant hemangiomas. Approximately 90% of these hemangiomas are capillary in type and likewise 80 to 90% involute by the fifth year.

Excision should not be performed before age 5, unless serious problems ensue (bleeding, blockage of an important orifice, ulceration, thrombocytopenia, etc.). Steroid treatment seems promising, and sclerosing agents occasionally useful.

The embryonal vascular endothelium of strawberry hemangioma is sensitive to irradiation, but even small doses may inhibit facial bone growth with severe sequelae.

B. Hemangioma of the Parotid Gland: It is the most common tumor of the parotid in infancy. Goldman advocates prompt surgical excision as soon as definite growth is recognized, while others suggest waiting until age 5.

C. Hemangioma of Bone: This lesion is found in the vertebral bodies, frontal and parietal bones, mandible, or maxilla; in females usually during the fourth decade. Slow progressive swelling is seen clinically, and a characteristic "honeycomb" or "sunburst" appearance is present radiographically. Massive hemorrhage may occur following tooth extraction in a mandible involved with a hemangioma. Surgical excision is the treatment of choice.

D. Hemangioma of the Larynx:
1. Subglottic Hemangioma of Infancy - The symptoms produced are of a croup-like syndrome with varying degrees of stridor, absence of hoarseness when crying, weight loss, and marked persistent cyanosis. The cyanosis may be worse when the patient is excited or cries. It is usually the cavernous type and usually located anteriorly. Ninety percent of patients develop symptoms before the age of three months, but only 50% have associated subcutaneous hemangiomas.

The diagnosis is made by laryngoscopy and tracheoscopy. Biopsy is generally contraindicated because of the possibility of severe hemorrhage. The treatment is tracheotomy to relieve the airway obstruction. Gradual involution of the hemangioma in 12 to 18 months is the usual course. Steroids occasionally seem to promote involution. Radiation is not recommended because of (a) absence of proof that in small doses of 300 to 600 r that any significant histologic effect occurs, (b) possible effects of radiation on the growth and development of the larynx, and (c) the possible cause of thyroid carcinoma years later.

2. Adult Laryngeal Hemangioma - The location is usually supraglottic or glottic and often polypoid or pedunculated in appearance. Adult hemangiomas of the larynx rarely cause respiratory embarrassment and generally should be left untreated.

REFERENCES

1. Bridger, G.P., Nassar, V.H. and Skinner, H.G.: Hemangioma in the Adult Larynx, Arch. Otol., Vol. 92, p. 493-498, 1970.

2. Cohen, S.R. and Wang, C.I.: Steroid Treatment of Hemangioma of the Head and Neck in Children, Ann. Otol. Rhinol. Laryng., 81:584, 1972.

3. Davis, E., and Morgan, L.: Hemangioma of Bone, Arch. Otol. Vol. 99, p. 443-445, 1974.

4. Feurstein, S.: Subglottic Hemangioma in Infants, Laryngoscope, Vol. 83, p. 466-475, 1973.

5. Goldman, R.L. and Perzik, S.L.: Infantile Hemangioma of the Parotid Gland, Arch. Otolaryngology, Vol. 90, p. 89-92, 1969.

6. Management of Hemangiomas in Infants, Pediatric Clinics of N. Amer., 6:511-28, May, 1969.

7. Overcash, K.E. and Putney, F.J.: Subglottic Hemangioma of the Larynx Treated with Steroid Therapy, Laryngoscope, Vol. 83, p. 679-682, 1973.

8. Stark, R.B. and Roth, R.F.: Hemangioma, Lymphangioma, and Arteriovenous Fistula, Chapter 27, p. 697-705, Plastic Surgery (Ed. Grabb and Smith), 1973.

HEMANGIOPERICYTOMA: Stout and Murray were the first to accurately describe and name this entity. The capillary pericyte of Zimmermann was the cell of origin of this tumor. It is about equally distributed in both sexes. It shows predilection for the 4th, 5th and 6th decades. Clinically, it presents as a slowly expanding asymptomatic mass. In bony cavities, pressure pain may be noted. With those in the nose and paranasal sinuses, epistaxis is a frequent complaint. Histologically, it features sheets or random distribution of ovoid or spindle-shaped cells with indistinct cytoplasm, large nuclei and rare mitoses. Silver reticulin stain is essential to establish the diagnosis. It is usually considered a malignant lesion with metastatic rates ranging from 35 to 57%. This tumor is radio-resistant. Wide excision is the treatment of choice.

REFERENCES

1. Stout, A.P. and Murray, M.R., Hemangiopericytoma: Vascular Tumor Featuring Zimmermann's Pericytes, Ann. Surg., 116: 26, 1942.

2. Walike, J.W. and Bailey, B.J.: Head and Neck Hemangio-pericytoma, Arch. Otolaryngol. 93:345, 1971.

LYMPHANGIOMA: This is a congenital, benign, unilocular or multilocular, endothelium-lined, fluid containing swelling of lymphatic origin. In 80% of the cases, the lesion is located in the neck. This condition is present at birth in 65% of the cases and would have manifested itself by age two in 90% of them. When symptomatic, they should be resected to prevent stridor and dysphagia in the infant. Resection should be performed carefully to spare all the vital structures. Lymphangioma has been said to be the most common tumor of the parotid gland in children. [1]

REFERENCE

1. Work, W.P. and Gates, G.A.: Tumors of the Parotid Gland and Parapharyngeal Space. Otol. Cl. of N. Am., October, 1969, p. 497.

MELANOMAS OF THE HEAD AND NECK: Melanocytes are believed to be derived from the neural crest cells that have migrated peripherally to the integument by the twelfth week of gestation. The melanocyte forms the pigment which is then transmitted to the malpighian cells of the basal layer of the skin.

Approximately 20% to 35% of melanomas occur in the head and neck region.[1,2] Conley reports the scalp to be the most frequent site, followed by the face, neck and ear. Melanoma occurs slightly more frequently in men except for superficial melanoma of the face which is more common in women. Less than 2% of melanomas occur before puberty. Predisposing etiologic factors are solar exposure, chronic infection, irradiation, friction irritation, thermal burns, and endocrine changes of puberty and pregnancy.

Nevi may be classified into three basic types depending upon the location of the melanocytes.[3]

1. Junctional Nevus - Melanocytes are present at the dermo-epidermal junction. Grossly, it is flat, light to dark brown or black, and non-hairy. Melanoma may arise from junctional nevi, but very rarely before puberty.

2. Compound Nevus - Melanocytes are present in both the epidermis and dermis. Grossly, it combines the features of a junctional and an intradermal nevus.

3. Intradermal Nevus - Melanocytes are exclusively in the dermis. Grossly, this is the common adult mole and may be papillary, pedunculated, or flat and is usually hairy.

Other varieties of nevi are the: (a) Spitz nevus = a dome shaped benign nevus, generally pink or red in color, primarily in children, usually measuring less than 1 cm in diameter. (b) Halo nevus = a central brown papule surrounded by a pale white circle of depigmentation. The regularity of the circle of depigmentation and benign-looking nevus in the center distinguishes it from melanoma. (c) Blue nevus = appears in infancy or childhood as a small black or dark blue, round dome-shaped hard papule with a smooth surface. These tend to appear on the face and on top of the hands and feet and persist unchanged through life. It is benign. The junctional nevus of childhood gradually matures into a compound and then an intradermal nevus. In pregnancy, new moles often appear and pre-existing ones become darker.

Only 25% of melanomas seem to arise from previously benign nevi, almost all junctional.[2] Signs of possible malignant change include: deepening pigmentation, spread of pigment beyond the gross confines of the lesion, ulceration, rapid growth, appearance of flat areas of depigmentation in a black mole, inflammation, satellite nodules, bleeding, and the presence of itching.

Melanoma may be classified into 3 basic types:

1. Superficial spreading melanoma: the surface is elevated, the margins are palpable, and the color variable. The prognosis is intermediate between lentigo maligna melanoma and nodular melanoma.

2. Lentigo maligna melanoma: (Melanoma in a Hutchinson's melanotic freckle) Hutchinson's freckle typically occurs on the cheek of elderly patients as a flat, slowly growing brown lesion.

Malignant melanoma frequently develops in Hutchinson's melanotic freckle and is characterized by thickening and development of black or amelanotic tumor nodules. It infrequently metastasizes and the prognosis is good.

3. Nodular melanoma: A palpable nodule with rapid growth is present in this variety with the poorest prognosis. A lateral flat component is not seen clinically or microscopically.[3,4,8]

The differential diagnosis also includes seborrheric keratosis, senile hemangioma, sclerosing hemangioma, pyogenic granuloma, and pigmented basal cell carcinoma. Eight percent of melanomas in Conley's series were non-pigmented.[1]

Biopsy: An excisional biopsy is performed if the lesion is small. When the location or size makes this impractical, a careful preoperative incisional biopsy is justified. Epstein found there was no evidence to indicate that incomplete removal of malignant melanoma followed by definitive surgery, even one week later, decreases the probability of survival.[5] A radical resection should obviously be made on only definite histologic proof. Frozen sections are highly diagnostic also.

Prognostic Factors: The two most important prognostic factors are type of melanoma and depth of invasion.[6,7] McGovern, et al[8] have classified depth of invasion as:

- Level 1 - Tumor confined to the epidermis
- Level 2 - Tumor invading the papillary dermis (80 to 90% 5-year survival)
- Level 3 - Tumor filling the papillary dermis (50% 5-year survival)
- Level 4 - Tumor invading the reticular dermis (30% 5-year survival)
- Level 5 - Tumor invading the subcutaneous tissue (less than than 20% 5-year survival)

Tumors less than 2 cm in size have a better prognosis than larger ones. Ulceration is associated with a poorer prognosis. Flat lesions have a better prognosis than pedunculated or polypoid lesions. Women of the premenopausal age have a better prognosis than men.[4]

Metastasis to regional lymph nodes varies greatly according to location of the primary (76% for melanoma of the scalp to 19% for primary superficial melanomas of the cheek). Diffuse hematogenous spread may occur to any organ but has a predilection for the brain, liver, and abdominal viscera. Spontaneous regression rarely occurs.

Treatment: Conley[1] divides surgical treatment into two basic categories:
1. Superficial melanomas of the cheek in females that arise in the lentigo nevus have little capacity for metastasis and should be treated with adequate local excision. Likewise, superficial melanomas of

the helix may be treated by wedge excision only because of the low rate of metastasis.[9]

2. Nodular melanomas or melanomas with significant invasion should be treated with wide resection of the primary lesion in continuity with the regional lymphatic drainage. Bilateral neck dissection is not justified and produces no cures for gross metastasis.

Melanoma is radio-resistant although an occasional patient may be palliated but rarely cured. Chemotherapeutic agents have produced only minimal short-term improvement.

Results: The five-year determinate cure rate in Conley's series of 200 patients with melanoma of the head and neck was 35%. Local excision alone produced a five-year cure rate of 62%, which rose to 76% with an elective neck dissection if no evidence of metastasis was found in the regional nodes. The cure rate abruptly drops to 25% if occult metastases were found in the lymph nodes. Composite resection when clinically palpable nodes were present reduced the five-year cure rate to 14%.[1]

REFERENCES

1. Conley, J.J.: Melanoma of the Head and Neck, Vol. 3, Chapter 53, Otolaryngology, (Ed. Paparella and Shumrick), 1973.

2. Knutson, C.O., Hori, J.M., and Spratt, J.S.: Melanoma, Curr. Probl. Surg., p. 3-55, 1971.

3. Ackerman, L.V., Rosai, J.: Surgical Pathology, p. 118-137, 5th ed., C.V. Mosby Co., St. Louis, 1974.

4. Davis, N.C., McLeod, G.R., Beardmore, G.L., Little, J.H., Quinn, R.L. and Holt, J.: Primary Cutaneous Melanoma: A Report from the Queensland Melanoma Project, CA-A Cancer Journal for Clinicians, Vol. 26, No. 2, p. 80-107, 1976.

5. Epstein, E., Bragg, K., and Linden, G.: Biopsy and Prognosis of Malignant Melanoma, JAMA, 208:1369-1371, 1969.

6. Mehnert, J.H. and Heard, J.L.: Staging of Malignant Melanomas by Depth of Invasion, Amer. Jour. Surg., 110:168, 1965.

7. Clark, W.H., Jr., From, L., Bernardino, E.A., and Mihrn, M.C.: The Histogenesis and Biologic Behavior of Primary Human Malignant Melanomas of the Skin, Cancer Res. 29:705-727, 1969.

8. McGovern, V.J., et al.: The Classification of Malignant Melanoma and Its Histological Reporting, Cancer 32: 1446-1457, 1973.

9. Pack, G.T., Conley, J., Oropeza, R.: Melanoma of the Extended Ear, Arch. Otol., Vol. 92, p. 106-117, 1970.

MELANOMA OF MUCOUS MEMBRANE: Melanoma of the mucous membrane comprises approximately 10% of the melanomas of the head and neck. The oral cavity is the site of approximately 50% of cases, the nasal and sinus cavities 35%, and the pharynx and larynx 15%. The most common sites are the palate and the inferior alveolus.

Mucosal melanomas are usually not related to junctional nevi and rarely occur in the olfactory area of the superior nasal recess where pigmentation is abundant. Mucosal melanomas are extremely rare in blacks and there is no apparent relationship to local irritation, chronic infection or allergy.

Nasal or paranasal sinus melanomas presented with epistaxis or nasal obstruction in 88% of patients. The nasal septum and maxillary sinus are the most common sites of origin.

The highest incidence occurs between ages 50 and 70. Grossly, the lesion often appears brownish-grey with a smooth, flat lacy pattern that appears deceptively benign. Nasal melanomas present usually as dark fleshy tumors that bleed easily. Conley advises the removal of all pigmented lesions of the mucous membranes in white patients for diagnostic purposes as well as prophylaxis.

Data by Conley showed metastasis to regional lymph nodes from mucosal melanoma had a lower incidence than melanoma of the skin. Local recurrence after excision varied from 25% in the pharynx to 40% in the nasal cavity and sinuses.

Treatment:

1. Local resection: A wide local resection (e.g. maxillectomy) is favored because of the relatively low incidence of regional metastasis and the discontinuity in the regional lymphatic system.

2. Electrodesiccation is used for superficial melanomas of the palate which gives localized control without extreme ablation.

3. Composite resection of the primary melanoma and the regional lymphatics is applied in continuity when the surgical anatomy permits. For melanomas of the inferior alveolus, lateral pharynx or floor of mouth, it is the treatment of choice.

4. Irradiation is almost universally ineffective against melanoma and should never be used as primary treatment. Some authors use it however pre-operatively or for palliation, especially in nasal or sinus lesions.

Prognosis: Conley reports a 15% five-year determinate cure rate; 11% living with melanoma beyond five years; and 74% dead within five years.

Melanoma of the nasal septum has a better prognosis than melanoma of the turbinates or sinuses.

REFERENCES

1. Barton, R.T.: Mucosal Melanomas of the Head and Neck, Laryngoscope, 85:93-99, 1975.

2. Conley, J. and Pack, G.T.: Melanoma of the Mucous Membranes of the Head and Neck, Arch. Otolaryngol., 99:315-319, 1974.

3. Friedman, H.M., DeSanto, L.W., et al: Malignant Melanoma of the Nasal Cavity and Paranasal Sinuses, Arch. Otolaryngol., 97:322-325, 1973.

CYSTS AND TUMORS OF MAXILLA AND MANDIBLE:

I. ODONTOGENIC TUMORS:

A. Ameloblastoma: (Adamantinomas, adamantine, epithelioma, soft odontoma, adamantoblastoma, epithelial odontoma) It is a very uncommon neoplasm that arises from odontogenic epithelium and comprises about 1% of tumors and cysts found in and around the maxilla and mandible. Rarely, ameloblastoma may arise from a dentigerous cyst. Eighty percent of these tumors are found in the mandible, especially in the molar-ramus region. In the maxilla, its predominant site is in the cuspid and periantral areas. The average age in reported series is 34 to 38 years old. The usual symptom is painless swelling with occasional pathological fracture. The radiographic picture is quite pathognomonic in that it presents multiple radiolucent compartments with a honeycomb arrangement. However, it could present as a unilocular cystic lesion. These are benign tumors though locally invasive, and are radio-resistant. Wide local surgical excision is the preferred treatment to prevent recurrence. Inadequate removal may cause wide local spread at a future date. A small number of cases have been reported with pulmonary metastasis. (The most frequent extraoral primary site is the pituitary gland).

B. Adenomatoid Odontogenic Tumor: The other name for this tumor is adenomeloblastoma which is unfortunate because it bears no relationship to ameloblastoma. It is usually located in the anterior teeth in the maxilla. It is usually related to unerupted teeth. The treatment of choice is locally shelling it out. Recurrence is rare.

C. Ameloblastic Fibroma: This tumor occurs mainly in the premolar-molar region of the mandible. Radiographically, it appears as a unilocular cyst. The age predilection is under 20. Treatment of choice is simple curettage with low recurrence rate. An ameloblastic fibroma with formation of dentin has been referred to as "Dentinoma".

D. Odontomas: It is a tumor of dentin and enamel in which pulp and cementum are also present. Depending upon its histological make-up, it can be subdivided into ameloblastic odontoma, ameloblastic dentinosarcoma, complex odontoma and compound odontoma. These are usually asymptomatic and identified at routine dental x-rays. Conservative removal is the treatment of choice.

E. Odontogenic Myxoma: These tumors occur only in the jaws and arise from connective tissue of the dental papillae. Painless swelling is the main symptom. Though benign, it is locally invasive. Hence, wide total local excision is essential. Radiographically, it is a unilocular or multilocular cyst. It is radio-resistant.

F. Odontogenic Fibroma: Unlike odontogenic myxoma, this is not locally invasive and can be shelled out uneventfully.

G. Cementoma: This is periapical cemental dysplasia. It is asymptomatic and is a routine dental film finding.

II. A. Tori Mandibularis: This is usually a bilateral osteoma occurring lingual to the lower canine or 1st premolar. This should be left alone unless symptomatic.

B. Tori Palatinus: This osteoma occurs in the midline of the palate. This should also be left alone unless symptomatic. Both Tori mandibularis and palatinus appear after puberty.

C. Arteriovenous Aneurysm: There are two varieties: (a) congenital and (b) traumatic. It usually presents as swelling, discoloration, pulsation and a murmur or thrill. Radiographically, a lytic lesion is noted and it is difficult to differentiate it from a benign cyst. Treatment is surgical. Pre-operative angiography may be helpful.

III. ODONTOGENIC CYSTS: It is derived from remnants of the dental lamina or from enamel organs. Symptomatically, it presents as a painless mass. It rarely causes any paresthesia or loosening of a tooth. Malignant degeneration of odontogenic cysts is rarely reported. Odontogenic cysts can be subclassified into:

A. Radicular Cyst: (Periapical or Apical Peridontal Cyst) Radicular cysts are more common in the anterior teeth; and more common in permanent dentition than deciduous dentition. Its etiology is usually acute followed by chronic inflammation of a tooth leading to cystic formation. The treatment is surgical removal of the cyst with possible preservation of the tooth.

B. Dentigerous (Follicular) Cyst: It arises from the enamel or dental lamina of a developing or developed tooth. Classically, it involves the crown of an unerupted tooth with the tooth inside the cyst wall; common sites include the third molar, cuspids, bicuspids, in that order of frequency. Surgical removal of the cyst is advised with possible preservation of the tooth.

C. Eruption Cyst is a dentigerous cyst associated with the erupting surface of a tooth.

D. Gingival and Palatal Cysts of Newborn: (Epstein's Pearl, Bohn's Nodules) The gingival cysts are remnants of the dental lamina. The palatal cysts result from epithelial invagination during development.

E. Lateral Peridontal Cyst is a cyst in bone along the root of a vital tooth.

F. Primordial Cyst forms from the enamel organ before any dental tissue develops. It usually occurs in the mandibular 3rd molar. Histologically, it has uniform epithelium covered with parakeratin and thick caseous debris.

IV. NON-ODONTOGENIC CYSTS: These are derived from epithelial remnants during developmental stage. The maxilla is the common site.

A. Globulomaxillary (Premaxilla-maxillary) Cyst arises from epithelial invagination between the globular process of the frontonasal bone and the maxillary processes of the palatine bone. Clinically, it occurs in the incisive suture between the premaxilla and maxilla (or between the lateral incisor and canine teeth). It is within the bone. The teeth remain vital but may be displaced by the cyst. The cyst is lined with squamous or respiratory epithelium.

B. Nasoalveolar (Nasolabial, Klestadt's) Cyst arises from epithelial rests between the globular, lateral nasal and maxillary processes. Unlike globulomaxillary cyst, it is on the bone with possible erosion of the bone. Ten percent of patients with nasoalveolar cysts have them bilaterally. It is epithelial lined and occurs on the floor of the vestibule anterior to the inferior turbinate.

Depending on the location, other cysts of the same type have been called nasopalatine, median anterior maxillary, median posterior palatine, median mandibular, and anterior lingual.

REFERENCES

1. Banovetz, J.D.: Cysts and Tumors of the Mandible and Maxilla, Otolaryngology, Ed. by Paparella and Shumrick, Vol. 3, Chap. 29, W.B. Saunders, Philadelphia, 1973.

2. Lash, M. and McCoy, G.: Ameloblastoma of the Mandible with Pulmonary Metastasis, Ann. Otol. Rhinol. Laryng., 78:430, 1969.

3. Richardson, J.F. and Greer, R.O.: Ameloblastoma of Mucosal Origin, Arch. Otolaryng., 100:174, 1974.

4. Ward, R.H., et al: Ameloblastoma - A Report of Three Cases, Laryngoscope, 78:2025, 1968.

CHAPTER 18

SYNDROMES AND EPONYMS

I. SYNDROMES AND DISEASES

AIDE'S SYNDROME: decreased pupillary reaction and deep tendon reflex. Etiology is unknown.

ALDRICH'S SYNDROME: Thrombocytopenia exzema and recurrent infections in the 1st year of life. It is inherited through a sex-linked recessive gene. The bleeding time is prolonged, the platelet count is decreased and the bone marrow megakaryocytes are normal in number.

AURICULO-TEMPORAL SYNDROME: (Frey's Syndrome) Characterized by localized flushing and sweating of the ear and cheek region in response to eating, this syndrome usually occurs after parotidectomy. It is assumed that following parotidectomy the parasympathetic fibers of the IX nerve innervate the sweat glands. It has been estimated that 20% of parotidectomy in children results in this disorder.

AVELLIS'S SYNDROME: Unilateral paralysis of the larynx and velum palati, with contralateral loss of pain and temperature sensitivity in the parts below the larynx. This syndrome is caused by involvement of the nucleus ambiguus or the vagus nerve along with the cranial portion of the XI nerve.

BARCLAY-BARON'S DISEASE: Vallecular dysphagia.

BARRETT SYNDROME: Esophagitis due to change of epithelium of the esophagus.

BASAL CELL NEVOID SYNDROME: This familial syndrome, non-sex linked, autosomal dominant with high penetrance and variable expressivity, manifests itself early in life. It appears as multiple nevoid basal cell epitheliomas of the skin, cysts of the jaw, abnormal ribs and metacarpal bones, frontal bossing and dorsal scoliosis. Endocrine abnormalities have been reported and it has been associated with medulloblastoma. The cysts in the jaw, present only in the maxilla and mandible, are destructive to the bone. The basal cell epitheliomas are excised as necessary and the cysts in the jaw rarely recur after complete enucleation. (Maddox, W.D., et al: Multiple Nevoid Basal Cell Epitheliomas, Jaw Cysts, and Skeletal Defects. JAMA 188:106, 1964).

BEHCET'S SYNDROME: Of unknown etiology, this disease runs a protracted course with periods of relapse and remission. It manifests as indolent ulcers of the mucous membrane and skin, stomatitis as well as anogenital ulceration, iritis, conjunctivitis. No definitive cure is known though steroids will help.

BESNIER-BOECK-SCHAUMANN'S SYNDROME: Sarcoidosis.

BOGORAD'S SYNDROME: This is also known as the syndrome of crocodile tears characterized by residual facial paralysis with profuse lacrimation during eating. It is caused by a misdirection of regenerating autonomic fibers to the lacrimal gland instead of to the salivary gland.

BONNIER'S SYNDROME: Due to a lesion of Deiter's nucleus and its connection, its symptoms include ocular disturbances, for example, paralysis of accommodation, nystagmus, diplopia, deafness, nausea, thirst, anorexia, as well as other symptoms referable to involvement of the vagal centers, VIII, IX, X, XI nerves, and the lateral vestibular nucleus. It can simulate Ménière's Disease.

BOURNEVILLE'S SYNDROME: Familial, its symptoms include polyps of the skin, harelip, moles, spina bifida, microcephaly.

BOWEN'S DISEASE: It is a precancerous dermatosis characterized by the development of pinkish or brownish papules covered with a thickened horny layer. Histologically, it shows hyperchromatic acanthotic cells with multinucleated giant cells. Mitoses are frequently observed.

BRIQUET'S SYNDROME: A shortness of breath, and aphonia due to hysterical paralysis of the diaphragm.

BRISSAUD-MARIE SYNDROME: Unilateral spasm of the tongue and lips of a hysterical nature.

CAFFEY'S DISEASE: (Infantile Cortical Hyperostosis). Of familial tendency, its onset is usually in the first year of life. It is characterized by hyper-irritability, fever, and hard non-pitting edema that overlies the cortical hyperostosis. Pathologically, it involves the loss of periosteum with acute inflammatory involvement of the intra-trabecular bone and the overlying soft tissue. Treatment is supportive consisting of steroids and antibiotics. The prognosis is good. The mandible is the most frequently involved.

CAISSON DISEASE: A symptom complex occurring in men working in high air pressures when too suddenly released to normal atmospheric pressure. Similar symptoms may occur in fliers when they suddenly go to high altitudes unprotected by counterpressure. It results from the escape from solution in the body fluids of bubbles (mainly nitrogen) originally absorbed at higher pressure. Symptoms include headache, pain in epigastrium, sinuses, tooth sockets, itchy skin, vertigo, dyspnea, coughing, nausea, vomiting, and sometimes paralysis. Peripheral circulatory collapse may be present. Nitrogen bubbles have been found in the white matter of the spinal cord. It can also injure the inner ear through the necrosis of the organ of Corti. There is a question of rupture of the round window membrane; hemotympanum and eustachian tube obstruction may occur.

CARCINOID SYNDROME: Symptoms include episodic flushing, diarrhea, ascites. The tumor secretes serotonin. The treatment is wide excision. The tumor may give a positive DOPA reaction.

CAROTID SINUS SYNDROME: (Charcot-Weiss-Barber's syndrome). When the carotid sinus is abnormally sensitive, slight pressure upon it causes a marked fall in blood pressure due to vasodilation and cardiac slowing. Symptoms include syncope, convulsions and heart block.

CAVERNOUS SINUS SYNDROME: The cavernous sinus receives drainage from the upper lip, nose, sinuses, nasopharynx, pharynx and orbits. It drains into the inferior petrosal sinus which in turn drains into the internal jugular vein. Cavernous sinus syndrome is caused by thrombosis of the cavernous intracranial sinus, 80% of which is fatal. The symptoms include orbital pain (V_1) with venous congestion of the retina, lids and conjunctiva. The eyes are proptosed with exophthalmos. The patient has photophobia and involvement of II, III, IV, VI, V_1 nerves. The treatment of choice is anticoagulation and antibiotics. The most common etiology for cavernous sinus thrombosis is ethmoiditis. (Ophthalmic vein and artery are involved as well. The nerves and veins are lateral to the cavernous sinus while the internal carotid artery is medial to it).

COGAN'S SYNDROME: (Nonsyphilitic Interstitial keratitis and vestibulo-auditory symptoms). Interstitial keratitis giving rise to rapid visual loss. Symptoms include episodic severe vertigo accompanied by tinnitus, spontaneous nystagmus, ataxia and progressive sensorineural hearing loss. There are remissions and exacerbations. It is believed to be related to periarteritis nodosa. Eosinophilia has been reported in this entity. Pathologically, it is a degeneration of the vestibular and spiral ganglia with edema of the membranous cochlea, semicircular canals and inflammation of the spiral ligament. Treatment with steroids has been advocated. (Cody, D. T. R. and Williams, H. L.: Cogan's Syndrome, Laryngoscope 70:447, 1960. Fisher, E.R. and Hellstron, H. R.: Cogan's Syndrome and Systemic Vascular Disease. Arch. Path. 72:96-116, 1961. Smith, J. L.: Cogan's Syndrome, Laryngoscope 80:121, 1970).

COLLET-SICARD SYNDROME: IX, X, XI, XII nerves are involved with normal sympathetic nerves. The etiology is usually a meningioma or other lesion involving the nerves in the posterior cranial fossa.

COSTEN'S SYNDROME: A temporal-mandibular-joint abnormality, usually due to impaired bite and characterized by tinnitus, vertigo, pain in the frontal, parietal and occipital areas with a blocked feeling and pain in the ear. After a careful work-up to rule out other abnormalities, the patient is treated with aspirin, heat and slow exercise of the joint. An orthodontist may help the patient. The TMJ differs from other joints by the presence of avascular fibrous tissue covering the articulating surfaces with an interposed meniscus dividing the joint into upper and lower compartments. The right and left TMJ's act as one functional unit. The condyle is made up of spongy bone with marrow and a growth center. The condyle articulates with the glenoid fossa of the temporal bone (squamosa). The squamotympanic fissure separates the fossa from the tympanic bone. The joint is a ginglymo-arthroidial joint with hinge and transverse movements. The key supporting ligament of the TMJ is the temporomandibular ligament. The boundaries of the glenoid fossa are:

Anterior = margins of the articular eminence
Posterior = squamosotympanic fissure
Lateral = zygomatic process of the temporal bone
Medial = temporal spine

The TMJ derives its nourishment from the synovial membrane which is richly vascularized and which produces a mucinous-like substance. The joint has a gliding motion between the meniscus and the temporal bone (upper compartment) while it has a hinge motion between the disc and the condyle (lower compartment). It is innervated by the auriculotemporal nerve, masseter nerve, lateral pterygoid nerve and the temporal nerve. It is supplied by the superficial temporal artery and the anterior tympanic branch of the internal maxillary artery. The lateral pterygoid muscle protracts the jaw while the masseter, medial pterygoid and temporalis muscles act as elevators. All these muscles are innervated by V_3. (See Chapter on Facial Trauma for muscles of the mandible). The sphenomandibular and stylomandibular ligaments have no function in the TMJ articulation.

CRI DU CHAT SYNDROME: Caused by a B group chromosome with a short arm, its symptoms are mental retardation, respiratory stridor, microcephaly, hypertelorism, midline oral clefts, laryngomalacia with poor approximation of the posterior vocal cords.

CROUZON'S DISEASE: See Chapter 6.

DANDY SYNDROME: Oscillopsia or jumbling of the panorama common in patients after bilateral labyrinthectomy. These patients are unable to focus while walking or moving.

DARIER'S DISEASE (KERATOSIS FOLLICULARIS): Autosomal dominant, a skin disorder of the external auditory canal characterized by keratotic debris in the canal. Some investigators have advocated the use of Vitamin A or steroids.

DOWN'S SYNDROME: (See Trisomy in Chapter 6).

DYSPHAGIA LUSORIA: Dysphagia secondary to abnormal right subclavian artery. The right subclavian arises abnormally from the thoracic aorta by passing behind or in front of the esophagus thus compressing it.

ECTODERMAL DYSPLASIA, HIDROTIC: (See Chapter 6).

ECTODERMAL DYSPLASIA, HYPOHIDROTIC: Hypodontia, hypotrichosis, hypohidrosis. Principally the structures involved are of ectodermal derivatives. X-linked recessive. Hypohidrosis can lead to severe hyperpyrexia.

EISENLOHR'S SYNDROME: Numbness and weakness in the extremities, paralysis of the lips, tongue, palate and dysarthria.

FANCONI ANEMIA SYNDROME: Aplastic anemia with skin pigmentation, skeletal deformities, renal anomalies and mental retardation. Death due to leukemia usually ensues within two years. It rarely occurs in adults. (A variant of this is congenital hypoplastic thrombocytopenia which is inherited autosomal recessively. It is characterized by spontaneous bleeding and other congenital anomalies. The bleeding time is prolonged, the platelet count is decreased and the bone marrow megakaryocytes vary from decreased to absent).

FELTY'S SYNDROME: Leukopenia, arthritis, enlarged lymph nodes and spleen.

FORDYCE'S DISEASE: Characterized by pseudocolloid of the lips, a condition marked by the presence of numerous, small yellowish white granules on the inner surface and vermillion border of the lips. Histologically, the lesions appear as ectopic sebaceous glands.

FOSTER-KENNEDY SYNDROME: Anosmia and optic atrophy ipsilateral to the frontal lobe tumor with contralateral papilledema.

FOTHERGILL'S DISEASE: Tic douloureux, anginose scarlatina.

FOVILLE'S SYNDROME: Alternating hemiplegia with abducens paralysis on one side and paralysis of the extremities on the other.

FREY'S SYNDROME:

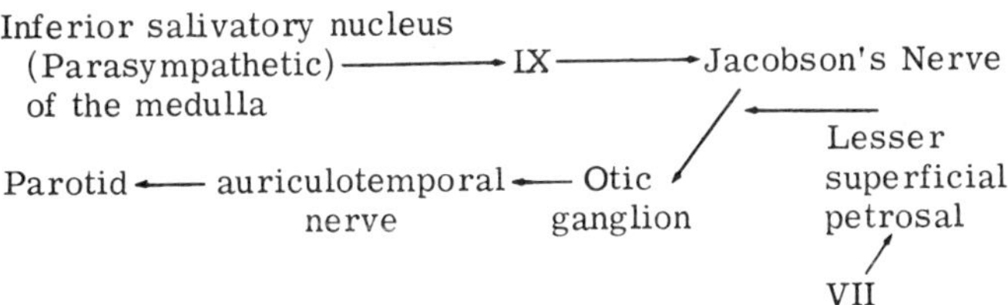

In the normal person, the sweat glands are innervated by sympathetic nerve fibers. After parotidectomy, the auriculotemporal nerve sends its parasympathetic fibers to innervate the sweat glands instead. The incidence of Frey's syndrome post parotidectomy in children has been estimated to be about 20%.

GARD-GIGNOUX SYNDROME: This syndrome involves paralysis of the XI nerve and the X nerve below the nodose ganglion. The cricothyroid function and sensation are normal. The symptoms include vocal cord paralysis and weakness of the trapezius and sternocleidomastoid muscles.

GARDNER'S SYNDROME: An autosomal dominant disease, its symptoms include fibroma, osteoma of the skull, mandible, maxilla and long bones with epidermoid inclusion cysts in the skin and polyps in the colon. (Arch. Derm. 90:20, 1964) These colonic polyps have a marked tendency towards malignant degeneration.

GARGOYLISM: (Hurler's Syndrome). See Chapter 6.

GERLIER'S DISEASE: With the presence of vertigo and kubisagari, it is observed among cowherds and is a disease marked by pain in the head and neck with visual disturbances, ptosis and generalized weakness of the muscles.

GOODWIN'S TUMOR: (Benign lymphoepithelial lesion). This is characterized by inflammatory cells, lymphocytes, plasma cells and reticular cells.

GRADENIGO'S SYNDROME: Due to extradural abscess involving the petrous bone, the symptoms are suppurative otitis, pain in the eye and temporal area, abducens paralysis as well as diplopia.

GUILLAIN-BARRÉ SYNDROME: Infectious polyneuritis of unknown etiology (? viral) causing marked paresthesias of the limbs, muscular weakness or a flaccid paralysis. CSF protein is increased without an increase in cell count.

HALLERMANN-STREIFF SYNDROME: It is characterized by dyscephaly, parrot nose, mandibular hypoplasia, proportionate nanism, hypotrichosis and bilateral congenital cataracts. There is no demonstrable genetic basis.

HEERFORDT'S SYNDROME OR DISEASE: It gives uveoparotid fever and is a form of sarcoidosis. (See Chapter 24).

HIPPEL-LINDAU DISEASE: Angioma of the cerebellum, usually cystic, associated with angioma of the retina and polycystic kidneys.

HORNER'S SYNDROME: The presenting symptoms are ptosis, miosis, anhidrosis and enophthalmos due to paralysis of the cervical sympathetic.

HUNT'S SYNDROME: (1) Cerebellar tumor, an intention tremor that begins in one extremity gradually increasing in intensity and subsequently involving other parts of the body. (2) Facial paralysis, otalgia and aural herpes due to disease of both motor and sensory fibers of the VII nerve. (3) A form of juvenile paralysis agitans associated with primary atrophy of the pallidal system.

INVERSED JAW WINKING SYNDROME: When there are supranuclear lesions of the V nerve, touching the cornea may produce a brisk movement of the mandible to the opposite side.

JACKSON'S SYNDROME: Unilateral paralysis of the larynx, velum palati and tongue.

JUGULAR FORAMEN SYNDROME: (Vernet's Syndrome). The IX, X and XI nerves are paralyzed while the XII is spared because of its separate hypoglossal canal. Horner's syndrome is not present since the sympathetic chain is below the foramen. This syndrome is most often caused by lymphadenopathy of the nodes of Krause in the foramen. Thrombophlebitis, tumors of the jugular bulb and basal skull fracture can cause the syndrome. Glomus jugulare usually gives a hazy margin of involvement while neurinoma gives a smooth, sclerotic margin of enlargement. The jugular foramen is bound medially by the occipital bone and laterally by the temporal bone. The foramen is divided into anteromedial (par nervosa) and postero-lateral (par vasculara) areas by a fibrous or bony septum. The medial area transmits the IX, X, XI nerves as well as the inferior petrosal sinus. The posterior compartment transmits the internal jugular vein and the posterior meningeal artery. The right foramen is usually slightly larger than the left foramen.

KALLMAN'S SYNDROME: Congenital hypogonadotrophic eunuchoidism with anosmia. It is transmitted via a dominant gene with variable penetrance.

KAPOSI'S SARCOMA: Multiple idiopathic, hemorrhagic sarcomatosis particularly of the skin and viscera. Radiotherapy is the treatment of choice.

KARTAGENER'S SYNDROME: Complete situs inversus associated with chronic sinusitis and bronchiectasis. This is also called Kartagener's triad.

KERATOSIS PALMARIS ET SOLARIS: Unusual inherited malformation. If these people live to 65 years old 50% to 75% of them would have developed carcinoma of the esophagus.

KLINEFELTER'S SYNDROME: This is a sex chromosome defect characterized by eunuchoidism, azoospermia, gynecomastia, mental deficiency, small testes with atrophy and hyalinization of seminiferous tubules. Usually XXY.

KLINKERT SYNDROME: Paralysis of the recurrent and phrenic nerves due to a neoplastic process in the root of the neck or upper mediastinum. The sympathetics may be involved. (The left side involvement is more common than right side involvement). This can be a part of the Pancoast syndrome.

LERMOYEZ'S SYNDROME: This is a variant of Ménière's Disease. It was first described by Lermoyez in 1921 as deafness and tinnitus followed by a vertiginous attack which relieved the tinnitus and improved the hearing.

LOFFLER'S SYNDROME: Pneumonitis characterized by eosinophiles in the tissues. This is possibly of parasitic etiology.

LOUIS-BAR SYNDROME: An autosomal recessive disease presenting ataxia, oculocutaneous telangiectasia, sinopulmonary infection, it involves progressive truncal ataxia, slurred speech, fixation nystagmus, mental deficiency, cerebellar atrophy, deficient immunoglobulin and marked frequency of lymphoreticular malignancies. The patient rarely lives past twenty years of age.

MARCUS-GUNN SYNDROME: (Jaw winking syndrome). There is increase in width of the eyelids during chewing. Sometimes the patient experiences rhythmic elevation of the upper eyelid when the mouth is open and ptosis when the mouth is closed.

MARIE-STRUMPELL DISEASE: Rheumatoid arthritis of the spine.

MELKERSSON-ROSENTHAL SYNDROME: A congenital disease of unknown etiology. It manifests as recurring attacks of unilateral or bilateral (see Chapter on Facial Nerve) facial paralysis, swelling of the lips and furrowing of the tongue.

MIDDLE LOBE SYNDROME: This is a chronic atelectatic process with fibrosis in one or both segments of the middle lobe. It is usually secondary to obstruction of the middle lobe bronchus by hilar adenopathy. The hilar adenopathy may be transient but the bronchiectasis that resulted persists. Treatment is by surgical resection.

MIKULICZ'S DISEASE: The symptoms characteristic of Mikulicz's disease (swelling of lacrimal and salivary gland) occur as a complication of some other disease such as lymphocytosis, leukemia, or uveoparotid fever (See Chapter 14).

MÖBIUS SYNDROME: Congenital facial diplegia (usually bilateral), with unilateral or bilateral loss of the abductors of the eye, anomalies of the extremities, aplasia of the brachial and thoracic muscles and frequently involves other cranial nerves. The etiology could be a primary muscle defect or neurogenic in nature.

MORGAGNI-STEWART-MOREL SYNDROME: It occurs in menopausal women characterized by obesity, dizziness, psychological disturbances, inverted sleep rhythm and hyperostosis frontalis interna. Treatment is supportive.

MYENBURG'S SYNDROME: (Familial myositis fibrosa progressive). Disease in which the striated muscles are replaced by fibrosis. Fibrosarcoma rarely originates from this disease.

NEUROFIBROMATOSIS: (von Recklinghausen's Disease)
Salient Features:

1. Autosomal dominant.
2. Mental retardation common in families with neurofibromatosis.
3. Arise from neurilemmal cells or Sheath of Schwann and fibroblasts of peripheral nerves.
4. Café au lait spots - giant melanosomes. (The presence of six or more spots greater than 1.5 cm. is diagnostic of neurofibromatosis even if family history is negative).

5. 4-5% of neurofibromatosis undergo malignant degeneration with sudden increase of growth of formerly static nodules. These may become neurofibrosarcomas. They may metastasize widely.

<u>External Features:</u>

1. Café au lait spots.
2. Fibromas

<u>Internal Features:</u>

1. Pheochromocytoma
2. Meningioma
3. Acoustic neurinoma - often bilateral
4. G.I. bleeding
5. Intussusception bowel
6. Hypoglycemia (intraperitoneal fibromas)
7. Fibrous dysplasia
8. Subperiosteal bone cysts
9. Optic nerve may be involved causing blindness and proptosis
10. May present with macroglossia
11. May involve the parotid or submaxillary gland
12. The nodules may be painful
13. Nodules may enlarge suddenly if bleeding of the tumor occurs or if there is malignant degeneration.

The treatment of this disease is only to relieve pressure from expanding masses. It usually does not recur if the tumor is completely removed locally.

NOTHNAGEL'S SYNDROME: The symptoms include dizziness, a staggering and rolling gait with irregular forms of oculomotor paralysis. Nystagmus is often present. This is seen in cases of tumor of the midbrain.

OCULOPHARYNGEAL SYNDROME: Hereditary ptosis and dysphagia. An autosomal dominant disease with equal incidence in both sexes, it is related to a high incidence of esophageal carcinoma. Its age of onset is between 40 and 50 years old and is particularly common among the French Canadians. Marked weakness of the upper esophagus is observed together with an increase in serum creatinine phosphokinase. It is a myopathy and not a neuropathy. Treatment includes dilatation and cricopharyngomyotomy.

OLLIER'S DISEASE: Multiple chondromatosis, 10% of which is associated with chondrosarcoma.

ORAL-FACIAL-DIGITAL SYNDROME I: (See Chapter 6 for Oral-Facial-Digital Syndrome II). A lethal trait in males, it is inherited as a X-linked dominant trait limited to females. Symptoms include multiple hyperplastic frenula, cleft tongue, dystopia canthorum, hypoplasia of the nasal alar cartilages, median cleft of the upper lip, asymmetric cleft palate, digital malformation, mild mental retardation. About 50% of the patients have hamartoma between the lobes of the divided tongue. This mass consists of fibrous connective tissue, salivary gland tissue, few striated muscle fibers and rarely cartilage. One-third of the patients present with ankyloglossia.

ORTNER'S SYNDROME: Laryngeal paralysis associated with cardiomegaly.

OSLER-RENDU-WEBER DISEASE: (Hereditary hemorrhagic telangiectasia). It is an autosomal dominant disease in which the heterozygous lives to adult life while the homozygous state is lethal at an early age. The patient has punctate hemangioma (elevated, dilated capillaries and venules) in the mucous membrane of the lips, tongue, mouth, G.I. tract, etc. Pathologically, these are vascular sinuses of irregular size and shape lined by a thin layer of endothelium. The muscular and elastic coats are absent. Because of their thin wall these vascular sinuses bleed easily and because of the lack of muscular coats, this bleeding is difficult to control. The patient has normal blood elements and no coagulation defect. The other blood vessels are normal as well. If a person with this disease marries a normal person, what are the chances that the offspring will have this condition? Since the patient with this disease is an adult, we can assume that he is heterozygous since the homozygous dies early in life. Therefore, the child will have a 50% chance of having this hereditary disease.

PAGET'S DISEASE: (Osteitis deformans - See Chapter 6). This term is also used to characterize a disease of elderly women with an infiltrated, eczematous lesion surrounding the nipple and areola associated with subjacent intraductal carcinoma of the breast.

PAGET'S OSTEITIS: This is related to sarcomas.

PANCOAST SYNDROME: (See Chapter 21).

PEUTZ-JEGHER'S SYNDROME: Pigmentation of the lips, oral mucosa, and benign polyps of the gastrointestinal tract. Granulosa-theca cell tumors have been reported in females with this syndrome.

PHEOCHROMOCYTOMA: Is associated with neurofibromatosis, cerebellar hemangioblastoma, ependymoma, astrocytoma, meningioma, spongioblastoma, multiple endocrine adenoma or with medullary carcinoma of the thyroid. Pheochromocytoma with or without the above tumors may be inherited as an autosomal dominant trait. Some patients have megacolon, others suffer neurofibromatosis of the Auerbach's and Meissner's plexuses.

PIERRE-ROBIN SYNDROME: (Glossoptosis, micrognathia, cleft palate). There is no sex predilection. The etiology is believed to be intrauterine insult at the 4th month of gestation or ? hereditary. Two-thirds of the cases are associated with ophthalmological difficulties (e.g. detached retina or glaucoma), one third are associated with otological problems (e.g. chronic otitis media and low-set ears). Mental retardation is present occasionally. If the patient lives past 5 years old, he can lead a fairly normal life. (See Chapter 6).

PLUMMER-VINSON SYNDROME: (Patterson-Kelly Syndrome). Symptoms include dysphagia due to degeneration of the esophageal muscle, atrophy of the papillae of the tongue, as well as microcytic, hypochromic anemia. Achlorhydria, glossitis, pharyngitis, esophagitis and fissures at the corner of the mouth are also observed. The incidence of this disease is higher in females than in males, usually present in patients who are in their 4th decade. Treatment consists of iron with esophagoscopy for dilation and to rule out carcinoma of the esophagus, particularly at the post-cricoid region. Pharyngo-esophageal webs or stenosing may be noted.

This disease is to be contrasted with Pernicious anemia which is a megaloblastic anemia with diarrhea, nausea and vomiting, neurological symptoms, enlarged spleen and achlorhydria. Pernicious anemia is secondary to failure of gastric fundus to secrete intrinsic factors necessary for B_{12} absorption. Treatment consists of IM B_{12} (Riboflavin).

Folic acid deficiency also gives rise to megaloblastic anemia, cheilosis, glossitis, ulcerative stomatitis, pharyngitis, esophagitis, dysphagia and diarrhea. No neurological symptoms and no achlorhydria are present. Treatment is through administration of Folic Acid.

REITER'S SYNDROME: Arthritis, urethritis, conjunctivitis.

SCALENUS ANTICUS SYNDROME: The symptoms are identical to those of cervical rib. In scalenus anticus syndrome, symptoms are caused by compression of the brachial plexus and subclavian artery against the first thoracic rib, probably as the result of spasms of the scalenus anticus muscle bringing pressure on the brachial plexus and the subclavian artery. Any pressure on the sympathetic nerves may cause vascular spasm resembling Raynaud's disease.

SCHAUMANN'S SYNDROME: Generalized sarcoidosis. (See Chapter 24).

SCHMIDT'S SYNDROME: Unilateral paralysis of a vocal cord, the velum palati, the trapezius, and the sternocleidomastoid muscles. The lesion is located in the caudal portion of the medulla and is usually of vascular origin.

SJÖGREN'S SYNDROME: (Sicca syndrome). Manifesting as keratoconjunctivitis sicca, dryness of mucous membranes, telangiectasias or purpuric spots on the face and bilateral parotid enlargement; this syndrome is often seen in menopausal women associated with rheumatoid arthritis, Raynaud's phenomenon and dental caries. Changes in the lacrimal and salivary glands resemble those of Mikulicz' Disease. Some attribute this syndrome to Vitamin A deficiency. A (+) L.E. prep, rheumatoid factor, an abnormal protein can be identified in this disorder.

STEVENS-JOHNSON SYNDROME: This is a skin disease (erythema multiforme) with involvement of the oral cavity (stomatitis) and the eye (conjunctivitis). Stomatitis may appear as the first symptom. It is most common in the third decade of life. Treatment is largely with steroid therapy and supportive therapy. This is a self-limiting disease but has a 25% recurrence rate. The differential diagnosis would include (a) herpes simplex, (b) pemphigus, (c) acute fuso-spirochetal stomatitis, (d) chicken pox, (e) monilial infection and (f) secondary syphilis.

STILL'S DISEASE: Rheumatoid arthritis in children (see pediatric textbook for more details).

STURGE-WEBER SYNDROME: This is a congenital disorder with no sex predilection and of unknown etiology. It is characterized by venous angioma of the leptomeninges over the cerebral cortex, ipsilateral port-wine nevi and frequent angiomatous involvement of the globe, mouth and nasal mucosa. The patient may have convulsions, hemiparesis, glaucoma and intracranial calcifications. There is no specific treatment.

SUBCLAVIAN STEAL SYNDROME: Stenosis or occlusion of the subclavian or innominate artery proximal to the origin of the vertebral artery causes the pressure in the vertebral artery to be less than that of the basilar artery, particularly when the upper extremity is in action. Hence, the brain receives less blood supply and may be ischemic. The symptoms consist of intermittent vertigo, occipital headache, blurred vision, diplopia, dysarthria, and pain in the upper extremity. The diagnosis, made through the patient's medical history, can be confirmed by the difference in blood pressure in the two upper extremities, by a bruit over the supraclavicular fossa and by angiography.

SUPERIOR ORBITAL FISSURE SYNDROME: (Orbital apex syndrome, optic foramen syndrome, sphenoid fissure syndrome). There is involvement of III, IV, VI, V_1 nerves, ophthalmic veins, and sympathetics of the cavernous sinus. This syndrome can be caused by sphenoid sinusitis or by any neoplasia in that region. Symptoms include paralysis of the upper lid, orbital pain, photophobia and paralysis of the above nerves. The optic nerve may be damaged as well.

SUPERIOR VENA CAVA SYNDROME: This is obstruction of the superior vena cava or its main tributaries by bronchogenic carcinoma, mediastinal neoplasm or lymphoma. Rarely, the presence of a substernal goiter causes edema and engorgement of the vessels of the face, neck and arms, as well as a non-productive cough and dyspnea.

TAPIA'S SYNDROME: Unilateral paralysis of the larynx and tongue is coupled with atrophy of the tongue while the soft palate and cricothyroid muscle are intact. This syndrome is usually caused by a lesion at the point where XII and X nerves together with the internal carotid artery cross one another.

TAY-SACH'S DISEASE: An infantile form of amaurotic familial idiocy with strong familial tendencies, it is of questionably recessive inheritance. It is more commonly found among those of Semitic extraction. Histologically, the nerve cells are distorted and filled with a lipid material. The juvenile form of this is called Spielmeyer-Vogt's Disease in which the patient is normal until after five to seven years of age. This juvenile form is seen in children of non-Semitic extraction as well.

TIETZE'S SYNDROME: Costal chondritis, chondropathia tuberosa; of unknown etiology; its symptoms include pain, tenderness and swelling of one or more of the upper costal cartilages (usually of the second rib). Treatment is symptomatic.

TREACHER-COLLINS' SYNDROME: (See Chapter 6).

TURNER'S SYNDROME: (See Chapter 6).

TUBE FEEDING SYNDROME: (See Chapter 31, II - 63).

VERNET'S SYNDROME: (See Jugular Foramen Syndrome).

VILLARET'S SYNDROME: This is the same as Jugular Foramen Syndrome except in that Horner's syndrome is present here suggesting more extensive involvement in the region of the jugular foramen, the retroparotid area, and the lateral pharyngeal space.

VOGT-KOYANAGI-HARADA SYNDROME: Spastic diplegia with athetosis and pseudobulbar paralysis associated with a lesion of the caudate nucleus and putamen, bilateral uveitis, vitiligo, deafness, alopecia, increased CSF pressure, retinal detachment.

WALLENBERG'S SYNDROME: (Syndrome of the posterior inferior cerebellar artery thrombosis or Lateral Medullary Syndrome). This is due to thrombosis of the posterior-inferior cerebellar artery giving rise to ischemia of the brain stem (lateral medullary region). Symptoms include vertigo, nystagmus, nausea, vomiting, Horner's syndrome, dysphagia, dysphonia, hypotonia, asthenia, ataxia, falling to the side of the lesion and loss of pain and temperature sense on the ipsilateral face and contralateral side below the neck.

WEBER'S SYNDROME: Paralysis of the oculomotor nerve on the side of the lesion and paralysis of the extremities, face and tongue on the contralateral side. It indicates a lesion in the ventral and internal part of the cerebral peduncle.

WILSON'S DISEASE: (Hepatolenticular degeneration). There are two chief types: one rapidly progressive which occurs in late childhood, the other slowly progressive occurring in the third or fourth decades. Familial, its symptoms are cirrhosis with progressive damage to the nervous system, brown pigmentation of the outer margin of the cornea called Kayser-Fleischer ring, and it can present with hearing loss as well.

WINKLER'S DISEASE: Arterio-venous anastomosis and nerve endings accumulation at the helical portion of the ear. It presents with pain. Ninety percent occur in males. The treatment is to excise it or treat it with steroids.

XERODERMA PIGMENTOSUM: (Autosomal recessive). Photosensitive skin with multiple basal cell epitheliomas. Squamous cell carcinoma or malignant melanoma can result from it. This condition occurs mainly in children. These children should be kept away from the sun.

II. EPONYMS

ADENOID FACIE: Crowded teeth, high arched palate, underdeveloped nostrils.

ADLER BODIES: Deposits of mucopolysaccharide found in neutrophils of the patients with Hurler's syndrome.

ANTONI TYPE A AND TYPE B: (See Chapter 31).

ARNOLD-CHIARI MALFORMATION:

- Type I = Downward protrusion of the long, thin, cerebellar tonsils through the foramen magnum.
- Type II = Protrusion of the inferior cerebellar vermis through the foramen.
- Type III = Bony occipital defect with descent of the entire cerebellum.
- Type IV = Cerebellar hypoplasia.

ABRIKOSSOFF TUMOR: (granular cell myoblastoma). Causes pseudoepithelial hyperplasia in the larynx, the site of predilection in the larynx being the posterior half of the vocal cord. Three percent of granular cell myoblastoma progress to malignancy. In order of decreasing frequency of involvement, the granular cell myoblastoma occurs in tongue, skin, breast, subcutaneous tissue, and respiratory tract.

ARNOLD GANGLION: Otic ganglion.

ASCHOFF BODY: Rheumatic nodule found in rheumatic disease.

BALLET'S SIGN: Paralysis of voluntary movements of the eyeball with preservation of the automatic movements. Sometimes this sign is present in exophthalmic goiter and hysteria.

BECHTEREW'S SYMPTOM: Paralysis of facial muscles limited to automatic movements. The power of voluntary movement is retained.

BEZOLD'S ABSCESS: Abscess in the sternocleidomastoid muscle secondary to perforation of the tip of the mastoid by infection.

BLANDIN, GLAND OF: A minor salivary gland situated in the anterior portion of the tongue.

BROOKE'S TUMOR: (epithelioma adenoid cystica). This originates from the hair follicles in the external auditory canal and auricle. It is of basal cell origin. Treatment is through local resection.

BROYLE'S LIGAMENT: Anterior commissure ligament of the larynx.

BRUDZINSKI'S SIGN: In meningitis, a passive flexion of the leg on one side causes a similar movement to occur in the opposite leg. Passive flexion of the neck brings about a flexion of the legs as well.

"BRUNNER" ABSCESS: Abscess of the posterior floor of the mouth.

BRUNS' SIGN: Intermittent headache, vertigo and vomiting, especially with sudden movements of the head. This occurs in cases of tumor of the fourth ventricle of the brain.

BRYCE'S SIGN: A gurgling is heard in a neck mass. It suggests a laryngocele.

CHARCOT-LEYDEN CRYSTALS: Crystals in the shape of elongated double pyramids, composed of spermin phosphates and present in the sputum of asthmatic patients. Synonyms are: Charcot-Newman's crystals, Charcot-Robin crystals.

CHARCOT'S TRIAD: Nystagmus, scanning speech, intention tremor seen in multiple sclerosis.

CHERUBISM: Familial, with the age of predilection between 2 and 5 years old. It is characterized by giant cell reparative granuloma causing cystic lesions in the posterior rami of the mandible. The lesions are usually symmetrical. It is a self-limiting disease with remissions after puberty. The maxilla may be involved as well.

CHVOSTEK'S SIGN: It is the facial twitch obtained by tapping the distribution of the facial nerve. It is indicative of hypocalcemia and is the most reliable test for hypocalcemia.

CURSCHMANN'S SPIRALS: Spirally twisted masses of mucous present in the sputum of bronchial asthmatic patients.

DEMARQUAY'S SIGN: Absence of elevation of the larynx during deglutition. This is said to indicate syphilitic induration of the trachea.

di SANT' AGNESE TEST: It measures the elevated sodium and chloride in the sweat of cystic fibrotic children.

DUPRE'S SIGN: Meningism.

EBNER, GUSTATORY GLANDS OF: These are the minor salivary glands near the circumvallate papillae.

ESCHERICH'S SIGN: In hypoparathyroidism, tapping of the skin at the angle of the mouth causes protrusion of the lips.

GALEN'S ANASTOMOSIS: An anastomosis between the superior laryngeal nerve and the recurrent laryngeal nerve.

GOODWIN'S TUMOR: (Benign lymphoepithelioma) - see Chapter 14.

GRIESINGER'S SIGN: Edema of the tip of the mastoid in thrombosis of the sigmoid sinus.

GUTTMAN'S TEST: In the normal subject, frontal pressure on the thyroid cartilage lowers the tone of the voice produced while lateral pressure produces a higher tone of the voice. The opposite is true in paralysis of the crico-thyroid muscle.

GUYON'S SIGN: The XII nerve lies directly upon the external carotid artery, whereby this vessel may be distinguished from the internal carotid artery. (The safer way prior to ligation of the external carotid artery is to identify the first few branches of the external carotid artery).

HENLE, GLANDS OF: These are the small glands situated in the areolar tissue between the buccopharyngeal fascia anteriorly and the prevertebral fascia posteriorly. Infection of these glands can lead to retropharyngeal abscess. Since these glands atrophy after the age of 5, retropharyngeal abscess is less likely to occur after that age.

HENNEBERT'S SIGN: (See Chapter on Congenital Deafness) The presence of a (+) fistula test in the absence of an obvious fistula is called Hennebert's sign. The patient has a normal appearing tympanic membrane and external auditory canal. The nystagmus is more marked upon application of a negative pressure. This sign is present in congenital syphilis and is believed to be due to an excessively mobile footplate or caused by motion of the saccule mediated by fibrosis between the footplate and the saccule.

HERING-BREUER REFLEX: (Respiratory reflexes from pulmonary stretch receptors). Inflation of the lungs sends an inhibitory impulse to the central nervous system via the vagus nerve to stop inspiration. Similarly, a deflation of the lungs sends an impulse to stop expiration. This is the Hering-Breuer reflex.

KERNIG'S SIGN: When the subject lies on his back, with the thigh at right angle to the trunk, straightening of the leg (extending the leg) will elicit pain, supposedly due to the pull on the inflamed lumbosacral nerve roots. This sign is present in meningitis.

KIESSELBACH'S PLEXUS: This is an area in the anterior septum where the capillaries merge. It is often the site of anterior epistaxis. It has also been referred to as the Little's area.

KRAUSE'S NODES: These are the nodes in the jugular foramen.

LITTLE'S AREA: (See Kiesselbach's Plexus).

LUDWIG'S ANGINA: (See Chapter 13).

LUSCHKA'S POUCH: (See Tornwaldt's Disease).

MARJOLIN'S ULCER: This is a carcinoma that arises at the site of an old burn scar. It is a well differentiated squamous cell carcinoma, aggressive, and metastasizes fast.

MECKEL'S GANGLION: Sphenopalatine ganglion.

MIKULICZ'S CELLS: These are macrophages in rhinoscleroma. (Russel bodies which are eosinophilic round structures associated with plasma cells are also found in rhinoscleroma).

MOLLARET-DEBRÉ TEST: This is a test performed for cat scratch fever.

MORGAGNI, SINUS OF: A dehiscence of the superior constrictor muscle and the buccopharyngeal fascia where the eustachian tube opens.

MORGAGNI, VENTRICLE OF: This separates the quadrangular membrane from the conus elasticus in the larynx.

NIKOLSKY'S SIGN: Detachment of the sheets of the superficial epithelial layers when any traction is applied over the surface of the epithelial involvement in pemphigus is characteristic of Nikolsky's sign. Pemphigus involves the intraepithelial layer while pemphigoid involves the subepithelial layer. The former is a lethal disease in many instances.

OLIVER-CARDARELLI'S SIGN: Recession of the larynx and trachea is synchronous with cardiac systole in cases of aneurysm of the arch of the aorta or in cases of a tumor in that region.

PAUL-BUNNEL TEST: It measures the elevated heterophile titer in infectious mononucleosis.

PSAMMOMA BODIES: These are found in papillary carcinoma of the thyroid.

RATHKE'S POUCH: (See Tornwaldt's disease)

REINKE TUMOR: This is a "soft" tumor variant of lymphoepithelioma in which the lymphocytes predominate. (In the hard tumor the epithelial cells predominate; this is called Schmincke's tumor.)

RHOMBERG'S SIGN: If a patient standing with feet together, "falls" when he closes his eyes, the Rhomberg test is positive. It is indicative of either abnormal propioception or abnormal vestibular function. It does not necessarily distinguish central from peripheral lesion. The cerebellar function is not tested in this test.

ROUVIER'S NODE: Lateral retropharyngeal node. It is a common target of metastases in nasopharyngeal carcinoma.

RUSSEL BODIES: Eosinophilic, round structures, associated with plasma cells found in rhinoscleroma.

SANTORINI CARTILAGE: Corniculate cartilage of the larynx, composed of fibroelastic cartilage.

SANTORINI FISSURES: Fissures in the anterior bony external auditory canal leading to the parotid region.

SCHAUMANN BODIES: Together with asteroids, they are found in sarcoid granuloma.

SCHMINCKE'S TUMOR: The "hard" variant of lymphoepithelioma in which the epithelial cells predominate. (See Reinke's tumor)

SCHNEIDERIAN MUCOSA: Pseudostratified ciliated columnar mucosa of the nose.

SEELIGMÜLLER'S SIGN: Contraction of pupil on the affected side in facial neuralgia.

SEMON'S LAW: A law stating that injury to the recurrent laryngeal nerve results in paralysis of the abductor muscle of the larynx (cricoarytenoid posticus) before paralysis of the adductor muscles. In recovery, the adductor recovers before the abductor.

STRAUS' SIGN: In facial paralysis, the lesion is peripheral if injection of pilocarpine is followed by sweating on the affected side later than on the normal side.

SULKOWITCH TEST: It determines an increase in calciuria.

TORNWALDT'S CYST: A depression exists in the nasopharyngeal vault which is a remnant of the Pouch of Luschka. When this depression gets infected a Tornwaldt's Cyst results. In the early embryo, this area has a connection between notochord and entoderm. The Tornwaldt's cyst is lined with respiratory epithelium with some squamous metaplasia. Anterior to this pit, the path taken by Rathke's pouch sometimes persists as the craniopharyngeal canal, running from the sella turcica through the body of the sphenoid to an opening on the undersurface of the skull.

TOYNBEE'S LAW: When CNS complications arise in chronic otitis media, the lateral sinus and cerebellum are involved in mastoiditis while the cerebrum alone is involved in the instances of cholesteatoma of the attic.

TROUSSEAU'S SIGN: In hypocalcemia, a tourniquet placed around the arm will cause tetany.

TULLIO'S PHENOMENON: (See Chapter on Congenital Deafness) This is said to be present when a loud noise precipitates vertigo. It can be present in congenital syphilis with a semicircular canal fistula or in a post-fenestration patient if the footplate is mobile. The tympanic membrane and ossicular chain have to be intact with mobile footplate.

WARTENBERG'S SIGN: Intense pruritis of the tip of the nose and nostril indicates cerebral tumor.

WARTHIN-FINKELDAY GIANT CELLS: These are found in the lymphoid tissues in measles.

WEBER'S GLAND: These are minor salivary gland in the superior pole of the tonsil.

WRISBERG CARTILAGE: This is the cuneiform cartilage of the larynx, made of fibroelastic cartilage.

XERODERMA PIGMENTOSA: Hereditary precancerous condition which begins in early childhood. These patients die at puberty.

ZAUFAL'S SIGN: Saddle nose.

CHAPTER 19

RADIOLOGY

I. RADIOGRAPHIC EXAMINATION OF THE TEMPORAL BONE

Radiographic examination of the temporal bone consists of standard projections (Law's, Schüller's, Mayer's, Owen's, Chausse's III, Stenvers', submentovertical and Towne's), tomography and polytomography (hypocycloidal or multi directional) and special studies (carotid arteriography, retrograde jugular venogram, posterior fossa myelography, combined polytome and posterior fossa myelography).

STANDARD PROJECTIONS: (Figure 19-1)[9,14,16,18,20,26,27,33]

1. Law's view is a lateral view of the mastoid obtained with the sagittal plane of the skull parallel to the film and with a 15° cephalocaudal angulation of the x-ray beam. The external and internal auditory canals are superimposed. An excellent view of the cellular development and disease of the mastoid portion of the temporal bone is obtained. It also shows the tegmen, the anterior wall of the lateral sinus, the external auditory canal, the temporomandibular joint, and the pneumatization of the anterior part of the squamous portion of the temporal bone. This view does not show the key area of the attic, aditus and antrum. (Figure 19-2).

2. Schüller's view (Runstrom) is a lateral view of the mastoid obtained with the sagittal plane of the skull parallel to the film and with a 30° cephalocaudal angulation of the x-ray beam.

This view is quite similar to the Law's view except that the x-ray tube is angled caudally 30° instead of 15°. Thus, it displaces the arcuate eminence of the petrous bone downward and shows the antrum and the upper part of the attic.

It also gives an excellent view of the extent of the pneumatization of the mastoid, the distribution and the degree of aeration of the air cells, the status of the trabecular pattern and the position of the vertical portion of the lateral sinus.

3. Mayer's view is obtained with the head of the patient rotated 45° toward the side under examination and the tube adjusted so that the central ray passes through the external auditory meatus nearest the film at an angle of 45° toward the feet.

This gives an axial view of the petrous bone and the mastoid cells. The mastoid antrum, the external auditory meatus and the upper part of the tympanic cavity are well shown. The obliquity of the Mayer's position, although necessary to free the key area from the shadow of the labyrinth, produces a distortion that may confuse the surgeon.

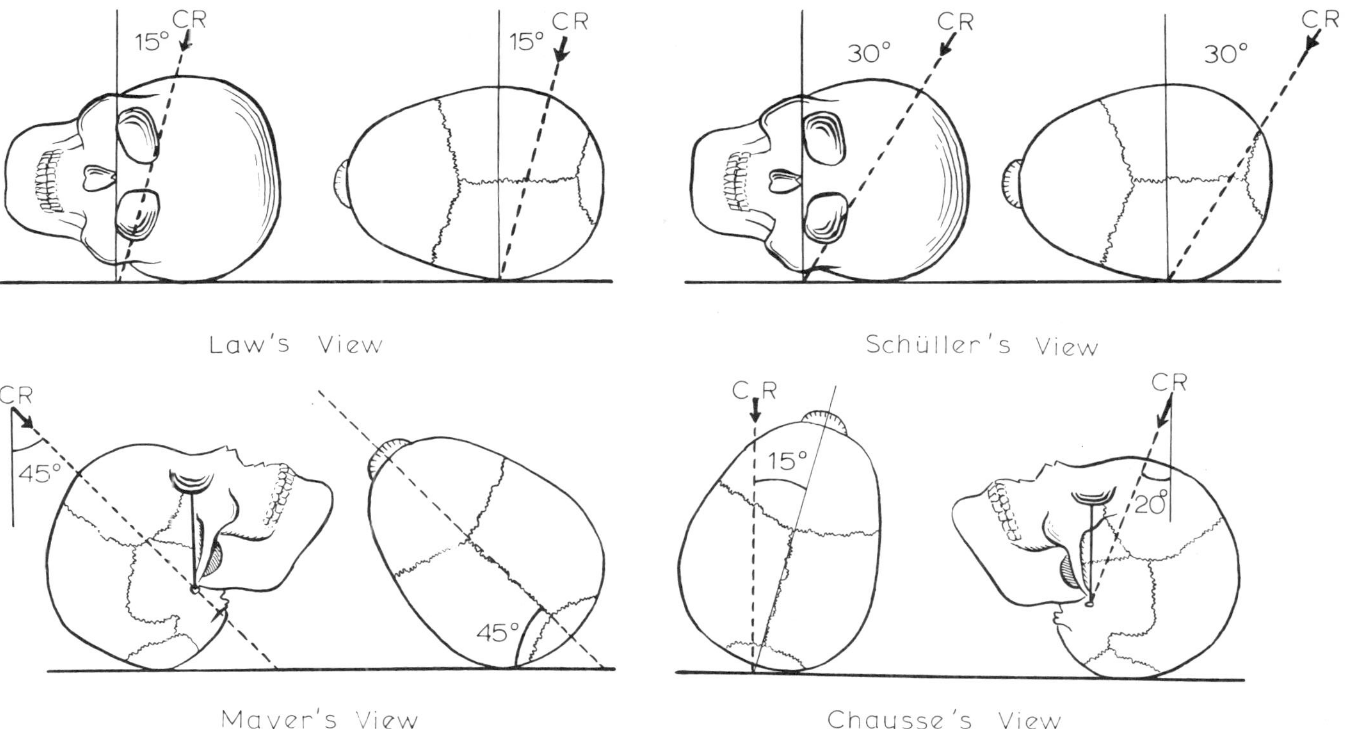

Figure 19-1A. Positions of the Skull for Temporal Bone X-rays.

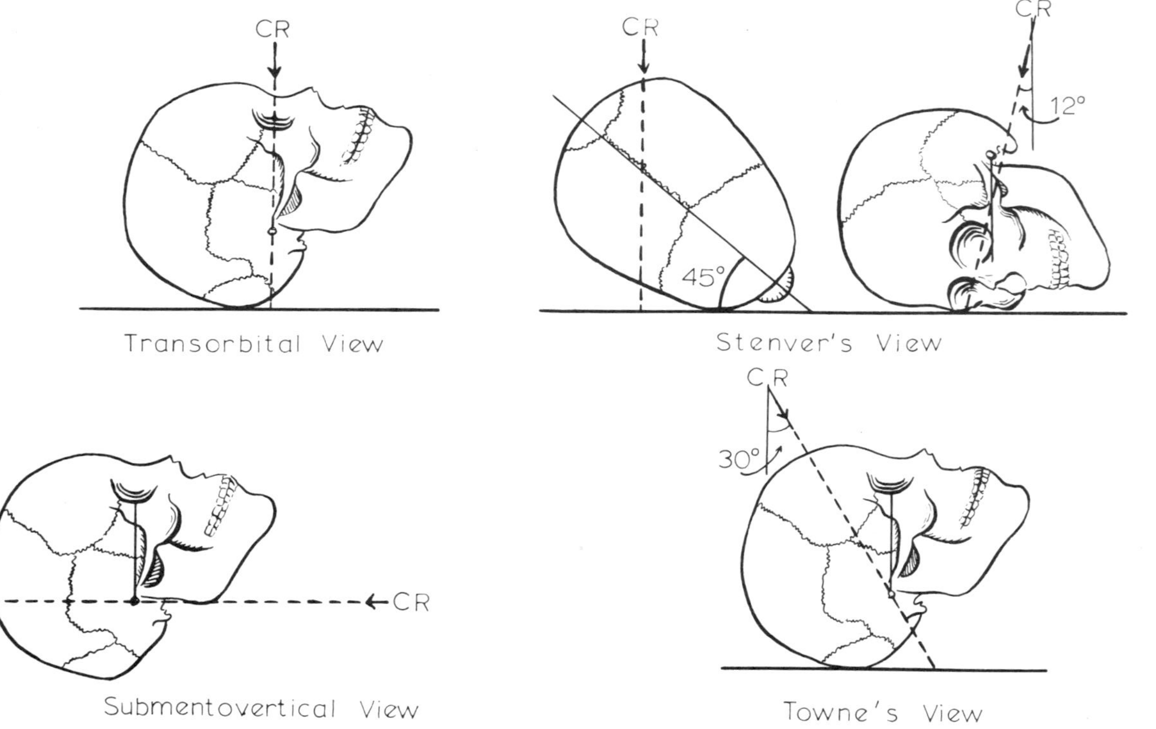

Figure 19-1B. Positions of the Skull for Temporal Bone X-rays.

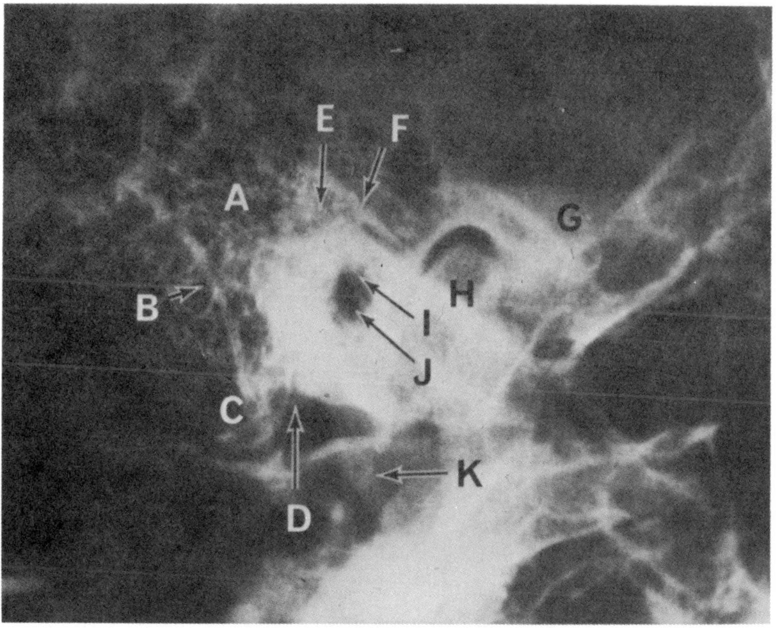

Figure 19-2. Law's view

A. Mastoid cells
B. Lateral sinus plate
C. Mastoid tip
D. Stylomastoid foramen
E. Antrum
F. Tegmen tympani
G. Zygomatic arch
H. Condyle of mandible
I. Malleus
J. External auditory canal
K. Styloid process

4. Owen's view resembles the Mayer's view but offers the advantages of less distortion. The patient's head is first positioned as for a Schüller's projection and it is then rotated with the face away from the film at an angle of approximately 30°. The x-ray beam is directed cephalocaudal with an angle of 35°.

This view gives a "surgeon's eye view" of the key area of the attic, aditus and antrum. It usually shows the malleus and the incus (a portion of it) in the natural position within the tympanic cavity.

5. Chausse's III view is obtained by positioning the occiput on the film, the head is rotated approximately 10 to 15° toward the side opposite to the one under examination and the chin flexed on the chest. There is no angulation of x-ray beam.

This view provides visualization of the attic, aditus, mastoid antrum and especially the anterior two-thirds of the lateral wall of the attic. In contrast, the Owen's view shows the posterior or aditus portion of the attic.

6. Transorbital view is obtained with the patient's occipit to the film in order to magnify the orbit. The chin is slightly flexed until the orbitomeatal line is perpendicular to the film.

In this view, the petrous pyramid, especially the internal auditory canal, is clearly visualized through the radiolucency of the orbit. It also shows the cochlea, vestibule and semicircular canals. (Figure 19-3).

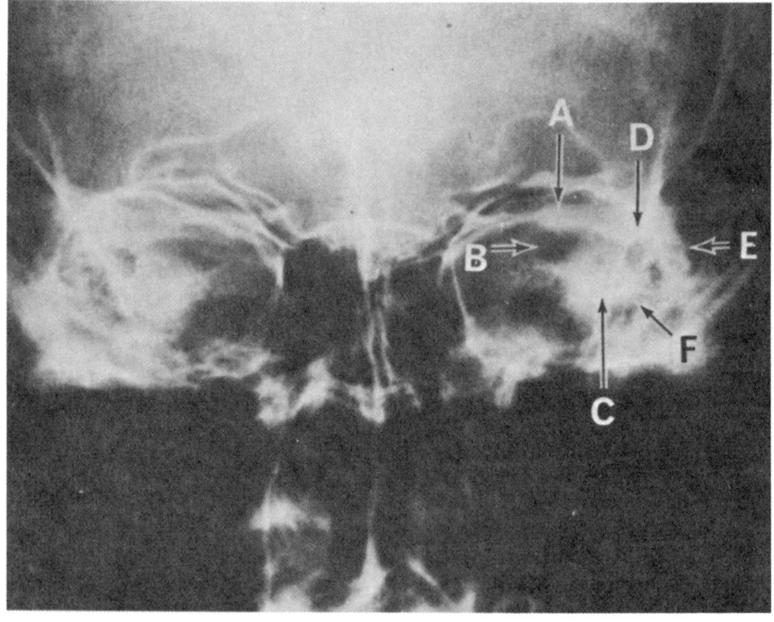

Figure 19-3. Transorbital view
A. Petrous pyramid
B. Internal auditory canal
C. Cochlea
D. Vestibule
E. Horizontal semicircular canal
F. Promontory

7. Stenvers' view is obtained with the patient facing the film with the head slightly flexed and rotated 45° toward the side opposite to the side under examination. The x-ray beam is angulated 14° caudad. The long axis of the petrous pyramid becomes parallel to the plane of the film and the entire pyramid is well visualized, including its apex.

This view clearly shows the entire pyramid, arcuate eminence, internal auditory canal, porus acusticus, horizontal and vertical semicircular canals, vestibule, cochlea, mastoid antrum and mastoid tip. The internal auditory canal may appear quite foreshortened because of rotation. (Figure 19-4).

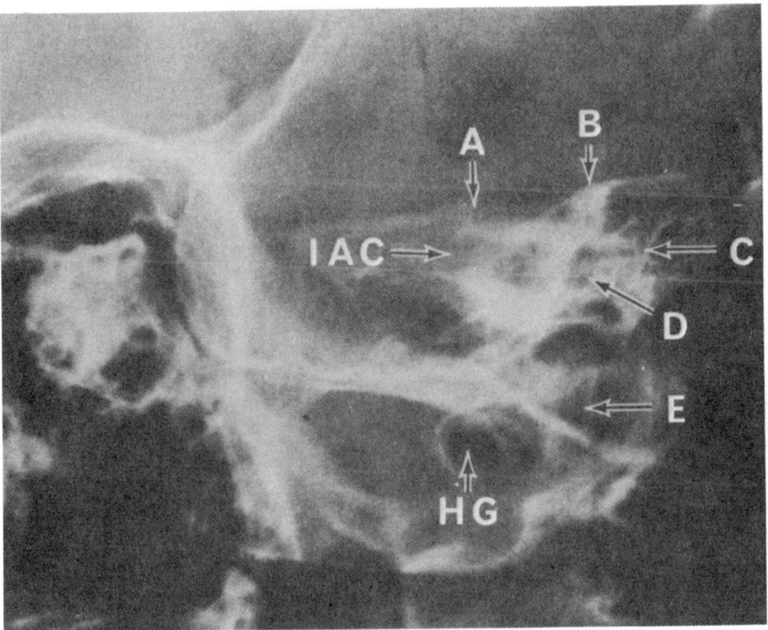

Figure 19-4. Stenvers' view
A. Petrous pyramid
B. Superior semicircular canal
C. Horizontal semicircular canal
D. Vestibule
E. Condyle of mandible
IAC Internal auditory canal
HG Hypoglossal canal

Heavy exposure will bring out details of the petrous apex, while a lighter exposure will permit visualization of details of the mastoid structure.

8. Submentovertical (axial, basal) view taken from "under the chin" has the advantage of showing both temporal bones on the same film so that comparison of both sides can be made.

This view shows the external auditory canal, the eustachian tube, the middle ear with the incus and the head of the malleus, the mastoid air cells, the styloid process, the internal auditory canal and the petrous apex. It also shows such structures of the base of the skull as foramen ovale, foramen spinosum and jugular foramen. (Figure 19-5). This view has the disadvantage of loss of clarity and detail of the ear structures because of increased antrum-to-film distance.

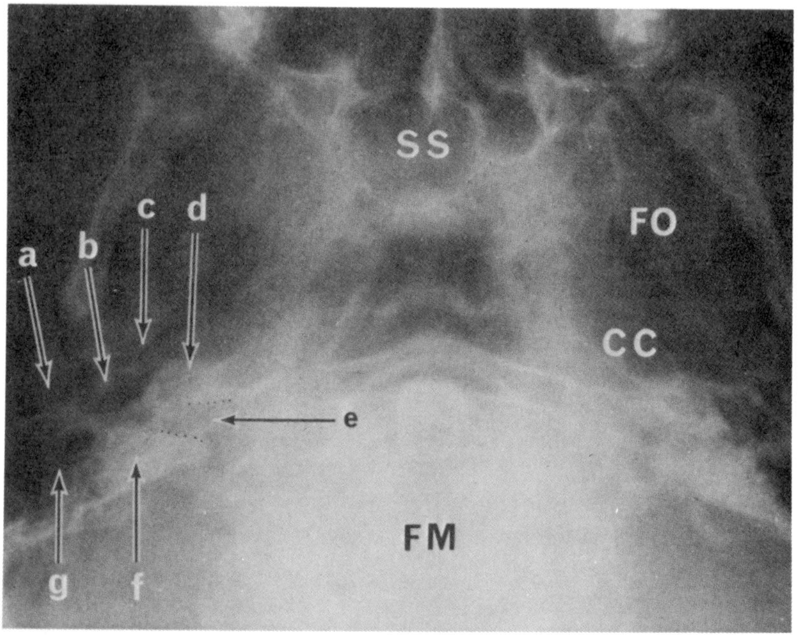

Figure 19-5. Submentovertical view

a. External auditory canal
b. Middle ear
c. Eustachian tube
d. Cochlea
e. Internal auditory canal
f. Labyrinth
g. Mastoid cells
SS Sphenoid sinus
FO Foramen ovale
CC Carotid canal
FM Foramen magnum

9. Towne's view is the anteroposterior projection with 30° tilt (from "above and in front"). As in the submentovertical view, this view allows comparison of both petrous pyramids and mastoids on the same film. The petrous apex, internal auditory canals, arcuate eminence, mastoid antrum, and mastoid process can be clearly identified. This is useful for evaluation of apical petrositis, acoustic neuroma and cerebellopontine angle tumor. (Figure 19-6).

TOMOGRAPHY AND POLYTOMOGRAPHY:[1,18,26] The use of special projections with various angulations of x-ray beam or of the patient's head, which are indispensable in conventional radiography in order to visualize certain structures, is not required in tomography. It has the following advantages: The positioning is simple and the projection easily reproducible; the ear structures can be visualized under the same angle of surgical approach; it can follow the same plane as used in histological section; and the cut of certain structures can be made at a right angle to the axis.

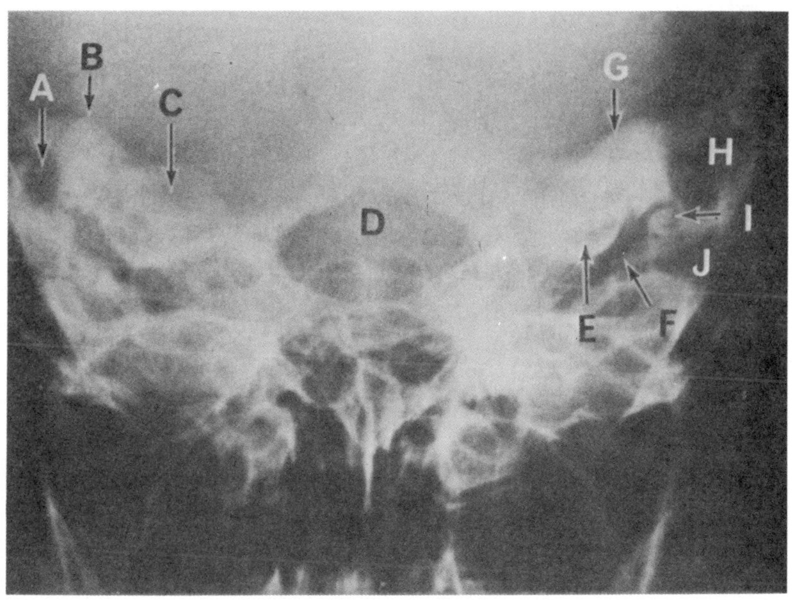

Figure 19-6. Towne's view

A. Antrum
B. Arcuate eminence
C. Internal auditory canal
D. Foramen magnum
E. Cochlea
F. Tympanic cavity
G. Superior semicircular canal
H. Mastoid cells
I. Ossicular mass
J. External auditory canal

Of the five tomographic projections, two of them, frontal and lateral are basic; the other three (axial, horizontal and Stenvers') are complimentary according to the area of pathology and examination desired. Tomography is a technique which allows visualization of a desired structure while obscuring those structures in front of and behind it. With the Phillips-Massiot polytome which furnishes a sufficiently thin cut and a high coefficient of distinction, it is possible to visualize clearly the small structures of the ear. The tomographic examination of the temporal bone consists of multiple sections obtained 1 or 2 mm. apart. In all projections both sides are examined so that the corresponding structures may be compared

This type of multidirectional or hypocycloidal tomography is excellent for the study of: (1) Congenital malformations; (2) Inflammatory processes (cholesteatoma) Figure 19-7); (3) Traumatic effects, (transverse and horizontal fractures, ossicular fracture and/or dislocation; (4) Neoplasm (glomus tumor, acoustic neuroma and carcinoma (Figure 19-8); and (5) Otodystrophy (otosclerosis, Paget's disease, osteogenesis imperfecta and fibrous dysplasia).

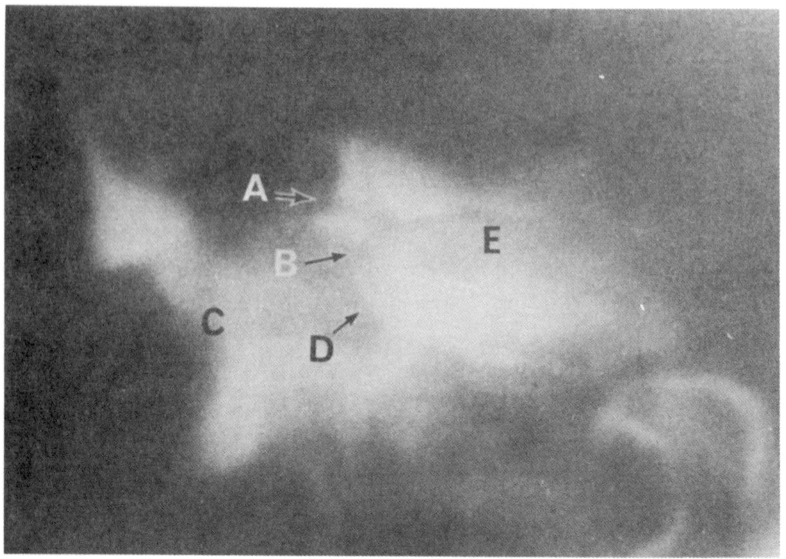

Figure 19-7. AP polytome showing a large cholesteatoma in the mastoid eroding the tegmen mastoideum and the roof of the external auditory canal.
A. Fistula of the horizontal semicircular canal
B. Oval window
C. External auditory canal
D. Promontory
E. Internal auditory canal

Carotid arteriography is useful in vascular anomalies of the temporal bone (glomus tumor, aneurysm, etc.). They may show soft tissue displacement or may show a tumor stain.

Retrograde jugular venogram. The jugular vein is catheterized and dye injected retrograde under pressure, filling the jugular vein and its tributaries. This is extremely useful in evaluation of collateral flow before ligation of the jugular vein, and for evaluation of the jugular bulb in anomalies and glomus tumors.

Posterior fossa myelography (cisternogram). Two to 3 cc. of Pantopaque (iophendylate) are injected in the subarachnoid space by lumbar puncture. Under fluoroscopic control the contrast media is then moved into the posterior cranial fossa in Trendelenburg position. This material outlines structures in the posterior fossa and is probably the most conclusive diagnostic test for acoustic neuroma. The absence of filling of the internal auditory canal and the demonstration of a filling defect in the cerebellopontine cistern are positive evidence of a space occupying lesion.

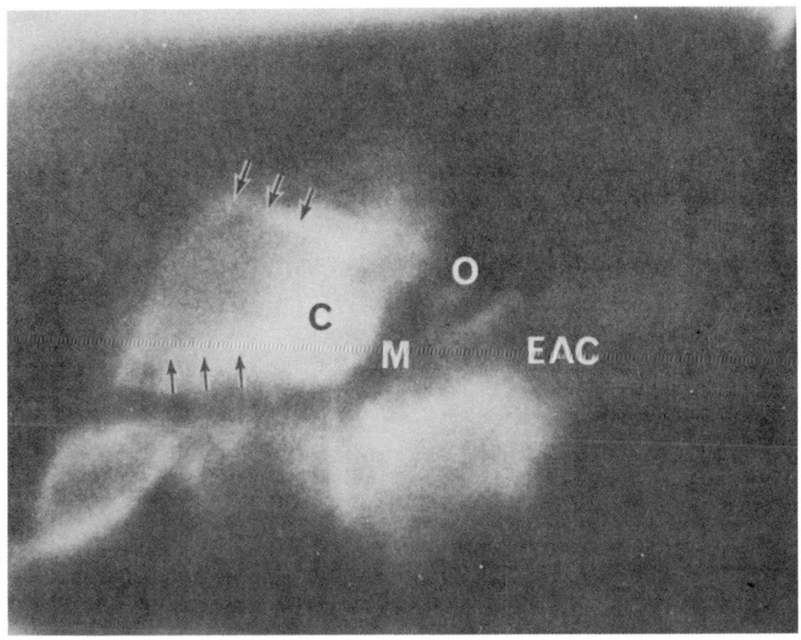

Figure 19-8. AP polytome showing marked enlargement of internal auditory canal indicative of acoustic neuroma.

O Ossicular mass
M Middle ear
EAC External auditory canal

Posterior fossa myelography is indicated: [24,25,26] (1) When the audiometric, vestibular, and tomographic studies are indicative of a retrocochlear lesion; (2) When the audiometric and vestibular tests are suggestive of a retrocochlear lesion, and a tomographic study is positive; and (3) Whenever the audiometric and vestibular tests consistently indicate a retrocochlear lesion in spite of a negative tomographic study to rule out the presence of a tumor limited to the cistern, or a tumor that is too small to produce changes in the bony outline of the internal auditory canal.

Combination technique. A combination of the polytomography and posterior fossa myelography is useful in the diagnosis of a small tumor within the internal auditory canal.

II. RADIOGRAPHY OF THE PARANASAL SINUSES

Radiographic examination of the paranasal sinuses consists of four standard projections (Waters, lateral, submentovertical and Caldwell), tomography, contrast radiography and angiography.

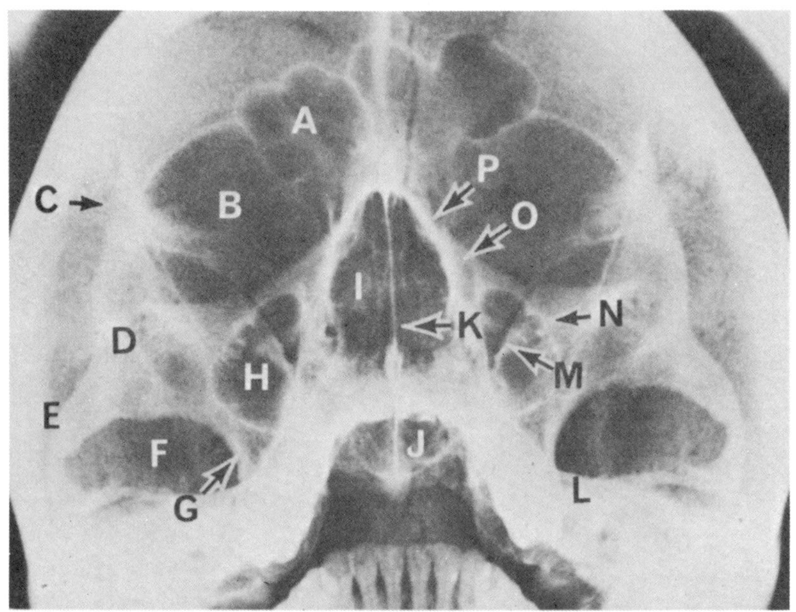

Figure 19-9. Waters' view

A. Frontal sinus
B. Orbit
C. Zygomaticofrontal suture
D. Zygoma
E. Zygomatic arch
F. Infratemporal fossa
G. Maxilla
H. Maxillary sinus
I. Nasal cavity
J. Sphenoid sinus
K. Septum
L. Petrous ridge
M. Superior orbital fissure
N. Infraorbital foramen
O. Frontal process of maxilla
P. Nasal bone

STANDARD PROJECTIONS:

1. Waters' view: (occipitomental, "chin-nose" position). This posteroanterior occipitomental projection is taken with the patient's head tilted upward so that his nose and chin are against the film surface. The petrous portion of the temporal bone is projected below the level of the maxillary sinus.

The maxillary sinuses are best shown in this view, followed by the frontal sinuses. The ethmoid sinuses are not well shown. A good view of the sphenoid sinus and its septum is obtained through the open mouth. (Figure 19-9).

This view also shows such maxillofacial structures as nasal bones, frontal process of the maxilla, zygoma of its arch, and mandible (especially coronoid process).

Other structures to be recognized include the oblique orbital line, the rim and floor of the orbit, superior orbital fissure (Cr. N. III, IV, V_1, VI, ophthalmic vein), foramen rotundum (V_2 maxillary N), foramen ovale (V_3 mandibular N.), zygomaticofacial foramen, infraorbital foramen, nasal ala and upper lip.

2. Lateral view. In this view the sphenoid sinuses are shown to best advantage followed by the frontal, ethmoidal and maxillary sinuses in that order. (Figure 19-10).

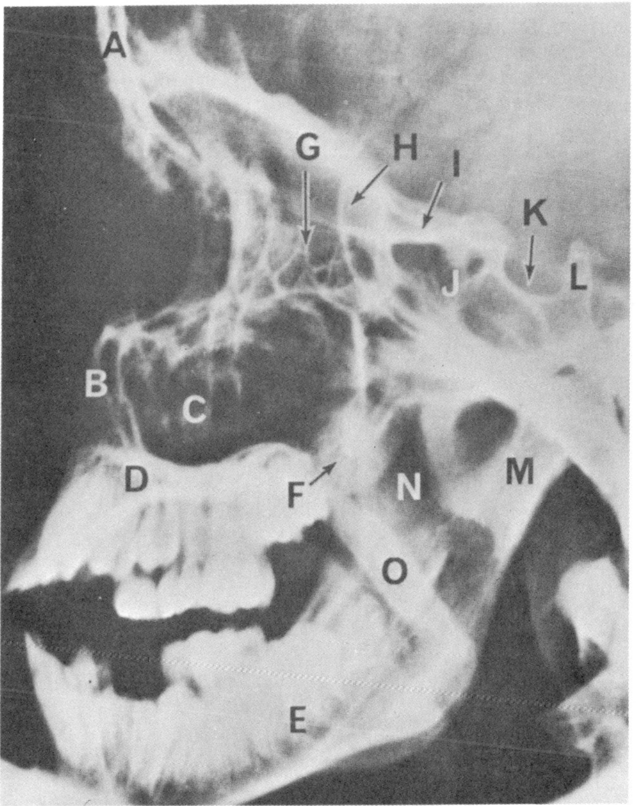

Figure 19-10. Lateral view

A. Frontal bone
B. Anterior wall of maxillary sinus
C. Maxillary sinus
D. Alveolar process of maxilla
E. Mandible
F. Posterior end of inferior turbinate
G. Ethmoid sinuses
H. Anterior wall of middle cranial fossa
I. Roof of sphenoid sinus
J. Sphenoid sinus
K. Sella turcica
L. Posterior clinoid process
M. Condyle of mandible
N. Nasopharynx
O. Soft palate

It also shows such maxillofacial structures as nasal bones, frontal sinus walls, the zygomatic process of the maxilla, the posterior wall of the maxillary sinus, the pterygoid plates, and the mandible. Other structures to be recognized in this view include anterior walls of the middle cranial fossa, the roof of the sphenoid sinus, the cribriform plate, the inferior turbinate, the coronoid process of the mandible, the zygomatic recess, the pterygomaxillary fissure, caroticoclinoid foramen, carotid sulcus and soft tissues (tonsils, adenoids, earlobe, soft palate, and base of the tongue).

3. Submentovertical view (Basal or base view). This view is obtained by passing x-rays at right angles through the base of the skull with the orbitomeatal line perpendicular to the central ray. In this view the sphenoid sinuses are shown to best advantage, followed by posterior ethmoidal, maxillary and frontal sinuses in that order. (Figure 19-11).

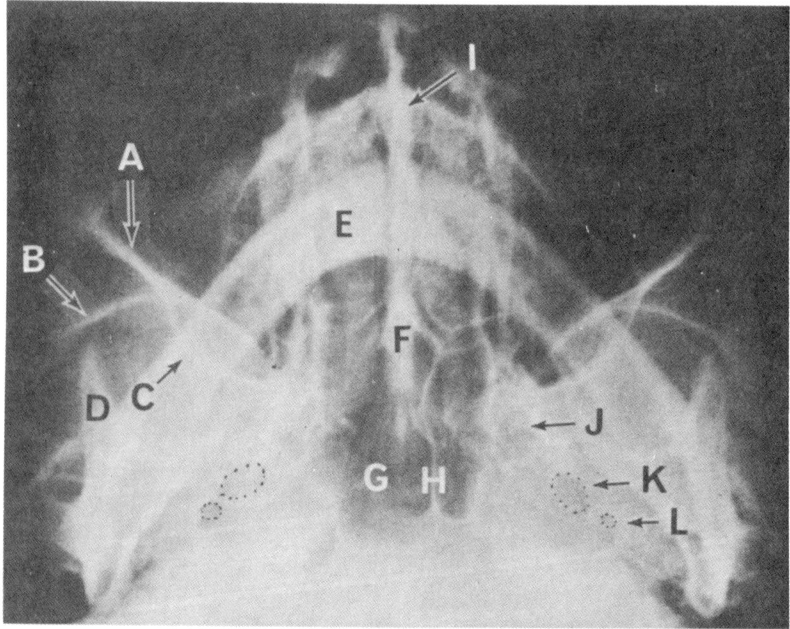

Figure 19-11. Submentovertical view
- A. Lateral wall of orbit
- B. Anterior wall of middle cranial fossa
- C. Posterolateral wall of antrum
- D. Coronoid process of mandible
- E. Body of mandible
- F. Vomer
- G. Sphenoid sinus
- H. Intraseptum of sphenoid sinus
- I. Nasal septum
- J. Pneumatized pterygoid process
- K. Foramen ovale
- L. Foramen spinosum

It shows such maxillofacial structures as zygomatic arch, the body of the zygoma, and the mandible (especially condyle).[29]

Other structures to be recognized include pneumatization of the pterygoid process and the greater wing of the sphenoid, the lateral three lines (1. Orbital line -- a straight line formed by the lateral wall of the orbit, 2. Antral line -- an "S" shaped line formed by the lateral wall of the antrum and 3. Middle cranial fossa line -- a "c" shaped curve with concavity backwards formed by the anterior wall of the middle cranial fossa), the pterygoid plate and pterygoalar bar, nasal cavity, the lacrimal canal, incisive foramen, greater and lesser palatine foramina, inferior orbital fissure, choana, foramen ovale (V_3 - mandibular N.), foramen spinosum (middle meningeal A.), foramen lacerum, carotid canals, eustachian tube, internal and external auditory canals and jugular foramen, and soft tissues (nasal turbinates, adenoids, uvula, lateral wall of the nasopharynx, and membranous external auditory canal).[30]

4. Caldwell view ("forehead-nose" position). This is obtained by positioning the nose and forehead against the cassette with the external auditory meatus and outer canthus of the eye forming a line perpendicular to the cassette. The x-ray tube is tilted caudally 15-20°.

In this view the frontal sinuses are best shown. The ethmoidal sinuses, particularly the orbital margin (lamina papyracea) are also well shown. The main cavity and lateral extensions of the sphenoid sinuses are recognizable. The posteromedial and inferolateral portion of the maxillary sinuses are usually visible. (Figure 19-12).

It shows such maxillofacial structures as the orbital margins, the zygoma, the zygomaticofrontal suture, the maxilla and the mandible.

Other structures to be recognized include the nasal cavity and its contents, floor and rim of the orbit, the infraorbital canal, the superior orbital fissure, the supraorbital foramen, Hyrtl's foramen (ophthalmomeningeal vein) lambdoidal suture, the foramen rotundum (always inferolateral to the lowermost portion of the superior orbital fissure) and soft tissues (palpebral fissures and "pony-tail" hair style).

Tomography:[6, 10, 19] It is of great value in determining the presence or absence of fractures or bone destruction in the paranasal sinuses and nasal structures, particularly in the planning of surgical or radiotherapeutic procedure. It is essential in the preoperative study of the diseases of the posterior ethmoid and sphenoid sinuses, and trans-sphenoidal hypophysectomy.

Multidirectional tomography (polytomography) is significantly superior to linear tomography.[19]

Contrast radiography: Radiopaque contrast media is used to outline anatomic or pathologic abnormalities within the paranasal sinuses, nasal cavity, and nasopharynx, such as cysts, polyps, neoplasms, oroantral fistula and choanal atresia.

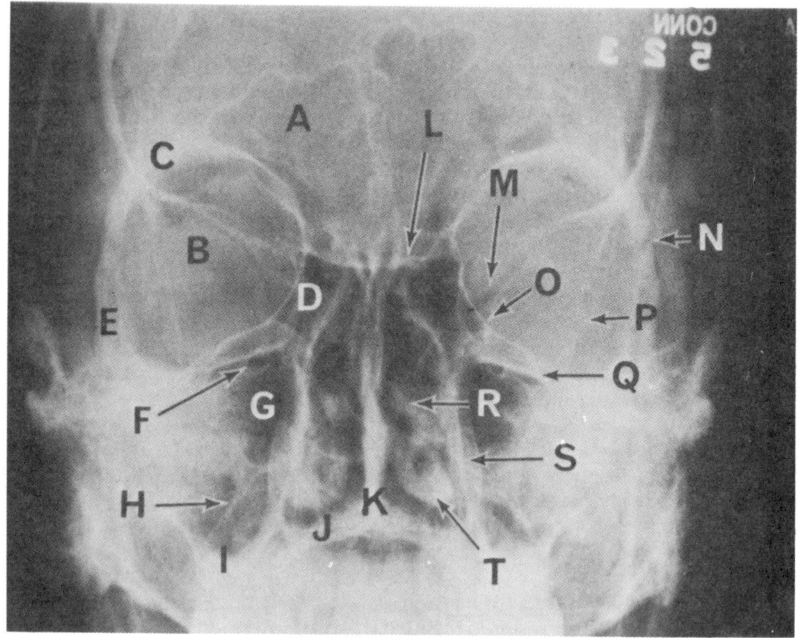

Figure 19-12. Caldwell View

A. Frontal sinus
B. Orbit
C. Superior orbital margin
D. Ethmoid sinus
E. Frontal process of zygoma
F. Foramen rotundum
G. Pneumatized pterygoid process
H. Lateral pterygoid plate
I. Floor of maxillary sinus
J. Floor of nasal cavity
K. Nasal septum
L. Limbus sphenoidalis
M. Superior orbital fissure
N. Frontozygomatic suture
O. Lamina papyracea
P. Oblique orbital line
Q. Floor of orbit
R. Middle turbinate
S. Lateral wall of nasal cavity
T. Inferior turbinate

Carotid arteriography may help delineate both benign and malignant lesions of the sinuses. In malignant lesions, soft tissue displacement, abnormal vascular pattern or a tumor stain may be shown. It is particularly useful for evaluation of angiofibromas of the nasopharynx. By the use of subtraction techniques, excellent visualization of occult extensions of the tumor with its vascular connections may be obtained.

Selective arteriography is extremely useful in the investigation and management of persistent and uncontrollable epistaxis prior to any surgical intervention.[2]

III. RADIOGRAPHY OF THE LARYNX

Radiographic examination of the larynx consists of conventional projections (anteroposterior and lateral), tomography, positive laryngography, air contrast laryngography and cinefluorography.

CONVENTIONAL RADIOGRAPHY: The antero-posterior (AP) and lateral views are commonly used.[16,27]

1. Anteroposterior view is of limited value in evaluation of the larynx itself because of the superimposition of the cervical spine. However, masses of the neck lateral to the larynx and distortion and/or displacement of the upper airway are shown.

2. Lateral view is of greater value and shows the outline of the base of the tongue and epiglottis, the vallecula, the hyoid, the aryepiglottic folds and arytenoids, the ventricles, the thyroid and cricoid cartilages, the subglottic space, and the prevertebral soft tissues. (Figure 19-13). This view is useful for evaluation of tumors and fractures of the larynx, a foreign body in the larynx, hypopharynx and upper esophagus, detection of calcification of normal and abnormal tissues, and evaluation of acute inflammatory conditions such as acute epiglottitis and retropharyngeal abscess. It is also useful for both pre-and postoperative evaluation of a thyrotomy and tracheotomy. The accuracy of the stent or mould placement for fractured larynx is also determined in this view.

Differential diagnosis of foreign body in the larynx, hypopharynx and upper esophagus include:

a. Sialolith
b. Tracheal rings
c. Semiopaque ear rings
d. Osteophytes of the cervical spine
e. Calcareous streaks in scar tissues
f. Ossification centers of the hyoid bone
g. Calcified cervical nodes
h. Residual dye from arteriography
i. Calcification in the laryngeal cartilages
j. Accessory ossification centers in the cervical spine
k. Calcified stylohoid ligaments
l. Sesamoid laryngeal cartilages
m. Calcification in the vessels of the neck

Tomography: Usually performed in the AP position and demonstrates laryngeal structures extending from the false cords to the upper trachea. The disadvantages of this technique are the amount of time consumed, difficulty of prevention of patients movement between or during exposures, and radiation exposure to the patient. The most useful information provided from this study is obliteration of the laryngeal ventricles or subglottic extension of neoplasms.

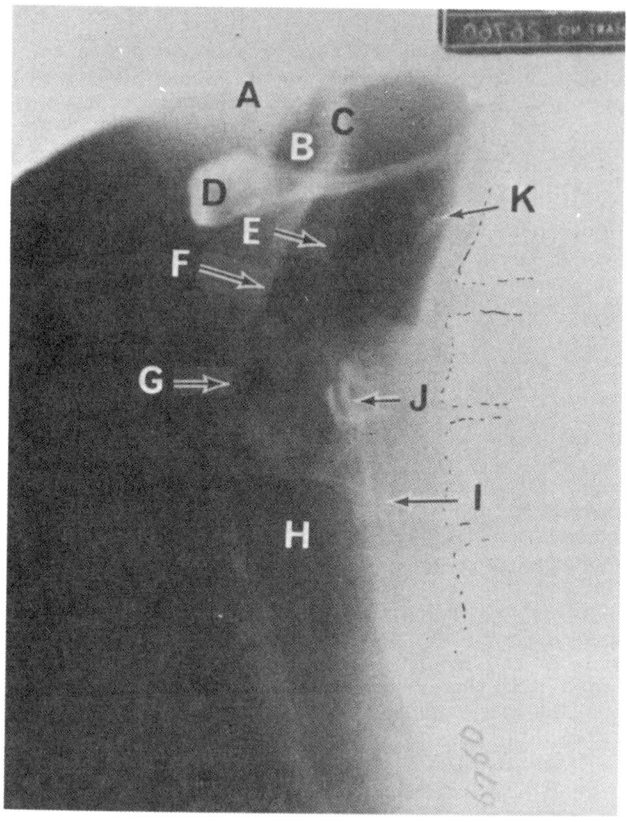

Figure 19-13. Lateral view of Larynx

A. Base of tongue
B. Vallecula
C. Tip of epiglottis
D. Hyoid bone
E. Aryepiglottic fold
F. Laryngeal surface of epiglottis
G. Ventricle
H. Trachea
I. Inferior cornu of thyroid cartilage
J. Calcified arytenoid cartilages
K. Cartilago triticea

Positive Contrast Laryngography: (Figure 19-14) Instillation of contrast media under fluoroscopic guidance provides a means of studying and recording on film or videotape the physiologic and pathologic processes. This diagnostic study is particularly useful in the selection of patients for conservation surgery of the larynx since it helps to outline the extent of the tumor and identify areas of involvement that cannot be directly or indirectly inspected.[6,15]

Under topical anesthesia the tip of the catheter is positioned in the pharynx just above the tip of the epiglottis. The contrast media

(Dionosil) is instilled slowly as the patient inspires, phonates, expires and executes the valsalva maneuver. Two major drawbacks are need for a topical anesthetic and the amount of time required for this study.

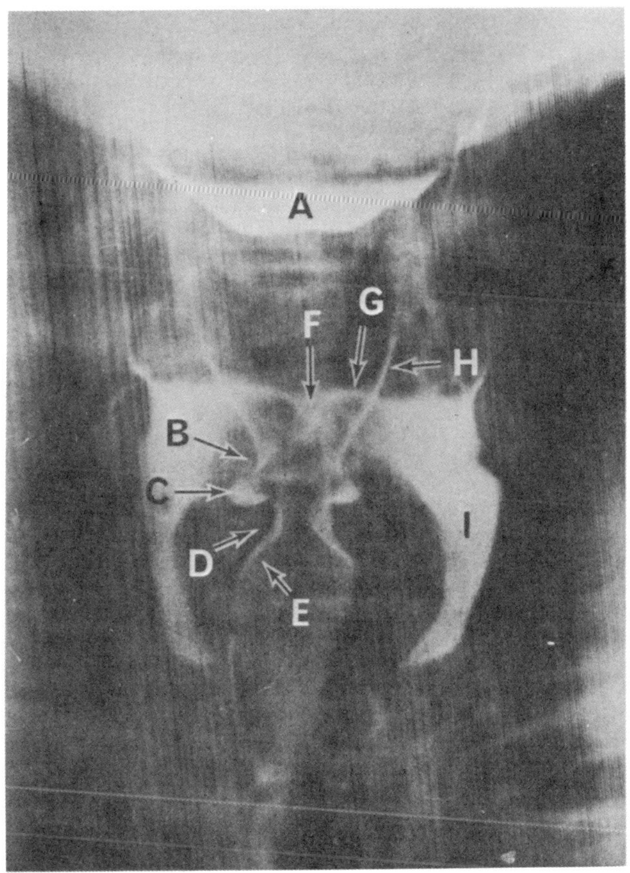

Figure 19-14. AP laryngogram

A. Vallecula
B. False cord
C. Ventricle
D. True cord
E. Subglottic angle groove
F. Interarytenoid groove
G. Arytenoid
H. Aryepiglottic fold
I. Pyriform sinus

Powdered tantalum has been used as a medium for laryngography.[35] Several features of powdered tantalum must be recognized: 1) it is potentially explosive; 2) particle size is not uniform; and 3) prolonged retention has been demonstrated in animal studies.

Air Contrast Laryngography: Laryngography using high kilo-voltage and heavy filtration provides information similar to positive contrast studies in the evaluation of laryngeal tumors. It is useful in the examination of patients with neoplasms who are unable to tolerate positive contrast study.

Xeroradiography: This technique, which is well accepted in mammography for its remarkable ability to record differences in soft tissue density, provides excellent images of soft tissues of the neck with great contrast in the lateral projection.[13]

Xeroradiography may be combined with zonography using the polytone machine (xeroradiographic zonography). It gives an excellent tomographic view of soft tissues of the larynx and hypopharynx in the frontal projection.[28]

IV. RADIOGRAPHY OF THE TRACHEOBRONCHIAL TREE

Conventional chest films and tomograms provide considerable information concerning the tracheobronchial tree. However, bronchography is far more fruitful. It offers valuable information concerning not only congenital, inflammatory and neoplastic lesions of the bronchi but provides information in certain parenchymal diseases such as alveolar lymphoma, alveolar cell carcinoma and organized or unresolved pneumonia.

Methods of bronchography. In those patients in whom the studies of all bronchial segments ("lung mapping") is desired. After suitable topical anesthesia, a soft rubber catheter is passed through the nose or the mouth into the trachea. When selective bronchography or brush biopsy of a lesion is desired, a transcricoid approach is used. The latter method is faster and less annoying to the patient. It requires a smaller amount of topical anesthetic and has the advantage of permitting selective studies of individual bronchi and allowing for brush-biopsy. Dionosil (oily or aqueous) is the contrast media of choice. Aqueous media is slightly more irritating to the bronchial mucosa and requires a greater amount of topical anesthetic. Recently, the use of barium sulfate and powdered tantalum for bronchography have been suggested. Both have the advantage of being chemically inert.

V. RADIOGRAPHY OF THE ESOPHAGUS

1. Radiographic examination of the esophagus is usually achieved by barium swallow, using both thick (better coating of the mucosa) and thin barium mixtures.

2. Fluoroscopy and spot films are often sufficient in fulfill the diagnostic needs. However, cineradiography improves the functional and anatomic evaluations especially in the study of pathophysiology of swallowing.

3. A small cotton pledget soaked in barium and swallowed may catch or hold on a foreign body. Capsules of various sizes filled

with barium and swallowed may demonstrate a stricture and its severity. A water-soluble contrast is used when an esophageal perforation is suspected.

4. The examination is conducted in both upright and recumbent positions, using posterior, anterior, lateral and oblique views. Inspiration, expiration, and the valsalva maneuvers are also used to note the esophageal position and intrathoracic dynamics.

VI. MISCELLANEOUS

1. Sialogram: Injection of radiopaque material into the salivary glands via the duct orifice will demonstrate abnormalities of the ductal system such as stricture, fistula, ectasia or neoplasm and abnormalities within the ductal system such as radiolucent calculi.

To perform sialography the duct orifices of the parotid (Stenson's) and/or submandibular glands (Wharton's) must first be topically anesthetized and dilated to permit a #60 P.E. catheter. Pantopaque is slowly injected into the catheter until the patient complains of discomfort in the gland. It is important to fill the duct to the patient's tolerance rather than to a predetermined volume. Usually, about 1 cc. will produce a satisfactory filling. After the x-ray examination the patient is instructed to chew on a fresh lemon for one minute. The normal gland will expell the contrast material within five minutes in response to this potent salivary stimulus.

The radiographs are taken with the patient seated in the P.A., tangential, and lateral projections. These same views are repeated following injection of contrast and again following emptying of the glands.

Stalography is helpful in determining if a lesion is inflammatory or neoplastic, whether it is an encapsulated or invasive lesion. The location of calculi in the duct or gland may be ascertained. Sialography is contraindicated in the presence of acute inflammatory disorders and when a history of sensitivity to iodine exists.

Plain films are made routinely to determine the adequacy of exposure and to detect radiopaque abnormalities in or around the salivary glands such as foreign bodies, calculi or calcifying disorders and to determine if abnormalities or adjacent osseous structures exist.

Radiosialography: (Salivary gland scanning). A salivary gland scan utilizes the same instrumentation and basic scintiscan techniques employed for thyroid scanning with 99 m technetium pertechnetate. This is a newer diagnostic technique and not yet widely adopted. Radiosialography is useful in the following situations:

a. Diagnosing a Warthin's tumor
b. Searching for occult primaries in cases of cervical metastasis
c. Confirming the presence and extent of neoplasm
d. Occasionally, to distinguish between benign and malignant disease

3. Tympanogram: (Tympanic clearance study) This is a method of eustachian tube function using radiopaque material in the middle ear.

Eustachian tube function can be determined by introducing not more than 1 cc. of radiopaque material such as pantopaque into the tympanic cavity through an intact or perforated tympanic membrane. A film is taken immediately in the Stenver's position. After ten minutes a second film taken in the same position will fail to show contrast material in the tympanic cavity if the eustachian tube function is normal. Retention of the dye indicates tubal disease.

4. Nasopharyngogram: (Contrast nasopharyngography) Examination consists of submentovertical and lateral projections. The submentovertical view demonstrates the lateral walls of the nasopharynx while the lateral projection demonstrates the roof and posterior walls of the nasopharynx as well as the nasopharyngeal surface of the soft palate. If tumor growth is suspected to involve the eustachian tube, additional films are taken during modified valsalva maneuver. This study is useful for precise location and extension of tumors of the nasopharynx and the adjacent structures. Premedication is not necessary. The patient is placed in a supine position with shoulders and trunk elevated to permit maximal extension of the neck, thus assuring a satisfactory submentovertical view of the base of the skull. The nostrils are sprayed with local anesthetic; contrast medium 15-20 cc for adults, is then utilized.

5. Evaluation of Facial Bone Injuries:[5,20,27,29] For the evaluation of the nasal bones, the right and left lateral, the superoinferior axial occlusal and the Waters' view are usually taken. Lateral views reveal depression or elevation of nasal bone fragments whereas superoinferior axial views show medial or lateral displacements of nasal fractures. The Waters' view will also show fracture and displacement of each nasal bone and the frontal process of the maxilla.

Facial bone series should include, in addition to the four standard sinus projections, an underexposed submentovertical view of zygomatic arches, and the exaggerated Waters' view to demonstrate fracture of the infraorbital rim and fracture-dislocation of the zygoma and zygomatic arch.

6. Pantomography: (Panoramic radiography) Panorex dental x-ray machine provides a panoramic view of the entire mandible and the anterolateral aspects of both maxillary sinuses. The x-ray beam has an aluminum filter and a narrow slit beam which moves horizontally from right to left (or vice versa) producing successive images on the film which in turn moves at a synchronized speed. The film is 12 inches long and requires approximately 24 seconds for total exposure. It is useful for evaluation of pathologic conditions of mandible and maxillae particularly for pre-and postoperative evaluation of mandibular fractures and tumors.

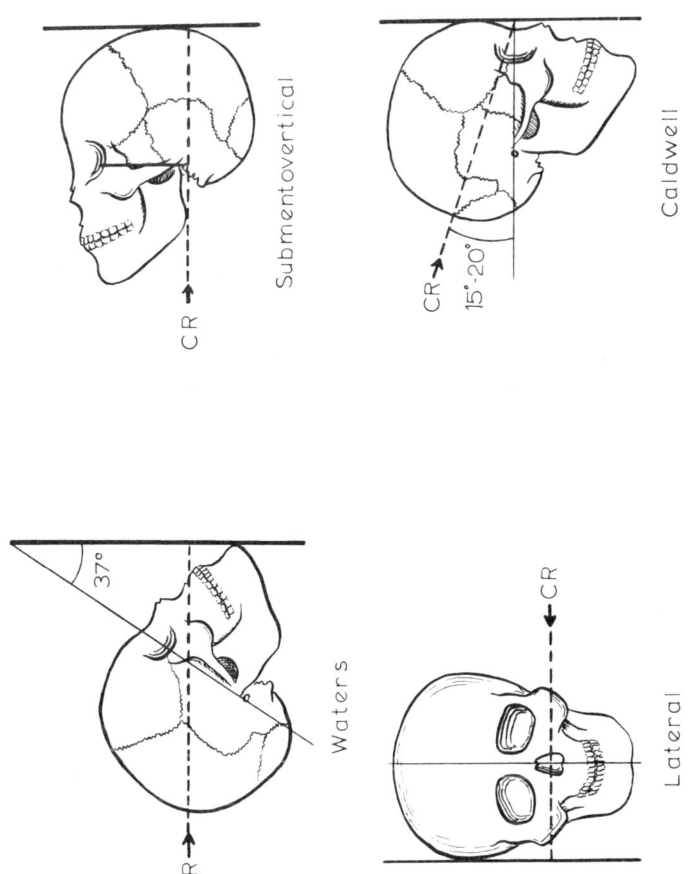

Figure 19-15. Positions on the Skull for Sinus X-rays.

7. Orbitogram: (Orbitography) This may be used for diagnosis of blowout fracture of the orbit. Five to ten cc. of water soluble contrast media (Hypaque) are injected into the extraconal space along the floor of the orbit in conjunction with hyaluronidase (Wydase). Typical orbitographic appearance of blowout fractures include demonstration of fluid level of contrast medium in the maxillary sinus, herniation of the orbital contents through the orbital floor and depressed bony fragments. Complications from this procedure include perforation of the eyeball, retrobulbar hemorrhage, central retinal artery spasm, drug idiosyncrasy, transient or permanent loss of vision, and excessive swelling of eye lid. This procedure is not recommended for evaluation of blowout fractures. Conventional Waters' view and laminogram are sufficient for diagnosis of blowout fractures.

8. Xerosialography. Sialography using xeroradiography is a superior method of examining the salivary glands, and affords better details, especially in ducts overlying bone, than does film recording. 12

9. Computerized axial tomography (CAT): Computerized tomography (CT): Computerized axial tomography (CAT, a new method for obtaining tomographic images), is a major advance in diagnostic radiology. Unlike conventional tomographic systems that use film both for the storage and display of transmitted x-rays, CAT makes use of sensitive scintillation detectors to detect x-rays that pass through a body section, and a digital computer is used to process this information. Tomographic images of selected planes through a subject are mathematically derived from a series of transmitted x-ray scan profiles, recorded from an x-ray tube head/detector assembly rotating about the subject. Alterations in tissue density in individual transverse cross sections are displayed on intensity modulated displays.

The EMI Scanner (named after the manufacturer of the first CAT unit in England) was specifically designed for the study of the skull and requires the use of the water absorber. The Automatic Computerized Transverse Axial Scanner (ACTA Scanner) was subsequently developed for the whole body and does not require the use of the water absorber.

Basically, an x-ray tube tracks across the body in the horizontal plane, passing a narrowly collimated beam of x-ray photons through the examined tissue slice. This "scan-pass" is repeated 180 times at one-degree intervals around a half-circle. Two sodium iodide crystals move in tandem opposite the x-ray source, detecting photon transmission through the slice. The data are analyzed by a computer and depicted on a television screen as a matrix of squares, each representing an absorption coefficient of the corresponding point in the tissue slice. Each absorption number is assigned a specific color or shade of gray and displayed on both color and black and white television monitors. Every scan consists of a pair of images representing tissue slices, 7.5-mm thick, separated by a space of 3 mm.

The CAT has proven to be of unique value in the study of orbital abnormalities, intracerebral and intraventricular hemorrhage, as well as other brain abnormalities. In the ENT area, the CAT may be useful to identify (1) large cerebellopontine angle tumors (it does not demonstrate intracanallicular tumors), (2) submucosal hematoma in the maxillary sinus (blood shows high density), (3) airfluid level in the paranasal sinuses, (4) upper airway tract, (5) tumors projecting into the lumen of the pharynx, larynx or trachea.

It is expected that CAT will play a dominant role in many other diagnostic areas as experience is gained.

FORAMINA IN BASE OF SKULL

Foramina	Contents	Veins which show best
Anterior Cranial Fossa:		
Foramen caecum	Emissary vein from nose to superior sagittal sinus	---
Anterior ethmoidal foramen	1. Anterior ethmoidal vessels 2. Nasociliary nerve	Lateral
Foramina in cribriform plate	Olfactory nerves	---
Posterior ethmoidal foramen	Posterior ethmoidal vessels and nerves	Lateral
Middle Cranial Fossa:		
Superior orbital fissure	1. Ophthalmic vein 2. Orbital branch of middle meningeal artery 3. Oculomotor nerve (3rd) 4. Trochlear nerve (4th) 5. Ophthalmic division of trigeminal nerve (5th) 6. Abducens nerve(6th) 7. Recurrent branch of lacrimal artery	1. Caldwell 2. Waters
Optic foramen	1. Optic nerve 2. Ophthalmic artery	Oblique orbital (Rhese)
Foramen rotundum	Maxillary division of trigeminal nerve (5th)	1. Caldwell 2. Waters

Foramen ovale	1. Mandibular division of trigeminal nerve (5th) 2. Accessory meningeal artery	1. Base 2. Waters
Foramen lacerum (carotid canal)	1. Internal carotid artery 2. Sympathetic carotid plexus 3. Superficial petrosal nerve 4. Vidian nerve 5. Meningeal branch of ascending pharyngeal artery	Base
Foramen spinosum	1. Middle meningeal artery 2. Recurrent branch of mandibular nerve	Base
<u>Posterior Cranial Fossa:</u>		
Internal auditory canal	1. Facial nerve (7th) 2. Auditory nerve (8th) 3. Internal auditory vessels	1. Stenvers 2. Trans-orbital 3. Towne 4. Base
Jugular foramen	1. Internal jugular vein 2. Inferior petrosal sinus 3. Transverse sinus 4. Meningeal branch from occipital and ascending pharyngeal arteries 5. Glossopharyngeal nerve (9th) 6. Vagus nerve (10th) 7. Spinal accessory nerve (11th)	1. Base 2. Towne
Stylomastoid foramen	1. Facial nerve (7th) 2. Stylomastoid artery	Base
Hypoglossal canal	1. Hypoglossal nerve (12th) 2. Meningeal branch of ascending pharyngeal artery 3. Emissary vein from transverse sinus	1. Stenvers 2. Towne

Foramen magnum	1. Medulla oblongata and spinal cord 2. Spinal accessory nerve 3. Vertebral arteries 4. Anterior and posterior spinal arteries 5. Membrana tectoria 6. Apical ligament	1. Base 2. Towne

REFERENCES

1. Buckingham, R.A. and Valvassori, G.E.: Tomographic anatomy of the temporal bone. Otolaryngol. Clin. N. Am. 6:337-362, 1973.

2. Coel, M.N. and Janon, E.A.: Angiography in patients with intractable epistaxis. Am. J. Roentgenol. 116:37-40, 1972.

3. Compere, W.E.: Radiographic atlas of the temporal bone, Book I. Am. Acad. Ophthal. Otol., 1964.

4. Compere, W.E.: Tympanic cavity clearance studies. Trans. Am. Acad. Ophthal. Otol. 62:444, 1958.

5. Dingman, R.O. and Natvig, P.: Surgery of facial fractures. Philadelphia, W.B. Saunders Co., 1964.

6. Dodd, G.D. (Editor): Symposium on diagnosis of tumor of the head and neck. Radiolog. Clin. N. Am., Vol. 8, No.3, 1970.

7. Dolan, K.D.: Radiographic anatomy of the nasal sinuses. Otolaryng. Clin. N. Am. 4:13-24, 1971.

8. Etter, L.E.: Atlas of roentgen anatomy of the skull. Springfield, Illinois, Charles C Thomas, Publisher, 1955.

9. Etter, L.E.: Roentgenography and roentgenology of the middle ear and mastoid process. Springfield, Illinois, Charles C Thomas, Publisher, 1965.

10. Fletcher, G.H. and Jing, B.S.: The head and neck. Chicago, Year Book Medical Publishers, Inc., 1968.

11. Gates, G.A.: Radiosialographic aspects of salivary gland disorders. Laryngoscope 82:115-130, 1972.

12. Glassman, L.M., O'Hara, A.E. and Cregar, D.: Xerosialography. Arch. Otolaryng. 100:341-343, 1974.

13. Holinger, P.H., Lutterbeck, E.F. and Bulger, R.: Xeroradiography of the larynx. Ann. Otol. 81:806-808, 1972.

14. Merrill, V.: Atlas of roentgenographic positions. 2nd ed. St. Louis, C.V. Mosby Co., pp. 384-385, 1959.

15. Ogura, J.H., Powers, W.E., Holtz, S., et al.: Laryngogram: their value in the diagnosis and treatment of laryngeal lesions. Laryngoscope 70:780-809, 1969.

16. Pendergrass, E.P., Schaeffer, J.P. and Hodes, P.J.: The head and neck in roentgen diagnosis. 2nd ed. Springfield, Illinois, Charles C Thomas, Publisher, 1956.

17. Petasnick, J.P.: Congenital malformations of the ear. Otolaryngol. Clin. N. Am. 6:413-428, 1973.

18. Petasnick, J.P.: Radiology of the temporal bone. In Maloney, W.H. (ed.): Otolaryngology. Hagerstown, Maryland, Harper & Row, Publishers, 1975, Ch. 5, pp. 1-40.

19. Potter, G.D.: Sectional anatomy and tomography of the head. New York, Grune and Stratton, 1971.

20. Samuel, E.: Clinical radiology of the ear, nose, and throat. London, H.K. Lewis & Co., Ltd., 1952.

21. Scanlan, R.L.: Positive contrast medium (Iophendylate) in diagnosis of acoustic neuroma. Arch. Otolaryngol. 80:698-706, 1964.

22. Shapiro, R. and Janzen, A.H.: The normal skull: A roentgen study. New York, P.B. Hoeber, Inc., 1960.

23. Twigg, H.L., Axelbaum, S.P. and Schellinger, D.: Computerized body tomography with the ACTA scanner. JAMA 234:314-317, 1975.

24. Valvassori, G.E.: The diagnosis of acoustic neuromas. Otolaryngol. Clin. N. Am. 6:391-400, 1973.

25. Valvassori, G.E.: Myelography of the internal auditory canal. Am. J. Roentgenol. Radium. Ther. Nucl. Med. 115:578, 1972.

26. Valvassori, G.E.: Radiography of the temporal bone. In Paparella M.M. and Shumrick, D.A. (ed.): Otolaryngology. Philadelphia, W.B. Saunders Co., 1973, Vol. 1, Ch. 45, pp. 1021-1042.

27. Valvassori, G.E. (ed.): Symposium on radiology in otolaryngology. Otolaryng. Clin. N. Am., Vol. 6, No. 2, 1973.

28. Woesner, M.E., Braun, E.J. and Sanders, I.: Xeroradiographic zonography of the larynx and hypopharynx. Ann. Otol. 83:42-48, 1974.

29. Yanagisawa, E., Merrell, R.A. and Myerson, M.: X-ray diagnosis of posterior displacement of zygoma. Arch. Otolaryng. 82:275-280, 1965.

30. Yanagisawa, E. and Smith, H.W., et al.: Radiographic anatomy of the paranasal sinuses. Arch. Otolaryng. I. Waters view. 87:184-195; II. Lateral view. 87:196-209; III. Submentovertical view. 87:299-310; IV. Caldwell view. 87:311-322, 1968.

31. Yanagisawa, E. and Smith, H.W.: Radiology of the normal maxillary sinus and related structures. Otolaryng. Clin. N. Am. 9:55-81, 1976.

32. Yanagisawa, E. and Smith, H.W.: Normal radiographic anatomy of the paranasal sinuses. Otolaryng. Clin. N. Am. 6:429-457, 1973.

33. Young, B.R.: The skull, sinuses and mastoids: a handbook of roentgen diagnosis. Chicago, The Year Book Medical Publishers, 1951.

34. Zizmor, J. and Noyek, A.M.: Radiology of the nose and paranasal sinuses, in Maloney, W.H. (ed.): Otolaryngology, Hagerstown, Maryland, Harper & Row Publishers, 1973, Ch. 4, pp. 1-52.

35. Zamel, N., Austin, J.H.M., Graf, P.D., Dedo, H.H., Jones, M.D. and Nadel, J.A.: Powdered tantalum as a medium for human laryngography. Radiology 94:547-553, 1970.

CHAPTER 20

ANESTHESIA

I. LOCAL ANESTHESIA

A. DEFINITIONS: Local Anesthesia is the loss of sensation in a circumscribed area. Local Anesthetics are drugs that block nerve conduction when applied locally to nerve tissue in appropriate concentrations. In addition, clinically useful local anesthetics have the following properties:

1. The nerve block is reversible.
2. The time of onset, and duration of blockade of the nerve fiber is predictable for common usage.
3. The drug is non-irritating to the tissue to which it is applied.
4. The drug is permeable and diffusable.
5. The drug has a high therapeutic index.
6. The drug is water soluble and chemically stable.

B. MECHANISM OF ACTION: Local anesthetics prevent the conduction of nerve impulses. They act by interfering with ionic exchange at the nerve cell membrane and stabilizing the membrane against the generation of an action potential.

C. CHEMISTRY: The local anesthetics consist of three parts: Aromatic lipophilic group, Intermediate chain, Hydrophilic group.

The common local anesthetics have as an intermediate chain either an ester (i.e. cocaine, procaine) or an amide linkage (i.e. Xylocaine, mepivicaine).

The terminal hydrophilic (amine) group is able to combine with an acid and form a water soluble salt.

BASE		SALT
$R_3 N + H^+ Cl^-$	$\rightleftarrows$	$R_3 NH^+ Cl^-$

The base unionized form is more lipid soluble and is the form that penetrates the neural membrane and produces anesthesia. The pKa of the particular drug and the pH of the solution determine the ratio of salt to base (as dictated by the Henderson Hasselbalch equation) and therefore, the amount of drug in the pharmacologically active form. When the tissues are acidotic into which a local anesthetic is introduced, a larger proportion of the drug is in the inactive (salt) form. This accounts for the diminished activity of local anesthetics in infected areas.

D. UPTAKE, METABOLISM AND EXCRETION: Most local anesthetic agents are absorbed rapidly into the bloodstream from the mucous membranes and subcutaneous tissues. Certain sites of particular interest to the otolaryngologist, such as the laryngeal and tracheal mucous membranes, are associated with such rapid uptake of local anesthetics that blood levels approach that achieved with intravenous administration.

Amide type drugs are metabolized by the liver in a complex series of steps beginning with N-dealkylation. Ester type drugs are hydrolyzed by cholinesterases in the liver and plasma. Both degradation processes depend on enzymes which are synthesized in the liver and therefore, both will be compromised in a patient with parenchymal liver disease.

Many of the end products of catabolism of both esters and amides are water soluble and are excreted to a large extent in the kidneys.

E. TOXICITY:

1. Local toxicity: reaction of tissue at the site of injection. These include reactions of the skin and mesenchymal tissues (cellulitis, ulceration, abscess formation, tissue slough) as well as lesions of the peripheral nerves (neuropathy). The commonest causes of local tissue reactions include:

   a. Faulty technique: contamination of the local anesthetic agents and traumatic administration.
   b. reactions from the local anesthetic agent itself.
   c. reactions from preservatives and vasoconstrictor agents added to the local anesthetic.

2. General toxicity: systemic reactions which occur due to absorption of a given drug into the general circulation. These may be due to an excessively high blood level, allergy, or miscellaneous causes.

a. A toxic blood level is the result of a drug overdose. This can be achieved by rapid absorption, excessive dose, and/or inadequate metabolism and redistribution. Most often a toxic overdose is a result of carelessness in exceeding the recommended dosage for a particular drug or inadvertant intravenous administration. Ninety-eight percent of systemic toxic reactions to local anesthetics are due to drug overdose.

Significant symptoms of toxic overdose of local anesthetic agents are confined to the central nervous system and cardiovascular system. The central nervous system responses to local anesthetic agents are biphasic with stimulation followed by depression. Clinically, patients may appear agitated with confused and rambling speech. This excitation may proceed to seizures and coma. The direct cardiovascular effects of local anesthetics are those of depression. Both myocardial performance and peripheral vascular tone are diminished by increasing levels of local anesthetic agents.

As in most iatrogenic complications, the most effective treatment of local anesthetic toxic overdose is avoidance. This requires care in the choice of agent and administration. When preliminary signs of overdose appear, O_2 should be administered and a venous cannula should be secured. Symptoms of excitement may be treated with hypnotics, (diazepam, barbiturates) although this should be done with caution so as not to exacerbate the subsequent cerebral depression. Likewise if seizures occur, anti-seizure medication should be employed but with the realization that the subsequent coma may be exacerbated. The physician should be prepared for general supportive measures in the case of ultimate cardiovascular and respiratory collapse. This may include endotracheal intubation, mechanical ventilation and intravenous fluid and pressor therapy.

b. True allergic reactions to local anesthetics are an infrequent occurrence (2% of reported complications), and most commonly occur with ester derivatives. These may present as any of the gamut of allergic syndromes from relatively innocuous dermatologic signs to anaphylactic shock. The treatment of allergic reactions to local anesthetic agents involves the same strategies as for any allergic reaction.

Trying to choose an anesthetic technique for a patient with a history of "allergy" to local anesthetics is a frequent clinical problem. A careful history with documentation, if possible, should help sort out those with reactions to toxic overdose (see above) or miscellaneous reactions (see below) from those with true allergy. If allergy is confirmed, some authors suggest that utilization of the opposite class of drug (i.e. amide if ester was previously used) is a relatively safe approach. Dyclonine, which is neither amide nor ester, may be safely used in some cases where allergy to both classes of drugs are suspected. If doubt exists, one must consider alternative techniques (i.e. general anesthesia).

c. Miscellaneous reactions: Included in this group are those adverse reactions which are not specific to the local anesthetic agent per se. An inappropriate response to the needle used for administration or an increased sensitivity to the preservative in the drug are examples. A unique adverse reaction occurs with the local anesthetic Prilocaine. When used in excess of 500 mg in an adult, a significant fraction of the patient's hemoglobin is reduced to the methemoglobin state. Methemoglobin has a diminished ability to transport oxygen to peripheral tissues. The treatment of methomobloginemia caused by prilocaine overdose is the slow intravenous administration of methylene blue, 1% solution, total dose 1-2 mg/kg.

F. LOCAL ANESTHETIC AGENTS: (See Table 1)

1. Cocaine was the earliest recognized local anesthetic and is the only agent that is naturally occurring. It was introduced into clinical practice for topical anesthesia by Sigmund Freud and Karl Koller in 1884 and for nerve trunk blockade by William Halsted in 1885.

Cocaine is unique among local anesthetic agents in its ability to block the reuptake of norephinephrine at adrenergic nerve endings. It is this metabolic action which accounts for its side effects of vasoconstriction, tachycardia, hypertension, "sensitization of the myocardium to catecholamines", mydriasis, cortical stimulation and addiction.

Other drugs which interfere with catecholamine catabolism, such as monoamine oxidase inhibitors (MAOI) may interact with cocaine and cause a hypertensive crisis.

Cocaine is an extremely potent topical anesthetic agent and an extremely toxic drug. The maximum permissible dose topically is 2-3 mg/kg. The onset of action is immediate, and the duration is 45 minutes. It is decomposed by autoclaving.

2. Procaine Hydrochloride (Novocaine) was first synthesized in 1905 by Einhorn as a result of a concerted effort to find a safer substitute for cocaine.

Procaine Hydrochloride is a relatively weak local anesthetic agent of the ester type. It is inactive when applied topically. When used for infiltration, it is associated with a rapid onset (2-5 minutes) and a brief duration of action (45-60 minutes). It has a relatively low toxicity, and a maximum recommended dose of 1000 mgm. It is commonly used in 2% solution for infiltration.

Procaine is rapidly hydrolyzed by intravascular cholinesterase. Procaine may prolong the effect of Succinylcholine (Anectine) which is also catabolized by cholinesterase.

3. Tetracaine Hydrochloride (Pontocaine) is a potent anesthetic of the ester family. Its potency and toxicity are approximately 10 times those of Procaine. It is effective when applied topically in a concentration of 1-2% and is associated with a rather delayed onset (6-12 minutes) and prolonged duration of action (1-1/2-2 hours). No more than 80 mgm should be used for topical anesthesia of the upper respiratory tract.

4. Chloroprocaine Hydrochloride (Nesacaine) is a halogenated derivative of procaine, and as such has similar pharmacologic properties. It is hydrolyzed more rapidly than procaine and is therefore less toxic. It is not useful for topical anesthesia. It is used in a 2% concentration for infiltration and the maximum recommended dose is 1 gm.

5. Hexyclaine (Cyclaine) is an ester having somewhat greater potency and toxicity than procaine. It is most frequently used for topical application, where it provides a rapid onset (2-3 minutes) and moderate duration of action. Infiltration use has been limited by a high incidence of local irritation. The solution is stable and may be autoclaved.

6. Lidocaine Hydrochloride (Xylocaine) is an aminoacetyl amide. It has excellent penetrating powers and is effective by all routes of administration, providing a rapid onset and a moderate duration of action (1 hour). The action may be prolonged by the addition of epinephrine in a concentration of 1:100,000 (1 mg of epinephrine per 100 cc of solution). For infiltration or nerve block, 1 and 2% solutions are used. A 4% solution is employed for topical anesthesia. The maximum recommended dose for topical anesthesia in an adult is 200 mgm (5 ml of the 4% solution) and for infiltration is 200 mgm (without epinephrine) and 500 mgm (with epinephrine).

The enhanced ability of lidocaine to suppress automaticity in ectopic myocardial foci has encouraged its use in the acute management of ventricular arrhythmia. A dose of 50-100 mgm as an intravenous bolus is used for the purpose.

7. Mepivacine Hydrochloride (Carbocaine) is an amide chemically related to lidocaine. It shares with lidocaine many clinical features. It is associated with less vasodilatation than that seen with lidocaine and has a slightly longer duration of action.

8. Prilocaine Hydrochloride (Citanest, Propitocaine) has similar clinical properties to those of lidocaine except that it is more rapidly metabolized. When the maximum dose of 500 mgm is exceeded, methemoglobinema may result (see miscellaneous reactions, above).

9. Bupivacaine (Marcaine) is an amide chemically related to lidocaine. It shares with Xylocaine many clinical features. It is associated with an extremely long duration of action (2-4 hours). It is tightly bound to tissue and plasma protein, and is not associated with high blood levels when appropriately administered. Bupivacaine is used for infiltration and nerve block in a 1-2% solution with a maximum recommended dose of 225 mgm. Its high potency and long duration of action make it a useful agent for prolonged procedures.

10. Dyclonine Hydrochloride (Dyclone) is neither an ester nor an amide. Therefore, it has been recommended for use in those patients who are allergic to both families of local anesthetics. It has a rapid onset of action (3-10 minutes) and a brief duration (30 minutes). It is used in a 0.5% solution for topical anesthesia and the recommended maximum safe dose is 300 mgm in an adult.

11. Dibucaine Hydrochloride (Nupercaine) is of the amide group. It is extremely potent for topical and infiltrative use. However, it has fallen out of common use because of a high reported incidence of local toxicity.

12. Piperocaine (Metycaine) is similar to procaine but more toxic and with a longer duration of action. The concentration used is 0.5 to 1% solution for infiltration and 2-10% solution for topical use.

13. Miscellaneous: Cetacaine is a mixture of tetracaine and ethyl and butyl aminobenzoate. Forestierre's solution is a mixture of cocaine (4%) phenol, potassium chloride and epinephrine, 1:1000. Bonnaine's solution is a mixture of cocaine (4%), methol and phenol.

G. PREMEDICATION: Drug premedication is only a supplement to a supportive and informative preoperative visit.

1. Hypnotics:
a. Barbiturates: The barbiturates are probably the most frequently employed of the hypnotics. They act principally by depressing cerebral cortical activity, but also may be associated with respiratory

and cardiovascular depression. Pentobarbital (Nembutal) and Secobarbital (Seconal) are the most commonly utilized of the short acting barbiturates. They are administered orally or intramuscularly in a recommended dose of 50-200 mgm for adult patients.

b. Chloral Hydrate is one of the oldest and safest hypnotics. It is especially useful in elderly patients in whom barbiturates may be contraindicated. The recommended dosage for adults is 0.5-1 gm by mouth.

c. Antihistamines: Antihistamines such as Hydroxyzine (Vistaril) and Diphenhydramine (Benadryl) are useful for their sedative, antihistaminic and antiemetic properties. They are commonly used to supplement the action of a narcotic premedicant. They are well tolerated and relatively safely administered to all age groups. Hydroxyzine and Diphenhydramine are administered in dosages of 25-100 mgm intramuscularly.

2. Narcotics: Morphine sulphate (10 mgm) and Meperedine (Demerol) (50-100 mgm) are commonly utilized in premedication. These drugs are especially useful when pain is a component of the pre-operative condition. Both these agents are associated with central nervous system and respiratory depression and on occasion nausea and vomiting.

3. Tranquilizers:
a. Phenothiazines are useful pre-operative medications, contributing excellent sedative, antiemetic, and antihistaminic properties. Many of the phenothiazines can be given orally as well as intramuscularly for pre-operative medication. Commonly utilized premedicants in this group include; Chlorpromazine (Thorazine) 15-50 mgm, Prochlorperazine (Compazine) 5-10 mgm, and Promethazine (Phenergan) 25-50 mgm.

b. Benzodiazepines are especially effective premedicants for local anesthesia because of the prophylactic protection they provide against seizures. Effective in both oral and intramuscular administration, Diazepam (Valium) 5-10 mgm, and Chlordiazepoxide (Librium) 25-50 mgm are the most frequently utilized of this family.

4. Belladonna Derivatives: Atropine sulphate (0.5 mgm) and Scopolamine (0.5 mgm) are the two most commonly employed belladonna agents. Used for their anti-muscarinic properties, their most beneficial action is that of drying of the secretions of the upper airway. Scopolamine is associated with more frequent central nervous system effects (sedation, excitation) ans is less effective in preventing reflex bradycardia than is atropine.

5. One of the authors (KJL) uses 100 mg seconal p.o. two hours pre-op.; 8- to 10 mg morphine IM, on call; 8- to 10 mg valium IM, on call. The use of valium also serves as an adjunct to protect against local anesthetic toxicity reactions, particularly in rhinoplasty or other procedures in which larger quantities of local anesthetic agents are used. The use of morphine causes pylorospasm, thus

preventing the absorption of the seconal if given simultaneously. Besides the pre-operative medication, it is essential to inform the patient pre-operatively of the procedure "step by step" and what to expect throughout. This pre-operative counseling has been referred to by Jackson as the "sermon".

H. INTRAVENOUS SEDATION:
1. Diazepam (Valium) (2.5 mgm - 5 mgm) given in slow intravenous increments, is a relatively safe and effective sedative. It is useful in supplementing local anesthesia to optimize clinical conditions. Its effectiveness for tranquilization and prophylaxis against local anesthetic induced seizures has been previously stressed. Very rapid administration is occasionally associated with transient respiratory depression.

2. Innovar is a mixture of droperidol (2.5 mgm per cc) and fentanyl (0.5 mg per cc). When given slowly in small increments (1/2 cc) it may enhance intraoperative sedation during local anesthesia. When given too rapidly, it may be associated with hypotension and chest wall spasm.

3. Barbiturates: Sodium Pentobarbital (Nembutal) and Secobarbital (Seconal) when given in small increments intravenously (25-50 mgm) may provide safe sedation to supplement local anesthesia. Too rapid administration may produce respiratory depression.

I. BLOCK TECHNIQUES: In virtually all blocks, eliciting an appropriate paresthesia prior to injection of the agent helps to insure success.

1. Laryngoscopy, Tracheoscopy: The larynx and trachea receive their sensory nerve supply from the superior and inferior laryngeal nerves, which are branches of the vagus nerve.

a. Anesthesia may be provided to the larynx by the topical application of local anesthesia (using a laryngeal syringe) to the mucous membrane of the pyriform fossa (deep to which runs the superior laryngeal nerve) and to the laryngeal surface of the epiglottis and the vocal folds. (Figure 20-1).

b. Local anesthesia of the larynx and trachea may also be accomplished by the percutaneous infiltration of local anesthetic solution around the superior laryngeal nerve and the trans-tracheal application of local anesthetic to the tracheal mucosa.

For percutaneous infiltration, the superior laryngeal nerve is located as it pierces the thyrohyoid membrane. (Figure 20-2)

1) Palpate the greater cornue of the hyoid bone.
2) Insert a 25 gauge needle approximately 1 cm caudal to this landmark.
3) The needle is inserted to a depth of approximately 1 cm until the firm consistency of the thyrohyoid membrane is identified.
4) 3 cc of local anesthetic solution are injected.

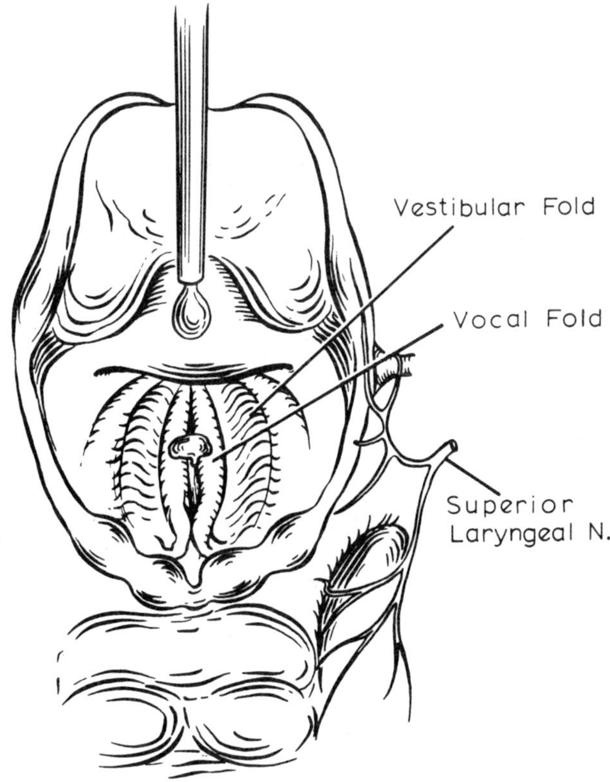

Figure 20-1. Topical Anesthesia to the Larynx.

The trans-tracheal application of local anesthesia requires the insertion of a 25 gauge needle through the cricothyroid membrane in the midline. (Figure 20-3)

1) Introduce the 25 gauge needle in the midline between the thyroid and cricoid cartilages.
2) Puncture the cricothyroid membrane. This is readily felt as a "pop". Free aspiration of air with the attached syringe verifies the intratracheal position of the needle tip.
3) Instill 4 cc of local anesthetic solution. In addition to anesthesia of the larynx and trachea (a. and b. above), the topical application of local anesthesia to the oropharynx is required for adequate visualization for laryngoscopy and tracheoscopy.

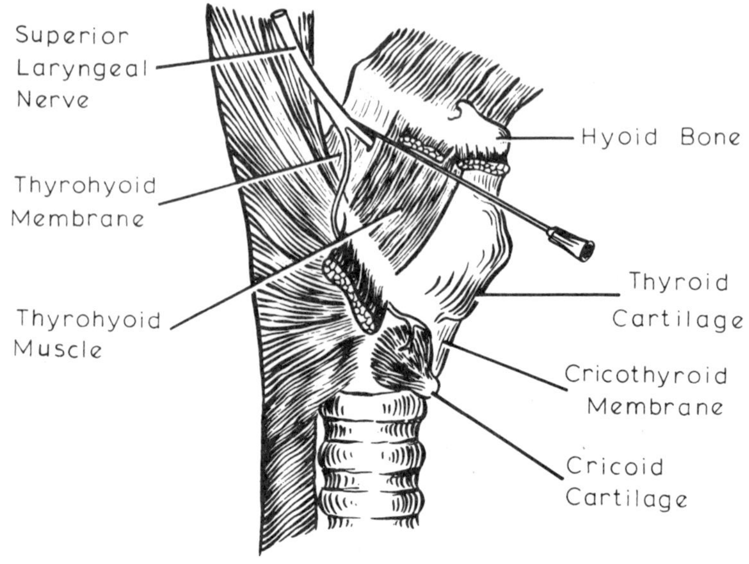

Figure 20-2. Infiltrating the Superior Laryngeal Nerve.

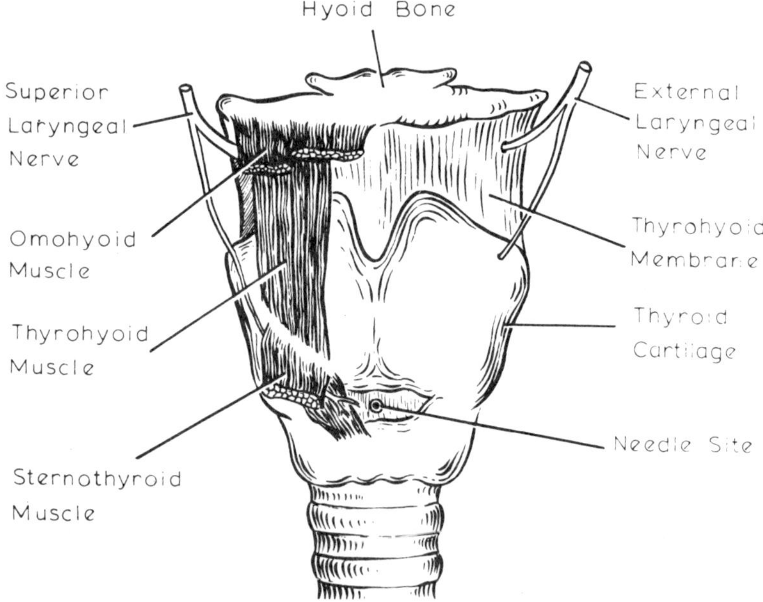

Figure 20-3. Trans-tracheal Application of Topical Anesthesia.

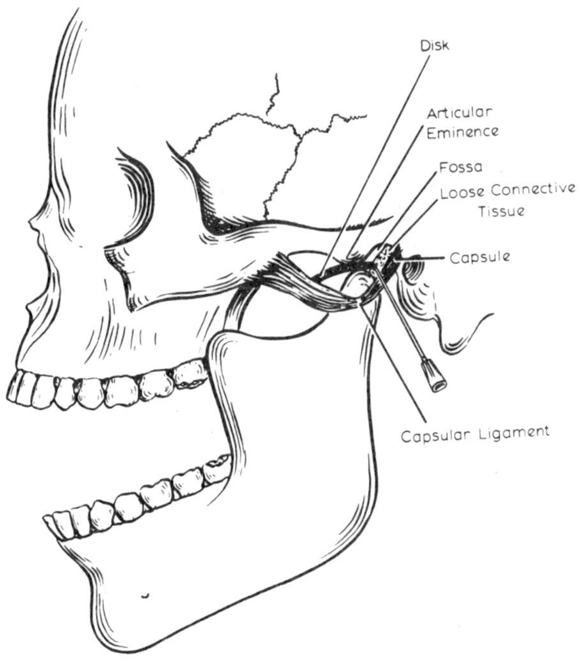

Figure 20-4. Local Block to the TMJ

2. Reduction of Dislocated Temporomandibular Joint: In the common presentation of temporomandibular dislocation, the condyle rests on the anterior slope of the articular eminence. (Figure 20-4) There is intense pain and severe spasm of the surrounding mandibular musculature. Reduction of this dislocation may frequently be accomplished by the unilateral, intracapsular injection of local anesthesia.

a. With the head of the condyloid process locked anteriorly, the depression of the glenoid fossa is easily palpated.
b. The needle is inserted into the depression of the glenoid fossa, and directed anteriorly towards the head of the condyloid process.
c. When the condyloid process is contracted, the needle is slightly withdrawn.
d. 2 cc of local anesthetic solution are instilled into the capsule.

3. Reduction and Fixation of a Mandibular Fracture: Complete anesthesia for reduction and fixation of a mandibular fracture requires adequate anesthesia of the maxillary and mandibular branches of the trigeminal nerve and superficial branches of the cervical plexus. (Figure 20-5)

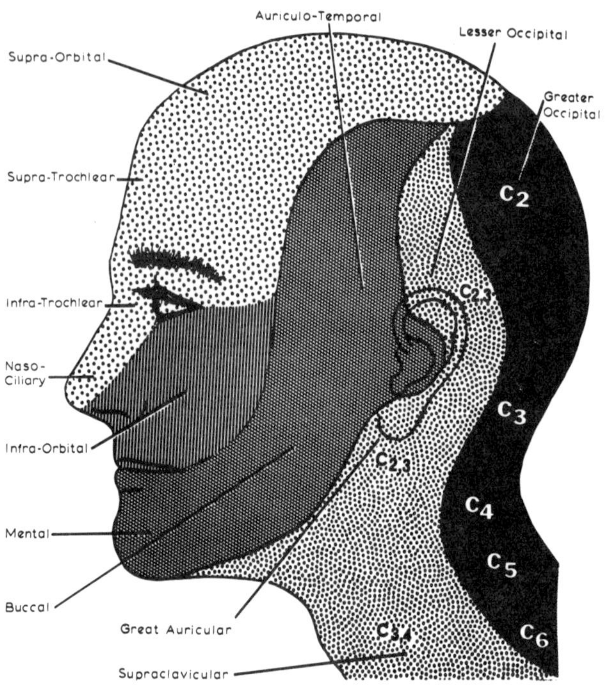

Figure 20-5. Cutaneous Innervation of the Head and Neck.

a. The mandibular branch of the trigeminal nerve is readily anesthetized near its exit from the skull through the foramen ovale. (Figure 20-6)

1. A skin wheal is raised at the mid point between the condyle and coronoid process of the mandible and just below the zygoma.
2. An 8 cm needle is introduced perpendicular to the skin until contact with the pterygoid plate occurs. This is usually at a depth of 4 cm.
3. The needle is withdrawn and then reinserted slightly posteriorly to a depth of approximately 6 cm.
4. When paresthesia in the mandibular division is elicited, the needle is fixed and approximately 5 cc of anesthetic solution are administered.

b. Anesthesia of the maxillary division of the trigeminal nerve may be accomplished in the pterygopalatine fossa near the foramen rotundum where the nerve exits from the skull. (Figure 20-7)

1. A skin wheal is raised just over the posterior inferior surface of the mandibular notch.
2. A 8 cm needle is inserted transversely and slightly anteriorly to a depth of 4-5 cm where it comes into contact with the lateral pterygoid plate.

3. The needle is withdrawn slightly and directed in a more anterior superior direction to pass anterior to the pterygoid plate into the pterygopalatine fossa.
4. The needle is advanced another 0.5-1.5 cm until paresthesia is elicited. A total of 5-10 cc of local anesthetic solution is deposited.

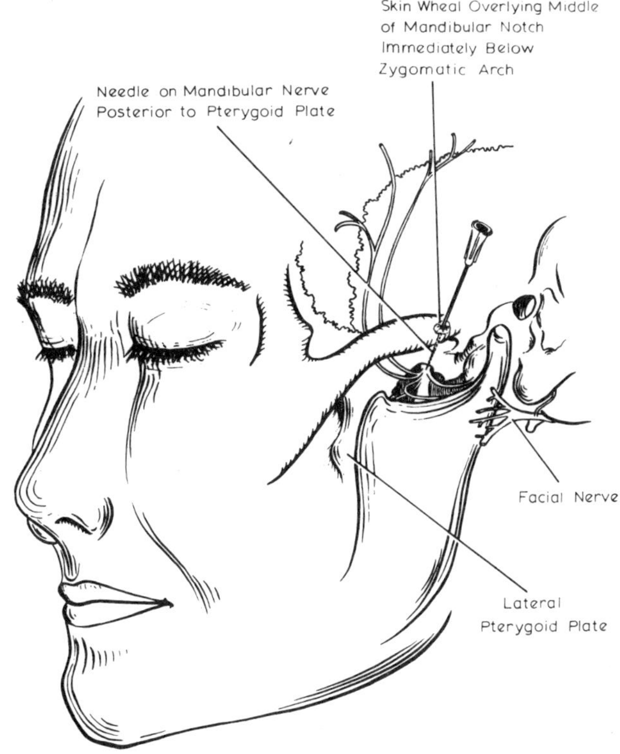

Figure 20-6. Mandibular Nerve Block

The most frequent complications of mandibular and maxillary nerve block is hemorrhage into the cheek. This is usually managed conservatively. Subarachnoid injections and facial nerve blocks are two other rarely reported complications.

c. The superficial branches of the cervical plexus are easily blocked as they emerge along the posterior margin of the sternocleidomastoid muscle. Starting at the mid point of the posterior margin of the sternocleidomastoid muscle, infiltration is accomplished along the posterior margin of this muscle using 10-15 cc of anesthetic solution.

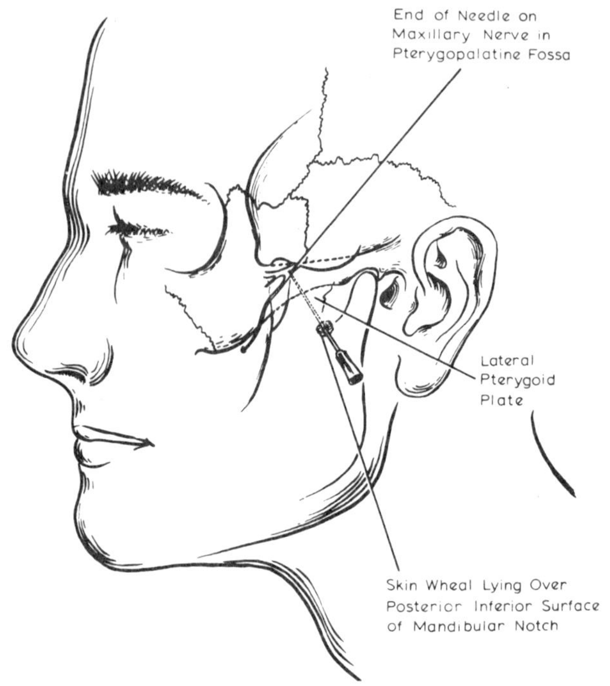

Figure 20-7. Maxillary Nerve Block.

4. OTOLOGY: The sensory innervation of the external ear is illustrated in Figure 20-8. The middle ear receives its sensory innervation through the tympanic plexus (V_3, IX, and X).

V_3 ⟶ Auriculotemporal nerve
IX ⟶ Jacobson's nerve
X ⟶ Auricular nerve

a. Myringotomy:

1) Inject the cartilaginous and bony junction of the external auditory canal.

2) Instead of introducing the local anesthetic through the classical 12 o'clock, 3 o'clock, 6 o'clock and 9 o'clock infiltration, infiltrate at 12 o'clock, 2 o'clock, 4 o'clock, 6 o'clock, 8 o'clock and 10 o'clock. In this manner, other than the first injection site, the subsequent injection sites are already anesthetized prior to the needle prick. The patient feels one needle prick instead of the classical four pricks. For myringotomy alone, it is not necessary to infiltrate the skin of the bony canal wall, thus no local anesthetic agent should infiltrate into the middle ear cavity. (See: complications of local anesthetic in Stapedectomy.)

b. Stapedectomy: In addition to the technique described for Myringotomy, it is necessary to infiltrate the tympanomeatal flap. Besides

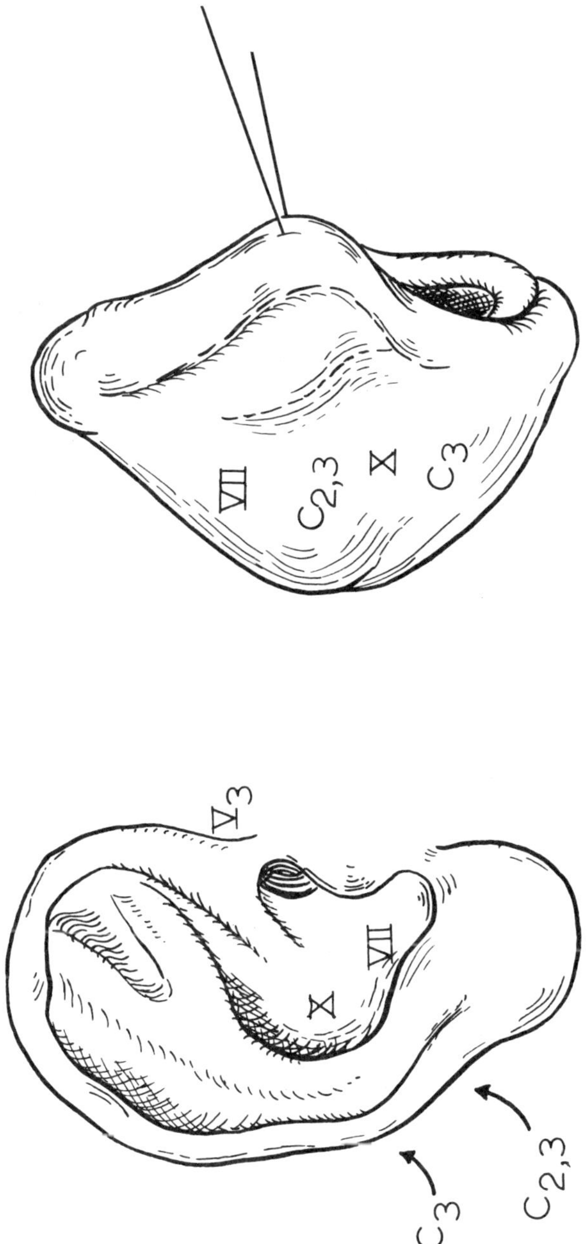

Figure 20-8. Sensory Innervation of the External Ear.

assuring adequate anesthesia, this provides vasoconstriction (1% Xylocaine with epinephrine 1:100,000) for hemostasis.

Complications: Two transient complications arising from the Xylocaine which migrated from the tympanomeatal flap to the middle ear cavity have been noted in local anesthetic infiltration for Stapedectomy:

1) Temporary facial nerve paralysis. This is due to the local anesthetic coming into contact with the dehiscent facial nerve. Patience and reassurance for a few hours will resolve the problem.

2) Violent vertigo with nystagmus (similar to Ménière's attack) can occur 45 minutes after the infiltration. Provided no damage has been done to the vestibular labyrinth, this is secondary to the effect of Xylocaine on the membranous labyrinth through the oval or round windows.

These two complications are particularly distressing if they occur after an office Myringotomy. Hence, it is the author's (KJL) advice that no infiltration in the skin of the bony canal wall is needed for Myringotomy. The infiltration at the junction of the bony and cartilaginous canal will not reach the middle ear cavity.

c. Tympanoplasty and Mastoidectomy: (Canal plasty, Meatoplasty) This procedure is usually performed under general anesthesia. However, it is quite possible to have it performed under local anesthesia. In addition to the Stapedectomy infiltration, post-auricular and conchal infiltration are necessary (See Figure 20-8 for the sensory innervation). The skin of the anterior canal wall needs to be anesthetized if surgery is to include that anatomical site.

5. NASAL SURGERY:

a. Nasal Polypectomy: Cocaine pledgets along the mucosal surfaces as well as in contact with the spheno-palatine ganglion supply adequate anesthesia for Polypectomy. Occasionally it is necessary to supplement this with external infiltration, as in Rhinoplasty.

b. Septoplasty and Rhinoplasty: The sensory innervation of the septum and external nose is illustrated in Figures 20-9, 20-10, 20-11, 20-12, 20-13. Besides local infiltration as shown in Figure 20-13, cocaine pledgets along mucosal surfaces and spheno-palatine ganglion are used. For best hemostasis and anesthesia results, it is wise to wait at least 20 minutes prior to performing the surgery.

6. SINUS SURGERY:

a. Caldwell-Luc: To achieve good anesthesia for this procedure, one needs to block the infra-orbital nerve, the spheno-palatine ganglion, and the posterior superior dental nerve. The posterior superior dental nerve exits from the maxillary nerve adjacent to the spheno-palatine ganglion. In order to block the spheno-palatine ganglion and posterior superior dental nerve, introduce the local anesthesia through the greater palatine foramen via a curved needle.

Further topical anesthesia is applied with cocaine pledgets intranasally against the spheno-palatine ganglion. Local infiltration of the mucosa in the canine fossa will supply the hemostasis needed over the line of incision.

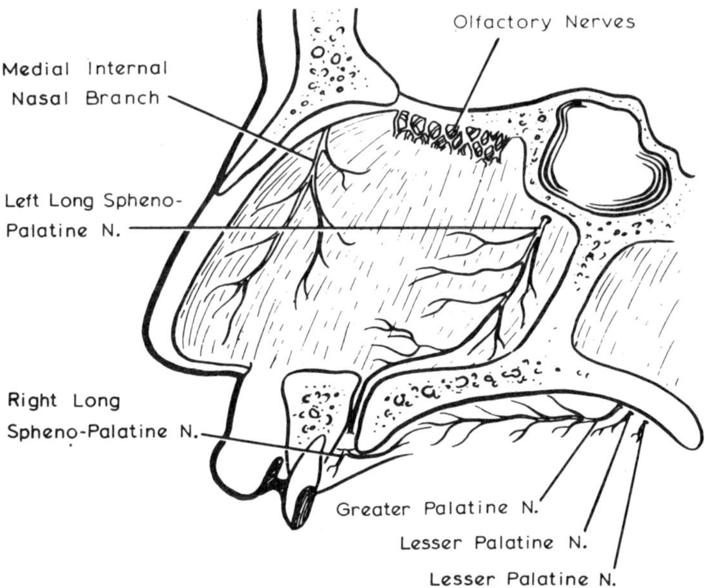

Figure 20-9. Sensory Innervation of the Nose.

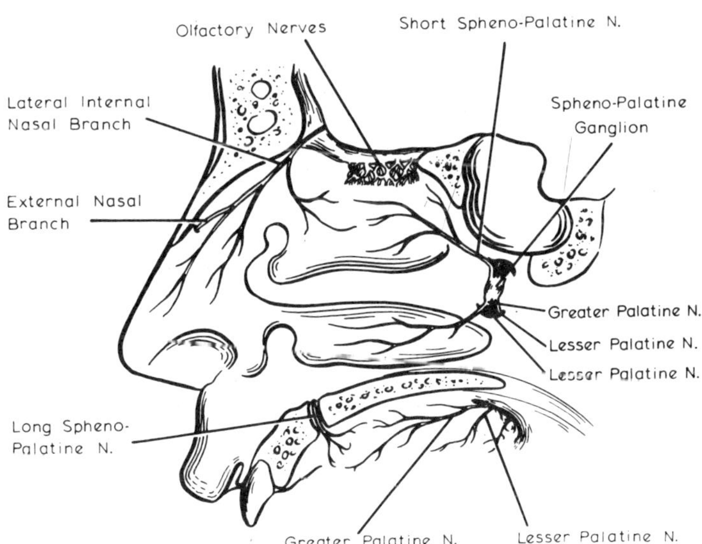

Figure 20-10. Sensory Innervation of the Nose.

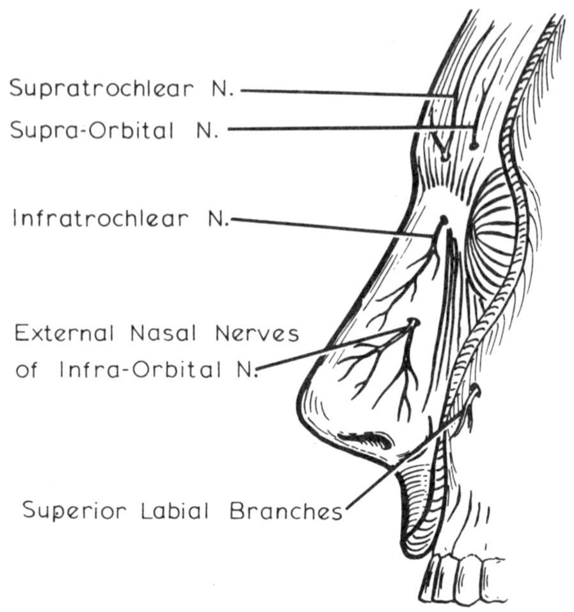

Figure 20-11. Sensory Innervation of the Nose.

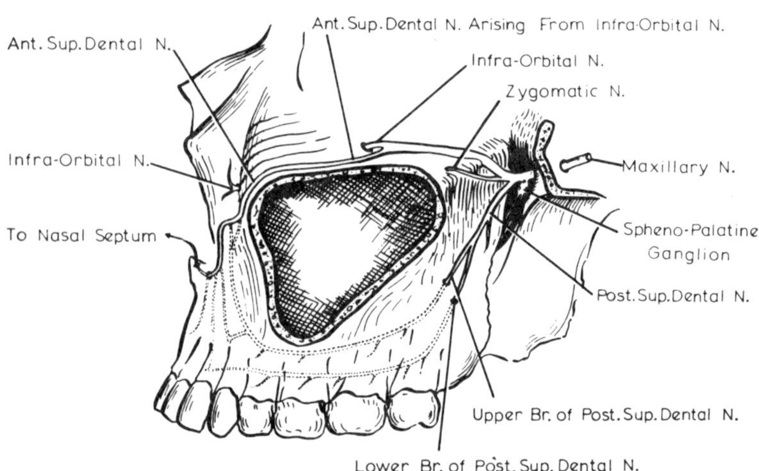

Figure 20-12. Sensory Innervation of the Nose.

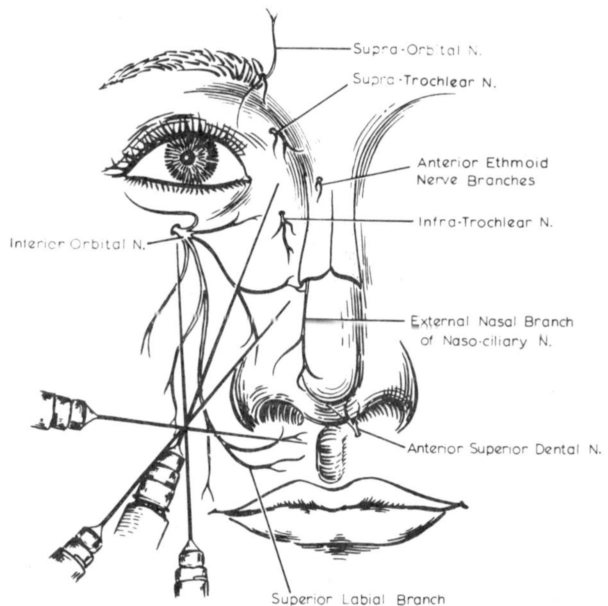

Figure 20-13. Infiltration for Rhinoplasty.

b. Ethmoid Sinuses: The sensory innervation of the ethmoid sinuses is intertwined with that of the nose and septum. In addition, it is innervated by the anterior ethmoid nerve (branch of the naso-ciliary, V_1) and the posterior ethmoid nerve (branch of infra-trochlear, V_1).

c. Sphenoid Sinuses: The sensory innervation is from the pharyngeal branch of the maxillary nerve as well as the posterior ethmoid nerve.

II. GENERAL ANESTHESIA

A. DEFINITION: General anesthesia is the chemically induced, reversible loss of consciousness.

B. MECHANISM OF ACTION: The mechanism of action of general anesthetics remains a controversial issue. Most likely, these agents block multisynaptic neuronal pathways, such as in the reticular activating system of the brain stem. General anesthetics act on virtually all cell membranes and therefore, affect all organs and systems.

C. GENERAL ANESTHETIC AGENTS:

1. Inhalation Anesthetic Agents: These anesthetics are administered via an inhalation route and absorption occurs through the alveolar-pulmonary capillary interface.

a. Nitrous Oxide is one of the oldest and remains one of the most useful of inhalation anesthetics. It is usually employed in an inspired concentration of 50-75% with oxygen. Nitrous oxide is a relatively safe but weak anesthetic agent.

b. Diethyl Ether is among the older of the clinically useful general anesthetics and remains a relatively safe and useful agent. One of the major advantages of diethyl ether is the ventilatory stimulation which occurs at anesthetic stages. This is in marked contrast to the respiratory depression seen with virtually all other general anesthetics. This property makes diethyl ether a useful agent for bronchoscopic examination. The flammability hazard with diethyl ether has limited its use in recent years.

c. Cyclopropane is a potent anesthetic, commonly used in inhalation concentrations from 6-20%. Its usefulness is also limited by its flammability characteristics.

d. Halothane is an example of the series of halogenated hydrocarbons that have been synthesized and introduced into clinical practice during the recent 2 or 3 decades. It is a potent agent providing profound anesthesia when administered in concentrations of 1-2%. It is associated with cardiovascular and respiratory depression.

e. Methyoxyflurane, Enflurane and Isoflurane are additional members of the halogenated hydrocarbon family having many properties and complications similar to those of halothane. Methyoxyflurane has been implicated in the production of a dose related high output renal failure.

2. Intravenous Anesthetics are administered via an intravenous route.

a. Thiopental is an ultra short acting thiobarbiturate. It has become one of the most widely used agents for the induction of anesthesia. Its use may be associated with profound cardiovascular and respiratory depression.

b. Ketamine is a newer intravenous anesthetic of the phencyclidine class of drugs. Ketamine induces a peculiar state, called dissociative anesthesia, in which patients are unresponsive to noxious stimuli but may appear to be awake with open eyes and spontaneous movement. Of significance, the pharyngeal and laryngeal reflexes remain intact until very deep levels of ketamine anesthesia are attained.

c. Innovar is a mixture of two drugs, droperidol (a major transquilizer) and fentanyl (a potent narcotic). It acts much like other so called "neuroleptic cocktails" (morphine and chlorpromazine, meperidine and diazepam) and is usually administered in combination with nitrous oxide and occasionally a short acting barbiturate drug.

d. Diazepam is a major tranquilizer of the benzodiazepine family. In large intravenous doses in combination with an inhalation agent such as nitrous oxide it is useful for the induction and maintenance of general anesthesia.

3. Neuromuscular Blockers act at the neuromuscular junction to induce a state of muscle paralysis. These are subclassified into the depolarizing agents (succinylcholine chloride) or the non-depolarizing drugs (d-Tubocurarine).

D. COMPLICATIONS: The discussion of the complications of general anesthetics will be confined to those of particular interest to otolaryngologists.

1. Aspiration pneumonitis may occur during general anesthesia as a consequence of the obtundation of laryngeal protective reflexes. Foreign matter which is permitted to accumulate in the pharynx (blood, gastric contents) will gain ready access to the pulmonary parenchyma. The result is the clinical syndrome of aspiration pneumonitis.

2. Cardiac arrhythmias: Most of the inhalation anesthetics are associated with a sensitization of the myocardium to catecholamines. In the presence of excess catecholamines, endogenously or exogenously produced, patients may develop ventricular arrhythmias and ventricular fibrillation. It is recommended that the exogenous administration of epinephrine be limited to a concentration of 1:100,000 and a total dose of 10 cc in any given 10 minute period when given in the presence of these anesthetics.

3. Hepatitis has been demonstrated to be a potential complication of virtually any anesthetic and surgical technique. A well publicized but poorly documented entity, so called "halothane hepatitis" has gained widespread notoriety. This type of hepatitis may be associated with an unusual metabolite of halothane to which certain sensitive individuals develop an allergic reaction. If this does exist as a unique entity it is extremely uncommon.

4. Malignant Hyperpyrexia is a rare adverse reaction to anesthetics (occurring in approximately 1 in 15,000 anesthetic administrations). It is associated with a rapid rise in temperature to as high as 112°F and cardiovascular collapse and shock. Treatment consists of rapid termination of surgery and anesthesia, submersion of the patient into an ice bath, and general supportive measures. The mortality of this complication of anesthesia remains at greater than 50%.

5. Nitrous Oxide induced elevation in middle ear pressure: Because of its large blood solubility relative to nitrogen, nitrous oxide is well known for diffusing into closed gas spaces and producing an elevation in intra-luminal pressures. In the case of tympanic surgery, diffusion of nitrous oxide into the middle ear may produce bulging of the tympanic graft. The distention is readily reversible if the nitrous oxide is discontinued and 100% oxygen is substituted.

TABLE I

Concentration and Maximum Safe Doses of Local Anesthetics

	TOPICAL		INFILTRATION	
	Concentration	Max Dose	Concentration	Max Dose
Esters				
Cocaine	4-10% *	3 mgm/Kg	NOT USED	
Procaine (Novocaine)	NOT EFFECTIVE		2-4%	14 mgm/Kg in adults 5 mgm/Kg in children
Tetracaine (Pontocaine)	0.5-2%	1 mgm/Kg	0.1-0.25%	1-1.5 mgm/Kg
Chloroprocaine (Nesacaine)	NOT EFFECTIVE		2%	14 mgm/Kg
Hexylcaine (Cyclaine)	5%	3 mgm/Kg	1-2%	7 mgm/Kg
Amides				
Lidocaine (Xylocaine)	2-4%	3 mgm/Kg	1-2%	3 mgm/Kg (Without Epinephrine) 7 mgm/Kg (With Epinephrine)
Mepivacaine (Carbocaine)	NOT EFFECTIVE		1-2%	7 mgm/Kg
Prilocaine (Citanest)	NOT EFFECTIVE		1-2%	7 mgm/Kg
Bupivacaine (Marcaine)	NOT EFFECTIVE		0.25-0.75%	3 mgm/Kg
Piperidine				
Dyclonine (Dyclone)	0.5%	4 mgm/Kg	NOT USED	
Epinephrine	1:1000-1: 100,000	1 mgm	1:1000-1: 100,000	1 mgm
	with Halothane anesthesia, 10cc of 1:100,000 (0.1 mgm) can be used over a ten minute period, or 30 cc over an hour (0.3 mgm).			

* (10% solution = 100 mgm per cc)
(1% solution = 10 mgm per cc)

TABLE 2

Local Anesthetic Toxic Symptoms

1. Central nervous system; Excitation:
   Cerebral cortex ──► excitement, disorientation, rambling speech ──► seizures
   Brain Stem ──► tachycardia, hypertension, vomiting, sweating

2. Central nervous system; Depression:
   Cerebral cortex ──► coma
   Brain Stem ──► bradycardia, hypotension, apnea

3. Cardiovascular system; Depression:
   Bradycardia
   Hypotension
   Shock

4. Cardiorespiratory Arrest

5. Death

TABLE 3

Prevention and treatment of toxicity

1. Prophylaxis
   a) Avoid overdose
   b) Valium premedication

2. Maintain verbal contact with patient throughout surgery; must be alert to early signs and symptoms of excitation.

3. Have an I.V. in place prior to administration of local anesthetics.

4. When toxic symptoms appear, stop surgery, give 0_2.

5. Maintain airway and ventilation.

6. Avoid giving further depressants if possible. However, I.V. Valium or Pentothal may be required to terminate seizure.

7. Fluid, pressor resuscitation as required.

TABLE 4

Rate of Topical Absorption in Decreasing Order

Tracheobronchial tree, nose, pharynx, larynx, esophagus

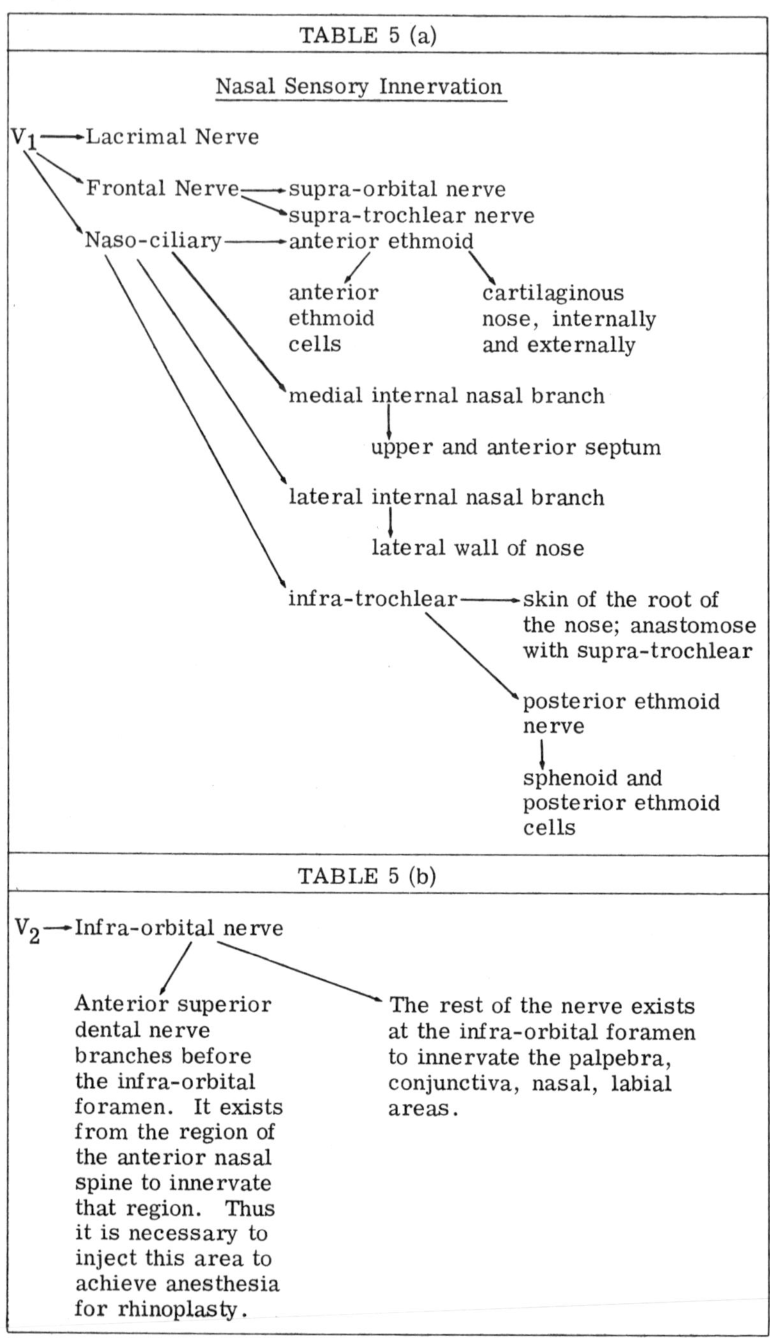
TABLE 5 (a)
Nasal Sensory Innervation
V1 → Lacrimal Nerve
Frontal Nerve → supra-orbital nerve
supra-trochlear nerve
Naso-ciliary → anterior ethmoid
anterior ethmoid cells
cartilaginous nose, internally and externally
medial internal nasal branch
upper and anterior septum
lateral internal nasal branch
lateral wall of nose
infra-trochlear → skin of the root of the nose; anastomose with supra-trochlear
posterior ethmoid nerve
sphenoid and posterior ethmoid cells
TABLE 5 (b)
V2 → Infra-orbital nerve
Anterior superior dental nerve branches before the infra-orbital foramen. It exists from the region of the anterior nasal spine to innervate that region. Thus it is necessary to inject this area to achieve anesthesia for rhinoplasty.
The rest of the nerve exists at the infra-orbital foramen to innervate the palpebra, conjunctiva, nasal, labial areas.

TABLE 5 (c)

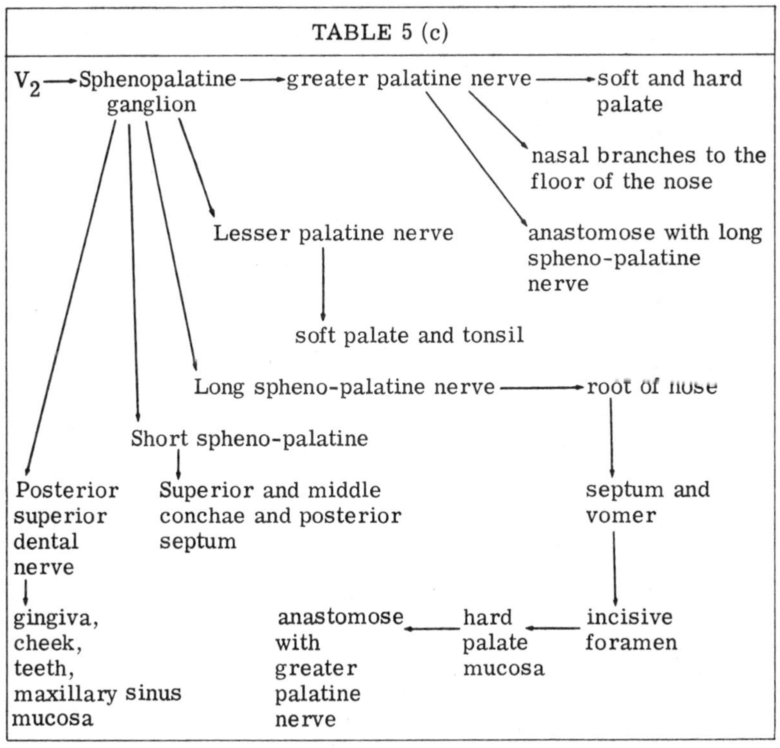

REFERENCES

I. LOCAL ANESTHESIA

1. General

Covino, B.: Local Anesthesia. NEJM 286:975-983, 1035-1042, 1972.

Jackson, C. & Jackson, C.L.: Bronchoesophagology. W.B. Saunders Co., Philadelphia, 1950.

Ritchie, J., Cohen, P.: "Cocaine, Procaine and Other Synthetic Local Anesthetics". The Pharmacologic Basis of Therapeutics. Edited by L.S. Goodman and A. Gilman. New York, 1975.

Snow, J.C.: Anesthesia in Otolaryngology and Ophthalmology. C.C Thomas, Springfield, 1972.

2. Complications and Treatment

Adriani, J., Campbell, D.: Fatalities Following Topical Application of Local Anesthetics to Mucous Membranes. JAMA 162: 1527-1530, 1956.

Ausinsch, B., et al.: Diazepam in the Prophylaxis of Lignocaine Seizures. Br. J. Anaesth. 48: 309-312, 1976.

Curran, J., et al.: Topical Analgesia Before Tracheal Intubation. Anaesthesia 30:65-768, 1975.

Campbell, D., Adriani, J.: Absorption of Local Anesthetics. JAMA 168:873-877, 1958.

Moore, D.S., Bridenbaugh, L.D.: Oxygen: The Antidote for Systemic Toxic Reactions from Local Anesthetic Drugs. JAMA 174:842-847, 1960.

Munson, E.S., Wagman, I.H.: Diazepam Treatment of Local Anesthetic Induced Seizures. Anesthesiology 37:523-528, 1972.

Fink, B.R.: Acute and Chronic Toxicity of Local Anaesthetics. Can Anaesth Soc J 20:5-16, 1973.

Kelly, J.F., Patterson, R.: Anaphylaxis: Course, Mechanisms and Treatment. JAMA 227:1431-1436, 1974.

3. <u>Clinical Application</u>

Johnson, W.B.: New Method for Reduction of Acute Dislocation of Temporomandibular Articulations. J Oral Surg 16:501-504,1958.

Moore, D.C.: Regional Block. Springfield, C. C Thomas, 1965.

II. GENERAL ANESTHESIA

1. <u>General</u>

Dripps, R.D., Eckenhoff, J.E., Vandam, L.D.: Introduction to Anesthesia. Philadelphia, W.B. Saunders Co., 1972.

Ngai, S.H., Mark, L.C., Papper, E.M.: Pharmacologic and Physiologic Aspects of Anesthesiology. N Engl J Med 282: 479-491, 541-556, 1970.

Snow, J.C.: Anesthesia in Otolaryngology and Ophthalmology. Springfield, C. C Thomas, 1972.

2. <u>Complications and Treatment</u>

Arens, J.F., McKinnon, W.M.P.: Malignant Hyperpyrexia During Anesthesia. JAMA 215:919-922, 1971.

Katz, R.L., Matteo, R.S., Papper, E.M.: The Injection of Epinephrine During General Anesthesia with Halogenated Hydrocarbons and Cyclopropane in Man. II Halothane. Anesthesiology 23:597-600, 1962.

McCormick, P.W.: Immediate Care After Aspiration of Vomitus. Anesthesiology 30:658-665, 1975.

Thomsen, K.A., Terkildsen, K., Arnfred, I.: Middle Ear Pressure Variations During Anesthesia. Arch Otolaryng. 82:609-611, 1965.

Van Dyke, R.A.: Biotransformation of Volatile Anaesthetics with Special Emphasis on the Role of Metabolism in the Toxicity of Anesthetics. Canad Anaesth Soc J 20:21-33, 1973.

CHAPTER 21

THE CHEST

PULMONARY VOLUMES AND CAPACITIES:

Tidal Volume (TV) = depth of breathing = volume of gas inspired or expired during each normal respiratory cycle = 0.5 litre on the average.

Inspired Reserve Volume (IRV) = maximum volume that can be inspired from end-inspiratory position = 3.3 litres on the average.

Expired Reserve Volume (ERV) = maximum volume that can be expired from end-respiratory level = 0.7 to 1 litre on the average.

Residual Volume (RV) = volume left in lungs after maximum expiration = 1.1 litre on the average.

Forced Expiratory Volume in 1 second = FEV_1 (FEV_1 should be 80% or more of predicted value from a normative chart).

Forced Vital Capacity = FVC (FVC should be 80% or more of predicted value from a normative chart).

The ratio of $\frac{FEV_1}{FVC}$ should be greater than 0.75 for young patients and 0.70 for older individuals.

Total Lung Capacity (6 litres for males 4.2 litres for females)	=	IRV + TV + ERV + RV (Total Volume contained in the lungs after maximum inspiration).
Vital Capacity (4.8 litres for males 3.1 litres for females)	=	IRV + TV + ERV (Maximum volume that can be expelled from the lungs by forceful effort following maximum inspiration).
Functional Residual Capacity (2.2 litres for males 1.8 litres for females)	=	RV + ERV (Volume in the lungs at resting expiratory level).
Physiological Dead Space (Dead space of upper airway by-passed by tracheotomy, 70-100 cc.)	=	Anatomical Dead Space + the volume of gas that ventilates the alveoli that have no capillary blood flow + the volume of gas that ventilates the alveoli in excess of that required to arteriolize the capillary blood.

MEAN NORMAL BLOOD GAS AND ACID BASE VALUES:

	Arterial Blood	Mixed Venous Blood
pH	7.40	7.37
pCO_2	41 mm Hg	46.5 mm Hg
pO_2	95 mm Hg	40 mm Hg
O_2 sat.	97.1%	75.0%
HCO_3^-	24.0 mEq/l	25.0 mEq/l

MISCELLANEOUS:

1. Silo-Filler's Disease (Bronchiolitis Obliterans) is a pathological entity consisting of a collection of exudate in the bronchioles obliterating the lumen. This complication often follows inhalation of nitrogen dioxide, exposure to open bottles of nitric acid and exposure to silos. The diagnosis is made on history of exposure, dyspnea, cough and x-ray findings similar to miliary Tbc. Treatment is symptomatic. Prognosis is poor since the majority of these patients eventually succumb to this disease.

2. Bronchogenic Cysts are congenital, arise from the bronchi and are lined with epithelial cells. Furthermore, their walls may contain glands, smooth muscles and cartilage. In the absence of infection they may remain asymptomatic; otherwise, they give a productive cough, hemoptysis, and fever. The recommended treatment is surgical excision.

3. Blebs or bulli -- These are air containing structures resembling cysts but their walls are not epithelium lined.

4. Anthracosilicosis -- Coal Miner's Pneumoconiosis.

5. Berylliosis -- This condition is characterized by an infestation of the lungs by beryllium. It is often found in workers at fluorescent lamp factories.

6. Bagassosis -- This condition is characterized by an infestation of the lungs by sugar cane fibers.

7. Byssinosis -- This condition is characterized by an infestation of the lungs by cotton dust.

8. Adenocarcinoma of the bronchus is the leading primary pulmonary carcinoma in females while bronchogenic (squamous cell) is most common in males.

9. Pancoast Syndrome (Superior Sulcus Tumor) is a syndrome caused by any process of the apex of the lung which can invade the pleural layers, infiltrate between the lower cords of the brachial plexus, and may involve the cervical sympathetic nerve chain, phrenic and recurrent laryngeal nerves. It is usually secondary to a benign or malignant tumor, however, a large inflammatory process may cause this syndrome as well. The symptoms are:

a. Pain in shoulder and arm, particularly in the axilla and inner arm.
b. Intrinsic hand muscle atrophy.
c. Horner's Syndrome (enophthalmos, ptosis of the upper lid, constriction of the pupil with narrowing of the palpebral fissure and decreased sweating homolaterally).

10. Congenital Agenesis of the Lung has been classified by Schneider as follows:

Class I	=	Total Agenesis
Class II	=	Only the trachea is present
Class III	=	Trachea and Bronchi are present without any pulmonary tissue.

11. Apnea can occur after tracheotomy. This is due to carbon dioxide narcosis causing the medulla to be depressed. Prior to the tracheotomy, the patient was breathing secondary to the lack of oxygen. After the tracheotomy this oxygen drive is removed and hence the patient remains apneic. Treatment for this is to ventilate the patient until the excess carbon dioxide level is reduced. Mediastinal emphysema and pneumothorax are the most common complications of tracheotomy. (For other complications, see Chapter 12).

12. Hypoxemia is defined as less than 75% oxygen saturation or less than 40 mm Hg pO_2. A level greater than 5 mg.% of Met-Hgb gives cyanosis.

13. Bronchogenic cyst is a defect at the 4th week of gestation. It constitutes less than 5% of all mediastinal cysts and tumors.

14. The bronchial tree ring is cartilaginous till it reaches 1 mm. in diameter. These small bronchioles without cartilaginous rings are held patent by the elastic property of the lung. The bronchial tree is lined by pseudostratified columnar ciliated epithelium as well as non-ciliated cuboidal epithelium.

15. The adult trachea measures 10-12 cm. and has 16 to 20 rings. The diameter is approximately 20 mm. x 15 mm.

16. The larynx descends on inspiration and ascends on expiration. It also ascends in the process of swallowing and in the production of a high-pitched note.

17. The esophageal lumen widens on inspiration.

18. The total lung surface measures 70 sq. meters. The lung contains 300 million aveoli. The lung secretes 200 ml. of fluid per day.

19. During inspiration the nose constitutes 79% of the total respiratory resistance, the larynx 6%, and the bronchial tree 15%. During expiration the nose constitutes 74% of the resistance, the larynx 3% and the bronchial tree 23%.

20. Tracheopathia osteoplastica is a rare disease characterized by growths of cartilage and bone within the walls of the trachea and bronchi that produce sessile plaques that project into the lumen. There is no specific treatment other than supportive. It is of unknown etiology. The serum calcium is normal and there are no other calcium deposits.

21. Calcification found in a pulmonary nodule usually implies that it is a benign nodule.

22. Middle lobe syndrome. (See Chapter 18).

23. The right upper lobe and its bronchus is the lobe that is most susceptible to congenital anomaly.

24. Cystic Fibrosis (Mucoviscidosis) is familial, may be autosomal recessive. The patient presents with multiple polyps, pulmonary infiltration with abscesses and rectal prolapse. The pancreas is afflicted with a fibrocystic process and produces no enzymes. Trypsin is lacking in the gastric secretion. Ten to 15% of the patients pass trypsin in the stool. There is general malabsorption of liposoluble vitamins. Treatment consists of high protein, low-fat diet with water soluble vitamins and pancreatic extracts. Many die of pulmonary abscesses.

25. If a person is ventilated with pure oxygen for 7 minutes, he is cleared of 90% of the nitrogen and can withstand 5 to 8 minutes without further oxygenation.

I. THE MEDIASTINUM

1. Suprasternal Fossa:

a. This is the region in which the sternocleidomastoid muscles converge toward their sternal attachments. Bound inferiorly by the suprasternal notch, they, however, have no superior boundary.

b. The deep cervical fascia splits into an anterior and a posterior portion. These are attached respectively to the anterior and posterior margins of the manubrium.

c. The space between these fascial layers is the small suprasternal space containing:

1) Anterior Jugular Veins
2) Fatty connective tissues

d. Behind this space lies the pretracheal fascia.

e. Laterally on each side are the medial borders of the sternohyoid and sternothyroid muscles.

2. In the adult, the innominate artery crosses in front of the trachea, behind the upper half of the manubrium. In the child, it crosses over the level of the superior border of the sternum.

3. The trachea enters the mediastinum on the right side.

4. The trachea bifurcates at T 4-5 or about 6 cm. from the suprasternal notch. As a person approaches 65 years of age or more, it is possible that the trachea bifurcates at T6.

5. To the left of the trachea are: Aorta, Left recurrent laryngeal nerve, Left subclavian artery.

To the right of the trachea are: Superior vena cava, Azygos vein, Right vagus, Right lung pleura.

6. The innominate and left carotid arteries lie anterior to the trachea near their origin. As they ascend, the innominate artery lies to the right of the trachea.

7. The pulmonary artery passes anterior to the bronchi and assumes a superior position to the bronchi at the hilus with the exception that the right upper lobe bronchus is superior to the right pulmonary artery.

8. The left main bronchus crosses in front of the esophagus. It presses on the esophagus and together with the aorta forms the broncho-aortic constriction. The 1st part of the aorta is to the left of the esophagus. As it descends it assumes a left postero-lateral position to the esophagus.

9. The course of the esophagus is as shown in Figure 21-1. The esophagus has four constricting points:

a. Cricopharyngeus muscle
b. Aorta crossing
c. Left main stem bronchus crossing
d. Diaphragm
($a < b=c < d$)

At the level of c the esophagus passes from superior mediastinum to the posterior mediastinum.

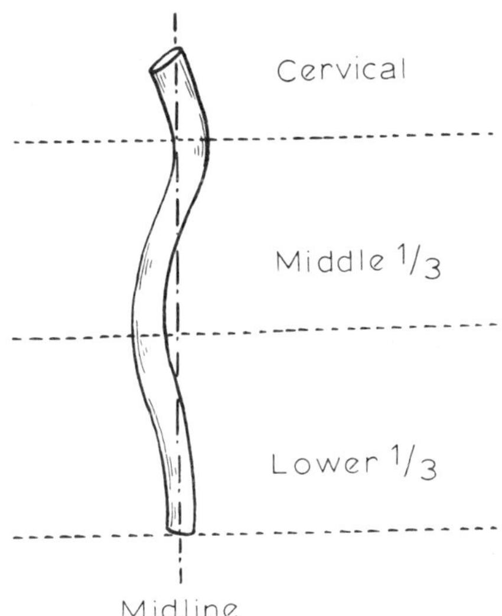

Figure 21-1. Diagrammatic representation of the course of the esophagus.

10. The following structures are found within the concavity of the aorta:
    a. Left main stem bronchus
    b. Left recurrent laryngeal nerve
    c. Tracheo-bronchial nodes
    d. Superficial part of the cardiac plexus

11. The right main stem bronchus is wider, shorter and follows a more vertical course than the left one.

12. The inferior thyroid vein is immediately in front of the trachea in its infraisthmic portion.

13. 10% of the population has a thyreoidea Ima artery. It arises from either the innominate artery or the aorta. It passes upwards along the anterior aspect of the trachea.

II. THE COURSE OF THE VAGUS

Left:

1. It passes inferiorly between the left subclavian and the left carotid.
2. It follows the subclavian to its origin.
3. Passes to the left of the arch of the aorta.
4. It gives off the recurrent laryngeal nerve which passes superiorly along the left border of the tracheo-esophageal groove. (Between the esophagus and trachea).
5. The main vagus continues to descend behind the left main stem bronchus.

Right:

1. It descends anterior to the subclavian where it gives off the recurrent laryngeal nerve which loops around the subclavian artery and ascends posteromedial to the right common carotid artery to reach the tracheo-esophageal groove. (Between the esophagus and the trachea).
2. The main trunk descends posteriorly along the right side of the trachea, between the trachea and right pleura.
3. It descends posterior to the right bronchus.

III. FASCIA OF THE MEDIASTINUM

The space between the various mediastinal organs is occupied by loose areolar tissues. The fascial layers of the mediastinum are a direct continuation of the cervical fascia. A portion of the cervical fascia, the perivisceral fascia, encloses the larynx, pharynx, trachea, esophagus, thyroid, thymus, and carotid sheath contents. This space enclosed by this perivisceral fascia extends to the bifurcation of the trachea. Anteriorly it is bound by the pretracheal fascia. The pretracheal fascia is an important landmark in mediastinoscopy in that dissection should be done only beneath this layer.

IV. BOUNDARIES OF THE MEDIASTINUM

1. Lateral - parietal pleural
2. Anterior - sternum
3. Posterior - vertebra
4. Inferior - diaphragm
5. Superior - superior aperture of the thorax

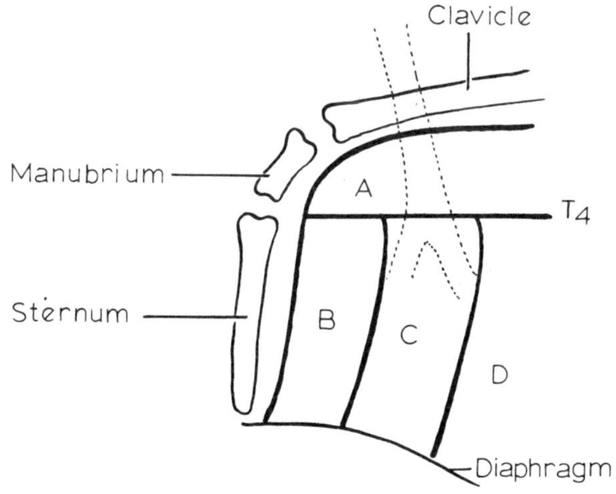

Figure 21.2. Diagrammatic Representation of the Various Chambers of the Mediastinum

SUPERIOR MEDIASTINUM:

Boundaries:
- Superior - superior aperture of the throat.
- Anterior - manubrium with sterno-thyroid and sternohyoid muscles.
- Posterior - upper thoracic vertebrae.
- Inferior - manubrium to IV vertebra.

Structures of the superior mediastinum: Thymus, Innominate veins, Aorta, Vagus, Recurrent laryngeal nerve, phrenic nerve, azygos vein, esophagus, thoracic duct.

ANTERIOR MEDIASTINUM: It lies between the body of the sternum and the pericardium and contains:

1. loose areolar tissues
2. lymphatics
3. lymph nodes
4. thymus gland

MIDDLE MEDIASTINUM: It contains the heart, ascending aorta, superior vena cava, azygos vein bifurcation of main bronchus, pulmonary artery trunk, right and left pulmonary veins, phrenic nerves, and the tracheal-bronchial lymph nodes.

POSTERIOR MEDIASTINUM: Anteriorly lies the bifurcation of the trachea, the pulmonary vein, the pericardium and the posterior part of the upper surface of the diaphragm. Posteriorly lies the vertebral column from T4 to T12. Laterally lies the mediastinal pleura.

The posterior mediastinum contains the thoracic aorta, azygos vein, hemiazygos vein, X nerve, splanchnic nerve, esophagus, thoracic duct, posterior mediastinal lymph nodes, and the intercostal arteries.

V. LYMPH NODES OF THE THORAX
FIGURE 21.3

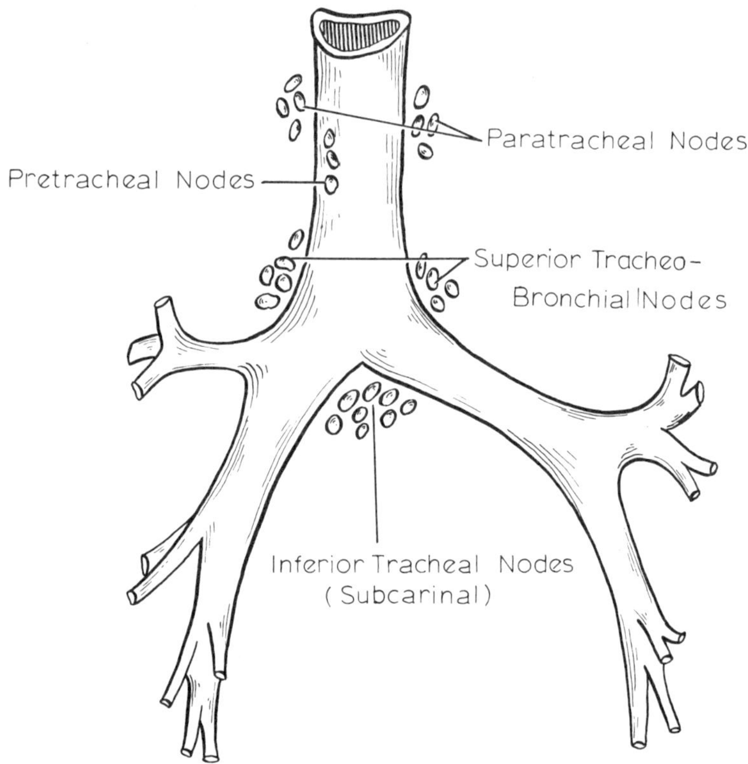

Figure 21.3. Thoracic Lymph Nodes

1. Parietal Nodes are inconsequential clinically. They are grouped into intercostal, sternal and phrenic nodes.

2. Visceral Nodes are of greater clinical importance. They are grouped as follows:

- a. Peritracheo-bronchial
  - 1) paratracheal
  - 2) pretracheal
  - 3) superior tracheo-bronchial
  - 4) inferior tracheo-bronchial
- b. Broncho-pulmonary (Hilar Nodes)
- c. Anterior mediastinal or prevascular
- d. Pulmonary
- e. Posterior mediastinal

LYMPHATIC DRAINAGE OF THE LUNG:

1. <u>Right:</u>

Superior Area (anteromedial area of the Right Upper Lobe)
Right paratracheal nodes

Middle Area (Posterolateral area of Right Upper Lobe, Right Middle Lobe and Superior Right Lower Lobe)
Right paratracheal nodes and Inferior tracheal-bronchial nodes.

Inferior area (Lower half of Right Lower Lobe)
Inferior tracheal-bronchial nodes and posterior mediastinal nodes.

2. <u>Left:</u>

Superior Area (Upper Left Upper Lobe)
Left paratracheal, anterior mediastinal and subaortic nodes.

Middle Area (Lower Left Upper Lobe and Upper Left Lower Lobe)
Left paratracheal, inferior tracheo-bronchial, and anterior mediastinal nodes.

Inferior Area (Inferior part of the Left Lower Lobe)
Inferior tracheo-bronchial nodes.

(The Left Inferior tracheo-bronchial nodes drain into the Right paratracheal nodes).

3. Right upper lung ——→ Right neck
Right lower lung ——→ Right neck
Left lower lung ——→ Right neck
Left upper lung ——→ Left neck
Lingular lobe ——→ Both sides of the neck

VI. PURPOSES OF MEDIASTINOSCOPY

(Barium Swallow and Tracheogram are usually obtained prior to mediastinoscopy if indicated).

1. Histological diagnosis
2. To determine which nodes are involved
3. To make the diagnosis of sarcoidosis

VII. MEDIASTINAL TUMORS

1. One third of all mediastinal tumors are malignant. Among the malignant ones, lymphoma is most commonly encountered.
2. Superior mediastinum = Thyroid, neurinoma, thymoma, parathyroid
   Anterior mediastinum = Dermoid, teratoma, thyroid, thymoma
   Low anterior mediastinum = Pericardial cyst
   Middle mediastinum = Pericardial cyst, bronchial cyst, lymphoma, carcinoma
   Posterior mediastinum = Neurinoma and enterogenous cyst

VIII. SUPERIOR VENA CAVA SYNDROME

1. Etiology: Malignant metastasis, mediastinal tumors, mediastinal fibrosis, vena cava thrombosis.

2. Signs and Symptoms include: Edema and cyanosis of the face, neck and upper extremities; venous hypertension with dilated veins; normal venous pressure of lower extremities; visible venous circulation of the anterior chest wall.

IX. ENDOSCOPY

SIZE OF TRACHEOTOMY TUBES AND BRONCHOSCOPES

Age	Tracheotomy	Bronchoscope
Premature	#000 x 26 to #00 x 33 mm	3 mm
6 months	#0 x 33 mm to #0 x 40 mm	3.5 mm
18 months	#1 x 46 mm	4 mm
5 years	#2 x 50 mm	5 mm
10 years	#3 x 50 mm to #4 x 68 mm	6 mm
Adult		7 mm

SIZE OF ESOPHAGOSCOPE

Child	5 x 35 or 6 x 35 mm
Adult	9 x 50 mm

During esophagoscopy, the average distance from the incisor teeth to the:

	Adult	3y.o.	1y.o.	Birth
Cricopharyngeus muscle:	16 cm.	10	9	7
Aorta:	23 cm.	15	14	12
Left Bronchus:	27 cm.	16	15	13
Hiatus:	38 cm.	23	21	19
Cardiac:	40 cm.	25	23	21
Greater curvature of the stomach:	53 cm.	30	27	23

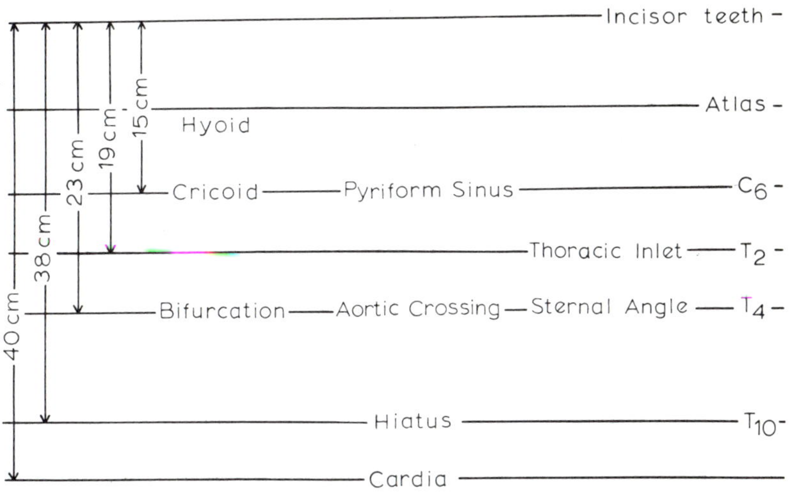

Figure 21.4. Relative Landmarks

LEFT LUNG:

Lobes	Segments
Upper Division of upper lobe	a. apical-posterior b. anterior
Lower Division of upper lobe	a. superior b. inferior
Lower Lobe	a. superior b. anterior-medial basal c. lateral basal d. posterior basal

RIGHT LUNG:

Lobes	Segments
Upper Lobe	a. apical b. posterior c. anterior
Middle Lobe	a. lateral b. medial
Lower Lobe	a. superior b. medial basal c. anterior basal d. lateral basal e. posterior basal

Relative contraindications for esophagoscopy:

1. Aneurysm of the aorta
2. Spinal deformities, osteophytes
3. Esophageal burns and being treated with steroids

Relative contraindications for bronchogram:

1. Acute infection
2. Acute asthmatic attacks
3. Acute cardiac failure

Etiologies for hemoptysis: (in order of decreasing frequency)

1. Bronchiectasis
2. Adenoma
3. Tracheobronchitis
4. Tbc
5. Mitral stenosis

Foreign bodies:

Right upper lobe bronchus = most common
Left upper lobe bronchus = second most common
Trachea = least likely

Most common site for esophageal foreign bodies is the cervical esophagus.

Most common foreign bodies in children are peanuts, safety pins, coins.

Most common foreign bodies in adults are meat and bone.

X. VASCULAR ANOMALIES

(See Chapter 8, Figure 2a, b, c)

1. Double Aortic Arch: This is a true vascular ring. It is due to the persistence of the right 4th branchial arch vessel. The symptoms include stridor, intermittent dysphagia and aspiration pneumonitis. The right posterior arch is usually the largest of the two arches.

2. Right aortic arch with ligamentum arteriosus: This is due to the persistence of the right 4th branchial arch vessel becoming the aorta instead of the left 4th arch vessel. This crosses the trachea causing an anterior compression.

3. Anomalous right subclavian artery: This is due to the right subclavian artery arising from the dorsal aorta giving a posterior compression of the esophagus. There is no constriction over the trachea.

4. Anomalous Innominate and/or left common carotid: The innominate arises too far left from the aorta. It crosses the trachea anteriorly causing an anterior compression. The left common carotid arises from the aorta on the right or from the innominate artery. It also causes an anterior compression of the trachea. In another variant of this anomaly, the innominate and the right common carotid arise from the same trunk and in dividing encircle the trachea and esophagus causing airway obstruction as well as dysphagia.

5. Patent ductus arteriosus.

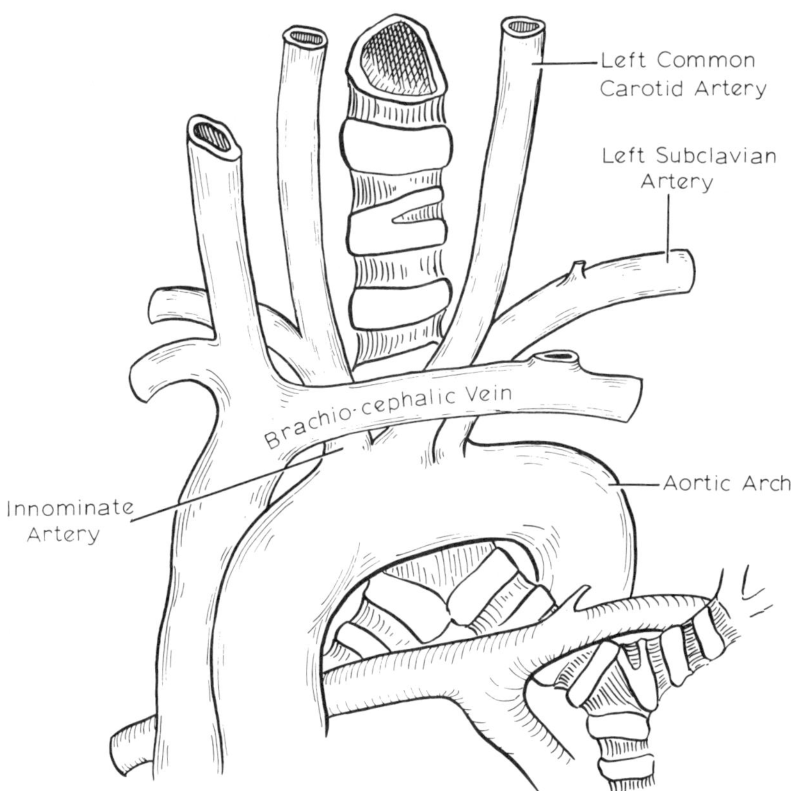

Figure 21.5. Diagrammatic representation of normal great vessels

6. Coarctation of the aorta.

7. An enlarged heart especially with mitral insufficiency can compress on the left bronchus.

8. Dysphagia Lusoria is a term used to include dysphagia caused by any aberrant great vessel. The common etiology is abnormal subclavian artery arising from the descending aorta.

9. Anomalous innominate arteries have been estimated to be the most common vascular anomaly. They cause an anterior compression on the trachea. During bronchoscopy if the pulsation is obliterated with the bronchoscope, the radial pulse on the right arm is reduced while the temporal pulse is also reduced. In the case of a subclavian anomaly the bronchoscope compressing the abnormal

subclavian produces a decrease of the radial pulse but the temporal pulse will remain normal. A bronchoscope compressing a double aortic arch pulsation will produce no pulse changes in either the radial or temporal pulse.

REFERENCES

1. Comroe, J.H., Jr.: Physiology of Respiration, 2nd ed., Year Book Medical Publishers, Inc., Chicago, 1974.

2. Hollinshead, W.H.: Anatomy For Surgeons: Volume 1, The Head and Neck, 2nd ed., Hoeber Medical Division, Harper & Row Publishers, New York.

CHAPTER 22

ALLERGY AND IMMUNOLOGY

THE IMMUNE SYSTEM: A bodily response mechanism for the detection and destruction of "foreigness".

MECHANISM OF IMMUNE RESPONSE:

A. NON-SPECIFIC IMMUNITY:

1. Phagocytes: The greatest number are monocytes, which become macrophages on stimulation. Those that are fixed comprise the reticulo-endothelial system of the bone marrow, lymph nodes, spleen, liver and lungs. Monocytes also circulate in the blood along with polymorphonuclear leukocytes, the most numerous phagocyte in circulation.

2. Interferon: Cells infected by virus rapidly produce a protein, interferon, which interacts with nearby non-infected cells. The effect of the interaction is to produce a second, intracellular, non-specific antiviral protein that is protective.

3. The Complement System: A group of nine heat-labile (56°C) proteins which react in series (much like the clotting proteins) and whose primary functions are to interact with IgG and IgM in the neutralization of foreign substances. Complement dependent antibody reactions in response to infection are: increased bacteriolysis (the whole chain of events viz. C1-9), opsonization or enhancement of phagocytosis (mainly C3b activity), and destruction of bacterial toxins. The completed complement response itself manufactures several other biologically active products including (C3a, C5a) or anaphylatoxin which enhances vascular permeability and (C3a, C5a, and C5-6-7) known as chemotactic factors that serve to attract phagocytic cells to the inflammatory site.

HANE (Hereditary Angioneurotic Edema): This condition has been shown to be due to a deficiency in the complement self-inhibiting system. The first component of complement, C1, a proesterase, is continuously converted to an esterase (C1 esterase), thereby, initiating the complement reaction. Normal serum contains a natural shut-off material, C1-esterase inhibitor, which prevents the reaction from going further. Those rare individuals with HANE are deficient in C1E inhibitor, and respond with overwhelming production of C1E following trauma. The edema is secondary to C3a and C5a, or anaphylatoxin production. This condition is life threatening when it occurs in the pharynx or larynx and tracheotomy may be required. HANE responds poorly to epincphrine or steroids. The definitive treatment is prophylaxis with epsilon aminocaproic acid.

B. SPECIFIC IMMUNITY:

1. Lymphatic system: This system originates from bone marrow stem cells which are processed in two ways.

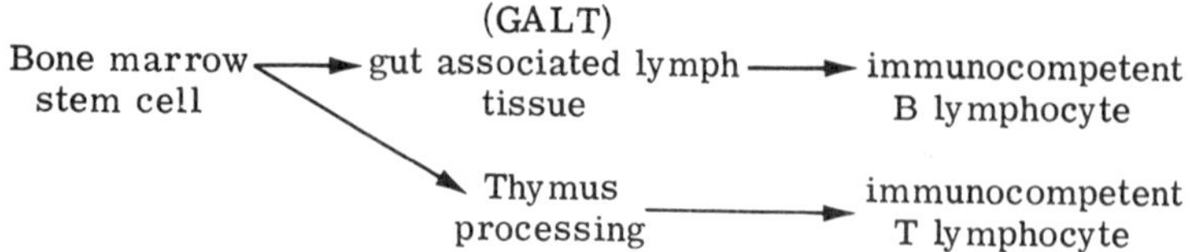

2. The responses of immunocompetent B and T lymphocytes to antigens:

a. B lymphocyte or the humoral (antibody) response: B lymphocyte + antigen + T lymphocyte "cooperation" - combine to produce the plasma cell, a mature B lymphocyte that produces antigen-specific antibodies. The clone theory: There exists one cell strain of lymphocytes with the genetic coding for each particular antigen; and, on combination with the antigen, the strain will begin to replicate immunocompetent daughter cells.

3. The Immunoglobulins:

a. The basic unit: IgG Molecule: four polypeptide chains, 2 heavy chains (H), and 2 light (L) chains, bound by non-covalent forces and disulfide bonds. The heavy chains have a mw 50,000-70,000, and are made up of a long strand of amino acids. More than half the heavy chain is constant, eg. the amino acids and their arrangement are the same, while the remaining 115 aa comprise the variable region. In IgG there are four genetically controlled subclasses of heavy chains. The light chains have a mw of 22,000 and approximately one-half the chain is constant and 1/2 variable (109 amino acids). There are two types of light chain found in all immunoglobulin classes, called kappa and lambda. Approximately 60% of humans have kappa light chains. Bence-Jones proteins represent abnormally increased production of either kappa or lambda short chains.

A model demonstrates the characteristics of the IgG molecule. (Figure 22.1) Enzymatic cleavage of the molecule with papain breaks the molecule into 3 parts, 2 Fab fragments and 1 Fc fragment. The Fab fragments of the molecule contain the variable portions of the light and heavy chains that are arranged in response to specific antigenic stimulation. They represent the antigen specific binding sites of this bivalent molecule. The Fc fragment is the portion of the molecule which binds to cell membranes and reacts with complement.

b. IgG: This immunoglobulin is the most abundant type of antibody both in the circulation and, very importantly, in the extra vascular regions. It crosses the placenta and provides a natural passive immunity in the infant for six to nine months. It will fix complement and fix to macrophages, enhancing phagocytosis.

c. IgA: IgA is produced in lymph tissue near the respiratory and G.I. tract in a form similar to IgG unit model (a monomer) with mw 170,000. Two IgA units are joined at the Fc terminals within the epithelial cells by a third protein, the secretory piece (50,000-60,000 mw) to form a dimer. The dimer is secreted into body fluids where it defends external surfaces. IgA does not fix complement. (Figure 22.2)

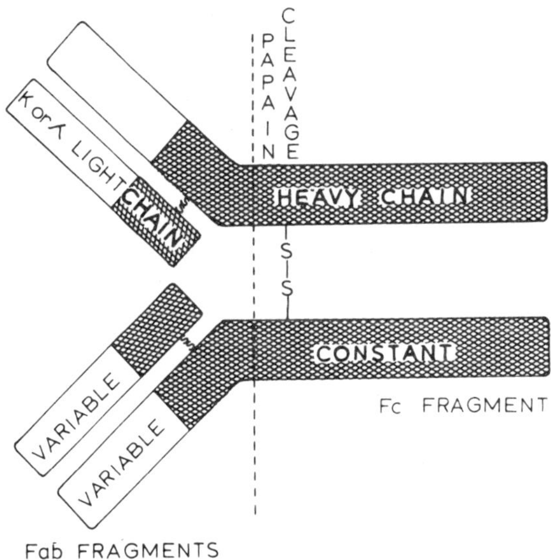

Figure 22.1. IgG Molecule

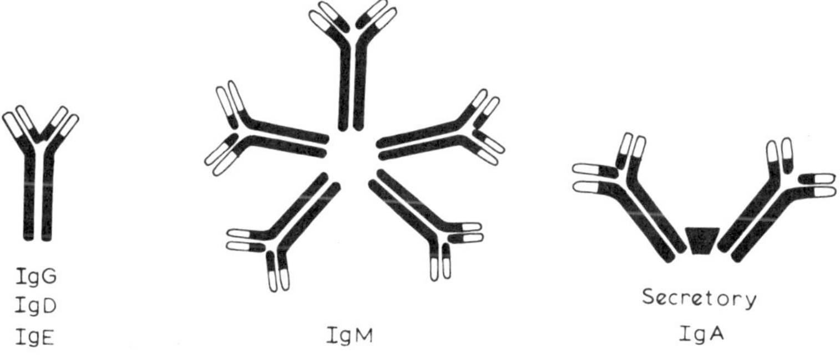

Figure 22.2.

d. IgM: The largest immunoglobulin molecule consists of five Y units connected at the Fc portions. The molecular weight is approximately 900,000 and the large size precludes passage through the placenta or out of the vascular system in large amounts. It is the first antibody formed in the newborn and it is the first antibody formed in response to antigenic challenge, but soon followed by higher concentrations of IgG. IgM participates in complement reactions and is an effective cytolytic antibody. Large size and multiple valancy make them effective agglutinators; in fact, the isoagglutinins, anti-blood group A or B, are mostly IgM.

e. IgE: This antibody is responsible for the type I immediate hypersensitivity (allergy) response in susceptible individuals. It has a mw 195,000 and has the same unit structure as IgG. Unlike the other immunoglobulins, however, it is produced in very small amounts by plasma cells. The serum concentration ranges from .000000040 gm/ml (40 nanograms) to .000002000 gm/ml in most allergic individuals. The values are usually given in international units that each equal 2 nanograms (eg 100 ng/ml=50 u/ml). IgE does not fix complement.

f. IgD: IgD comprises about one percent of total immunoglobulins and has no known function.

T LYMPHOCYTE AND CELL MEDIATED IMMUNITY: 70-80% of circulating lymphocytes are T lymphocytes and function as surveillance cells circulating throughout the body. These cells are also found in the paracortical portion of the lymph nodes; the B lymphocyte is located in the cortical lymphoid follicles. When specifically sensitized T cells make contact with an antigen, they recognize the foreign material, cooperate with B lymphocytes in antibody synthesis, and are capable of releasing eight or more biologically active substances known as <u>lymphokines</u>. Some of the more important lymphokines include: <u>macrophage inhibitory factor (MIF)</u> which inhibits the migration of macrophages inducing them to stay at the site of injury; several <u>chemotactic factors</u> which cause granulocytes or macrophages to migrate toward the released lymphokine; <u>mitogenic factor</u> causes blast formation in lymphocytes; <u>interferon</u> (see above); and <u>transfer factor</u> (see Type IV immune reaction).

Hypersensitivity diseases have been artificially catergorized into four groups according to pathological mechanism by Gell and Coombs. (Table I) This method of classifying immune disorders has been useful thus far. There are increasing numbers of diseases listed under each category and many diseases have more than one mechanism. The following discussion will emphasize the mechanisms and treatment of Type I hypersensitivity responses, namely, allergy.

<u>Type I Hypersensitivity Response</u>: For the otolaryngologist, allergic rhinitis with associated sinus, otologic, and laryngo-pharyngeal disorders are of primary interest. Bronchial asthma, and gastrointestinal allergy are other examples of type I reactions. Approximately 15 to 20% of the population is atopic, or in other words have hereditary tendency to nasal allergy, asthma, or atopic eczema. The mode of inheritance is multifactorial and has not been precisely determined.

TABLE I

CLASSIFICATION OF HYPERSENSITIVITY DISEASE

(After Gell and Coombs)

		Immunoglobulin	Mechanism	Disease Examples
Type I	Immediate hypersensitivity	IgE	mast cell or basophil vasoactive amines	allergic rhinitis, asthma, g.i. allergy
Type II	Cytotoxic-antibody Induced hypersensitivity	IgG, IgM	cell death secondary to antibody reacting with cell surface antigen, complement aided	blood group incompatabilities; ABO and Rh, autoimmune diseases, Hashimoto's thyroiditis, hemolytic anemia
Type III	Antigen-antibody complex	IgG, IgM IgE	abnormal Ab-Ag complexes result in inflammation secondary to complement and Hageman factor activity	Arthus reaction serum sickness
Type IV	Delayed hypersensitivity (cell mediated immunity)		24-48 hour infiltration of lymphocytes and macrophages	contact dermatitis, sensitivity to fungi, bacteria, transplant rejection syndromes

1. Mechanism: In response to antigenic stimulation such as ragweed, IgE antibodies are formed in high levels and persist in atopic persons. IgE is present in very low titers in sera, but also fixes by the Fc portion, to the surface of the vasoactive amine mediator cells, eg. the basophils in circulation or the mast cells in the skin and sub-mucosal tissues of the respiratory and G.I. tracts. The reaction of antigen with the Fab portion of IgE antibodies on the cell surface initiates a complicated chain of events which decreases the intracellular cyclic 3'-5' AMP and results in the release of vasoactive substances primarily histamine, and SRS-A (slow reacting substance of anaphylaxis). Basically, the reaction of

$$\text{ATP} \xleftrightarrow{\text{adenyl cyclase}} \text{C 3'-5' AMP} \xleftrightarrow{\text{phospho diesterase}} \text{5' AMP}$$

is modulated by two enzymes. The activity of the first, adenyl cyclase, is intimately related to cell surface events, and this activity is decreased by the IgE-antigen interaction. The result is decreased amounts of C 3'-5' AMP, the subsequent release of vasoactive amines, followed by typical allergic inflammation. Conversely, increased intracellular levels of C 3'-5' AMP inhibits the release of these substances. C 3'-5' AMP is the ubiquitous "secondary messenger" found in cells throughout the body.

2. The vasoactive amines: Histamine activity includes; vasodilitation of arterioles and venules, increased vaso-permeability in venules and capillaries, smooth muscle contraction, stimulation of exocrine glands and vasoconstriction of arteries.

SRS-A: Produces slow contraction of smooth muscle, but its importance in nasal allergy is undetermined. The kinins, prostaglandins, and perhaps, serotonin, may also be involved in nasal allergic response.

3. The skin tests: Introduction of antigen into the skin of sensitized individuals results in activation of the IgE and mast cell histamine reaction. It is manifest clinically as a wheal that forms in 10 minutes and subsides in 30 minutes. Intradermal testing (as opposed to scratch and prick tests) is the most sensitive skin testing method and correlates highly to direct measurement of specific IgE levels (RAST test). Many otolaryngologists favor the intradermal serial dilution titration method developed by Rinkel. P-K (Prausnitz-Kunstner) test - This test demonstrated the existence of reagin or IgE for the first time. Serum of a sensitive individual is injected (passively transferred) into the skin of a non-allergic individual. The response is destroyed by pre-heating the serum to 56°C. After a 24 hour wait, while the injected IgE fixes to the recipient's mast cells, the subject will respond with an allergic wheal challenge with the proper antigen at the injection location.

4. Radioimmunoassays: (RIST & RAST TESTS) Both are radioisotope assisted assays used to measure serum IgE antibodies which are present in extremely low concentrations (nanograms). The RIST (radioimmunosorbent test) measures total serum IgE while RAST, the (radioallergosorbent test), measures IgE antibodies to a specific allergen, such as ragweed, Timothy grass, etc. RAST testing has been used experimentally to test for food sensitivities and to standardize the potency of allergenic extracts. (Table II)

TABLE II

INTERPRETATION OF RIST TEST VALUES

1. Serum IgE Levels	# Total Normals	# Total Allergic Patients
less than 20 u/ml	64%	0
20-100 u/ml	34%	40%
more than 100 u/ml	2%	60%

Johansson, S.G.O., Advances in Diagnosis of Allergy, RAST: pg. 9, Evans, R. ed. Symposia Specialists, Miami, 1975.

2. Relative Serum IgE Levels

Lowest	-	Nasal allergy - normal to 5 times normal range
Mid Range	-	Asthma - mean 5 to 7 times normal range
Higher Range	-	Atopic Dermatitis
Highest	-	Intestinal parasites (Helminthiasis)

5. Nasal Allergy:

a. Typically perennial nasal allergy patients have low normal to moderate elevations of IgE. In general, serum IgE levels are of limited use in the diagnosis of nasal allergy.

b. Nasal pollenosis: "hayfever" - antigens vary widely over the USA, but for the Northeast, Middle Atlantic, and Midwest, the pollen seasons are early spring - March, April, May - tree pollens, May, June - grass pollens, mid-August through September - summer weeds, especially ragweed. Symptoms include marked nasal obstruction, profuse clear nasal discharge, itchy palate, allergic conjunctivitis (red, itchy, watery eyes). There is an increased serum IgE during the season, plus an increased nasal eosinophil count.

c. Perennial nasal allergy: chronic nasal obstruction, thickened post nasal drainage, headaches, intermittent or complete loss of smell, associated allergic sinusitis. May or may not be associated with pollenosis. Most commonly it is secondary to dust, mold, or epithelial allergy. There may also be an associated food sensitivity, as well as endocrine imbalances.

d. Nasal polyposis: hyperplastic nasal disease is commonly, but not exclusively, associated with allergy. Probably represents an underlying abnormality of nasal mucous membrane that in co-existence with allergy, chronic infection, or disorders such as cystic fibrosis, results in polyps.

1) Aspirin Intolerance: A chemical sensitivity that can occur at any age, but often in middle age, in persons who have previously tolerated ASA without difficulty. Usually begins with a watery nose,

followed by obstruction, polyp formation, and often the explosive onset of bronchial asthma. There is a high eosinophil count in nasal and bronchial mucus. No skin sensitivity to ASA or passive transfer can be demonstrated. Other implicated drugs are indomethacin and tartrazine (USD+C yellow food dye #5).

6. Treatment of Nasal Allergy:

a. Antihistamines: This type of medication competes with histamine for H_1 receptor sites in the nasal vasculature. They work best to prevent the allergic response. Patients find individual preferences. Drowsiness and dryness are the most troublesome side effects.

1) Examples of 3 types of antihistamines that are effective in nasal allergy:

Chlor: or brom-pheniramine - Chlortrimeton[R] and Dimetane[R]
Triprolidine: Actidel[R]
Tripelenamine: Pyribenzamine[R]

b. Vasoconstrictors: Types of adrenergic receptors: Alpha - constriction of smooth muscle of blood vessels of skin, mucous membrane, and viscera. Beta 1 - cardiac stimulation. Beta 2 - relaxation of smooth muscle (bronchodilation).

1) Systemic:

pseudoephedrine (Sudafed[R]) affects both alpha and beta 2 receptors. Nasal decongestant and bronchodilator.

ephedrine: stimulates both alpha and beta receptors, same effects as epinephrine, but is effective orally and longer acting.

2) Topical: All nose drops or sprays cause rebound with overuse.

phenylephrine: (Neosynephrine[R]) differs from epinephrine by one -OH. Alpha stimulator with little B_1 effect. Effective only for 7-10 days because depends on norepinephrine stores for activity.

1% ephedrine solution: (as above)

Imidazoline derivatives: Are long acting vasoconstrictors.

oxymetazoline: Afrin

xylometazoline: Otrivin

c. Steroids: (occasionally used)

1) Topical:

Dexamethasone - (Decadron[R]) nasal spray is a long acting steroid, absorbed in part. Beclomethasone diproprionate has not been released in U.S. as yet (4/1/76). Advantage - not systemically absorbed in topically therapeutic doses (400 micrograms per day).

2) Systemic: (rarely necessary) Prednisone 20 mg. early AM in alternate day doses over a short period.

d. Others: Cromolyn sodium: (Aarane[R], Intal[R]). Not approved for nasal use, but has a prophylactic effect of stabilizing the membranes of sensitized mediator cells, thus preventing histamine release.

e. Hyposensitization: Injection (.05 to .50 cc) of properly selected antigens by a gradual build-up from very dilute concentrations 1:100,000 to the 1:10 wt/vol. range.

Many otolaryngologists prefer treatment with dosage schedules based on individual sensitivities (Rinkel method). Hyposensitization generates IgG production against the injected antigen ("blocking antibody"). This antibody is thought to react with the antigen before it reaches the IgE - mast cell complex, thereby providing improvement. Symptomatic improvement, however, does not correlate well with blocking antibody levels. Hyposensitization also causes a decrease in amount of histamine released by WBC's in an immunologic reaction. Finally, hyposensitization causes an initial increase in IgE levels, but they gradually decrease to below the starting level as therapy. proceeds.

Type II Immune Reaction: A reaction which occurs secondary to antibodies directed against cell surface antigens. The combination of antibody + antigen + complement results in lysis of the cell, and in the instance of auto-antibodies against specific tissues, target organ destruction. Conditions include transfusion reactions, autoimmune hemolytic disease, Hashimoto's thyroiditis, and bullous pemphigus.

Type III Immune Reaction: The Arthus reaction and serum sickness represent examples of a local and generalized Type III reaction. Other diseases generally included in this category are lupus erythematosus, scleroderma, poststreptococcal acute glomerulonephritis.

1. Arthus reaction: Injection of antigen into the skin of a previously sensitized animal with a high serum titer of precipitating, complement-fixing antibodies produces a rapid local erythematous and edematous response which culminates in 3 to 8 hours, but may go on to local necrosis. This inflammatory reaction is due to the intravascular precipitation of ag-ab complexes, the initiation of the complement reaction, (especially the release of anaphylatoxin (C3a-C5a), platelet aggregation, release of vasoactive amines, and the appearance of neutrophils.

2. Serum sickness: IgG, IgM and at times IgE immunoglobulins are formed against serum proteins (as in antitoxin therapy for tetanus or in the now more common instance of drug allergy), and form disseminated intravascular ag-ab complexes on exposure to the antigen excess. The urticarial response in drug allergy is due to an immediate IgE type reaction. The other symptoms are thought due to a type III hypersensitivity response described above under Arthus reaction. Serum sickness occurs one week or more following

injection of a large amount of antigen and results in fever, urticaria, pruritis, arthritis, myalgia, lymphadenopathy, splenomegaly and hematuria. The disease is usually self-limited.

Type IV: Characterized by the onset of symptoms 24 to 48 hours after exposure to an antigen (delayed hypersensitivity). T cells are responsible for surveillance and recognition of foreign substances and respond by release of lymphokines. This mechanism does not depend on an antibody response. Contact dermatitis and transplant rejection are examples of a functioning system whereas malignancy may be a failure of T cell recognition or response to new foreign antigens.

Transfer factor: a very low molecular weight (700-4, 000) polypeptide which is obtained from the dialyzable portion of an extract of sensitized lymphocytes. It may represent a double stranded RNA. Its biologic behavior is poorly understood; however, it is capable of transferring delayed sensitivities of the donor to a recipient. Given by injection, it is non-antigenic, and causes a generalized response within 24 to 48 hours, most probably by transmitting information from the surface to the nucleus of T lymphocytes. Thus incorporated into a cell it is replicated. This substance has been used experimentally as an adjunct in the treatment of certain anergic conditions such as Wiskott-Aldrich Syndrome, mucocutaneous candidiasis, as well as malignant melanoma and osteogenic sarcoma to name a few.

CHAPTER 23

RELATED OPHTHALMOLOGY

I. ANATOMY:

1. The orbit forms a quadrilateral pyramid: floor, roof, medial wall, and lateral wall.

Roof	=	orbital process of the frontal bone lesser wing of the sphenoid
Floor	=	orbital plate of maxilla orbital surface of zygoma orbital process of palatine bone
Medially	=	frontal process of maxilla lacrimal bone sphenoid bone lamina papyracea of the ethmoid bone
Laterally	=	lesser and greater wings of the sphenoid, zygoma

2. The trochlea, a pulley through which runs the tendon of the superior oblique muscle, is located between the roof and the medial wall. A displaced trochlea will give diplopia on downward gaze.

3. The inferior orbital fissure is in the floor of the orbit. It is bound by the greater wing of the sphenoid, orbital surface of the maxilla, and orbital process of the palatine bone. It transmits the infraorbital nerve, infraorbital vessels, zygomatic nerve, twigs from the sphenopalatine ganglion to the lacrimal gland, ophthalmic vein branch.

4. The anterior and posterior ethmoid foramina are situated at the junction between the frontal and ethmoid bone (but they are on the frontal bone per se).

5. The superior orbital fissure lies between the roof and the lateral wall of the nose. It is a gap between the lesser and the greater wings of the sphenoid. It transmits III, IV, VI, V_1, the superior orbital vein, ophthalmic vein, orbital branch of middle meningeal artery and recurrent branch of lacrimal artery.

6. The optic canal runs from the middle cranial fossa into the apex of the orbit. It is formed by the two roofs of the lesser wing of the sphenoid. It transmits the optic nerve and the ophthalmic artery.

7. The upper lid contains:
   a. orbicularis oculi
   b. levator palpebrae superioris
   c. sweat glands
   d. Meibomian glands
   e. Wolfring glands
   f. Tarsal plate

8. The lower lid contains:
   a. Tarsal plate
   b. orbicularis oculi
   c. sweat glands
   d. Meibomian glands
   e. Wolfring glands

9. The lateral ends of the tarsi unite to form the lateral palpebral ligament which fixes onto the orbital surface of the zygomatic bone. A displaced lateral canthal ligament may give an inferiorly displaced canthus or slight ptosis.

10. The medial ends join to form the medial palpebral ligament which is attached to the frontal process of the maxilla immediately in front of the lacrimal fossa. Displacement of the medial palpebral ligament gives rise to a rounding of the medial canthus or pseudohypertelorism. The medial palpebral ligament sends a few fibers to be attached to the posterior lacrimal crest. This is believed to keep Horner's muscle in place which in turn maintains the lacrimal puncta against the globe. Hence, displacement of Horner's muscle may lead to epiphora.

11. The septum orbitale is the orbital periosteum which extends into the lid to attach to the tarsal plates. It separates the orbital contents from the lacrimal apparatus. Medially, it is fused with the palpebral ligament leading towards the posterior lacrimal crest.

12. The suspensory ligament of Lockwood is a continuous band of fibrous tissue slung beneath the eye-ball from side to side. The ends of the suspensory ligament blend with the check ligaments and with the medial and lateral horns of the aponeurosis of the levator palpebral superioris.

II. 1. The upper eyelid is opened by the levator palpebral superior (III Nerve) and the smooth muscles (sympathetic fibers). It is closed by the orbicularis oculi (VII Nerve). The ophthalmic division of the V Nerve is responsible for the sensory innervation to the upper lid while the lower lid is innervated by the first 2 divisions of the V nerve.

2. Entropion = turning in of the lid margin.
   Ectropion = turning out of the lid margin.

3. Horner's Syndrome = paralysis of the sympathetic nerve, especially the superior cervical sympathetics, giving rise to ptosis, miosis, and anhidrosis.

III. 1. The 6 extra-ocular muscles and their functions are:

Lateral rectus	to	abduct
Medial rectus	to	adduct
Superior rectus	to	elevate (and intort)
Inferior rectus	to	depress (and extort)
Superior oblique	to	intort (and depress)
Inferior oblique	to	extort (and elevate)

2. LR$_6$ (SO$_4$), the rest by III

The lateral rectus is innervated by the VI nerve.
The superior oblique is innervated by the IV nerve.
The rest of the extraocular muscles are innervated by the III nerve.

3. The inferior rectus muscle is the most commonly trapped muscle in a Blow-out fracture, the second being the inferior oblique. When these muscles are trapped, the patient may experience difficulty looking upwards. This condition is not due to paralysis but rather to the trapping of the 2 muscles mentioned above. To differentiate paralysis of the elevators from trapping of the inferior rectus and the inferior oblique muscles, the "forced duction test" is performed under local or general anesthesia. The "forced duction test" consists of grasping the globe adjacent to the limbus with small forceps and rotating it up, down, in, and out. If the globe moves freely, there is no entrapment of these muscles.

4. There are 6 cardinal directions of gaze, each controlled by a set of 2 muscles:
Eyes to right: Right lateral rectus and left medial rectus
Eyes to left: Right medial rectus and left lateral rectus
Eyes up and right: Right superior rectus and left inferior oblique
Eyes down and right: Right inferior rectus and left superior oblique
Eyes up and left: Right inferior oblique and left superior rectus
Eyes down and left: Right superior oblique and inferior rectus

When diplopia occurs it may exist in more than one direction. The muscles suspected of being involved are those controlling the direction of gaze in which the images of the diplopia are furthest apart. It is usually obvious as to which eye is involved. However, when such is not the case, each eye should be covered in turn and tested. The eye that sees the peripheral image is the one injured.

IV. LACRIMAL SYSTEM:

1. The lacrimal gland (a serous gland predominantly) is located in a fossa within the zygomatic process of the frontal bone. The lacrimal sac lies in a fossa bound by the lacrimal bone, the frontal process of the maxilla, and by the nasal process of the frontal bone.

2. The lacrimal gland secretes tears through 17 to 20 openings. Although the gland is developed, secretion of tears does not take place till 2 weeks after birth.

3. When cannulating the inferior and superior canaliculi, it is important to remember that each canaliculus has a vertical portion (about 2 mm) and a longer horizontal portion (about 8 mm). The lacrimal sac is about 12 mm long and the duct about 17 mm in length. The nasolacrimal duct empties into the anterior portion of the inferior meatus. This area is to be avoided when creating a nasoantral window. The most common site of obstruction in the lacrimal system is the upper portion of the nasolacrimal duct giving rise to dacrocystitis, the symptoms of which are epiphora and pain.

4. A lacerated canaliculus should be sutured together if possible. If not, a silk string or polyethylene tube should be passed from one canaliculus to the other.

5. A lacerated nasolacrimal duct can be sutured primarily over a polyethylene stent passing from the canaliculus to the nose. If the lacerated ends cannot be identified, then a polyethylene tube passing from the canaliculus into the nose can be left in place for two to three weeks.

V. 1. Malignant exophthalmos is caused by an endocrine disorder. One of the etiologies is an over secretion of "exophthalmos factor" by the anterior pituitary. This factor is possibly linked to TSH. The more severe form of exophthalmos is caused by excessive orbital edema giving rise to an increase in bulk of the extraocular muscles and adipose tissues. These adipose tissues are found at such time to contain a greater amount of mucopolysaccharides.

2. The exophthalmos is not only esthetically undesirable but can lead to:

a. Corneal abrasions (due to an inability to properly close the eye).
b. Chemosis secondary to venous stasis.
c. Fixation of the extraocular muscles causing ophthalmoplegia. The earliest limitation noted is in the upward gaze.
d. Retinal venous congestion leading to blindness.

3. Since the consequences of malignant exophthalmos are grave, many surgical corrections have been devised.

a. <u>Kronlein Procedure</u> removes the lateral orbital wall to allow the orbital contents to expand into the zygomatic area.
b. <u>Naffziger Procedure</u> removes the roof of the orbital cavity to allow expansion of the orbital contents into the anterior cranial fossa. It does not expose any of the paranasal sinuses and it preserves the superior orbital rim. Postoperatively, the cerebral pulsations may be noticed in the orbit.
c. <u>Sewell's Procedure</u> consists of an ethmoidectomy and removal of the floor of the frontal sinus for expansion.
d. <u>Hirsch's Procedure</u> removes the orbital floor to allow decompression into the maxillary sinus. A ridge of bone around the infraorbital nerve is preserved to support the nerve.
e. <u>Ogura</u> has described a method in which the floor and the medial wall of the orbit are removed to allow expansion into the ethmoid and maxillary sinus. As complete an ethmoidectomy as possible is performed.

CHAPTER 24

RELATED NEUROLOGY

I. MULTIPLE SCLEROSIS

Multiple sclerosis is a chronic disease characterized physiologically by the presence of numerous areas of demyelinization in the central nervous system, and clinically, by a variety of neurological signs and symptoms which have a tendency toward remission and exacerbation. It is primarily a disease of the young adult. The most common symptoms in multiple sclerosis are weakness and paresthesias. Vertigo is the presenting symptom of this disease in 7 to 10% of the patients and it eventually appears during the course of the disease in up to 1/3 of the cases. Deafness, on the other hand, is rare while involvement of the extraocular muscles gives diplopia. Nystagmus is present in about 70% of all cases of multiple sclerosis. The nystagmus, most commonly of the horizontal type, is observed only on lateral gaze. Vertical nystagmus is present in about 33% of the cases. While oscillopsia (rapid oscillations of the eyes in the horizontal plane) is occasionally seen, internuclear ophthalmoplegia is a common ocular manifestation of this disease. In internuclear ophthalmoplegia, the internal rectus on one side is paralyzed while the external rectus on the opposite side is weak, thus producing nystagmoid jerks of the outwardly deviating eye (monocular nystagmus or ataxic nystagmus). Internuclear ophthalmoplegia rarely occurs in other diseases, hence its presence is pathognomonic of multiple sclerosis.

Multiple sclerosis has an inherited predisposition although not inherited according to Mendelian laws.

Charcot's Triad in multiple sclerosis includes nystagmus, scanning speech and intention tremor.

II. MYASTHENIA GRAVIS

Myasthenia Gravis is a disease characterized by weakness and abnormal fatigability of the striated muscles. Its pathophysiology is believed to be impaired transmission across the myoneural junction. The usual age of involvement varies from 5 to 40. Children born of a myasthenia gravis mother may have neonatal myasthenia gravis symptoms. Their chief symptom is an inability to suck and swallow. The cricopharyngeus muscle which is not involved in poliomyelitis is involved in myasthenia gravis. Like multiple sclerosis, remissions and exacerbations are characteristic of this disease. Ocular muscle involvement is present in 40% of the cases. Facial, laryngeal and pharyngeal muscles are often involved. A distinctive trait of this disease is that the weakness is greatest after exercise and at the end of the day. Nystagmus and vertigo seldom occur.

The diagnosis is made from the patient's medical history together with the Prostigmin or Tensilon Test.

(From the PDR, 1976).
TENSILON: (edrophonium chloride) Tensilon is a short and rapid-acting cholinergic drug. Chemically, edrophonium chloride is ethyl (m-hydroxyphenyl)-dimethylammonium chloride.

10-ml vials: Each ml contains, in a sterile solution, 10 mg edrophonium chloride compounded with 0.45% phenol and 0.2% sodium sulfite as preservatives, buffered with sodium citrate and citric acid, and pH adjusted to approximately 5.4

1-ml ampuls: Each ml contains, in a sterile solution, 10 mg edrophonium chloride compounded with 0.2% sodium sulfite, buffered with sodium citrate and citric acid, and pH adjusted to approximately 5.4.

Actions: Tensilon is an anticholinesterase drug. Its pharmacological action is due primarily to the inhibition or inactivation of acetylcholinesterase at sites of cholinergic transmission. Its effect is manifest within 30 to 60 seconds after injection and lasts an average of 10 minutes.

Indications: Tensilon is recommended for the differential diagnosis of myasthenia gravis and as an adjunct in the evaluation of treatment requirements in this disease. It may also be used for evaluating emergency treatment in myasthenic crises. Because of its brief duration of action, it is not recommended for maintenance therapy in myasthenia gravis.

Tensilon is also useful whenever a curare antagonist is needed to reverse the neuromuscular block produced by curare, tubocurarine, gallamine triethiodide or dimethyl-tubocurarine. It is not effective against decamethonium bromide and succinylcholine chloride. It may be used adjunctively in the treatment of respiratory depression caused by curare overdosage.

Contraindications: Known hypersensitivity to anticholinesterase agents; intestinal and urinary obstructions of mechanical type.

Warnings: Whenever anticholinesterase drugs are used for testing, a syringe containing 1 mg of atropine sulfate should be immediately available to be given in aliquots intravenously to counteract severe cholinergic reactions which may occur in the hypersensitive individual, whether he is normal or myasthenic. Tensilon should be used with caution in patients with bronchial asthma or cardiac dysrhythmias.

DOSAGE:
Intravenous Dosage (Adults): A tuberculin syringe containing 1 ml (10 mg) of Tensilon is prepared with an intravenous needle, and 0.2 ml (2 mg) is injected intravenously within 15 to 30 seconds. The needle is left in situ. Only if no reaction occurs after 45 seconds is the remaining 0.8 ml (8 mg) injected. If a cholinergic reaction (muscarinic side effects, skeletal muscle fasciculations and increased muscle weakness) occurs after injection of 0.2 ml (2 mg), the test is discontinued and atropine sulfate 0.4 mg to 0.5 mg is administered intravenously. After one-half hour the test may be repeated.

Intramuscular Dosage (Adults): In adults with inaccessible veins, dosage for intramuscular injections is 1 ml (10 mg) of Tensilon. Subjects who demonstrate hyperreactivity to this injection (cholinergic reaction) should be retested after one-half hour with 0.2 ml (2 mg) of Tensilon intramuscularly to rule out false-negative reactions.

Dosage (Children): The intravenous testing dose of Tensilon in children weighing up to 75 lbs. is 0.1 ml (1 mg); above this weight, the dose is 0.2 ml (2 mg). If there is no response after 45 seconds, it may be titrated up to 0.5 ml (5 mg) in children under 75 lbs, given in increments of 0.1 ml (1 mg) every 30 to 45 seconds and up to 1 ml (10 mg) in heavier children. In infants, the recommended dose is 0.05 ml (0.5 mg). Because of technical difficulty with intravenous injection in children, the intramuscular route may be used. In children weighing up to 75 lbs., 0.2 ml (2 mg) is injected intramuscularly. In children weighing more than 75 lbs., 0.5 ml (5 mg) is injected intramuscularly. All signs which would appear with the intravenous test appear with the intramuscular test except that there is a delay of two to ten minutes before a reaction is noted.

Tensilon Test for Evaluation of Treatment Requirements in Myasthenia Gravis: The recommended dose is 0.1 ml to 0.2 ml (1 mg to 2 mg) of Tensilon, administered intravenously one hour after oral intake of the drug being used in treatment. Response will be myasthenic in the undertreated patient, adequate in the controlled patient, and cholinergic in the overtreated patient.

III. MIGRAINE HEADACHE

Migraine headache can take various forms. It is usually severe, periodic, unilateral and lasts for hours. The patient is free of headache between attacks. There is familial tendency with onset at adolescence and prevalence in females.

The headache can be localized at the temporal, retro-orbital or frontal region. It is preceded by an aura, usually visual. Associated with the headache, the patient may have photophobia, pallor, dizziness, tinnitus, paresthesias, nausea, vomiting and diarrhea.

It is believed that the etiology is "vascular" and the symptoms precipitated or aggravated by stress. Ergotamine tartrate (Cafergot) has been used to treat the attacks, while Sansert (methysergide maleate) is used for the prevention or reduction of their intensity and frequency. However, Sansert has been reported to cause severe complications, e.g. retroperitoneal fibrosis, pleuropulmonary fibrosis and cardiac complications.

IV. CLUSTER HEADACHES (HISTAMINE CEPHALGIA, HORTON'S SYNDROME, NASOCILIARY NEURALGIA)

Cluster headache is typified by bouts of attacks for a few days between months or years of remission. It often occurs in young adults. The headache is severe, unilateral, lasts less than an hour and often awakes the patient from a sound sleep. It may be associated with scleral injection, lacrimation, ipsilateral rhinorrhea and nasal congestion. The treatment is similar to that for Migraine headache.

V. TEMPORAL ARTERITIS

Temporal Arteritis mainly strikes those in their 50's and 60's. Its pathology is similar to that of periarteritis nodosa except for a more severe inflammatory reaction around the vessels and for the presence of many multinucleated giant cells in the media (giant cell arteritis). It is usually restricted to the temporal arteries.

The patient suffers severe pain along the arteries, feels lethargic, and has a low grade fever. Temporal arteritis is usually a self-limiting disease unless the central artery of the retina is involved in which case residual blindness would be present. The treatment for this disease consists of steroid administration.

VI. SARCOIDOSIS

Sarcoidosis is a multifaceted disease of unknown etiology. Pathologically, epitheloid cell tubercles are found without evidence of necrosis or caseation. Giant cells containing calcified bodies are identified in these tubercles. The usual age of onset is between 20 and 50 years old. The organs possibly involved, in order of decreasing frequency, are the lymph nodes, lungs, skin, eyes and bones. In the practice of otolaryngology, the nose, tonsil and larynx are sites of predilection. Localization of sarcoidosis in the respiratory tract and in the salivary gland happens in only about 3% of all cases. The most common ophthalmic manifestations are iridocyclitis, keratitis, conjunctivitis, and episcleritis.

<u>Uveoparotid fever of Heerfordt</u>, a variant of sarcoidosis, is characterized by fever, parotid involvement, uveitis, facial paralysis (usually bilateral and transient).

The frequency of hypercalcemia in sarcoidosis ranges from 3 to 20% and ranges from 45 to 70% for hyperglobulinemia. Leukopenia is encountered quite frequently while eosinophilia occurs in 20% of the cases.

VII. PITUITARY ADENOMA

1. The pituitary (hypophysis) has two divisions in the human. The anterior pituitary is termed the adenohypophysis from which a variety of hormones are released, including prolactin, ACTH, TSH, growth hormone, FSH and LH. The posterior pituitary is termed the neurohypophysis and releases antidiuretic hormone (ADH or vasopressin)

and oxytocin (both are actually formed in the hypothalamus, from whence they are transported to the neurohypophysis for storage and release). Anatomically, the important features in regard to the trans-sphenoidal approach to the sella turcica include the following: (a) Inferiorly, there is a dural covering over the pituitary gland. (b) Superiorly, there is the diaphragma sella, through which the infundibulum of the pituitary passes. (c) Anteriorly, the venous circular sinus is located within the dura. (d) Posteriorly, the dorsum sellae may be palpated on intrasellar exploration. (e) Located on either side laterally is the cavernous sinus, which contains the carotid artery, third, fourth, and sixth cranial nerves, as well as the first and second divisions of the fifth cranial nerve.

2. The cell types of the anterior pituitary include the chromophobe cells (comprising 50% of the total cell population), acidophils (also termed alpha cells; containing 40% of the pituitary cells), and basophils (also termed beta cells; containing 10% of pituitary cell population). The glial cells of the posterior pituitary are termed pituicytes. Using various histochemical techniques, finer classification of this division of cell types has been made, but as yet the final terminology of the finer cell types has remained unsettled.

3. Types of tumors: The differential diagnosis of sella and parasellar tumors should include the following:

a. Pituitary adenoma:
   1) Chromophobe: 80% of pituitary adenomas.
   2) Acidophilic adenomas: 15% of pituitary tumors.
   3) Basophilic: 5% of pituitary tumors.
b. Craniopharyngioma
c. Aneurysm of the internal carotid artery
d. Empty sella syndrome - may be primary or secondary, with or without enlarged third ventricle.
e. Metastatic tumors
f. Optic and/or hypothalamic glioma
g. Hamartomas of the hypothalamus
h. Ectopic pinealoma, teratoma, dermoid
i. Meningioma (tuberculum sellae, diaphragma sellae)
j. Prepontine lesions - chordoma, meningioma
k. Mucocele of the sphenoid sinus
l. Sella abscess secondary to sphenoid sinusitis
m. Chronic granulomas, especially sarcoidosis and tuberculosis

4. Symptoms of pituitary tumors may be divided into three broad categories:

a. Endocrine:

1) Chromophobe pituitary adenoma: Hypogonadism including sterility, impotence and/or amenorrhea may be seen in as many as 3/4 to 4/5 of cases. Hypoadrenalism may be seen in as many as 1/3 of cases. Evidence of hypothyroidism is relatively infrequent except in extreme cases of panhypopituitarism.

2) Acidophilic adenoma: Gigantism may be seen in childhood before the epiphyses of the long bones have been closed. In adults acromegaly is seen. However, the histological type of pituitary tumor seen in many, if not most, cases of acromegaly is that of a chromophobe adenoma.

3) Basophilic Adenoma: Clinically demonstrable tumors of the pituitary which are present in about 10% of patients with Cushing's Disease are found to be basophilic adenomas. Classically these tumors are microscopic. In cases of Cushing's syndrome after bilateral adrenalectomy, Nelson's syndrome may be seen (hyperpigmentation with increasing sella size). Basophilic adenomas tend to occur in a younger age group and are more likely to be seen in females than other pituitary adenomas.

Pituitary adenomas may occur as part of pluriglandular adenomatosis, a rare syndrome of adenomas of the pituitary, parathyroids and pancreatic islets.

b. Visual Symptoms: The classic visual symptom associated with enlarging suprasellar extension of pituitary adenomas is that of bitemporal hemianopsia. However, a variety of other field cuts may be seen. With further growth of tumor, there is a progressive decrease in visual acuity. A syndrome of pituitary apoplexy may also be seen in pituitary tumors. This is a sudden loss of vision associated with hemorrhage within a pituitary tumor. These are relative emergencies, which particularly lend themselves toward a transsphenoidal approach for removal of the hematoma if these patients are seen relatively soon after their apoplexic episode.

c. Headache: Headache is a common symptom associated with pituitary adenomas. Initially the headache may be due to pressure by growth of the tumor along the dural covering of the cavernous sinus and/or stretching of the dura fibers of the diaphragma sellae. With further suprasellar extension of tumor, obstruction of the foramena of Monro may occur with associated hydrocephalus and increased intracranial pressure. This latter development is usually a late symptom.

Preoperative Evaluation of Pituitary Tumors: The team approach is essential in evaluation of lesions in and about the pituitary. This should include the following:

1. Complete neurological examination.
2. Complete otolaryngological evaluation, including examination of the gums and teeth.
3. Neuro-ophthalmological examination.
4. Endocrinological workup (as indicated below).
5. Neuroradioiogical evaluation including:
   a. Skull films
   b. Tomography of the sphenoid sinus and sella turcica
   c. Radio-isotope scans
   d. Computerized tomography scan
   e. Arteriography and/or pneumo-encephalography
6. Nose and throat culture
7. Antibiotics as indicated
8. Preoperative and intraoperative steroids with continuance into the postoperative period.

Preoperative Endocrine Studies for Pituitary Adenomas: Complete endocrinological evaluation is required for pituitary adenomas. Endocrine studies should include serum cortisol levels (AM and

PM), growth hormone levels, Prolactin, complete thyroid evaluation (including PBI, T3, T4, T7, radio-active iodine uptake), FSH and LH levels (urinary), and serum and urine osmolalities. In addition, further tests such as metapyrone test, insulin tolerance test, arginine infusion test and glucose stimulation test may be required. (The normal values for many of these tests vary from laboratory to laboratory.)

Postoperative Endocrine Care: Many cases undergoing pituitary surgery will have at least a transient diabetes insipidus. In a few cases this may be permanent. Hourly monitoring of urine output and specific gravity is required in the immediate postoperative period. In addition, close monitoring of serum and urine electrolytes and osmolality is required. Acutely, if there is prolonged urine output of greater than 250 cc. per hour with a specific gravity of 1.005 or less, one may assume that the patient has diabetes insipidus. Therapy may initially include intravenous fluids at a rate to replace the previous hour's urinary output. However, if the volume of urinary output becomes too excessive and/or prolonged, one may give pitressin. There are two preparations, an in-oil preparation or aqueous pitressin, the latter having a shorter duration of action than the former. In cases of chronic diabetes insipidus, pitressin snuff may include the requirement of steroid and thyroid maintenance, especially in cases of preoperative panhypopituitarism. In such instances a total of 37.5 mg. of cortisone acetate each day and two grains of dessicated thyroid each day will be sufficient. This dosage is required in hypophysectomy cases and in cases of pituitary adenoma presenting with hypopituitary function.

Rationale for Hypophysectomy in Cases of Carcinoma of Breast: The indications for hypophysectomy in cases of carcinoma of the breast include that of advanced disease with evidence of a previous objective response to endocrine manipulation. Of great interest is a new test, estrogen binding factor, which may be made upon primary breast or metastatic tissues. In 30% of cases of carcinoma of the breat, estrogen binding factor will be present. In such cases there is approximately a 90% response rate to endocrine manipulation.

VIII. DIFFERENTIAL DIAGNOSIS OF CEREBELLOPONTINE ANGLE TUMORS

1. ACOUSTIC NEUROMA: Hearing loss (retrocochlear pattern) is an early symptom, usually associated with tinnitus. With a progressive increase in tumor size, involvement of the fifth (decreased corneal reflex, facial hypesthesia) and seventh (peripheral facial paresis) cranial nerves occurs. Further tumor growth may involve the cerebellum (gait ataxia, dysmetria, nystagmus, etc.) brain stem (hemiparesis, Babinski response, etc.) and/or jugular foramen (ninth, tenth and eleventh cranial nerves). Bilateral acoustic neuromas may be seen in von Recklinghausen's disease.

X-rays, including skull films, Stenver's views and tomography of the internal auditory meatus usually reveals enlargement of the internal auditory meatus. Brain scan is usually negative in smaller lesions.

It is positive in up to 60% of larger tumors. Computerized tomography scanning may be positive in larger tumors. Both studies are negative in intracanalicular lesions. Angiography may reveal displacement of the anterior inferior cerebellar artery and/or the petrosal vein, as well as other vascular displacement in larger lesions.

Pneumoencephalography reveals nonfilling of the cerebellopontine angle cisterns. There is displacement of the fourth ventricle with associated hydrocephalus with larger acoustic neuromas.

Cerebellopontine myelography reveals nonfilling of the internal auditory meatus.

2. MENINGIOMA: This is the second most common primary cerebellopontine angle mass lesion. Hearing loss tends to occur later in the clinical course of these lesions as compared to acoustic neuromas. Multiple cranial nerve palsies, brain stem, and cerebellar signs may be present with further tumor growth.

X-rays may reveal abnormal calcification and/or local hyperostosis involving the petrous ridge, but the internal auditory meatus will be normal in size.

Brain scan and computerized tomography scan are more likely to be positive in these lesions as compared to acoustic neuromas.

Angiography will reveal local vessel displacement and tumor stain may also be seen (usually not seen with acoustic neuromas).

Pneumoencephalography is usually not performed, but if done, findings similar to those seen in acoustic neuromas are noted. CSF protein, as in cases of acoustic neuromas, is usually elevated.

Cerebellopontine angle myelography, if performed, reveals nonfilling of the cerebellopontine angle.

3. EPIDERMOID: This is the third most common primary cerebellopontine angle mass lesion. Hearing loss, if present, tends to occur late in the patient's clinical course. Multiple cranial nerve palsies, with or without brain stem and/or cerebellar signs may be found.

Plain skull films and laminograms are usually within normal limits. The internal auditory meatus is normal in size.

Brain Scan is usually negative. Computerized tomography scan may also be negative.

Angiography may reveal local vascular displacement without tumor stain.

Pneumoencephalography is usually diagnostic, revealing air filling the finger-like interstices of an angle mass lesion. CSF protein may be elevated.

Cerebellopontine angle myelography, if performed, reveals an irregular angle mass lesion with Pantopaque irregularly filling the interstices of the tumor.

4. METASTATIC NEOPLASM: Metastatic tumors (lung, breast, etc.) have a more rapid clinical course than the first three diagnostic possibilities. Multiple, bilateral lower (and upper) cranial nerve palsies usually evolve as a manifestation of meningeal carcinomatosis. Most often a previous history of neoplasia is obtained. Evidence of metastatic disease elsewhere is often present. Plain skull films and laminograms of the internal auditory meati are normal.

Brain Scan and computerized tomography scan are often positive in larger lesions.

Angiography will reveal local vessel displacement with or without a tumor stain.

Pneumoencephalography and Cerebellopontine angle myelography are usually not performed. CSF protein may be elevated and tumor cells may be noted on CSF cell analysis.

5. GLIOMA: Occasionally brain stem or cerebellar gliomas (astrocytoma, subependymoma, etc.) may "escape" into the subarachnoid space and grow out toward the cerebellopontine angle. In such cases they may present with symptoms of a lesion in this area. Examination may reveal a predominantly brain stem or cerebellar lesion. Plain x-rays are usually normal.

Brain Scan is often negative. Computerized tomography scan may be helpful in revealing a cerebellar lesion.

Angiography reveals local tumor displacement.

Pneumoencephalography is often diagnostic, especially of brain stem lesions. CSF protein may or may not be elevated. Despite the above noted findings, on occasion the diagnosis may be unsuspected and diagnosed only at the time of surgery.

6. ANEURYSMS AND OTHER LESIONS: Aneurysms are diagnosed by angiography. Chordoma and other bony lesions are usually diagnosed by appropriate x-rays, including laminography.

IX. MISCELLANEOUS

1. Parosmia = perverted sense of smell
   Hyperosmia = over sensitive sense of smell
   Hyposmia = impaired sense of smell
   Anosmia = total loss of smell
   Cocosmia = a sense of foul smell when none is present

2. Diphenylhydantoin (Dilantin) and Carbamazepine (Tegretol) have been used to treat Trigeminal neuralgia.

3. Vitamin A has been used to treat Anosmia. (See Chapter 11).

4. Ammonia stimulates the V cranial nerve and not the I cranial nerve. Hence, it can be used when a psychogenic cause of anosmia is suspected.

CHAPTER 25

THYROID AND PARATHYROID

THYROID GLAND

1. FUNCTION:

1. Anatomy: The thyroid is a 20-25 gram bi-lobed structure, the lobes being connected across the midline by an isthmus. The lobes lie on either side of the trachea extending from the lower third of the thyroid cartilage downwards to about the fifth tracheal ring. The isthmus crosses anterior to the 2nd, 3rd, and 4th tracheal rings. The latter is an important point to remember in the performance of a tracheostomy. Embryologically, the gland arises as an offshoot of the primitive alimentary tract as a median anlage from the pharyngeal floor in the region of the foramen cecum at the base of the tongue. From this point it descends down to its position in the anterior neck. The course of this descent is marked in about 80% of patients by a pyramidal lobe, a narrow projection of thyroid tissue extending from the isthmus upward towards the hyoid bone. During embryonic development, the descending thyroid is joined by a pair of lateral components originating from the 4th and 5th branchial pouches.

Opinions differ as to the nature of unattached thyroid tissue occasionally found lateral to the gland proper. True lateral aberrant thyroid rests do occur but are apparently extremely rare. In all probability, most such tissue represents metastatic papillary carcinoma replacing a lymph node.

2. Blood Supply: The abundant blood supply of this highly vascular gland is derived from paired superior thyroid arteries, the first branches of the external carotids, which enter the upper poles of each lobe, and paired inferior thyroid arteries which, arising from the thyrocervical trunk of the subclavian course upwards then turn downwards and medially to enter the lateral aspect of the lobes at the junction of the lower and middle thirds. In most subjects, a fifth vessel, the thyroid ima, arises from the arch of the aorta and ascends to enter the isthmus.

3. Lymph Drainage: The lymph drainage of the central segment of the thyroid gland is mainly to the prelaryngeal nodes on the cricothyroid membrane and to the pretracheal nodes anterior to the trachea and below the isthmus. From the lateral parts of the lobes, lymphatics pass laterally to the deep cervical nodes.

4. Important Anatomic Relationships: The recurrent laryngeal nerves arise from the vagi, passing from before backwards around the subclavian artery on the right and the aortic arch on the left, then turning and proceeding upwards in the tracheo-esophageal groove on either side ultimately to enter the larynx behind the articulation of the inferior cornu of the thyroid cartilage with the cricoid. They supply all of the intrinsic muscles of the larynx except the cricothyroid, and the mucous membrane below the vocal fold. These

almost always lie in close relationship to the inferior thyroid artery, running either over, beneath or between a bifurcation of this vessel. This vessel is an important aid in the location of the nerve during thyroid surgery. It is important to remember that in a fair percent of subjects the nerves at this level lie slightly more anteriorly in an exposed position on the anterolateral aspect of the trachea.

The external branch of the superior laryngeal nerve destined to innervate the cricothyroid muscle lies in close proximity to the superior thyroid artery just above the upper pole of the thyroid and unless caution is used, may be damaged in division of this vessel in thyroidectomy.

The parathyroid glands will be discussed below.

5. Physiology: The basic physiologic functions of thyroid hormone are concerned with calorigenesis of heat production, embryonic growth and differentiation and metabolic processes including those of various foodstuffs and minerals. The exact mechanism of action of thyroid hormone at the subcellular or molecular level has not been fully elucidated. It is postulated that it influences energy transport mechanisms within the cell.

Hormone biosynthesis. The normal human requires about 50 mcg. of iodide per day. Intake is normally far greater (10 grams of iodized salt contain 750 mgms). The bulk of the excess of ingested iodide is excreted in the urine. A small pool of extra-thyroidal iodide, about 400 mgms, is retained in the body. Circulating plasma iodide is rapidly taken up by the cell of the thyroid follicle and is oxidized to form iodine. In the cell, this active form iodinates the amino acid tyrosine to form moniodotyrosine (MIT) and diiodotyrosine (DIT). Two molecules of DIT then join to form one molecule of thyroxine (T4) and one molecule of DIT plus one molecule of MIT may join to form one molecule of triiodothyronine (T3). These are held in peptide linkage with a specific thyroprotein, thyroglobulin, and are stored as intrafollicular colloid.

Release of the active thyroid hormones T3 and T4 is under direct control of the thyroid-stimulating hormone of the anterior pituitary regulated by a negative feedback system, which is in turn governed by influences from the cerebral cortex and the hypothalamus via its thyrotropin-releasing factor (TRF) as well as by sensors in various tissues sensitive to changes in blood level of thyroid hormone. Stimulation then causes enzymatic breakdown of the thyroglobulin complex and results in the release of T3 and T4 into the circulation. These are then bound by plasma proteins TBG (thyroxine-binding globulins) and TBPA (thyroxin binding pre albumin). Such "protein bound iodine" containing compounds can be measured in the serum and form the basis for one of the tests of thyroid activity. In the blood, the ratio of T4 and T3 is from 10 to 20:1. T3 is much more active and is more loosely bound to protein and accounts for approximately 50% of the effect of the secreted hormone. An excess quantity of T3 or T4 added to a test tube of blood will saturate TBG and spill over onto albumin or red cells. The amount of spillover depends upon the amount of TBG present in the blood sample and the degree of saturation of the TBG. Hence, in hypothyroidism, spill-over is less and RBC uptake of T3 is less while in hyperthyroidism the reverse is true. This is used as a clinical test (RBC-T3 uptake). Thyroxine is readily extractable from serum protein with butanol, so that butanol extractable iodine (BEI) is a good measure of circulating iodine.

II. DISEASES OF THE THYROID GLAND: Diseases of the thyroid gland include those involving increased or decreased hormone secretion with or without changes in the size of the gland and those which may merely involve enlargement or changes in consistency of the gland or a portion thereof.

1. Tests of Thyroid Function: In the evaluation of thyroid disease certain common tests of thyroid function are of basic importance. These include the following:

a. Basal metabolic rate: A time-honored and now obsolete method involving a spirometric measurement of oxygen uptake under controlled conditions. It is subject to variation depending upon preparations for the test, body composition and habit, state of nutrition and other diseases besides those of the thyroid such as blood dyscrasias, tumors of the lymphoid series and anxiety states. Variations of ± 15% are considered within normal limits.

b. Radioactive isotope studies: A variety of radioactive isotopes are available, radioactive iodine being the most widely used. When I^{131} is given orally or intravenously it is cleared by the thyroid and the kidney. Almost none remains in the plasma after 24 hours. After a small dose (5 to 50 micro C.) the mean thyroidal uptake in 24 hours is approximately 30% (range 15 - 40%). Values greater indicate hyperthyroidism and lower, hypothyroidism. Expansion of body stores of iodine may cause a lowering of I^{131} uptake. In clinical medicine, this is most commonly seen after administration of organic iodinated compounds used in radiographic studies such as pyelography and cholecystography. Too early use of I^{131} uptake after one of these studies may yield falsely low results.

c. Scanning: A scintigram may be obtained by moving a scintillation counter over the gland after administration of a radioactive isotope. This will chart the localization of iodine accumulation in the gland or in ectopic thyroid tissue. Scans are of particular value in the assessment of solitary or multiple nodules which, as a result, can be classified as "hot" or hyperfunctioning, "warm" - function equal to that of the remainder of the gland, or "cold" - non-functional, concentrating no radioactivity. The latter are accepted to exhibit a higher incidence of malignancy other than thyroid nodules.

In hyperthyroidism, the scan may be of value in determining the presence of hyperfunctioning thyroid tissue not in the usual location, such as in a lingual thyroid or in thyroid tissue in a substernal position.

In view of the therapeutic implications, scans may be of real value in determining the presence or absence of function in a carcinoma or metastases therefrom.

d. Protein-bound iodine (PBI): Serum proteins may be washed, precipitated and the iodine measured chemically. This is essentially a measurement of T-4. The normal range is 4-8 micrograms percent. Values above indicate hyper while those below, hypothyroidism. Recently administered iodides in any form (the list grows longer each year, e.g., BSP, iodides, Floraquin, vitamins with iodine, syrup of hydriatic acid, roentgenographic contrast materials, estrogens, etc.), may increase the measured PBI. For this reason the test is now of doubtful value.

e. Butanol extracted iodine (BEI): Thyroxine is extracted from the serum and the iodine content is measured. (Normal 3.5 - 7.5 micrograms percent). This test eliminates errors due to ingestion of inorganic iodides, but exogenous organic iodides may interfere.

f. T-3: Red blood cell uptake of added I^{131} labeled T-3 is measured (normal 12-20%). This is a valuable test as it is modified only by conditions affecting serum proteins (e.g. pregnancy, nephrosis, etc.).

g. T-4: A recently developed measurement of thyroxine using chromatographic separation gives normal values of two micrograms percent.

h. T-7: The product of T-3 and T-4 levels. (Not another thyroxine-like molecule). Certain compounds (estrogens, for example) alter thyroxine binding globulin in such a way that misleading results are obtained from standard T-3 and T-4 testing. Using the product of T-3 and T-4, the deviations balance one another and the product gives a relatively accurate reading of the state of thyroid activity.

i. Thyroxine binding globulin (TBG). Abnormalities of thyroxine binding capabilities of certain proteins may be congenital or acquired. These are of no clinical significance but may suggest erroneous diagnoses of thyroid abnormalities based on other testing.

j. Thyroid-stimulating hormone (TSH) -- measured by radioimmunoassay. Normal, up to 10 μ U per c.c. No known factors cause a significant and persistent rise in TSH levels other than primary hypothyroidism.

k. Radioimmunoassays of T-4 (normal range 4.5 to 11.5 ng/ 100 c.c.) and of T-3 (normal 70 - 160 ng. per 100 c.c.) are extremely accurate and reproducible. In the evaluation of the hyperthyroid state, these will probably replace all other tests.

l. Blood cholesterol: This is increased in primary myxedema while the value is usually normal in hypothyroidism due to pituitary failure. The concentration is influenced by a multitude of factors but may be of value in determining response to therapy.

m. Thyroid autoimmunity: In Hashimoto's disease, antibodies to thyroid antigen are present in the serum. Antibody titre can be evaluated by one of several methods. A greatly increased titre in a euthyroid or hypothyroid patient with goitre is suggestive of Hashimoto's Disease. In a patient with exophthalmos, an increased titre suggests thyrotoxicosis.

2. Hypothyroidism: This may be infantile or adult. In infants, known as cretinism, it may occur endemically in areas known as "goitre belts" where the water and soil are deficient in iodine or it may occur less frequently and sporadically and be associated with an atrophic thyroid gland. Of vital importance is recognition early in infancy before lasting deficiencies of growth and mental development occur.

In adult life, hypothyroidism, known as myxedema, may result from a number of causes. Among these are the following:

a. Replacement of the thyroid gland by nonfunctioning goitre or multiple adenomas.
b. A sequel to thyroiditis or Hashimoto's Disease.
c. Surgical removal of the gland for thyrotoxicosis, goitre or malignancy.
d. Treatment of thyrotoxicosis with radioactive iodine (very common).
e. Overtreatment of thyrotoxicosis with antithyroid drugs.
f. Secondary to panhypopituitarism.
g. Idiopathic (usually in women in the 4th to 5th decade).
   Clinical manifestations (in adults) include:
   1) Fatigue or apathy with retardation of mental and physical processes as well as dulling of intellectual function and impairment of speech.
   2) Skin: thickened, puffy and dry.
   3) Hair: dry, brittle and falls out easily.
   4) Tongue: enlarged, may fill the mouth
   5) Muscle cramps.
   6) Headaches: may be severe and occur daily. May suggest CNS diseases.
   7) Abdominal manifestations - constipation, distention, changes in bowel habits and cramps. Remarkable dilatation may be seen on x-ray.

Tests of major value in establishing the diagnosis of hypofunction. (Note: The basal metabolic rate is notoriously inaccurate in this respect. Often gives a falsely high result).

a. Index of circulating thyroxine (PBI, BEI or RBC - I^{131} uptake).
b. Determination of etiology of deficiency (TSH stimulation test or antithyroglobulin antibody titre).

Treatment involves the use of dessicated thyroid (60 - 120 mgms daily). This substance may apparently lose its potency on storage after three to four months. Fresh extract is advisable.

3. Hyperthyroidism: In 1835 and 1843, Graves and Basedow independently reported illnesses characterized by diffuse thyroid enlargement, exophthalmos and thyrotoxicosis. It became well accepted that this disease is due to accelerated metabolism of most body tissues due to an excess of circulating thyroid hormone and the cause was for years assumed to be the result of increased stimulation of the thyroid by pituitary thyroid stimulating hormone (TSH). More recently it has been demonstrated that TSH levels are not increased in these individuals and that a long acting thyroid stimulator (LATS), a gamma globulin with many characteristics of an antibody directed against thyroid antigen, is present in the plasma of most patients with thyrotoxicosis. It is possible that this disease is therefore, the result of some sort of autoimmune mechanism.

Hyperthyroidism may present in one of three forms, namely, diffuse hyperplasia (Graves' or Basedow's disease), multinodular toxic goitre, or as a single, toxic nodule. Diffuse hyperplasia is much more common in females. Exophthalmos with other eye signs may or may not be present in thyrotoxicosis. By the same token in thyrotoxicosis with exophthalmos thyroid enlargement may be absent.

Clinical features include nervousness, tremor, increased sweating, a sense of heat and intolerance to heat, increased appetite but paradoxical loss of weight, muscle weakness and palpitation. Restlessness, excitability, irritability, insomnia and emotional instability are common features. Intermittent diarrhea is common and in females menses may be scant or absent. On exam, the skin will be warm and moist, the pulse rapid, a fine tremor may be present and nail softening sometimes with clubbing of the fingers is not uncommon. The hair is fine and may readily fall out on combing. Eye signs are common with Graves' disease but are unusual with multinodular goitre or toxic solitary nodule. These include retraction of the upper lid (manifested by lid-lag),external ophthalmoplegia, exophthalmos with proptosis, periorbital swelling, congestion and edema and signs of weakness of extraocular muscles.

Cardiac problems, on the contrary, are more common with toxic adenomata either single or multiple. These include atrial fibrillation at first paroxysmal but later continuous and congestive failure (with an increased circulation time) controlled with difficulty with digitalis. The pulse pressure may be greatly increased.

Local examination of the neck may reveal diffuse enlargement, enlargement with multiple nodules, or a single palpable adenoma.

Laboratory tests of greatest value include the PBI, BEI, RBC-T3 uptake and the I-131 uptake and scan. The marked increase in these values seen in Graves' disease is less striking in multinodular toxic goitre or single adenoma. These latter two diseases can be shown to demonstrate autonomous hyperfunction and are thus independent of TSH and LATS stimulation.

Methods of treatment include antithyroid drugs, radioactive iodine or surgery and will vary depending upon the pathology and age of the patient.

Antithyroid drugs (propylthiouracil 100-300 mgms. t.i.d. or methimazole (Tapazole) 5-15 mgms. t.i.d.) block hormone formation by inhibiting the oxidation of iodide to iodine and also by inhibiting the coupling of iodotyrosines. Improvement usually occurs within two weeks and the patient will be euthyroid within six to eight weeks. Treatment should be continued one to two years and the drug should then be gradually withdrawn. If a relapse occurs, as it will in approximately one half the patients, some feel that another course of therapy should be started while others think surgery is indicated. Toxic reactions which require cessation of treatment include agranulocytosis, aplastic anemia, urticaria and pruritis. Reaction to one drug does not necessarily imply that a similar reaction to others will occur.

A fact well recognized by clinicians of former years and now often forgotten is that most patients with thyrotoxicosis would, if they could be kept alive long enough, sooner or later go into remission and that relapses seldom occur. An interesting question arises in a patient with Graves' disease who responds well to treatment and does not have a recurrence after cessation of the drug, namely was it the drug that effected the lasting remission or was it the natural course of the disease taking place during treatment? If it can be shown to be the latter, it would seem to be a strong argument in favor of a trial of a second or even a third course of drug therapy.

Radioactive iodine therapy is becoming an increasingly popular mode of treatment. Major reservations regarding this method have been the possible genetic effect in women in the child-bearing age and the threat of carcinogenesis or the development of leukemia in younger individuals. To date, there has been no solid evidence that this is a real hazard but until the matter has been settled caution is urged. Most clinicians avoid the use of therapeutic I^{131} in patients under 40. Approximately 160 microcuries are given per gram of estimated gland weight. Response is slow, a disadvantage in severe cases, and it may take from 3 to 18 months to reach a euthyroid state. Unfortunately, myxedema develops in a high percent of cases and figures are beginning to suggest that this may occur in 100% of patients if they live sufficiently long after treatment.

Subtotal thyroidectomy (80-85%) until very recently was the method of choice in therapy. It eliminates hyperthyroidism (in about 95% of cases) and goitre rapidly and the mortality rate in skillful hands is almost nil. An easily correctable myxedema develops in about 10% of cases. The major flaws in this technique relate to recurrent laryngeal nerve damage and inadvertent resection or devascularization of the parathyroids. The frequency of occurrence of these complications depends almost entirely upon the experience and technical ability of the surgeon. In good hands, nerve injuries might be expected in 0 to 3% of the cases, and in the vast majority should only be temporary due to manipulation, stretching or edema. Actual removal of too much parathyroid tissue should be avoided if careful attention is given to careful preservation of the postero-lateral aspect of the capsule of the gland as well as prior identification of the parathyroids.

In rare instances of huge irregular glands (most often seen with multiple adenomatous colloid goitre or malignancy) the recurrent laryngeal nerves or parathyroid glands may be so removed from their normal positions that injury is a possibility. (For treatment of acute hypoparathyroidism - see under Parathyroid Glands).

It should be mentioned here that with Graves' disease, depending on age and sex, treatment with antithyroid drugs or I^{131} is the method of choice. Patients with multiple toxic nodular goitre respond less well to medical therapy and are difficult to bring into a well controlled euthyroid state. When surgery has been necessary in this condition, it has been the experience of the author that near total extra capsular thyroidectomy is required, and myxedema is prone to develop.

In the case of the hyperfunctioning ("hot") nodule, surgery is so simple and so definitive and, if done properly, so completely without complication, that barring unusual contraindications it should be regarded as the treatment of choice. Another point in favor of removal is the fact that while at one time all of these lesions were regarded as benign, it is now well known that a solitary hyperfunctioning nodule may be malignant.

4. Multiple Adenomatous or Diffuse Colloid Goitre: These probably represent the commonest causes of thyroid enlargement seen by surgeons. They may be familial as exemplified by a genetic metabolic enzymatic defect affecting iodide to thyroxine metabolism and as a result, many such patients will become hypothyroid, requiring treatment. Endemic goitre occurs in areas where iodine ingestion is less than required or where goitrogens are ingested. Iodine prophylaxis, for example as administered in iodized salt, has been a most effective preventive measure. Lacking a steady normal intake of iodine or lacking ability to use iodine properly the gland goes through intermittent periods of hyperplasia and involution, not all areas in the gland reacting in the same way at the same time. During hyperinvolution, areas develop which contain multiple large follicles surrounded by low cuboidal or flat epithelium, filled with colloid. These follicles may enlarge to become colloid filled cysts, resulting in areas of multinodularity representing areas of colloid rich nodules intermingled amongst areas of normal thyroid tissue and other areas of lymphocytic infiltration. In the nodular areas hemorrhage is not uncommon and under the microscope, cholesterol clefting and areas of calcification are frequently seen. These lesions are most frequently seen in females, are asymptomatic and their development over the years is insidious. Malignancy, usually papillary carcinoma, develops in a relatively small number of patients (5% or less). An occasional case is allowed

to continue to grow to such enormous proportions, that a huge "museum piece" goitre develops. In this situation, distortion of the normal course of the recurrent laryngeal nerves may prove to be a vexing problem for the surgeon.

Aside from suggestive malignant changes, the indications for surgical therapy are cosmetic disfigurement and tracheal and esophageal pressure symptoms, including choking, hoarseness, nocturnal breathing problems and rarely a Horner's syndrome. A complicating hyperthyroidism may rarely develop. Subtotal thyroidectomy, with an attempt to leave an adequate remnant of normal functioning gland, is indicated.

One complication to be borne in mind is that of tracheomalacia, a destruction or softening of the normal cartilagenous tracheal rings that may result from years of compression. After removal of the thyroid such trachea can flatten completely resulting in acute airway obstruction. A temporary tracheostomy allows restoration and fixation of the normal tracheal configuration.

5. The "solitary" nodule: As mentioned previously, such a solitary palpable nodule on I^{131} scanning may be "hot" or hyperfunctioning, "warm" or exhibiting function similar to the surrounding normal thyroid tissue or "cold" that is to say with little or no function. It is the cold nodule that has been the subject of hot debate over the past twenty years for in these the incidence of malignancy is significant. Although there have been isolated instances of solitary hot nodules proving to be malignancies, in general, the vast majority of carcinomas will take up less I^{131} than the para-nodular tissue.

In many cases, a solitary palpable nodule will be found at surgery simply to be the only discretely palpable portion of a gland otherwise afflicted by multiple adenomatous colloid disease and the nodule will prove to be a colloid adenoma or cyst. This group probably represents the majority of the solitary palpable nodules. Ultrasound studies have now been shown to be of real value in differentiating cystic from solid nodules. The remainder are true neoplasms approximately four-fifths of which will be benign and will be labeled by the pathologist as embryonal, fetal, follicular, Hurthle cell or papillary adenomas. (It has been suggested that the Hurthle cell adenoma may have slightly more ominous significance in terms of development of future malignancy). Of the neoplastic group, approximately 20% will prove to be carcinomas.

A significant number of solitary nodules will reduce in size and may occasionally disappear when the patient is given dessicated thyroid to suppress TSH. Based on this fact, many clinicians feel that the treatment of choice is a trial of TSH suppression.

Each case should be evaluated on its own merits; age and sex are important. Solitary nodules in younger individuals, particularly males,are more apt to be malignant. Nodules in children are very likely to be cancer. Rate of growth, nodule consistency and sensation of fixation all must be carefully evaluated. Resection for benign nodules is simple, definitive, and should be without complication. In the author's opinion, both schools of thought regarding therapy should be explained to the patient.

If suppressive therapy is selected, it should be carried on for about three and certainly no more than six months. If the nodule has not then disappeared, surgery is indicated. Even if the nodule gets much smaller or disappears, the patient must be carefully watched for a considerable period of time. Some malignant nodules will respond remarkably, but temporarily to suppression. The fear of using suppressive therapy in malignancy, the simplicity and definity of surgery, and the much greater peace of mind on the part of the patient all persuade the author to favor early surgery.

6. Thyroiditis: This term covers several disease entities in the thyroid gland exhibiting varying types of inflammation.

a. Acute suppurative thyroiditis: This is an extremely rare disease in which an abscess develops in the substance of the thyroid gland following an acute upper respiratory infection. The onset is sudden with local pain, swelling and tenderness along with chills, fever and dysphagia. Treatment consists of proper surgical drainage.

b. Subacute thyroiditis: This entity is also known as De Quervain's disease or non-suppurative thyroiditis. The cause is unknown. It is most frequently seen in young or middle aged females and in most cases follows an upper respiratory infection. Sore throat, neck pain radiating posterior to the ear, hoarseness, dysphagia, and low-grade fever are features. The thyroid will be tender and the disease may be diffuse. Microscopically, one sees diffuse acute inflammation, fibrosis, disruption of acini with spill of colloid and foreign body reaction with giant cells. Tests of thyroid function will generally be on the low side of normal with return to normal when the disease subsides. A transient hyperthyroidism may occur early in the course. If symptoms are severe, the most effective treatment involves the use of steroids. In most cases, aspirin, an ice collar and propylthiouracil are effective. Small doses of x-ray therapy may be necessary.

Granulomatous ("pseudotuberculous") thyroiditis is probably a variant of the subacute disease. Microscopically one sees a subacute inflammatory response accompanied by an accumulation of giant cells of the epithelial foreign body type and later an eosinophilic infiltration. Thyroid extract is the treatment of choice.

c. Hashimoto's Thyroiditis: (Struma Lymphomatosa). This is the commonest type of thyroiditis and in it there is some evidence of genetic predisposition. It is an autoimmune process and almost all patients will be shown to have circulating antithyroid antibodies as demonstrated by red cell agglutination and compliment fixation tests.

Clinically, the disease is characteristically seen in young to middle aged females. It is a common cause of thyroid enlargement in children. It generally presents with enlargement, pain and tenderness in the region of the thyroid and is often accompanied by cough and difficulty in breathing and swallowing. Overt symptoms of hypothyroidism are common. The gland is generally diffusely enlarged and firm. A significant number of patients (20-25%) will manifest symptoms of coexistent connective tissue disease such as rheumatoid arthritis, fibrositis, lupus and others.

Microscopically, there is a diffuse or focal lymphocytic infiltration with disruption of the acini. Some of the remaining epithelial cells show oxyphilic changes. In a variant of this disease, a remarkable fibrosis may develop.

Early in Hashimoto's Disease tests may show mild thyroid hyperfunction but later, as the disease progresses the results of testing will be normal or subnormal. The diagnosis is established by the finding of a high titre of thyroid antibodies in the serum.

If compression symptoms are lacking, treatment should be restricted to the use of suppressive doses of thyroid hormone. One hundred and eighty to three hundred milligrams daily may be required. If nodules develop, resection is indicated. Carcinoma rarely develops. It is generally felt that this disease is of a self-limiting type, reaching a stage of maturity then remaining static. Progressive fibrosis can occur but is generally not severe.

d. Reidel's Struma: This is a rare chronic inflammatory fibrosing condition which may involve both lobes and may extend to surrounding fascia, muscles, nerves and trachea. The cause is unknown and biopsy is necessary to differentiate the rocky hard tissue from carcinoma. Patients are usually middle-aged and thyroid function is depressed or normal. Microscopically, a dense infiltrative fibrous tissue extends through the gland and into surrounding structures. Acini are few and far between. Surgery is confined to attempts to relieve tracheal or esophageal obstruction simply by removing what tissue seems necessary, the thyroid isthmus for example. A tracheostomy may be necessary. Treatment is otherwise confined to the use of thyroid extract. This disease is sometimes seen with retroperitoneal fibrosis causing ureteral obstruction.

7. Carcinoma of the Thyroid: To the casual reviewer of surgical literature no topic could appear more hopelessly muddled than that of thyroid cancer. On one hand one gains the impression that these are in most instances virtually benign diseases if properly treated with TSH suppression and that if the palpable primary is removed as best as possible and if such nodes as seem grossly involved are extricated, (the rationale supporting the plucking out of such nodes has always eluded the author) the patient will survive ad infinitum. On the other hand, there are those who advocate total or near total thyroidectomy with radical neck dissection on one or both sides for all cancers of the thyroid. The reason for this divergence of opinion hinges largely on the fact that the most common of the thyroid cancers, the papillary adenocarcinomas, are indeed, hormone dependent or are, at any rate, dependent for many years upon the growth stimulating effect of the thyrotropic hormone of the anterior pituitary (TSH). The production of this hormone is readily suppressed by the

administration of thyroid extract. Logical argument against this somewhat laissez-faire attitude obtains when one considers the facts that not only are thyroid carcinomas, even papillary, often multi centric rather than unicentric in origin, but that of even greater importance, many which are papillary on microscopic examination in one area may prove to be a mixed papillary-follicular type in another or on careful study may even exhibit a neoplasm of much more ominous significance. For those of a more simplistic persuasion who feel that for a patient's ultimate well being, if a cancer is present it is far preferable to have it removed completely, the more radical approach within bounds of reason seems far more acceptable. Here the phrase "within bounds of reason" refers to the delicate balance of long term life expectancy against the odds of tetany, recurrent laryngeal nerve paralysis and gross disfiguration. With the latter reservations in mind, the author prefers the "radical" to the "ultraconservative" approach.

a. Papillary carcinoma: A slow growing and readily "curable" type of cancer that accounts for approximately two thirds of all thyroid cancers. It occurs at any age but is seen frequently in children and young adults. It metastasizes to regional lymphatics. The most common sign is goitre varying in dimensions from tiny to huge. Local symptoms of pain or pressure are rare. There is some evidence that papillary cancers may persist for years as a primary cell type then dedifferentiate in some areas into a more malignant cell type. Papillary and follicular cell types (or worse) may coexist in the same tumor at the same time of original discovery. Operation should include total (subcapsular) lobectomy on the side of the lesion with removal of the isthmus and three-fourths of the medial aspect of the opposite lobe. This should be accompanied by a modified neck dissection on the side of the primary, sparing the sternocleidomastoid muscle, the spinal accessory nerve, and the jugular vein. Thyroid extract (at least 180 mgms. daily) may be initiated immediately if extensive nodal involvement is reported microscopically, or may be withheld until evidence of palpable recurrence occurs. Prognosis for long-term survival (15 - 20 years) is probably about 80 - 90%.

b. Follicular Carcinoma: This is a slightly more malignant variety of cancer which accounts for about one-fourth of all thyroid malignancies. It is more common in females and in patients older than the average of those with papillary carcinoma. It metastasizes much more frequently via the blood stream than via lymphatics. The blood borne metastases in lung or bone often retain the microscopic appearance of normal thyroid tissue, hence the term "benign metastasizing goitre". Hurthle cell variants are often seen microscopically. Clinically one may obtain a long history of goitre (up to ten years) with pain or pressure symptoms a late manifestation. In many cases, symptomatic metastatic disease calls attention to the primary. Surgery includes removal of the involved lobe and the isthmus and if palpable nodes are present, a modified neck dissection. If distant metastases are present, total thyroidectomy has been advocated in order to enhance the avidity of the metastatic deposits for a therapeutic dose of radioactive iodine. The survival rates are slightly less than those anticipated with papillary carcinoma.

c. Medullary Carcinoma: This entity has been only recently described. It differs from all other types of thyroid cancer in its ability to produce amyloid. It represents only 5 - 10% of all thyroid cancers and occurs in patients about the age of 35 to 50. It is considerably more malignant than papillary or follicular carcinomas (a 50% five-year mortality) but does not carry the same grave outlook that characterizes the undifferentiated carcinomas. This interesting growth seems to show considerable familial predisposition and is often associated with one or more other endocrine disorders. The coincidental finding of pheochromocytoma, parathyroid adenoma, Cushing's syndrome and neurofibromatosis, carcinoid-like syndromes, extra thyroidal malignancies and multiple mucosal neuromas have all been demonstrated.

One of the most fascinating aspects of this growth is that it originates from the para-follicular cells. It has been suggested that medullary carcinomas of the thyroid are indeed, tumors of the parafollicular cells for extremely high concentrations of thyrocalcitonin have been measured in medullary carcinoma tissue. Of particular interest is the speculation into the cause and effect relationship between parathyroid adenomas and their accompanying hypercalcemia and the calcium lowering effect of thyrocalcitonin produced by medullary carcinomas of the thyroid when the two lesions coexist in the same individual.

Proper surgical treatment involves near total thyroidectomy and modified neck dissection on the side of origin.

d. Anaplastic Carcinoma: Under this heading are included undifferentiated carcinomas as well as spindle cell and giant cell carcinomas. These are amongst the most lethal of all tumors known to man. Occurring later in life (average age about 65) and slightly more frequently in women, these tumors are unencapsulated and extend and infiltrate widely beyond the confines of the gland. A disturbing feature has been recently emphasized, namely that this type of cancer is associated with differentiated thyroid carcinomas in a considerable percentage of cases. They are also associated with long-standing undiagnosed "goitre" which presents with a sudden acceleration in growth rate. The woeful results of any type of treatment of anaplastic thyroid cancer emphasize the real importance of adequate early initial treatment of the more differentiated cancers.

Extensive resection should be attempted but efforts rarely meet with success. Tracheostomy is often necessary. Radiation therapy coupled with pituitary suppression should be tried. Future success may lie with chemotherapy, but an effective agent has not yet been discovered.

PARATHYROID GLANDS

I. FUNCTION:

1. Anatomy: A discussion of the anatomy of the parathyroid glands requires a brief review of their embryological development. The upper parathyroids arise from the fourth branchial pouch along with the previously mentioned lateral thyroid anlage. They descend slightly and gain their normal adult position along the lateral or posterolateral aspect of the capsule of the upper lobe of the thyroid gland. Unless enlarged they are apt to be relatively fixed and may usually be identified in the expected position. The lower parathyroids on the other hand, arise with the thymus gland from the third pouch and descend with that gland to a more inferior position, lying usually on the capsule of the posterolateral aspect of the lower lobe of the thyroid often below, but in close proximity to the inferior thyroid artery. Much more variable in position than the upper glands, they may be found anywhere along the line of descent of the thymus, that is from the mandibular angle down to the mediastinum in a position anterior to the adult thymus gland. Probably due to the effects of gravity, enlarged inferior parathyroids are often found at or below the level of the sternoclavicular junction.

Most humans have four glands, but a finding of three or five glands is not rare. Occasionally one or more glands may be entirely embedded in the substance of the thyroid lobe. The glands are dark brown in color and measure approximately 6 by 3 by 2 mm in size. The upper glands are usually slightly larger than the lower ones and the total weight of parathyroid tissue is approximately 130 to 150 mgms. This is an important figure to remember in the performance of subtotal parathyroidectomy in the treatment of hyperplasia.

2. Calcium and phosphorus metabolism and the parathyroid hormone: The metabolism of calcium and phosphorus is a fascinatingly complex study but can be presented only in brief outline here. The homeostatic mechanism for the regulation of serum calcium levels is one of the most highly developed feedback control systems in the body and is largely under control of the parathyroid glands. A significant deviation of the serum calcium above or below normal levels of 8 to 10.5 mgms percent for any significant time is poorly tolerated by the human being and under most circumstances the deviation can be rapidly and efficiently corrected by parathormone.

The dietary source of calcium is milk or milk products and due to the relative insolubility of most calcium compounds calcium is poorly absorbed from the intestinal tract. Phosphates on the other hand are well absorbed except in the presence of excess oral calcium, in which case insoluble calcium phosphate is excreted in the feces. The intestinal absorption of calcium and phosphorus takes place in the mucosal epithelium of the duodenum and jejunum. The most important effect of Vitamin D is the enhancement of transport of calcium through the membrane of the epithelial cell. The most common Vitamin D compounds are calciferol (D_2) and 7 dihydro-cholesterol (D_3), the latter being formed in the skin as a result of irradiation by the ultraviolet rays of sunlight. As Vitamin D increases calcium absorption it secondarily increases the rate of phosphorus absorption. With even minute drops in serum calcium ion concentration the parathyroid glands are prompted to secrete parathormone (PTH) and this hormone greatly increases the rate of calcium absorption in the gastrointestinal mucosa. Increased serum calcium concentration results in a decreased PTH production and a reduction in the rate of intestinal calcium absorption.

The body contains slightly more than 1000 grams of calcium of which 11 grams are in the cells, 4 grams are exchangeable in bone, 1 gram is in the extracellular fluid and all of the remainder is stable in the bone. In the plasma, 50% of the calcium is bound to plasma protein and hence is non-diffusible through capillary membranes. Five percent is bound to organic anions such as citrate and phosphate and is diffusible and the remaining 45% is ionized, freely diffusible and is the fraction vitally important for most calcium functions in the body.

The average adult intake is in the neighborhood of 1 gram per day, 800 mgms. of which are excreted in the feces and the excretion of the remaining 200 mgms, is divided about half and half between urine and sweat. An additional 600 mgms. are secreted by the intestinal glands and mucosa and are largely resorbed. An additional important mechanism for calcium homeostasis relates to PTH control of calcium resorption by the renal tubules. A decrease in plasma ionic calcium signals the parathyroids which oblige by the production of increased PTH. This then increases tubular resorption of calcium and the plasma level rises. The converse is true with an elevation of the serum calcium. One of the most important effects of increased PTH is to decrease tubular resorption of phosphorus and to increase urinary excretion of this substance. Hence, the decreased serum phosphorus and greatly increased phosphaturia in hyperparathyroidism.

The third major effect of parathyroid hormone on calcium homeostasis relates to the metabolic flux in bone. Bone is made up of an organic matrix of collagen fibers, a small amount of ground substance composed of mucoprotein, chondroitin sulfate and hyaluronic acid and of large quantities of crystalline salts deposited in and around the organic matrix. These salts are formed principally by calcium and phosphate and are called hydroxyapatites. Other ions, particularly magnesium, are also present. Approximately 70% of the dry weight of bone is mineral. The collagen matrix of bone is covered by a layer of bone cells, some of which are osteoblasts which lay down new bone, and others, osteoclasts which cause bone resorption. In bone a continuous process of deposition and absorption takes place which generally adjusts to strength needs, bone stress, and as in many tissues, to aging where as bone becomes older, it becomes weak and brittle and must be injected with new life.

Germane to this discussion is the fact that the absorption activity of bone osteoclasts is to a degree under the control of the parathyroid hormone. Indeed, it is felt that PTH has the property of converting osteoblasts and osteocytes into osteoclasts. The activity of these cells then causes bone resorption with the release of calcium into the circulation.

Bone provides an extremely important additional factor in calcium homeostasis, namely, an almost instant buffering of hypocalcemic states independent of parathyroid activity, which is due to the level of readily available 4 grams of "exchangeable" calcium in bones. It is known that the maximum effect of injected (or released) PTH on calcium concentration is reached in approximately eight hours and lasts approximately 34 to 36 hours. This is not a sufficiently rapid defense mechanism to protect thoroughly against the lethal effects of radical changes in calcium ion concentration which may under certain conditions take place rapidly. For example, in very severe diarrhea several grams of calcium can be lost into the intestinal tract in a very few hours. By the same token under certain dietary situations a person could easily ingest large quantities of calcium and might absorb a gram or more in one hour. Adding or subtracting a gram of calcium rapidly to the extracellular pool which in itself contains about one gram could rapidly result in a fatal excess or deficiency state.

Approximately 0.5 to 1% of all bone calcium exists as exchangeable calcium, probably not under the control of the parathyroid hormone, and located in surface positions in and on bone rather than fixed in matrix. This calcium is in reversible equilibrium with the calcium and phosphate in extracellular fluids. With great rapidity an increase in the product of plasma calcium and phosphate ion concentrations can result in an immediate deposition of calcium in or on bone while a decrease in the product can result in an extremely rapid dissolution of bone salts with the release of ionized calcium.

Calcitonin inhibits the resorption of bone. It presumably acts at the same site as does PTH but its exact mechanism is unknown. Within minutes after administration it can cause almost total cessation of bone salt resorption and accordingly the serum calcium concentration falls rapidly. The hypocalcemic action of calcitonin is much more rapid than the hypercalcemic action of PTH and it is hoped that this hormone may prove of therapeutic benefit in certain potentially lethal hypercalcemic states.

In summary, parathormone exerts its influence on the serum calcium level in three ways. It increases the rate of absorption of calcium in the gastrointestinal tract, it increases tubular resorption of calcium in the kidney, and by control of osteoclastic activity it can promote the resorption of bone with the liberation of calcium.

II. HYPO AND HYPERPARATHYROID STATES:

Most of the acute symptoms of reduced or excessive function of the parathyroid glands are readily explained if one considers the abnormal physiological effect of decreases or elevation of the serum calcium levels. Neuronal permeability depends to a degree on extracellular fluid concentration of calcium. When this concentration falls below normal, permeability increases and nervous system excitability progressively increases. This occurs in both the central nervous system and in the peripheral nerves, although it is the peripheral nervous manifestations which are most pronounced clinically. The nerve fibers become so excitable that they begin to discharge spontaneously, initiating impulses which on passage to peripheral muscles cause tetanic contraction. Signs of latent tetany can be elicited by tapping the facial nerve over the ramus of the mandible. In most patients with acquired postoperative or idiopathic hypoparathyroidism this will produce a contraction of the facial muscles known as Chvostek's sign. In advanced tetany carpopedal spasm may develop. In this the patient exhibits marked flexion of the hand on the wrists and of the fingers at the metacarpophalangeal joints. In latent tetany, the elicitation of this deformity by reduction of circulation with the use of a tourniquet is known as Trosseau's sign. Hyperventilation which decreases the PCO_2 and increases the pH of blood thus increases nerve irritability and can likewise bring out overt signs in latent tetany. Tetany usually develops when the concentration of serum calcium drops below 7 mgms. %.

It is of scant comfort to the human victim to know that acute hypocalcemia causes essentially no other serious effects because tetany kills the patient before other effects can develop.

When serum calcium concentration in extracellular fluid increases above the normal range, the reverse neuromuscular and other diverse consequences are noted. The central nervous system is depressed and reflex activities become sluggish. The muscles become weak, perhaps due to the effect of increased calcium concentration on muscle cell membrane. Increased calcium concentration likewise decreases the QT interval in the heart, and results in lack of appetite and chronic constipation, presumably due to depressed contractibility of the muscular walls in the gastrointestinal tract.

1. Hypoparathyroidism: Idiopathic or primary hypoparathyroidism is a very rare disease. It may fall into the autoimmune classification inasmuch as antibodies to parathyroid tissue have been demonstrated in this condition. In this disease the parathyroids are usually absent or atrophied. It has been reported to develop after I^{131} therapy for thyrotoxicosis. This is a treatable disease (see below) and as such must be differentiated from two closely related apparently genetic disorders, namely, pseudohypoparathyroidism and pseudopseudohypoparathyroidism in which there is an end organ resistance to the action of parathyroid hormone.

The commonest cause of hypoparathyroidism is inadvertent removal of the glands during surgery on the thyroid gland. A frequent accident in the days before awareness of the importance of the parathyroids, nowadays it is a distinct rarity and when seen is usually transient. Operative trauma to the parathyroids or removal of one or two glands will occasionally result in temporary hypoparathyroidism which corrects itself with supportive treatment in days or weeks after surgery. In rare instances a period of months may go by before symptoms become manifest. This lag period is not clearly understood, but it has been suggested that it is due to vascular trauma with gradually progressive ischemia of the glands leading to hypofunction.

Should signs of tetany develop postoperatively intravenous calcium chloride or calcium gluconate (10%) should be started immediately and therapy continued with 5 to 15 grams of calcium lactate powder and 50,000 to 100,000 units of Vitamin D (calciferol or 7 dihydrocholesterol) daily. The patient should be placed on a high calcium low phosphorus diet. Treatment can usually be tapered gradually and ceased. In rare cases parathormone and dihydrotachysterol (AT 10) may be necessary. To date, transplantation techniques have proven to be disappointing.

2. Hypercalcemia: In consideration of a diagnosis of hyperparathyroidism, the various other causes of hypercalcemia include:

a. Extraparathyroid neoplasms which themselves produce para-thormone or a PTH - like substance. Common among these are tumors of breast, lung, kidney, skin, liver, pancreas and neoplasms of the lymphatic series. These are common causes of hypercalcemia and the diagnosis can almost always be made after appropriate investigation.

b. Sarcoidosis: In this disease hypercalcemia presumably results from increased absorption of calcium from the gastrointestinal tract secondary to an exaggerated sensitivity to Vitamin D, hence the increase in calcium levels in these patients during the summer months when the effect of sunlight on Vitamin D synthesis in the skin is most intense. The diagnosis can generally be made by chest films, node biopsy, blood studies and the Kveim skin test.

c. Multiple Myeloma: Here elevated calcium levels are seen in approximately 40% of the patients and are probably due to bone erosion by the tumor cells. X-rays, bone marrow examination and serum electrophoresis will usually give the diagnosis.

d. Malignant Disease: Malignancies, not in themselves producing PTH but with bone metastases may give hypercalcemia. As in multiple myeloma, this is due to bone erosion. Breast, kidney, lung, prostate and thyroid are frequent offenders. Serum calcium will be elevated and as in hyperparathyroidism bone alkaline phosphatase (which must be distinguished from the enzyme produced by the liver) may be elevated, but serum phosphorus will be normal or elevated. A thorough work up with metastatic series and/or bone scan should provide the diagnosis.

e. Vitamin D Intoxication: Hypercalcemia usually develops after a long period of excessive ingestion of this vitamin and the effect is exerted due to increased bone resorption and excessive gastrointestinal absorption of calcium. A careful history should provide the diagnosis.

f. Idiopathic Hypercalcemia of Infancy: This is thought to be due to a hypersensitivity to Vitamin D as in sarcoidosis. It is often seen in association with multiple congenital cardiovascular lesions and mental retardation.

g. The Milk-Alkali Syndrome: This is a rare cause of hypercalcemia and renal failure, due to the excessive ingestion of milk or calcium containing antacids and absorbable antacids such as bicarbonate of soda for peptic ulcer. Renal damage with failure is usually preceded by hypercalcemia for a considerable period of time. Nephrocalcinosis or renal stones may develop. This is now much less prevalent since the use of non-absorbable antacids in ulcer therapy. Again a careful history should provide the clue.

h. Immobilization of patients with or without fractures may lead to atrophy or disuse osteoporosis and calcium loss from the bones at a rate that exceeds the kidneys' ability to excrete calcium. Immobilization is particularly apt to cause this problem in Paget's Disease.

i. Thyrotoxicosis: Significant hypercalcemia is rare in this disease. The cause is not certain although it is probably due to increased bone resorption. Phosphorus and bone alkaline phosphatase will be normal. The diagnosis is usually obvious.

j. Adrenal insufficiency: Hypercalcemia has been reported in Addison's Disease, and particularly in acute adrenal failure. The cause has not been determined but the calcium level may be expected to return to normal with adrenal replacement therapy.

3. Hyperparathyroidism: Primary hyperparathyroidism is caused by either single or multiple adenomas of the parathyroids, hyperplasia or carcinoma. Approximately four-fifths of the cases are due to a single adenoma, about 12 to 14% are due to hyperplasia of all four glands, and the remaining cases are found to be due to two or more adenomas or to carcinoma, roughly 3% each. Approximately three-fourths of the cases come to the attention of a physician due to renal stones and most of the rest with bone pain or pathologic fractures. The diagnosis should be considered in patients with peptic ulcer, pancreatitis, and unexplained CNS mental abnormalities.

Most of the symptoms and signs are directly due to the effects of hypercalcemia or to the action of PTH on bone. Symptoms due to the elevated calcium may of course, be seen in any patient with hypercalcemia regardless of the cause. These might include renal stones or nephrocalcinosis with or without hypertension or renal failure, depression, fatigue and muscle weakness, peptic ulcer, constipation and possibly pancreatitis. Eye changes include band keratitis and calcium in the palpebral fissures but ectopic calcification in skin and subcutaneous tissues is rare in primary hyperparathyroidism. Increased urinary output is manifested by polyuria and excessive thirst. Secondary to bone resorption caused by excessive PTH are bone pain, cysts and pathologic fractures.

Particular mention should be made of "hypercalcemic crisis" for in this relatively rare situation emergency therapeutic measures may be life saving. Equally urgent are the differential diagnostic studies. Crisis is apt to occur when the calcium level rises above 17 - 18 mgms.% and is most often seen in patients with some degree of renal failure with nephrocalcinosis. The onset is insidious with progressive increase in severity of symptoms. Predominant symptoms include weakness, nausea and vomiting, fatigue, lethargy, drowsiness and confusion, bone pain, abdominal pain, constipation and renal colic. One fourth of the patients will be in or near coma.

The mainstay of treatment is the emergency removal of the parathyroid tumor but during the period when certain measures are undertaken to exclude hypercalcemic crisis on a basis other than hyperparathyroidism, (carcinoma of the breast is the commonest) certain steps should be taken to improve the patient's condition. The most important of these is intravenous saline to restore hydration and to increase urinary output. Sodium citrate, sodium sulfate, and inorganic phosphate (500 cc of 0.1M phosphate intravenously in 4 hours) have been used with some success. Thyrocalcitonin has attractive possibilities. Dialysis may be necessary.

Diagnostic studies of value in the diagnosis of hyperparathyroidism include serial evaluation of the serum calcium and phosphorus levels for hypercalcemia and hypophosphatemia and the serum alkaline phosphatase (the "bone" type of enzyme may be elevated if osseous changes are present). A test for the tubular resorption of phosphate may be indicative,for with increased PTH levels resorption should be low. Urinary calcium and hydroxyproline levels may be indicative of hypercalcemia but are not of course specific for hyperparathyroidism. X-rays of the kidneys for stones or nephrocalcinosis and of the bones, particularly of the hands to show terminal phalangeal bone resorption, may be helpful. Distortion on inferior thyroid arteriography has been described in the presence of large adenomas. Isotope scanning has been disappointing. The most useful of all the tests has been the recently developed method of plasma parathormone radioimmunoassay. Selective jugular venous catheterization with assay of samples has been of value in localization of tumors.

In brief, the surgical treatment includes careful exploration of all four parathyroids and removal of the adenoma or adenomas if present. If hyperplasia is discovered, three glands and a portion (usually one-half) of the fourth are removed. Postoperatively, a transient hypothyroidism may develop and require treatment for several days or weeks.

4. <u>Secondary Hyperparathyroidism:</u> In certain diseases such as renal disease with calcium wasting or in conditions which decrease calcium absorption from the intestinal tract as in rickets, the chronically lowered serum calcium results in increased secretion of parathormone. The compensatory response by the parathyroids may result in a chief cell hyperplasia. Here the compensatory increase in parathormone output occurs in response to a stimulus

(low extracellular fluid calcium concentration) while in primary hyperparathyroidism the secretion is uninfluenced by stimulation and the glands function in an autonomous fashion.

The signs of secondary hyperparathyroidism are therefore, the renal and bone changes secondary to excess parathormone secretion. Metastatic tissue calcification occurs much more commonly in the secondary type.

The treatment of secondary hyperparathyroidism depends upon removal of the cause. Parathyroidectomy has been suggested for those with renal failure who have developed severe bone pain. A few such patients have had dramatic relief.

5. Tertiary Hyperparathyroidism: In rare cases of secondary hyperparathyroidism the chief cell hyperplasia may become autonomous either as chief cell hyperplasia or with an adenoma, a situation then known as tertiary hyperparathyroidism. In the secondary disease if a cure is effected by removing the cause e.g. correcting the renal disease or improving calcium malabsorption or even by renal transplant for renal failure, then the lack of stimulus of low calcium concentration should result in the regression of hyperplasia and calcium levels should become normal. In tertiary autonomy after "cure" of the secondary state the calcium will rise to abnormal levels. The adenoma or seven-eighths of the hyperplastic tissue should be removed.

REFERENCES

1. Wells, C., Kyle, J., and Dunphy, J.E.: Scientific Foundations of Surgery, W.B. Saunders Co., Philadelphia and Toronto.

2. Symposium on Graves' Disease. Mayo Clinic Proceedings, 47: Nos. 11-12, 1972.

3. Schwartz, S.I.: Principles of Surgery, McGraw-Hill, New York and Toronto, 1969.

4. Wang, Ghiu-an: The Use Of The Inferior Cornu of the Thyroid Cartilage In Identifying The Recurrent Laryngeal Nerve. Surg. Gynecol. Obstet., 140:91, 1975.

5. Katz, Alfred D., and Zager, Warren J.: The Lingual Thyroid, Arch. Surg. 102:582, 1971.

6. DeGroot, Leslie J., and Ochi, Yukio: Long Acting Thyroid Stimulator of Graves' Disease. New Engl. J. Med. 278:718, 1968.

7. Lindem, Martin C., and Clark, John H.: Indications for Surgery in Thyroiditis, Am. J. Surg., 118:829, 1969.

8. Hamlin, Edward, Jr., and Vickery, Austin, L.: Struma Lymphomatosa (Hashimoto's Thyroiditis) New Engl. J. Med., 264:226, 1961.

9. Comings, David E., Skubi, K.B., Van Eyes, J., and Motulsky, Arno G.: Familial Multifocal Fibrosclerosis, Ann. Int. Med., 66:884, 1967.

10. Smith, Frederick, W.: The Case For Thyroidectomy For Nodular Goiter, Surgery, 65:503, 1969.

11. Hurxthal, Lewis M., and Heineman, Arthur, C.: Nodular Goiter and Thyroid Cancer, New Engl. J. Med., 258:457, 1958.

12. Kantounis, Stratos, and Brown, Lowell: The Thyroid Nodule, Am. J. Surg., 129:532, 1975.

13. Wooner, Lewis, B., Beahrs, Oliver H., Black, Marden B., McConahey, William M., and Keating, Raymond F.: Classification and Prognosis of Thyroid Carcinoma, Am. J. Surg., 102:354, 1961.

14. Beahrs, Oliver H., Sanfelippo, Peter M., and Hayles, Alvin B.: Indications for Thyroidectomy in The Pediatric Patient, Am. J. Surg., 122:472, 1971.

15. Mustard, Robert A.: Treatment of Papillary Carcinoma of the Thyroid with Emphasis on Conservative Neck Dissection, Am. J. Surg., 120:697, 1970.

16. Tollefsen, Randall, H., Shah, Jatin P., and Huvos, Andrew G.: Follicular Carcinoma of the Thyroid, Am. J. Surg., 126:523, 1973.

17. Block, Melvin A., and Horn, Robert C.: Medullary Carcinoma of the Thyroid: Surgical Implications, Arch. Surg., 96:521, 1968.

18. Thomas, Colin G. Jr., and Buckwalter, Joseph A.: Poorly Differentiated Neoplasms of the Thyroid Gland, Ann. Surg., 177:632, 1973.

19. Cope, O.: The Story of Hyperparathyroidism at the Massachusetts General Hospital, New Engl. J. Med., 274:1174, 1966.

20. Hunt, P.S., Poole, M., and Reeve, T.S.: A Reappraisal of the Surgical Anatomy of the Thyroid and Parathyroid Glands, Brit. J. Surg., 55:63, 1968.

21. Sherwood, L.M.: Relative Importance of Parathyroid Hormone and Thyrocalcitonin in Calcium Homeostasis, New Engl. J. Med., 278:663, 1968.

22. Black, W.C., III, and Utley, J.R.: The Differential Diagnosis of Parathyroid Adenoma and Chief Cell Hyperplasia, Am. J. Clin. Pathol., 49:761, 1968.

23. Egdahl, R.H., Canterbury, J.M., Reiss, E.: Measurement of Circulating Parathyroid Hormone Concentration Before and After Parathyroid Surgery for Adenoma or Hyperplasia, Ann. Surg., 168:714, 1968.

24. Krementz, E.T., Race, J.L., Sternberg, W.H. and Hawley, W.D.: Parathyroid Adenoma: Problems in Diagnosis and Management, Ann. Surg., 165:681, 1967.

CHAPTER 26

FLUIDS, ELECTROLYTES AND ACID-BASE BALANCE

BODY FLUID: The total fluid content of the human can be estimated on the basis of 60-70% of the body weight. The intracellular water represents 40-50% of the total weight. The circulatory blood volume may be estimated as 7% of the body weight in normal man and 6.5% in women. Thus in a 70 kg. man the various estimated volumes are:

Blood volume	-	4900 ml.
Intracellular water	-	32 liters
Total body water	-	49 liters

The maintenance of a normal circulating blood volume is all important to maintain the normal function of the heart as a pump and deliver adequate blood and nutrients to all organs but particularly to the lungs and kidneys for their regulatory functions.

Hypovolemia or decreased circulating blood volume may be recognized clinically by:

1. Decreased urinary output - less than 30 ml/hour with an increased specific gravity of the urine.
2. Low central venous pressure 0-5 cm. H_2O.
3. Increased pulse rate. Pulse may be soft and thready.
4. Decreasing systolic blood pressure.
5. Thirst and dry skin as it becomes well established.

The ill effects of the hypovolemic state are related to the lack of circulation to all systems but impairment of cardiac function and the development of metabolic acidosis are of greatest concern. Impaired tissue perfusion causes anaerobic metabolism of carbohydrates with formation of lactic acid and increased acidosis. Acute hypovolemic states may also precipitate acute tubular necrosis of the kidney.

The ideal treatment of the hypovolemic state is the replacement of the fluid that has been lost - not only in quantity but in quality. If hemorrhage is responsible then whole blood should be replaced. Other fluid losses should be replaced with solutions of similar electrolyte content. The speed of such replacement depends on the need.

Hypervolemia or increased circulating blood volume may be recognized by:

1. Increased urinary output of a dilute urine.
2. High central venous pressure - above 15 cm. and rising.
3. Ascites, basal pulmonary rales and peripheral edema.
4. Distended neck veins.
5. Bounding pulse; increased cardiac rate and blood pressure.

The ill effects of the hypervolemia are related primarily to the overloading of the heart with precipitation of failure and pulmonary edema. The local edema in operative wounds is undesirable because of impairment of healing and increased infection.

Treatment plans are adjusted on the apparent need to correct the overload. Simple withdrawal of intake may be sufficient but the use of diuretics, digitalization and phlebotomy may be indicated.

MAJOR ELECTROLYTES IN BODY FLUIDS: The electrolyte content of the intracellular and extracellular fluids are shown in the table:

Substance	Extracellular fluid (mEq/liter)	Intracellular fluid (mEq/liter)
Sodium	140	10
Potassium	4	150
Magnesium	1.7	40
Chloride	105	10
Bicarbonate	28	10
Phosphate and sulphate	3.5	150
Protein anions	15	40

The osmolality of the serum is an expression of the osmotic pressure capability of the ionic constituents of the serum and/or extracellular fluid generated against cell membranes. It is dependent primarily on the sodium ions and the anions, chloride and bicarbonate which accompany it with a significantly less contribution by glucose and protein. The urea diffuses so freely that it contributes very little to osmotic pressure. The normal osmolality of serum is about 285 milliosmoles/liter. The sodium ions provide about one half. The body regulatory mechanisms adjust to control the serum osmolality and not the level of serum sodium.

The composition of the intracellular fluids is quite different. The greatest ionic effect is provided by the high potassium and magnesium concentrations. The main anions within the cells are phosphate, sulfate and protein.

For all practical purposes the body cells maintain perfect osmotic balance between the intracellular and extracellular fluids at all times. Hypo-osmolality may be produced by either sodium depletion, potassium depletion or excess of water or a combination of the three. Hyperosmolality is produced by sodium or potassium excess or by body water depletion.

The control of the osmolality of the serum is accomplished by several factors. The intake and output of water is under CNS control. A small increase in the concentration stimulates the thirst center as well as production of antidiuretic hormone (ADH). The ADH acts on the distal tubules of the kidney causing water to be reabsorbed thus producing maximally concentrated urine. Fluid loss also occurs in sweating, via the lungs and gastrointestinal tract.

SODIUM: The control of sodium loss through the kidney is another powerful mechanism. The variation in the amount of sodium filtered through the glomerulus is influenced greatly by many factors, particularly circulatory factors. The resorption of the sodium in the distal tubule is controlled by the hormone aldosterone from the adrenal.

The aldosterone causes the cells of the distal tubule to conserve the sodium and excrete potassium. Although the body constantly secretes some aldosterone in a circadian rhythm the known stimuli include:

1. Changes in extracellular fluid volume including acute hemorrhage.
2. Diets low in sodium or high in potassium.
3. Acute heat stress.

Hyponatremia may develop with the following clinical derangements:

1. Loss from the gastrointestinal tract with vomiting, diarrhea, and fistulae. Excessive water loss also occurs.
2. Starvation states including prolonged surgical illness.
3. Cardiac, hepatic and renal diseases in which there is over-expanded extracellular fluid volume:
   a. Right sided heart failure.
   b. Cirrhosis of the liver with portal hypertension.
   c. Nephrotic syndrome.
4. Acute tubular necrosis or other renal states in which excess fluid has been given to encourage renal output.
5. Inappropriate secretion of anti-diuretic hormone after major surgical operations.
6. Certain malignant tumors produce anti-diuretic hormone resulting in water retention and sodium dilution.

Hypernatremia may occur under the following conditions:

1. Stuporous patient fails to take sufficient water.
2. Inadequate or inappropriate water replacement after operation. Solutions with high salt content given by tube feeding or intravenously may increase the obligatory urinary loss.
3. Renal disease states in which there is abnormal water loss.

POTASSIUM: Most of the body potassium is intracellular, only about 75 mEq. being in the extracellular fluid. The normal range in the plasma is 3.5 - 4.8 mEq/l. Daily urinary losses of 50 mEq are usual. The required intake averages 50-60 mEq/day. Unfortunately the plasma concentration doesn't give an accurate reflection of the intracellular concentration but is the best available for clinical use.

The greatest clinical effect of hypokalemia is muscle weakness. All muscles are affected, myocardial most severely and respiratory muscles minimally. The involvement of the intestinal musculature may be clinically manifested by gastric dilatation or paralytic ileus. Renal damage may occur with prolonged depletion. This is manifested by the inability of the kidney to concentrate urine by the absorption of water - tubular cells having been damaged.

Hyperkalemia is life threatening by its action on the heart. Muscle cells are depolarized and serious impairment of the conductive tissue results. There is a sudden onset of ventricular fibrillation. The heart stops in diastole. The voluntary muscles of the extremities may become painful and weak.

Common causes of hypokalemia:

1. Abnormal loss of gastrointestinal fluids - vomiting, aspiration, diarrhea, fistula, diseases with ulceration or malabsorption.
2. Loss of fluids in burns or other large granulating wounds.
3. Excessive urinary loss - many renal diseases, hyperaldosteronism, alkalosis and diuretics.
4. Metabolic disorders as diabetes mellitus, starvation and severe trauma.

Causes of hyperkalemia:

1. Renal failure.
2. Rapid hemolysis of red blood cells as in hemolytic crisis.
3. Dehydration - particularly with acidosis of diabetes.
4. Adrenal failure - lack of aldosterone secretion.

CHLORIDE ANION: The chloride in the body is the predominant anion in the extracellular fluid. The plasma chloride level is normally between 100 and 106 mEq/liter. Most of the chloride is in the extracellular fluid. The plasma concentration is obviously affected by the state of hydration and a high concentration may be due to water loss only. The primary role of the chloride anion seems to be related to the acid - base regulation exercised by the kidneys. Depending on the metabolic state and in order to have electrical neutrality the cations excreted in the urine must be balanced by anions, mainly chloride, bicarbonate and phosphate. Thus in a state of alkalosis with a high bicarbonate, the urinary loss of chloride will be reduced and the bicarbonate loss increases. This is one of the main methods of control of the pH of the blood.

The disease state resulting from the derangement of chloride concentration is invariably associated with other related metabolic problems - acute dehydration, hypokalemia, hyponatremia, etc. Symptoms or physiologic changes cannot be attributed to the abnormality of the chloride only.

Hypochloremia occurs frequently in surgical patients with:

1. An excess of water without loss of chloride due to action of anti-diuretic hormone after operation or similar stress.
2. Abnormal loss of fluid from the gastrointestinal tract - vomiting, diarrhea, fistulae, etc.
3. Renal losses - diuretics, kidney disease.
4. Chronic respiratory acidosis.

Hyperchloremia is a relatively uncommon clinical problem due to:

1. All forms of excessive water loss.
2. Operative procedures for urinary diversion into the colon. The resorption of the sodium and chloride results in hyperchloremic acidosis.
3. Administration of ammonium chloride to acidify the urine.

ACID-BASE BALANCE: The extracellular fluids are maintained at a pH of 7.4 or in close range thereto. This figure represents the hydrogen ion concentration or the acid ion in the balance. When there is neutrality in water the hydrogen ion concentration is $10^{-6.8}$ the same as the concentration of OH^-. The pH designation refers to minus the log of the hydrogen ion concentration; thus the pH = 6.8 at neutrality. The plasma pH of 7.4 means that the base is slightly in excess. In plasma the predominant bases are chloride and bicarbonate ions. Phosphate and protein ions are bases of lesser importance. Bicarbonate, phosphate and proteinate anions are buffer bases since they can modulate the effects of an increase in hydrogen ions by removing them from solution.

The measurement of the respiratory component of the acid-base balance is best accomplished by measuring the pCO_2 of plasma. A rise means that the carbon dioxide is not being cleared adequately by the lungs and a fall indicates excess removal. It may be complicated when metabolic changes also occur but it remains the best evaluation.

The kidney controls the concentrations of the acids other than the carbonic acid which is eliminated through the respiratory tract. The other acids are for the most part metabolic products of all types of foods. The kidney eliminates these products by various metabolic and excretory functions.

Respiratory alkalosis: This occurs as a result of excessive ventilation. The pCO_2 is low. It may be caused by:

1. Over breathing - either voluntary or involuntary
2. Involuntary excessive respiratory exchange - excessive blood ammonia or lesions of the central nervous system may stimulate the respiratory center.

If the compensatory mechanism does not operate quickly enough the pH will rise and symptoms of tetany will develop.

Respiratory acidosis: This occurs as a result of subnormal respiration. The blood pH is either low, or normal if compensated. It may be caused by:

1. Parenchymal disease of the lungs interfering with gaseous exchange.
2. Impairment of respiratory movements - as with drugs, muscle paralysis, fixation of chest wall by disease, chest wall trauma.
3. Deficient circulation through the lung by cardiovascular failure, embolism.
4. Inadequate respiratory exchange under anesthesia particularly with high oxygen concentration.

The ill effects of the acidosis are primarily cardiac arrhythmias, increased susceptibility to shock and increased vulnerability to drugs.

Metabolic alkalosis occurs commonly with:

1. Loss of chloride in prolonged vomiting, gastrointestinal fistulae, diarrhea.
2. Diuretics, particularly mercurials and chlorothiazide.
3. Excessive potassium loss with large bowel tumors.
4. Alkali overdosage as in ulcer therapy.

The significant loss of potassium which frequently accompanies the chloride loss is the chief concern of this metabolic state. The dehydration may also be of significance.

Metabolic Acidosis is one of the most common and serious derangements in the surgical patient. Frequent causes include:

1. Low blood flow with impaired tissue perfusion - shock, cardiac decompensation, hypovolemia.
2. Renal failure
3. Diabetes mellitus

The various metabolic processes produce acids which under normal conditions may be buffered and eliminated. With poor tissue perfusion anaerobic metabolism of carbohydrate produces an excess of lactic acid adding to the acid load which must be buffered by the bicarbonate buffer system. The lungs cannot remove the other acids produced in normal or abnormal metabolism. Only the normal kidney can effectively offer a complete control or resolution of metabolic acidosis.

The ill effects of the acidosis are the same whether the origin is respiratory or metabolic.

TABLE I

	pH	pCO_2	HCO_2	Rx
Metab. Acidosis	↓	↓	↓	HCO_2 ventilate
Metab. Alkalosis	↑	↑	↑	THAM
Resp. Acidosis	↓	↑	↑	Tracheotomy
Resp. Alkalosis	↑	↓	↓	5% CO_2

CHAPTER 27

HEMOSTASIS AND BLOOD VOLUME

When a blood vessel wall is damaged, hemostasis occurs as a result of interaction of platelets, plasma factors, the vessel wall and surrounding tissue. Defects or deficiencies of any of these can substantially interfere with adequate hemostasis. Pressure from surrounding tissue such as muscle, and constriction of the blood vessel wall, play a role but a minor one. However, activating factors are present in both the blood vessel wall and surrounding tissue which are very important in initiating coagulation. As a result of this activation, plasma factors and platelets play the most important role in hemostasis.

It appears that trauma to the vessel wall and surrounding tissue initiates an immediate reaction resulting in hemostasis, and additional control so that clotting is limited to the immediate area of trauma. The first reaction to damage to a blood vessel wall is the accumulation of a number of platelets forming a loose plug. This clumping which is referred to as platelet aggregation can be activated by adenosine diphosphate and can be measured. Aggregation is probably initiated by collagen fibers and later accelerated by ADP. After clumping, the platelets release a number of substances into the surrounding plasma including serotonin, calcium, ADP, ATP and possibly an antiheparin factor, as well as numerous enzymes. Table 27-I is a list of the presently identified plasma factors which are involved in production of fibrin. The Roman numerals were agreed upon to identify the different factors after a proliferation of synonymous names for each factor resulted in great confusion. All of these, except calcium, may potentially be so deficient that a bleeding disorder may result. Hemostatic plasma factors are present in an inactive state in circulating blood. In the method of their activation is the story of the formation of the fibrin clot. Coagulation is accomplished by two routes: an intrinsic system initially activated by exposure of the circulating plasma factors to collagen in the vessel wall similar to that described for platelets, and an extrinsic system activated by a tissue factor (thromboplastin).

Table 27-II[1] outlines the sequence of events of coagulation initiated through the intrinsic and extrinsic pathways. The activation of Factor XII principally by collagen fibers[2] results in further activation of XI by the active XII, and then in the presence of minute amounts of calcium the rest of the intrinsic sequence occurs. The phospholipid involved in the conversion of Factor X to activated X and prothrombin to thrombin is provided in the intrinsic system by platelets and in the extrinsic system by the tissue factor itself. Thrombin plays a potent role in accelerating the breakdown of platelets and in further accelerating a number of the other steps in the intrinsic pathway. Factor XII can also be activated by exposure to glass and this is the principle upon which the whole blood clotting time is based.

TABLE 27-I

NOMENCLATURE AND SYNONYMS FOR COAGULATION FACTORS

Roman Numerals	Preferred Descriptive Name	Synonyms
I	Fibrinogen	
II	Prothrombin	
III	Thromboplastin	
IV	Calcium	
V	Proaccelerin	Labile factor, Accelerator Globulin (AcG) Thrombogen
VII	Proconvertin	Stable factor, Serum prothrombin conversion accelerator (SPCA), Autoprothrombin I
VIII	Antihemophilic factor (AHF)	Antihemophilic globulin (AHG), Antihemophilic factor A, Platelet co-factor I, Thromboplastinogen
IX	Plasma thromboplastin	Christmas factor, Antihemophilic factor B, Autoprothrombin II, Platelet co-factor 2
X	Stuart factor	Prower factor, Autoprothrombin C, Thrombokinase
XI	Plasma thromboplastin antecedent (PTA)	Antihemophilic factor C
XII	Hageman factor	Glass factor, Contact factor
XIII	Fibrin stabilizing factor	Laki-Lorand factor (LLF), fibrinase

(VI has been deleted by the Committee.)

CONTACT SYSTEM
XII —Surface→ XIIa
XI → XIa
Tissue Factor
+
VII —Ca++— "complex"
ACTIVATION OF FACTOR X
IX —XIa / Ca++— IXa
X —VIII, Ca++ / Lipid— Xa
PROTHROMBIN CONVERSION
Prothrombin —Xa, Lipid / V, Ca++→ Thrombin
FIBRIN FORMATION
Fibrinogen —Thrombin→ Fibrin monomer
FIBRIN STABILIZATION
FSF —Thrombin / (Ca++)→ FSF*
Fibrin monomer —FSF*→ Cross-linked fibrin

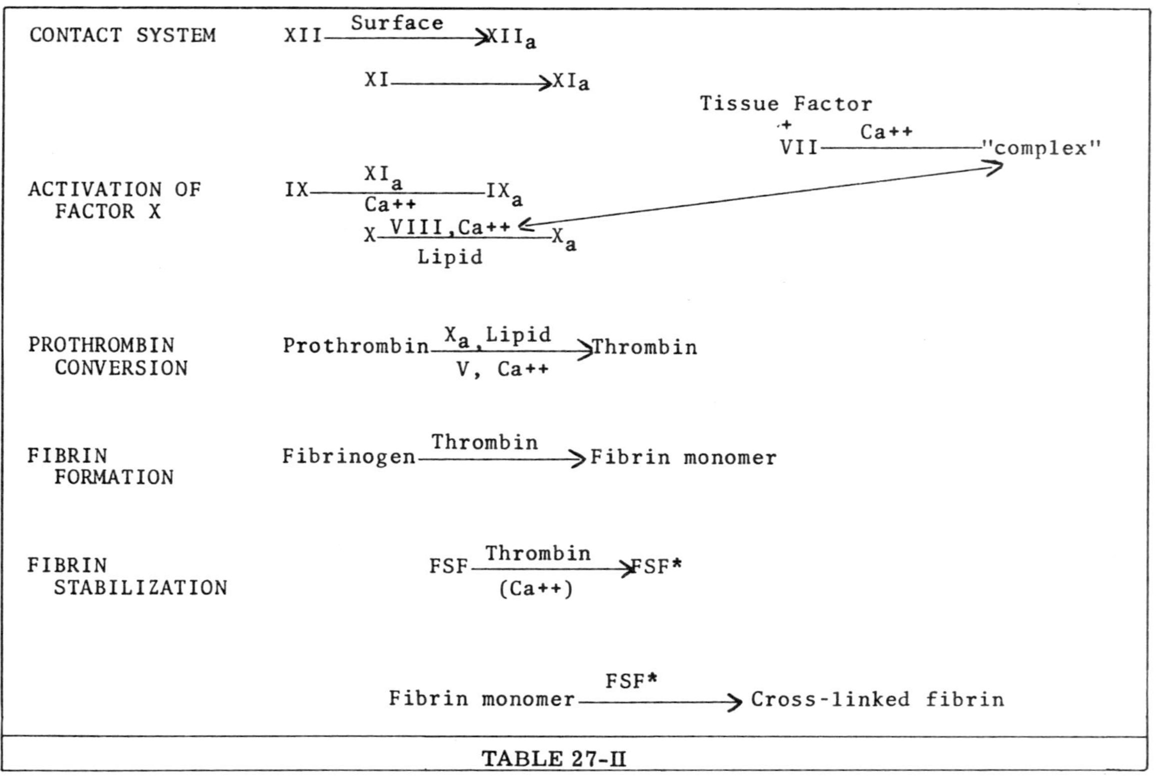

TABLE 27-II

TABLE 27-III

THERAPY OF CONGENITAL COAGULATION DEFECTS

DEFICIENT FACTOR	EFFECTIVE PLASMA LEVEL % NORMAL	THERAPEUTIC AGENT	LOADING DOSE	MAINTENANCE DOSE
			Per Kg.	Body Weight
I	50 (100 mgm/ml)	FFP *	25 ml	15 mgm. q.d.
		Cryoppt. ***	ppt. from 100 ml	ppt. from 14.20 ml. q.d.
			100 mgm	7-10 ml. q.d.
II	15-20	S. ** Plasma	10-15 ml bid	5-10 ml. q.d.
V	5-20	FFP	10-15 ml	10 ml. q.d.
VII	5	S. Plasma	5-10 ml	5 ml. q.d.
VIII	25	FFP	30 ml	15 ml. bid
			30 W	15 u. bid
		Cryoppt	ppt. from 70 ml	35 ml. ppt. bid
IX	15-20	S. Plasma	60 ml	7 ml. bid
X	15	S. Plasma	15 ml	10 ml. q.d.
XI	<10	S. Plasma	10 ml	5 ml. q.d.
XII	<10	S. Plasma	5 ml	5 ml. q.d.
XIII	2-3	S. Plasma	2-3 ml.	0

* FFP = Fresh Frozen Plasma
** S. = Stored
*** Cryoppt. = Cryoprecipitate

TABLE 27-IV

THE CLINICAL DISTINCTION BETWEEN DISORDERS OF VESSELS AND PLATELETS AND DISORDERS OF BLOOD COAGULATION

Findings	Disorders of Coagulation	Disorders of Platelets or Vessels ("Purpuric" disorders)
Petechiae	Rare	Characteristic
Deep dissecting hematomas	Characteristic	Rare
Superficial ecchymoses	Common; usually large and solitary	Characteristic; usually small and multiple
Hemarthrosis	Characteristic	Rare
Delayed bleeding	Common	Rare
Bleeding from superficial cuts and scratches	Minimal	Persistent; often profuse
Sex of patient	80-90% of hereditary forms occur only in males	Relatively more common in females
Positive family history	Common	Rare

The intrinsic system is capable of clot formation alone, but this occurs very slowly, taking as long as 20 minutes. When the extrinsic system participates also, a mere 12 seconds is required for the formation of a clot. This is the basis of The Quick I-Stage prothrombin time[3] in which thromboplastin is added to calcified plasma. The equivalent of activation of the extrinsic system occurs and the in vitro coagulation process is markedly accelerated. The "prothrombin complex", Factors II, V, VII and X are measured by the prothrombin time. The partial thromboplastin time[4] is performed by adding a synthetic platelet substance which simulates the activation of Factor XII and also provides the phospholipid necessary for later steps reproducing the intrinsic system.

The interaction between the intrinsic and extrinsic systems is not clearly understood, but it has been demonstrated that the combination of tissue factor (thromboplastin) and Factor VII may at times activate the intrinsic system also.

HEMORRHAGIC DISORDERS: Hereditary disorders of coagulation have been described relating to defects or deficiencies in Factors I, II and V through XII. By far, the most important, is Factor VIII deficiency, hemophilia A, (sex-linked recessive). Factors IX (Christmas disease, Hemophilia B, sex-linked recessive) and XI are the next most frequent with vonWillebrand's disease, while congenital deficiencies of the other factors are relatively rare. Factor XI deficiency (Hemophilia C) is autosomal recessively inherited and is very rare.

Although in some instances these diseases are the result of deficient synthesis of the particular compound, the majority of cases are due to defective synthesis. The result of the latter is a product which is enzymatically inactive or is incapable of being transformed into an active product. The severity of the disease depends upon the level of deficiency or the degree of defective activity. Table 27-III lists the effective plasma levels of the various substances and indicates the very small amounts of some that are necessary for effective clotting.

The clinical characteristics of Factor VIII deficiency have been extensively described, and in general, apply to all the other hereditary disorders when they are comparable in severity. As indicated in Table 27-IV deep hematomas and involvement of the joints are common. Delayed bleeding following surgical procedures or trauma is another characteristic.

von Willebrand's disease may very well be the most common of all bleeding disorders. No accurate figures are available concerning the incidence of this disease. It is characterized by a prolonged bleeding time and by a deficiency in Factor VIII. The clinical picture is similar to hemophilia. At one time it was thought that the prolonged bleeding time was due to either a vascular defect or a qualitative disorder of platelets. Subsequently, it has been shown that such is not the case, but that functional defects in the platelets occur in these patients. These defects and the prolonged bleeding time may possibly be due to an abnormality in a humoral factor which is apparently related to Factor VIII. Raising the Factor VIII levels in these patients satisfactorily controls bleeding. The treatment of Factor VIII deficiency and of individuals of vonWillebrand's disease is accomplished by the administration of cryoprecipitate or Factor VIII concentrate or fresh frozen plasma. Table 27-III lists an effective dose and time schedule for the management of all of these disorders.

ACQUIRED COAGULATION DISORDERS: The acquired coagulation disorders are more common than congenital ones. The synthesis of prothrombin and Factors VII, XI and X is dependent upon the presence of vitamin K. A deficient intake or absorption of vitamin K or the administration of drugs which antagonize the action of vitamin K (e.g. coumarin) will result in deficiencies in any or all of these four clotting factors with resultant bleeding tendency. Since these and most of the other clotting factors are synthesized in the liver, severe liver disease can also result in defects in coagulation, as well as in thrombocytopenia. Circulating anticoagulants which inhibit the action of just about every one of the clotting factors have been described. Individuals with lupus erythematosus frequently develop a coagulation inhibitor referred to as "lupus anticoagulant."

A recently recognized severe acquired bleeding disorder is disseminated or diffuse intravascular coagulation. As a complication of a wide range of infections, neoplasms, vascular disorders, tissue injury and obstetrical complications, both the intrinsic and extrinsic coagulation systems are activated, resulting in widespread clotting and fibrin deposition throughout the intravascular system. This coagulation is so widespread that all of the clotting factors and platelets are utilized more rapidly then they can be replaced, resulting in extensive and multiple coagulation factor deficiencies. As a result, there is extensive hemorrhage from all orifices, from recent phlebotomy sites and, in postoperative patients, generalized oozing from the operative site and bleeding from tubes, catheters and drains. The management of this particular acquired coagulation disorder requires first, control of the underlying disease process. While that is going on, two other approaches are possible. Since the bleeding problem is primarily due to excessive coagulation, many of these patients have been treated with heparin. If this course is to be followed, adequate anticoagulant therapy should be provided. Heparin can be given either every 4 hours in intermittent doses or as a continuous drip. An initial loading dose in the neighborhood of 10,000 units is advisable and thereafter the equivalent of 5,000 units every 4 hours at least. Most patients with DIC are in shock and severely anemic due to the loss of blood. Packed red cell or whole blood transfusions are, therefore, indicated. Thrombocytopenia is usually not severe enough to justify platelet concentrates. The most effective way to replace the plasma clotting factors is by the administration of fresh frozen plasma. A combination of such replacement therapy with or without heparin depending on the individual situation is probably the best management while the underlying pathology is being corrected. At one time, replacement therapy was felt to be contraindicated because it would increase the amount of fibrin deposits; however, many of these people, if not most, have an associated plasminogen activation resulting from the same factors which precipitate the clotting mechanism. This results in excessive plasmin formation and fibrinolysis, preventing the deposition of large amounts of fibrin.

As with DIC, the management of other acquired coagulation defects involves both replacement and correction of the underlying disorder. (Calcium levels low enough to produce coagulation disorders are incompatible with life).

THROMBOCYTOPENIC DISORDERS: The most common form of thrombocytopenia is idiopathic thrombocytopenic purpura (ITP). The acute form is most prominent in children following an antecedent infection. Petechial bleeding in the skin plus bleeding from the gums and the nose occur suddenly. The platelet count is usually below 20,000 and the bone marrow shows an increased production of megakaryocytes. This disease is usually self limited and rarely lasts longer than 6 to 8 weeks. In case of severe bleeding, steroid therapy is indicated to prevent complication until the remission occurs.

Chronic ITP occurs more commonly in adults with a female to male ratio of 3:1. It is not related to infection. The onset is insidious and may be recurrent over a period of years. Platelet counts are found sometimes below 20,000 resulting in spontaneous bleeding and at other times, about 50,000, but rarely if ever at normal levels. The bone marrow here also contains a megakaryocytic hyperplasia. On physical examination, except for purpura, there are no distinguishing findings. The spleen is so rarely enlarged that the findings of splenomegaly should raise a serious question of some other underlying disorder, such as a lymphoma. Steroid therapy over a short period of time can be used to control bleeding, but eventually most of these patients require splenectomy. Platelet survival time is greatly reduced and, therefore, platelet transfusions are of little value.

Thrombocytopenia is found very commonly in the course of many leukemias, of metastatic carcinoma, myeloma and other disorders which may invade and replace bone marrow. Pernicious anemia and severe iron deficiency anemia may also be accompanied by thrombocytopenia. Disorders of the spleen can stimulate that organ to destroy increased numbers of platelets resulting in peripheral thrombocytopenia and bone marrow megakaryocytic hyperplasia. Many infections are accompanied by thrombocytopenia. A variety of commonly used drugs can result in either toxic damage to the bone marrow or peripheral destruction of platelets resulting in severe thrombocytopenia. In those disorders in which no humoral factor is involved platelet transfusions are sometimes lifesaving.

THE DIAGNOSIS OF BLEEDING DISORDERS: A careful history is perhaps the most important diagnostic test. A history of excessive bleeding requiring transfusions following tooth extraction or a tonsillectomy or of delayed bleeding occurring 5 to 8 days after the procedure are strongly suggestive of a coagulation defect. A family history of bleeding disorders may be helpful. For all patients being prepared for surgery whether the history is suggestive or not, the preoperative laboratory workup should include a CBC, platelet count, prothrombin time, and partial thromboplastin time. If these are all normal, a significant coagulation defect is extremely unlikely and surgery may proceed. (The PTT and Prothrombin Time will detect over 90% of coagulation defects.) If an abnormality in the prothrombin time or partial thromboplastin time is found, individual factor assays should be done to determine the reason and appropriate replacement measures taken. If a thrombocytopenia is found, a bone marrow examination is indicated.

ESTIMATION OF BLOOD VOLUME: In the physiology laboratory it is possible to measure blood volume accurately with radioactive isotopes or with dye. However, in a clinical situation the following formulas will help the surgeon estimate the blood volume quickly.

1. Blood volume of children in cc = 7.5% to 8.5% of body weight in grams

2. Blood volume of adult male in cc = 6% to 7.5% of body weight in grams

3. Blood volume of adult female in cc = 5.5% to 7% of body weight in grams

For example: A 75 Kilogram male has:

$$\frac{7}{100} \times 75000 \text{ gm} = 5250 \text{ cc}$$

20% to 30% loss of total blood volume is significant and may need replacement. No blood or plasma transfusion is needed for any blood loss under 20% of total blood volume.

REFERENCES

1. Nemerson, Y. and Pitlick, F.A., pp. 1-37, Progress in Hemostasis and Thrombosis. Vol. 1, 1972.

2. Wilner, G.D., Nossel, H.L. and LeRoy, E.C., J. Clin. Invest. 27:2608, 1968.

3. Quick, A.J. Am. J. Med. Sci. 190:501, 1935, Am. J. Med. 246:517, 1963.

4. Proctor, R.R. Rapaport, S.I. Am. J. Clin. Path. 36:212, 1961.

5. Wintrobe, M.M., et al. Clinical Hematology, Vol. 7, 1974.

CHAPTER 28

MEDICATIONS

I. ANTI-HISTAMINE

Anti-histamine acts as a competitive antagonist by occupying the "receptor site" on the effector cells. It does not prevent the release of histamine nor does it destroy the histamine. The basic formula for anti-histamine is:

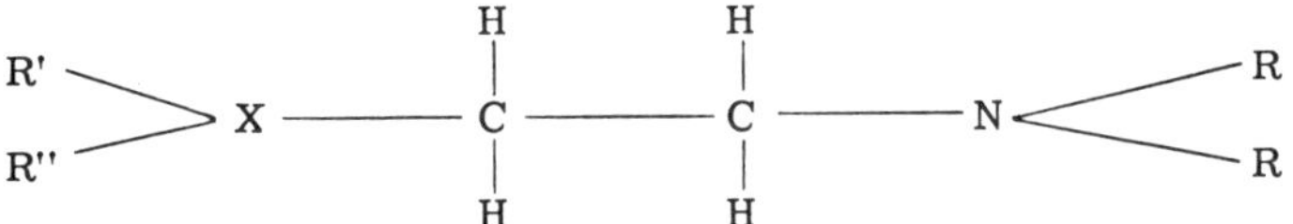

There are many derivatives sharing the same pharmacological action and side effects. In general, anti-histamine blocks the histamine effect on smooth muscles of the gastrointestinal tract and respiratory tract, inhibits the histamine vasoconstricting effect of major vessels and vasodilating effect of venules and arterioles. It also inhibits the increase in capillary permeability caused by histamine. Anti-histamine has no effect on gastric secretion secondary to histamine stimulation. Since it acts by competitive inhibition and has no direct effects on the smooth muscles of the vasculature or the bronchial muscles, it has little therapeutic benefits in anaphylactic shock. Anti-histamine also has no pharmacological effects on other autacoids and hence it is not used in the treatment of bronchial asthma.

Anti-histamine can either cause CNS depression or stimulation depending on the dose and the individual. Depressive symptoms include somnolence, lassitude and fatigue. The aminoalkyl ethers (e.g. diphenhydramine) are particularly prone to giving this side effect. CNS stimulative symptoms may include restlessness, nervousness, insomnia and focal seizures in patients with previous cerebral lesions.

Anti-histamine also suppresses motion sickness. The diphenhydramine, promethazine and piperazine derivatives are particularly effective in this regard. Promethazine and pyrilamine have mild local anesthetic effects.

All anti-histamines produce atropine-like activity giving rise to dry mouth, possible micturition problems and impotence. It is possible to experience blurred vision, diplopia, euphoria, elevated B.P., anorexia, constipation or diarrhea and epigastric distress from anti-histamines. Anti-histamines seldom cause allergic reactions although when used topically they may produce urticaria. Leukopenia and agranulocytosis have been reported. Piperazine compounds (e.g. cyclizine, chlorocyclizine, meclizine) have demonstrated teratogenic effects in experimental animals and hence should be avoided during pregnancy. Anti-histamine is usually contraindicated in patients taking MAO inhibitors.

When taken orally, anti-histamine's onset of action is about 15 to 30 minutes lasting 3 to 6 hours. It is metabolized mainly in the liver.

Acute poisoning particularly in children can be lethal. The patient may experience CNS stimulatory symptoms to include convulsions, ataxia, athetosis and hallucinations. He may then elapse into coma and cardio-respiratory arrest in 2 to 18 hours. Treatment of anti-histamine poisoning is supportive.

Commercial preparations have combined anti-histamine with decongestive medications (e.g. phenylephrine hydrochloride). Sometimes preparations contain stimulants such as caffeine to counteract the depressive effects.

TABLE I

Ethanolamines (Diphenhydramine)	Benadryl, Dramamine	4+ sedative effects 4+ atropine-like effects
Ethylenediamines (Pyrilamine)	Pyribenzamine	2+ sedative effects 4+ GI symptoms
Alkylamines (Chlorpheniarmine)	Chlortrimeton Dimetane	1+ sedative effects 2+ stimulation effects
Piperazines (Chlorcyclizine)	Cyclizine HCl Marezine HCl Meclizine HCl Bonine HCl	2+ sedative effects
Phenothiazines (Promethazine)	Phenergan	4+ control motion sickness

Drixoral contains Dexbrompheniramine maleate and d-isoephedrine sulfate.
Dimetapp contains Dimetane and vasoconstrictors (phenylephrine hydrochloride and phenyl-propanolamine).
Actifed contains Actidil (triprolidine HCl and Sudafed (Pseudoephrine HCl).
Ornade contains Teldrin (chlorpheniramine maleate) phenyl-propanolamine and isopropamide iodide (drying agent).
Ornex contains no anti-histamine. It has acetaminophen, salicylamide, caffeine, phenylpropanolamine.
(The rest can be found in the PDR)

II. ANTICHOLINERGIC DRUGS

This group of drugs is considered by some to be the best established agents for the prevention of motion sickness. The mechanism of action is blocking of acetylcholine from its receptor sites. This action produces both peripheral and central effects such as blocking of the parasympathetic system, depression of smooth muscle activity and depression of cerebral and medullary centers. Experiments with DFP (di-isopropylfluorophosphate, a potent anticholinesterase) provide evidence to suggest that the vestibular receptors are cholinergic.

Drugs in this category include scopolamine (hyoscine); atropine and the synthetic agents, (amphenadrine, cycrimine, and trihexyphenidyl). The most effective one is scopolamine. Scopolamine has less side effects than atropine and the synthetic belladonna drugs. A dose of 0.6 mg of scopolamine appears to be best for suppression of motion sickness with minimal side effects. The side effects are:

1. dry mouth
2. increase in pulse rate
3. drowsiness
4. headache
5. stomach awareness
6. nightmares
7. blurred vision
8. vertigo

The addition of 10 mg of d-amphetamine to 0.6 mg of hyoscine may decrease the side effect of drowsiness. The onset of therapeutic action is approximately one hour after the medication is given, the duration of action is approximately four hours.

III. PHENOTHIAZINES

This group includes prochlorperazine (Compazine), chlorpromazine (Thorazine), promethazine (Phenergan), perphenazine (Trilafon), trifluoperazine (Stelazine) and promazine (Sparine). Phenergan is the best in this group for controlling motion sickness. It can also be classified as an anti-histamine. It is also a hypnotic which means its side effect is drowsiness. The duration of action of phenergan is about six hours. An amphetamine can be added to combat the drowsiness.

IV. VASOCONSTRICTORS

1. EPINEPHRINE:
   a. It stimulates the sympathetic nervous system.
   b. It increases tone and vasoconstriction as evidence by marked pallor and shrinkage of the mucous membrane.
   c. It is vagolytic and antagonistic towards the parasympathetic nervous system.
   d. It is a bronchial dilator.
   e. Its onset of action is only a few minutes after subcutaneous injection. Its action lasts 1 hour.
      <u>Dosages:</u>
      0.05 cc to 0.1 cc infants
      0.15 cc to 0.25 cc up to 8 years old
      0.3 cc to 0.5 cc older children and adults
   f. It is irritating to nasal mucosa. Neosynephrine and ephedrine are less irritating.
   g. It cannot be given orally.

2. EPHEDRINE:
   a. It stimulates the peripheral sympathetic system and the CNS. It thus produces insomnia, palpitation and nervousness
   b. It can depress the heart giving rise to extrasystoles.
   c. It may cause urinary retention.
   d. It can be given orally.

3. NEOSYNEPHRINE: (Phenylephrine) is a synthetic ephedrine.

4. ISUPREL: (isoproterenol)
   a. It does not have the excitatory and pressor effects of epinephrine.
   b. It can be given sublingually, orally and it can be inhaled.
   c. Overdosage can cause bronchial spasm instead of bronchial dilation.

5. TOPICAL VASOCONSTRICTORS include:
   Propylhexedrine (Benzedrex)
   Naphazoline (Privine)
   Oxymetazoline (Afrin)
   Tetrahydrozoline (Tyzine)
   Xylometazoline (Otrivin)

V. STEROIDS

1. The adrenal cortex secretes:
   a. Glucocorticoids e.g. hydrocortisone
   b. Mineralocorticoids e.g. aldosterone
      1) Glucocorticoids have the following properties:
         (a) Increase gluconeogenesis
         (b) Decrease the sensitivity of tissues to the action of insulin
         (c) Increase protein catabolism
         (d) Increase diuresis of water
         (e) Delay wound healing
         (f) Retard growth centers
         (g) Inhibit formation of fibroblasts and tissue vascularization
         (h) Alter the union of Antibody and Antigen
         (i) Increase the plasma level of oxidase enzyme which degrades histamine.
         (j) Suppress the secretion of ACTH from the anterior pituitary gland.
      2) Mineralocorticoids have no anti-inflammatory properties and cause Na retention and K secretion: e.g. Aldosterone.

2. Clinically, it is better to administer glucocorticoids than ACTH because the patient may be allergic to the ACTH extract and further ACTH depresses pituitary function.

3. When indicated, the use of corticosteroids should not replace the use of epinephrine since corticosteroids are not effective till 60 to 120 minutes after administration even when given IV.

4. Normal daily secretion of glucocorticoids is 20 mg. of cortisone a day or 5 mg. prednisone a day.

TABLE 28-II					
	Trade Name	Relative Dosage	Anti-Inflam-matory Properties	Cushingoid or Gluconeo-genic	Na Retention
Hydrocortisone	Solu Cortef Cpd F.	20 mg	1	1	1
Cortisone	Cpd E	25 mg	0.8	1	1
Prednisone		5 mg	3-5	5	0.8
Prednisolone	Delta Cortef	5 mg	3-5	5	0.8
Triamcinolone	Aristocort Kenacort	4 mg	20	20	0
Dexamethasone	Decadron	0.75 mg	20-30	20	0
Methylpred-nisone	Medrol or Solu Medrol	4 mg	10	10	0
Betamethasone		0.6 mg	25	20	0

VI. ANTIBIOTICS

1. COMPETITIVE ANTAGONIST: e.g. Sulfonamide is a structural analog of PABA and PABA is needed for Folic Acid Synthesis in the bacteria.

2. INHIBITION OF CELL WALL SYNTHESIS: e.g. Penicillin, Keflin, Bacitracin, Vancomycin, Novobiocin, Cycloserine.

3. INHIBITION OF CELL MEMBRANE FUNCTION: e.g. Polymyxin on Gram negative organisms, Polyene on Fungi.

4. INHIBITION OF PROTEIN SYNTHESIS: e.g. Chloramphenicol, Tetracycline, Streptomycin and Erythromycin.

5. INHIBITION OF NUCLEIC ACID SYNTHESIS: e.g. Actinomycins and Griseofulvin.

6. Sulfonamides: Bacteriostatic
   - Penicillin: Bacteriocidal in high concentrations and bacteriostatic in low concentrations.
   - Cephalosporin: Bacteriocidal
   - Streptomycin: Bacteriocidal
   - Tetracycline: Bacteriostatic and Rickettsiostatic
   - Chloramphenicol: Bacteriostatic
   - Bacitracin: Bacteriocidal (when used systemically, it is toxic to the kidney causing tubular and glomerular necrosis).
   - Neomycin: Bacteriocidal
   - Kanamycin: Bacteriocidal
   - Polymyxin B and E: Bacteriocidal (Colistin)
   - Vancomycin: Bacteriocidal
   - Erythromycin: Bacteriostatic or Bacteriocidal
   - Lincomycin: Bacteriostatic or Bacteriocidal
   - Cleocin: (Clindamycin) Bacteriostatic or Bacteriocidal

7. Sulfa drugs and H. streptococcal infections can give rise to secondary anemia.

8. Phenylalanine helps to combat the agranulocytosis encountered in patients receiving chloromycetin.

9. Tetracycline potentiates the hypoglycemic effects of oral hypoglycemic agents.

10. Benemid (Probenecid) inhibits the tubular secretion of penicillin thus increasing the plasma levels.

11. Lincocin may cause severe diarrhea with blood and mucous in the stool. Fatal colitis may ensue. The same applies to cleocin.

12. Chloromycetin may cause aplastic anemia, hypoplastic anemia, thrombocytopenia and granulocytopenia. There are reports of aplastic anemia following administration of chloromycetin that terminated in leukemia. Blood dyscrasias have been reported following short and long term therapy.

VII. OTOTOXICITY

1. SALICYLATES: Salicylates cause a reversible hearing loss and tinnitus. It has been postulated that salicylates exert an uncoupling action on oxidative phosphorylation. They inhibit various transaminases and dehydrogenases. In humans, discontinuation of high doses of the drug will cause the salicylate level to fall as the drug is excreted and the hearing reverts to normal within 24-72 hours. No histological changes have been demonstrated. To get toxicity, 6 to 8 gm. per day have to be taken. Salicylates are rapidly metabolized in tissues and approximately 50% of it is eliminated in 24 hours. Within 48 to 72 hours all salicylates would have been excreted in the urine.

Twenty mg% or higher of salicylates serum level will cause hearing loss. The higher the serum level (up to 50 mg%) of salicylate, the greater the hearing loss.

2. DIHYDROSTREPTOMYCIN: Dihydrostreptomycin can cause severe and erratic hearing loss even as long as 2 months after the medication has been stopped. The hearing loss is unpredictable and not dose related. Since this drug has no advantage over streptomycin sulfate, it should never be used. In the United States, it has been taken off the market.

3. STREPTOMYCIN: Streptomycin sulfate causes vertigo prior to the onset of tinnitus and hearing loss. Its affinity for the vestibular over the auditory system has been capitalized to treat intractable bilateral Menière's Disease. For this purpose an average dosage of 2 gm a day is given until no caloric response is obtained upon stimulation with ice water.

The vestibular toxic effect of streptomycin sulfate is dose related. 1 gm Q.D. for 10 days does not give vestibular symptoms. However, 2 gm Q.D. for 14 days has been reported to give vestibular symptoms in 60 to 70% of the patients.

Fifty to sixty percent of streptomycin sulfate is excreted unchanged by the kidneys in the first 24 hours. The larger the dose the faster the excretion by a normal kidney. Hence, any renal impairment will build up the serum level very fast. A very small amount is secreted by the liver to be excreted through the G.I. tract.

Peak plasma level is detectable within 1 or 2 hours after IM injection and diminishes by about 50% in 5 hours. The antibiotic can be detected in the plasma for at least 0 to 12 hours after administration. Recommended doses for children are 15-30 mg/kg/day.

Histological findings following ototoxicity due to streptomycin are:

a. Minimal scattered loss of outer hair cells in the upper basal turn of the cochlea. Normal supporting cells.
b. Severe damage to the sensory epithelium of the cristae of all canals. Severe hair cell loss and flattening of the sensory epithelium of the cristae and saccule. The utricular macula is involved but least so in the vestibular end organs.
c. Stereocilia in the canal ampullae are swollen and are twice their normal diameter.

4. KANAMYCIN: Kanamycin may not be as ototoxic as neomycin. However, in patients with poor renal function, its administration has to be justified and the minimal dosage necessary used. In adults with good renal function, 15 mg per kg per day will cause no hearing loss, or a mild loss.

Kanamycin is poorly absorbed orally. IM administration of 1 gm yields a peak plasma level of 20 to 35 μ g/ml in about 1 hour. In 12 hours, the level falls to 1.2 μ g/ml. Fifty to eighty percent of this drug is excreted by the kidney in 24 hours. In patients with normal kidney function, repeated injections of Kanamycin should not lead to accumulation of the drug. Kanamycin is nephrotoxic as well.

Histological findings following ototoxicity due to Kanamycin are:

a. Destruction of inner and outer hair cells. The latter are believed to be destroyed first. A more severe hair cell degeneration is found in the basal turn, the apical turn being less involved.
b. The supporting cells are usually not altered. Hence, neural degeneration is insignificant.
c. Normal semi-circular canal cristae and maculae of the utricle and saccule.

5. NEOMYCIN: Neomycin is not absorbed well topically or orally. Therefore, using Neomycin orally to sterilize the bowel carries little risk of ototoxicity. However, repeated use of Neomycin over inflamed GI mucosa has caused irreversible deafness.

Five to eight grams given parenterally over 4 to 6 days have caused tinnitus and irreversible hearing loss. A 1 gm parenteral dose will give a plasma level of 20 μ g per ml for 6 to 8 hours. Neomycin is secreted by the kidneys. Hence, when renal disease is present, Neomycin should be withheld due to its potential for nephrotoxicity.

Neomycin, dihydrostreptomycin, and Kanamycin are eliminated more slowly from the inner ear than from the rest of the body, resulting in delayed ototoxicity. Hearing loss as a result of Neomycin ototoxicity may occur as late as 1 to 2 weeks after the drug is stopped. The following histological findings have been noted in Neomycin ototoxicity:

a. Destruction of inner and outer hair cells, the outer ones being slightly less involved. Apical and basal turns are both involved, the basal turn being more so that the apical turn.
b. Some destruction of pillar cells is present with some atrophy of the stria vascularis.
c. A minimal loss of Deiter's cells and Hensen's cells.
d. Maculae and cristae remain normal.

6. ETHACRYNIC ACID: This diuretic has been demonstrated to cause destruction of the intermediate layer of the stria vascularis and outer hair cells of the Organ of Corti, most severe in the basal turn. The hearing loss can be transient or permanent.

7. QUININE: Quinine is readily absorbed when taken orally. Ninety-five percent of the drug is metabolized in the liver so no untoward effects are feared in the event of renal disease. Most of the drug is excreted in 24 hours. The usual dosage is 0.3 to 0.6 gm Q.I.D. The ototoxic effects of Quinine are hearing loss and tinnitus, both of which are reversible. The ingestion of quinine in therapeutic doses may not give rise to hearing loss in the mother, but may affect the fetus,giving rise to severe bilateral sensori-neural hearing loss. Histologically, the external hair cells, and stria vascularis have been noted to be atrophied. The brain stem vestibular and cochlear nuclei have been noted to be normal. Taking chloroquinine in pregnancy is similarly hazardous to the fetus.

8. GENTAMICIN: Gentamicin affects the vestibular rather than the auditory system. If used at serum levels of 10-12 μ g per ml, it does not cause any ototoxicity. The recommended dosage is 1 mg per kg per day. In patients with renal damage, this dose should be adjusted.

9. NITROGEN MUSTARD: Nitrogen Mustard causes destruction of hair cells giving rise to sensory hearing loss.

10. OTHER OTOTOXIC DRUGS INCLUDE: Polymyxin B, Colistin, Viomycin, Vancomycin, Restocetin, Arsenicals, Oils of Chenopodium, Chloroform, Iodoform and Alkaloids (Strichnine, Opiates, Pilocarpine, Scopolamine), Tetanus Antitoxin.

VIII. NEUROLOGICAL MEDICATIONS

1. Dilantin (sodium diphenylhydantoin). It stabilizes seizure activities and prevents the spread of seizure activities.

2. Soma (Carisoprodol) is a muscle relaxant. It acts by blocking the interneuronal activity in the descending reticular formation and spinal cord.

3. Sansert (Ergotamine tartrate) selectively constricts cerebral vessels thus relieving the headache from cerebral vascular dilation.

4. Tegretol (Carbamazepine) is used for genuine Trigeminal neuralgia. Death from aplastic anemia (agranulocytosis, thrombocytopenia, leukopenia) has been reported. Its mechanism of action is unclear.

REFERENCES

1. Himwich, W.A., et al.: Isolation and Injection of Selected Arterial Areas of the Brain, J. Appl. Physiol. 15:303, 1960.

2. Physicians Desk Reference (PDR) 30th Edition, 1976, Medical Economics Company, Oradell, New Jersey.

3. Schuknecht, H.F.: Pathology of the Ear, Chapter 4, Page 183, Boston, Harvard University Press, 1974.

4. Wood, C.D. and Graybiel, A.: The Antimotion Sickness Drugs, The Otolaryngologic Clinics of North America, Vol. 6: No. 1, Ed. Wolfson, R.J., February, 1973, W.B. Saunders, Philadelphia.

CHAPTER 29

BASIC INFORMATION ON FLAPS AND GRAFTS

SKIN GRAFTS: (Figure 29-1)

1. Thiersch graft = 0.008" to 0.010"
2. Split-Thickness graft = 0.010" to 0.018"
3. Dermal graft = dermis only
4. Full-Thickness graft = epidermis + dermis

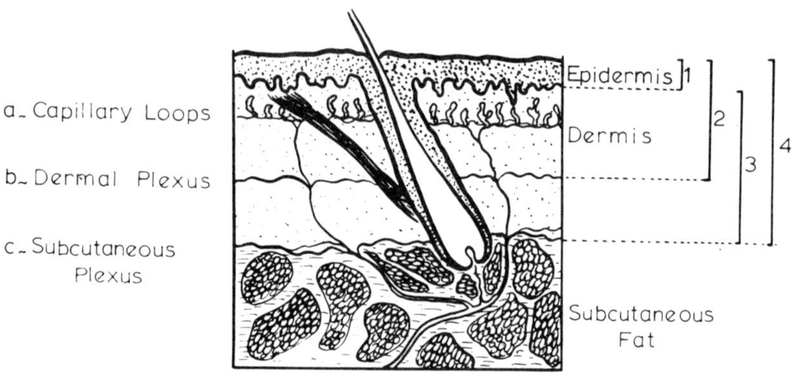

Figure 29.1. Diagrammatic Cross Section of the Skin.

A. THIERSCH AND SPLIT THICKNESS GRAFTS:

Advantages:

1. High percentage of take
2. Donor site heals without a graft
3. Gives excellent immediate cover

Disadvantages:

1. No tensile strength
2. Poor color match
3. Contraction on healing
4. Lacks bulk

B. FULL-THICKNESS GRAFT:

Advantages:

1. Less contracture
2. Better color
3. Greater bulk

Disadvantages:
1. Small areas
2. Poorer take

C. DERMAL GRAFT:

Advantages:
1. Strong - will take in irradiated tissue
2. High resistance to infections

Uses:
1. For carotid artery cover following neck dissection in irradiated patients.
2. For pharyngeal suture line cover in irradiated patients.

PHYSIOLOGY OF GRAFT NUTRITION:

0 - 12 hrs.	Plasma circulation, nutrition to graft by imbibition of exudate from host bed.
12 - 24 hrs.	Inosculation - direct connection of graft and blood vessels.
24 - 48 hrs.	Host vessels grow into graft.
48 hrs. on	Peripheral cellular union of graft and host with epithelialization.

Plasmatic circulation works as follows: the hydrostatic pressure at the capillary end of the skin's capillary-venule glomerulus drives crystalloids through the inter-endothelial cement substance into the tissues where they become tissue fluid. This tissue fluid flows between the fibers of collagen and elastin, embedded in mucopolysaccharides of the ground substance. To re-circulate or to return to the donor circulation, the tissue fluid can do so by lymphatic circulation or by the blood circulatory system directly. An open wound does not have a plasmatic circulation and hence the tissue fluid escapes through the portal of the wound and is not re-circulated. A wound covered with a skin graft permits restoration of vascular and tissue fluid balance, returning plasmatic and hemic circulation to normal.

Hemic circulation of the graft depends on capillary buds that grow from the donor towards the graft's circumference by seemingly purposeful orientation. Blood flow can be detected microscopically in new capillary buds by the 4th day.

Once the transplant has a vascular purchase on the host bed, peripheral cellular union of graft and host is accomplished by epithelization. The rate of epithelization is about 0.5 mm. per day.

VASCULARIZATION AND GRAFT TAKE DEPENDS ON:

1. Healthy host bed with adequate blood supply
2. Adequate fixation and immobilization
3. No infection
4. Graft over bone or cartilage requires intact periosteum or perichondrium

CAUSES OF FAILURE OF GRAFT TAKE:

1. Graft
   a. Tension
   b. Inadequate immobilization
   c. Inaccurate approximation of graft to host bed and the margins

2. Host Bed
   a. Infection
   b. Poor hemostasis (hematoma seroma)
   c. Fibrosis of bed
   d. Irradiation of host bed
   e. Lack of perichondrium or periosteum over cartilage and the bone

MAJOR FLAPS IN HEAD AND NECK RECONSTRUCTIVE SURGERY:
(Pedicle Flaps)

Classification:

Forehead
Medially-based Chest Flap
Laterally-based Chest Flap
Nape of Neck

Definition: Pedicle Flap (Vascular attachment to the body at all times by transferred tissue)

Basic Concepts:

1. Based on arterial supply
2. A flap is an island. The width of the base of the flap is unimportant beyond the necessity to contain a vascular pedicle.
3. Tubing of flap is useful if only the distal portion is used in the transfer (Prevents infection and granulation)
4. Delay of flaps:
   a. Decision based on need.
   b. Will increase chances of survival.
   c. Effects dermal and subdermal vessel hypertrophy and hyperplasia with a 7-14 day delay.
   d. Allows greater length of flap for use.
5. Transfer of blood supply from graft site to distal useful end of flap -- approximately 14 days.
6. Flaps die of congestion, rarely from anemia.
7. The patient's blood pressure, hemoglobin and hematocrit are vital to flap survival.
8. A clean, well-vascularized bed required for transfer.
9. No tension at suture line.
10. No twisting of pedicle or pressure on pedicle allowed or impairment of flap circulation will occur.

ADVANTAGES AND DISADVANTAGES OF THE FLAP:

1. Capable of carrying tissues other than skin.
2. Carries its own blood supply, therefore, more likely to "take".
3. Less tendency to discolor, more resistant, more elastic, more movable, and less likely to contract. (Although a 25% leeway should be kept in mind in the planning of a pedicle flap).
4. More adaptable to weight bearing.
5. Capable of bridging a defect.
6. Can be used on a host bed of questionable nutrition.
7. No pressure dressing necessary.
8. One disadvantage is that it usually needs many stages.

FOREHEAD FLAP:

Arterial Base: Superficial temporal artery and postauricular artery. (Note: flap can be based on scalp vessels should the external carotid be tied in a previous major procedure).

Delay: Rarely necessary but can be achieved by isolation and ligation of the supratrochlear and supraorbital vessels on both sides.

Uses: Buccal cavity, oropharynx, hypopharyngeal reconstruction, chin and neck skin reconstruction.

Methods of Entry:

1. Beneath or above the zygoma
2. Through a cheek incision to the buccal cavity.

Disadvantages: Cosmetic deformity.

Special Uses: A bipedicle bucket handle forehead flap for chin reconstruction.

Donor Site: Closed by immediate or delayed skin grafting.

SPECIFIC FOREHEAD FLAPS:

1. Forehead Island Flap: The flap is based on the supraorbital or supratrochlear artery. It is a full-thickness skin flap with a subcutaneous pedicle carrying the artery. It is transferred subcutaneously and is used as a full thickness skin graft over the nasal bridge.

2. Indian Forehead Flap: It is based on the superficial temporal artery. It is used for nasal reconstruction. The disadvantage is a minor cosmetic defect. Closure of the donor site is with split-thickness skin graft.

3. Median Forehead Flap: Based on supratrochlear-supraorbital artery, its donor site is closed primarily.

MEDIALLY-BASED CHEST FLAP:

Arterial Base: Includes four perforated arteries of the internal mammary artery.

Delay: Advisable. Allows greater length and greater reliability.

Staged Delay: Increases length possibilities and reliability.

Uses: Buccal cavity, oro-hypopharyngeal and cervical esophageal reconstruction following major head and neck resections. Reliable, particularly following delay.

Donor Site: Closed with split-thickness skin graft, immediate or delayed.

LATERALLY-BASED CHEST FLAP:

Arterial Base: Acromiothoracic artery.

Delay: Preferable but not necessary. Will increase both length and reliability.

Disadvantage: Disfiguring in females (Nipple in the neck)

Uses: Buccal-oral cavity, hypopharyngeal and laryngopharyngeal reconstruction.

Donor Site: Covered by split-thickness skin graft, immediate or delayed.

NAPE OF NECK:

Arterial Base: Occipital artery.

Delay: Essential.

Uses: Neck skin replacement, cervical esophageal reconstruction, oral cavity and hypopharyngeal reconstruction.

Disadvantages: One of the least reliable of major head and neck flaps.

Donor Site: Covered with split-thickness skin graft, delayed or immediate.

THE USE OF FLAPS AND PHARYNGOSTOMES IN IRRADIATED PATIENTS: In using flaps for head and neck reconstructive surgery, careful planning is essential. Such planning allows preparation for possible complications. In initial surgery on irradiated patients, discretion is always the better part of valor. It is often desirable to create a pharyngostome to be sure of adequate carotid coverage and healing prior to planned reconstruction at a later date. Prepared delayed chest flaps with greater length and reliability prior to definitive surgery decreases the risks of failure of the flap on reconstruction.

TRANSPOSED, ADVANCEMENT AND INTERPOSED FLAPS:
Definition: Use of local viable tissue to close a defect, with simultaneous staggering of the inevitable scar line.

Types:
1. Z-plasty
2. Simple advancement
3. Bilobe advancement
4. V-Y closure

Advantages:
1. Viable graft tissue with excellent blood supply.
2. Tissue close to defect, subsequently excellent color and texture match.
3. Good scar camouflage.
4. Adequate thickness, hence less contracture.
5. Necrosis rare with correct planning.

Disadvantage: Limited by local available tissue.

Uses:
1. To correct contracted linear scar.
2. To reposition malposed tissue.
3. To close facial cutaneous defects.

Z-PLASTY:
Definition: Classically, the Z-plasty is based on a Z figure. The central limb and arms are of equal length. The arms are at opposite ends of the central limb and parallel. Therefore, the two angles so formed are equal.

Principle:
1. The greater the angle the greater the amount of gain. Inevitably, the greater the angle the more difficult the flap transposition.
2. In general, the 60° Z-plasty is the most widely used, giving good lengthening and a reasonable margin of safety for flap survival.
3. When faced with a long scar revision, multiple Z-plasties are preferable to large Z-plasties.
4. A 60° angle Z-plasty gives a 73% increase in scar length.

Uses:
1. To prevent scar contracture.
2. To change plane of scar.
3. To reposition poorly placed tissue.
4. To remove webbing.
5. To close cutaneous defects.
6. To remove "dog ears".
7. To augment tissue.
8. To correct defects at the commissure of the mouth, eye, etc....
9. To enlarge a constricting tracheostome.

COMPOSITE GRAFTS:

Definition: Graft which contains two layers of tissue, e.g. skin and cartilage.

Uses: Ear, nose, eyelid and trachea.

Principles:

1. Handle with care.
2. Always use sharp instruments when taking a graft.
3. Use no electrocautery to graft or vessel ligation.
4. Never allow the periphery of the graft to be at a greater distance than 1.5 cm from the center. The length is irrelevant.
5. Fine sutures (6-0) when suturing in place.

Bed:

1. To have well-nourished recipient site.
2. To have no infection.

METHODS OF INCREASING GRAFT SURVIVAL:

1. Cooling of graft to decrease metabolic requirements. This appears to allow increase in size of periphery to center of up to 2 cm.

Disadvantage: Edema of graft appears to last for a longer period of time.

2. Treatment of donor site with histamine dichloride.

3. Galvanic current stimulation to donor site one day prior to surgery.

REFERENCES

Shumrick, D.A.: Reconstructive Flaps in Head and Neck Surgery, The Otolaryngologic Clinics of North America, Edited by Ogura, J.H., Vol. 5:685, October, 1969, W.B. Saunders, Philadelphia.

Tardy, M.E., Jr.: Editor, Symposium on Reconstructive Plastic Surgery of the Head and Neck, The Otolaryngologic Clinics of North America, Vol. 5, October, 1972, W.B. Saunders, Philadelphia.

CHAPTER 30

ELECTROPHYSIOLOGICAL MEASURES OF HEARING AND BALANCE

The auditory and vestibular systems are such that it is possible to elicit an electrophysiological response from these systems and make quantitative measurements. The adequate stimulus for the auditory system is sound (pressure variations) and the adequate stimulus for the vestibular system is motion (e.g. visual tracking, whole body rotation and positioning, and caloric stimulation). Responses from such stimulations are presently being recorded electronically and have become part of a technique used in the assessment of auditory and vestibular disorders.

I. AUDITORY IMPEDANCE TESTING. (or impedance audiometry) is a technique used to test the functional status of the middle ear (including tympanic membrane) and certain neural pathways associated with the tensor tympani and stapedius muscles. Impedance testing may be divided into three areas: (1) tympanometry; (2) Eustachian tube function; and (3) stapedius muscle activity (acoustic reflex).

Acoustic impedance testing is based upon the principle that a change in mass or stiffness of the middle ear conductive system will cause a change in the impedance of the tympanic membrane, that is, the transmission properties of the middle ear change. Such changes may be observed by measuring the variation of sound pressure in the external auditory meatus when the external auditory meatus is heremetically sealed. Changes in the transmission properties of the middle ear will occur when the atmospheric pressure in the external auditory meatus is varied, or through contraction of the intra-aural muscles. The magnitude of the change will likewise be affected by existing middle ear conditions.

1. TYMPANOMETRY: (Figure 30-1) is a means of assessing middle ear compliance (mobility). This is accomplished by measuring the changes in sound pressure level at the tympanic membrane as a function of atmospheric pressure changes in the external auditory meatus. There are three types of tympanograms that have been classified according to abnormalities in the conductive system.

Type A: Normal Conductive mechanism. If the peak is reduced by more than half, but clearly present, then stapes fixation may be present.

Type B: Typical of fluid-filled ears and/or extensive ossicular fixation. This is characterized by a flattening of the curve with little or no peak present.

Type C: Demonstrates the presence of negative middle ear pressure. Occasionally there will be a slight amount of fluid. A valsalva maneuver should correct this condition if the Eustachian tube is functioning properly. Often times a Type C tympanogram will indicate initial or final stages of otitis media.

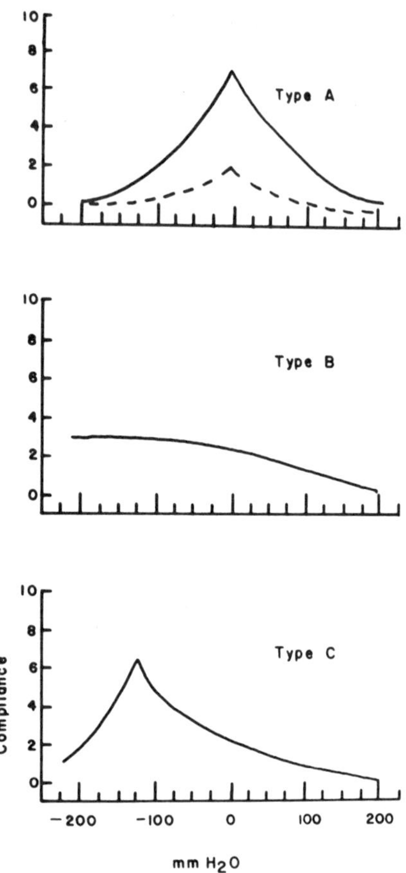

Figure 30-1. Type A, B, and C Tympanograms.

It is not unusual to see Type B or C tympanograms in patients who have normal hearing and no air-bone gap. This measure is not affected, nor dependent on, sensorineural hearing level. However, since it is assessing middle ear function, conductive losses are generally present with abnormal tympanograms.

2. STAPEDIUS REFLEX RESPONSES: may be elicited by acoustic or tactile stimulation. The stapedius reflex is a bilateral phenomenon. That is, if a stimulus causes the stapedius muscle to contract, (e.g. acoustic reflex testing) the muscle in both middle ears will simultaneously respond. Since, upon activation, the stapedius muscle changes the impedance of the middle ear, a change in sound pressure level of a probe tone in the external auditory canal will occur. For purposes of our discussion, the stapedius reflex will be activated through the use of auditory stimuli. In general, the contraction of the stapedius muscle in response to auditory stimuli is referred to as the acoustic reflex. The response characteristics are:

(A) Acoustic Reflex Threshold: The purpose of the acoustic reflex test is to determine the intensity at which the acoustic reflex is elicited, and whether or not it is present in both ears. The probe tone is placed in one ear and the reflex is stimulated with an auditory stimulus presented to the ear contralateral to the probe. The threshold of the acoustic reflex, depending upon the frequency of stimulation, will occur at an intensity level of 70 to 90 dB above auditory threshold for the respective auditory stimulus.

There are four possible results that may be obtained from this test: (1) the thresholds of the acoustic reflex may be elicited at normal levels; (2) the acoustic reflex may be absent due to the presence of middle ear pathology or the inability to stimulate the reflex at a high enough intensity level due to equipment limitations; (3) the threshold is elicited at a higher than normal intensity sensation level; and (4) the acoustic reflex is elicited at a lower than normal sensation level. Cochlear disorders may be suspected when the threshold of the acoustic reflex is 15 to 50 dB above auditory thresholds for the respective auditory stimulus. Although not a test of recruitment, the presence of a reduced sensation level for the threshold of the acoustic reflex is a common finding associated with recruitment, and found in cochlear hearing losses.

Except in the case where middle ear pathology is present, the ear under test is the ear in which the acoustic stimulus is presented; not the ear in which the probe is located. Consequently, if the test ear has an elevated threshold, the threshold of the acoustic reflex will be elevated. This occurs in both cochlear, retrocochlear and conductive hearing losses. Therefore, the presence of conductive hearing loss must be ruled out prior to the utilization of the acoustic reflex threshold test. The acoustic reflex will generally not occur in the presence of conductive pathologies for the probe ear, or, if the pathology is in the test ear, an elevated threshold will be noted. When the acoustic reflex has been stimulated at a lower than normal sensation level, it indicates the presence of cochlear involvement.

(B) Acoustic Reflex Decay: The acoustic reflex response, upon continuous stimulation, tends to decay at 2000 Hz and 4000 Hz in normal ears. However, at 500 Hz and 1000 Hz such decay does not occur in normal ears. Therefore, if the reflex decays to 1/2 amplitude at 500 Hz or 1000 Hz within a ten-second period at 10 dB above the threshold of the acoustic reflex, the test is positive and indicates a retrocochlear (8th nerve) disorder (Figure 30-2).

The test is administered in the same manner as described in the acoustic reflex threshold. That is, the stimulus is presented to the ear contralateral to the probe. Again, the presence of middle ear pathologies will invalidate this test.

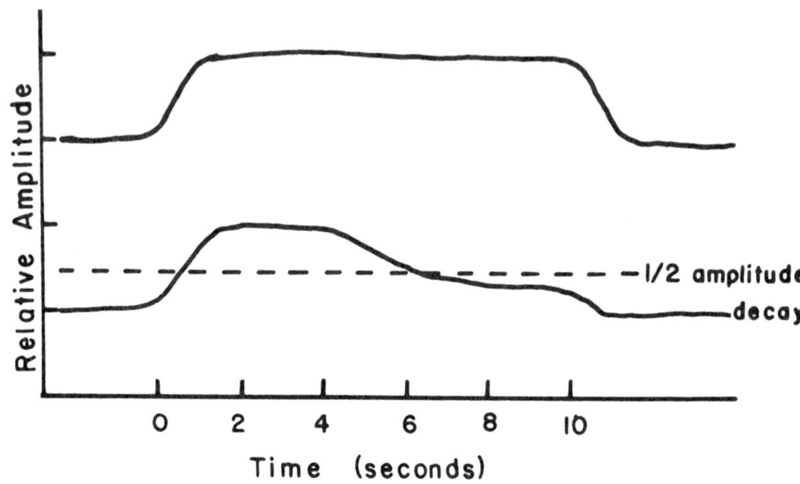

Figure 30-2. Relative Amplitude of Acoustic Reflex as a Function of Time.

(C) Ipsilateral Acoustic Reflex Test: This is the uncrossed acoustic reflex whereby the probe tone and stimulus are presented in the same ear. Excluding the presence of any middle ear anomalies there are three possibilities when the ipsilateral reflex is not elicited:

1) The ear under test has an 8th nerve disorder. This is highly suspect in the presence of acoustic reflex decay.
2) There is a contralateral facial nerve dysfunction, and pure tone thresholds are within normal limits for the ear under test.
3) There is a brain stem disorder. Additionally, pure tone thresholds are within normal limits and there is an absence of the acoustic reflex when stimulated contralaterally.

Although the contingency of pure tone thresholds within normal limits has been stated, it is possible for two conditions to exist (e.g. cochlear and retrocochlear involvement). Precise interpretations may only be done in light of contralateral stimulation and pure tone thresholds. For example, it is possible that a reflex is not elicited because the reflex threshold exceeds the limits of the audiometers or middle ear pathological conditions exist.

3. EUSTACHIAN TUBE TESTING: is most easily accomplished in patients with perforated tympanic membranes or myringotomy tubes. However, an indirect method of determining Eustachian tube function is also possible with intact tympanic membranes. The two most common methods are:

(A) Swallow test: The swallow test is accomplished (in patients with perforated tympanic membranes) by placing the probe in the ear and causing first a negative pressure of -200 mm H_20 in the external auditory meatus and then asking the patient to swallow small amounts of water. The test is then repeated using +400 mm H_2O. The change on the manometer is then observed and recorded for each successive swallow. In patients with normal Eustachian tube function pressure equilization should occur within a total of six swallows. The absence of the ability of the patient to perform this task is indicative of abnormal Eustachian tube function.

(B) Negative Peak Pressure: In patients with intact tympanic membranes, Eustachian tube malfunction may be suspected when a type C tympanogram is observed.

II. EVOKED RESPONSE AUDIOMETRY (ERA): is a means of recording the electrophysiological responses to auditory stimuli of the auditory system. Presently, three recording sites are used which include measurement of eighth nerve activity, brain stem activity and cortical activity.

1. GENERAL CONSIDERATION: Common to all three procedures are:
   A) The further the electrodes are placed from the nerve (or core conductor), the smaller the response amplitude seen at the electrode, and the longer the latency (frequently the latency parameter is the most stable measure).
   B) Amplitude decreases and latency increases as: 1) the repetition rate increases; 2) as intensity decreases; and 3) as frequency of stimulation increases (Figure 30-3 shows a typical waveform).
   C) Electrical and myogenic artifacts may influence the quality of recording. Also, they may be misinterpreted as actual responses by those not familiar with such electrophysiological recording techniques and procedures. ERA requires the use of an averaging computer. The abilities and resolution for each type of recording varies somewhat; however, equipment requirements are beyond the intent of this chapter.

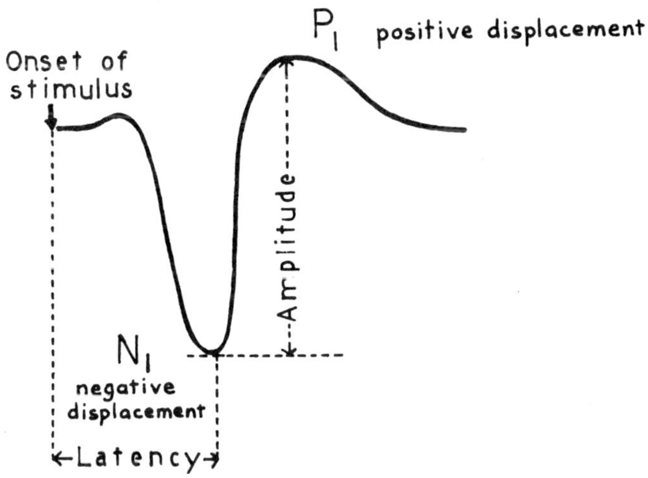

Figure 30-3. Typical ECOG Waveform.

2. ELECTROCOCHLEOGRAPHY (ECOG): relates to the measurement of the cochlear potentials (CP) and 8th nerve action potentials (AP). Presently, the AP is being used as a clinical measure of auditory function.

In addition to those previously mentioned, the following are specific considerations to ECOG:

a) Three electrode positions have been used and include: (1) a needle electrode on the promontory (transtympanic; (2) a ball electrode placed on or near the tympanic membrane; and (3) a vertex-mastoid disc electrode. The preferred electrode location is the transtympanic electrode. The ear canal electrode and vertex-mastoid electrodes may be used satisfactorily if the equipment is of superior quality. However, there will be a significant decrease in the recorded amplitude of the response and some increase in latency.

b) The latency of the first negative wave (N_1) occurs between 1.2 and 2.8 msec depending on: 1) repetition rate; 2) frequency of stimulation; and 3) intensity. Regardless of electrode location, latency measures have been found to be the most stable parameter (Figure 30-4).

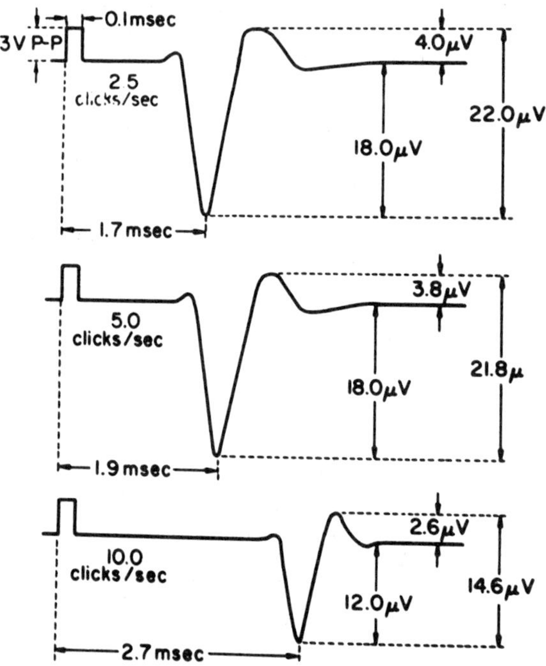

Figure 30-4. Amplitude and Latency Characteristics of the Whole Nerve Action Potential (ECOG).

c) Depending upon the electrode and stimulus parameter listed in 2-b the amplitude of individual response will be between 0.1 and 10.0 microvolts.

It is not possible to discuss absolute changes in magnitude of responses since each facility must establish its own normative data. However, the following trends relate to various pathologies:

d) Middle ear disease will cause a shift of amplitude and latency (see Figure 30-5 for example of normal function) equal to the shift in auditory thresholds. That is, if there is a 30 dB shift in auditory threshold, the amplitude and latency parameters of the N_1 will show a similar shift. As such, the most efficiency means of reporting the results is in reference to dB above threshold (dB SL).

e) Cochlear hearing loss may be similar to that described for middle ear pathology or, in many cases, a steeper growth of the intensity function seen in Figure 30-4 (similar to recruitment) may be observed. Qualitatively there may be some distortion of the waveform, but it is easily identified.

f) Eighth nerve disorders (space occupying lesions, demyelinization, etc.) are characterized by a sensitivity loss, little or no amplitude-latency growth and a qualitative broadening and flattening of the waveform. Frequently, there is no classical N_1-P_1 (first positive wave) but a shallow N_1 wave. Latency is increased with respect to the SL of the stimulus.

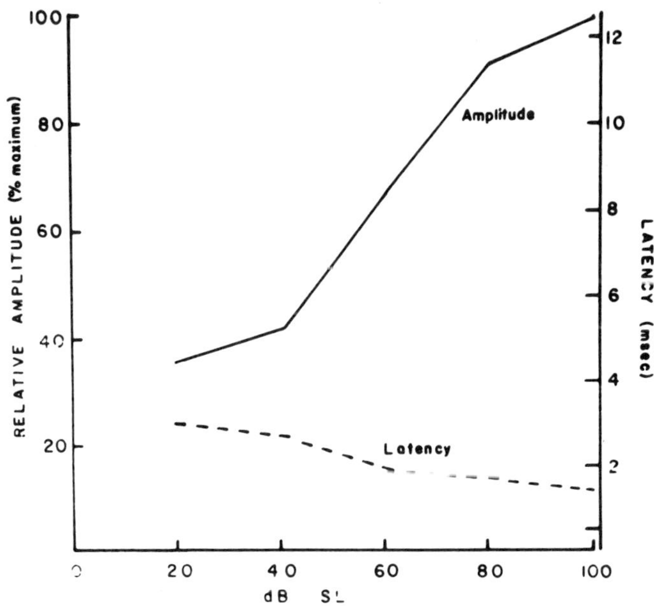

Fig. 30-5. Normal Growth Curve of the Amplitude and Latency of the Eighth Nerve Action Potential as a Function of Intensity Above Threshold.

3. BRAINSTEM EVOKED RESPONSE: (BER) audiometry refers to the recording of the auditory neural activity as it passes through the brainstem to the cortex. Although five waveforms are identifiable (wave I being the auditory nerve) wave V, being the brain stem response, is the most stable and consequently the one used for clinical measures. Waves II, III, and IV are not used for clinical measures.

a) Electrodes are used in a forehead-mastoid or vertex-mastoid configuration. The latency occurs between 6 and 10 msec depending upon stimulation rate and intensity. Since amplitude is quite variable between subjects, and latency much more stable, the latency-intensity function is used for clinical interpretation (Figure 30-5).
b) Middle ear anomalies influence these recordings in the same manner as discussed for ECOG (2-d).
c) Cochlear hearing loss influences these recordings in the same manner as discussed for ECOG (2-e).
d) Eighth nerve disorders (peripheral to the brainstem) are characterized by a sensitivity loss and flattening of the growth in the latency-intensity curve (see Figure 30-5). There will be an increase in latency with respect to the sensation level of the stimulus. There will be an elongation of the waveform but not to the extent noted for ECOG.
e) Brainstem disorders are characterized by an increase in latency. The waveform broadens and there is oftentimes no distinguishable peak.

4. CORTICAL EVOKED RESPONSE: first described in 1963 by Davis. It is a polyphasic waveform with latencies of P_1 occurring around 50 msec and N_2 occurring at about 300 msec depending upon stimilus parameters. Originally, this was thought to be a good means of assessing auditory threshold. However, the state of the subject (e.g. attention, sedation, etc...) affects these measures and it is not well suited for such assessment. Presently, it is being researched as a means to study certain auditory and non-auditory behavior (e.g. habituation, expectancy).

III. ELECTRONYSTAGMOGRAPHY (ENG): a technique used to objectively record eye movement (EOG) during vestibular testing.

1. CALIBRATION: critical for accurate reading of the ENG. Generally a 10 mm deflection for 10° of eye movement will give acceptable resolution. Linearity should be examined by comparing waveforms produced by 20° and 40° displacement. The waveforms should be essentially a square wave with twice the deflection noted on the recorder for twice the number of degrees displaced (Figure 30-6). Electrodes are placed as shown in Figure 30-7 and should have an impedance less than 50,000 ohms. The following order of testing provides for efficiency in administering the test:

2. SPONTANEOUS NYSTAGMUS: tested in the eyes closed condition for approximately 30 to 60 seconds with the head in the neutral (upright) position.

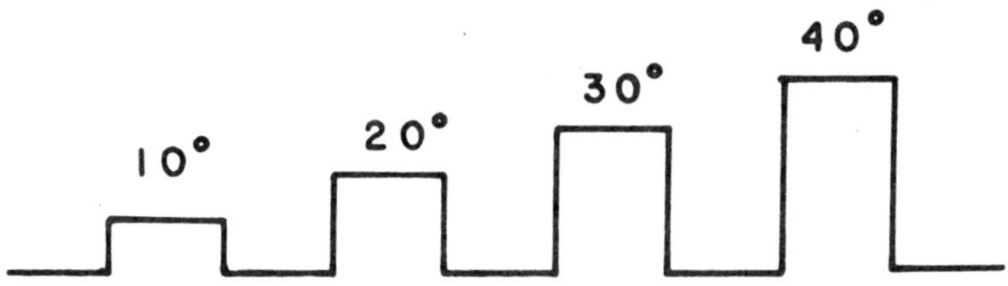

Figure 30-6. Calibration Waves for ENG at 10, 20, 30 and 40° Variation in one Direction.

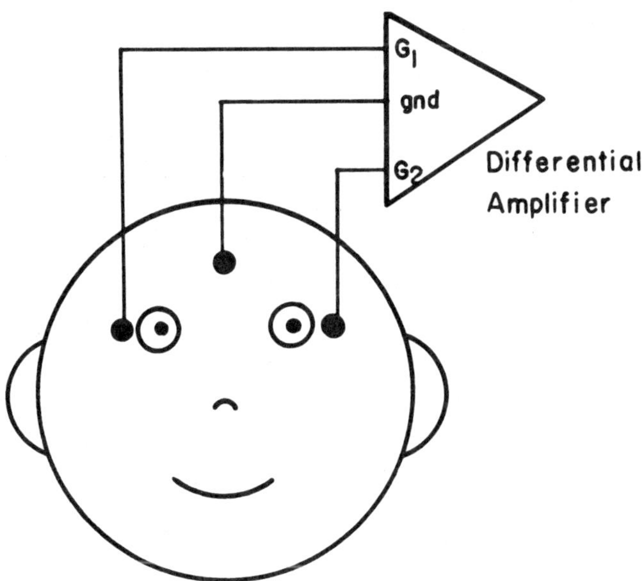

Figure 30-7. Electrode Placement Used in ENG Recordings.

3. GAZE NYSTAGMUS: tested in the eyes open condition with eyes placed at center, left 30° and right 30° for approximately 30 to 60 seconds. The head is in the neutral position. Results are presented as either gaze nystagmus present or absent in each position.

4. POSITIONAL NYSTAGMUS: testing is done in four basic head positions with the eyes closed. A recording is made for each position lasting approximately 30 to 60 seconds. Four common positions are head right, head left, head back and head down. Results are classified according to Aschan et al (1957) which is a modification of Nylen's classification.

Type I (persistent) nystagmus in one or more directions for some positions, and in the other direction for other positions and continues for 60 seconds.

Type II (persistent) nystagmus beats in the same direction regardless of position for 60 seconds.

Type III (transitory) diminishes within 60 seconds after the patient is placed in position.

Other test positions include (1) sitting, (2) supine, (3) right lateral, (4) left lateral and (5) head hanging.

5. OPTOKINETIC NYSTAGMUS: (OKN) occurs when the patient's visual field is centered on a moving pattern consisting of two extreme contrasts (usually black and white strips). The stimulus is moved at a uniform velocity for about 20 to 30 seconds and the direction reversed. The two trials are then compared and reported as symmetrical (normal) or asymmetrical (abnormal).

6. VISUAL TRACKING: or eye tracking is the eye movement caused by tracking a sinusoidal moving object (usually following a pendular path). There are four types of responses (Figure 30-8):

a. Type I Sinusoidal response.
b. Type II Disruptive and irregular tracking response.
c. Type III Sinusoidal but presence of saccadic activity noted.
d. Type IV inability to accurately track.

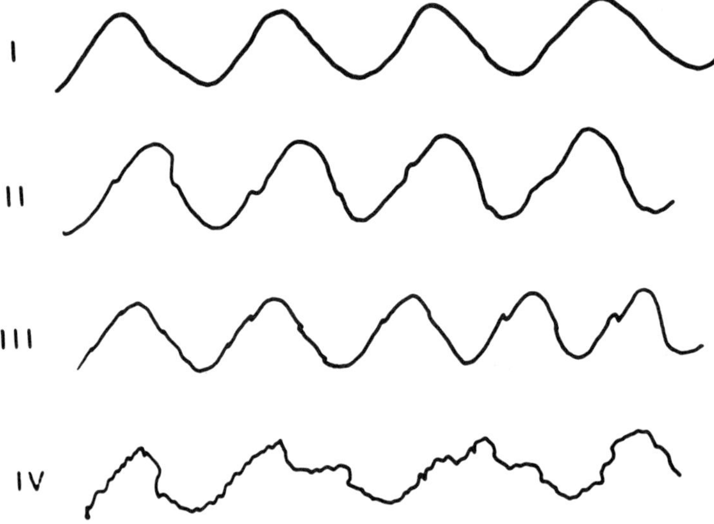

Figure 30-8. Waveform for Type I, II, III, and IV Eye Tracking.

7. CALORIC STIMULATION: (bithermal stimulation). The patient is placed in the supine position with the head elevated 30° placing the horizontal semicircular canal in a vertical attitude. Each ear is irrigated for 45-60 seconds at 30°C and 40°C. A 5 to 10 minute rest period is given between irrigations and between ears. (Figure 30-9) The slow phase of the nystagmus is used as a reference for quantifying and describing the results (this is true for all ENG measurements).

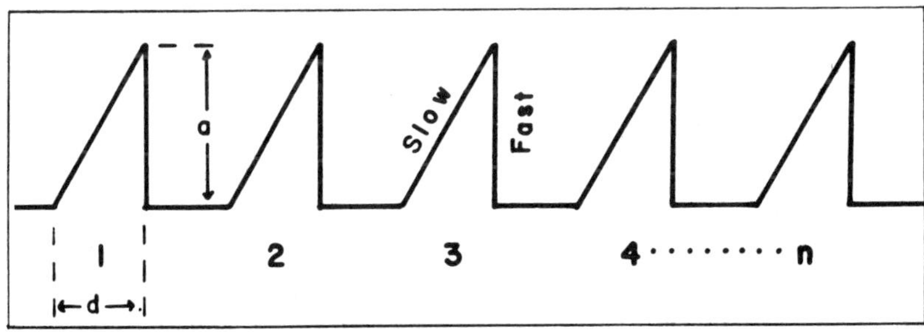

Figure 30-9. Schematized Waveform in Response to Caloric Stimulation

8. NYSTAGMUS: may be classified as left beating or right beating and is in reference to the slow component. Respective to caloric stimulation, the cold (30°C) stimulus will result in beats toward the non-stimulated side, and warm (40°C) stimulation will result in beats toward the stimulated side (COWS: Cold Opposite; Warm Same).

a. Slow component velocity (SCV) is the most stable and therefore most accepted response for clinical evaluation. The SCV is calculated by dividing the duration of each nystagmus (d) into the amplitude (a): scv = a/d

It is best to determine an average SCV or summed slow component (SSC) by measuring the total duration (d) and total amplitude (a) for a given number (N) of waveforms usually 10. Therefore:

$$\text{SSC} = \frac{\Sigma a/n}{\Sigma d/n} = \frac{\Sigma a}{\Sigma d}$$

and is in units of degrees/second.

b. Unilateral weakness (UW) is a comparison of the right ear vestibular response to the left ear vestibular response. It is calculated by:

$$\text{UW} = \frac{\text{SSC right ear - SSC left ear}}{\text{Total SSC}}$$

and this multiplied by 100 to obtain a percentage. In practice, the computation is:

$$UW = \frac{(RC + RW) - (LC + LW)}{RC + RW + LC + LW} \; 100$$

Where RC, RW, LC and LW are the SSC for right cold, right warm, left cold and left warm responses respectively. If UW is greater than 20% then there is a canal paresis on the weaker side.

c. Directional preponderance (DP) (left or right beating nystagmus) is a comparison of left versus right beating nystagmus:

$$DP = \frac{\text{Right beating SSC - left beating SSC}}{\text{Total SSC}}$$

and multiplied by 100 to obtain a percentage. In practice the computation is:

$$DP = \frac{(RW + LC) - (RC + LW)}{RC + RW + LC + LW} \times 100$$

If the DP is 30% or greater then there is directional preponderance towards the stronger beating direction.

9. CLINICAL INTERPRETATION: must be done in light of other clinical tests and patient history. However, Table 30-1 gives an overview of the possible clinical interpretations.

TABLE 30-1

	Peripheral	Central
1. Spontaneous Nystagmus	stronger with eyes closed than eyes opened	Vice versa
2. Positional nystagmus	Aschan Type III (may be Type II)	Type I (may be Type II)
3. Optokinetic	Symmetrical	Asymmetrical
4. Visual Tracking (questionable significance at this time)	Type I	Type IV
5. Caloric	Paresis	

REFERENCES

1. Bradford, L.: Physiological Measures of the Audio-Vestibular System. New York: Academic Press, 1975.

2. Jerger, J.: Clinical experience with impedance audiometry. *Archives of Otolaryngology*, 99, 409-413, 1974.

3. Jerger, J.: *Handbook of Clinical Impedance Audiometry,* New York: American Electromedics Corporation, 1975.

4. McPherson, D.: Impedance Audiometry. *Archives of Otolaryngology,* 93: 338-340, 1971.

5. McPherson, D., Miller, J. and Axelson, A.: Middle ear pressure: Effects on the auditory periphery. *Journal of Acoustical Society of America,* 59:135-142, 1976.

6. Rubin, W. and Norris, C.: *Electronystagmography*. Springfield: Charles C Thomas, publisher, 1974.

CHAPTER 31

MISCELLANEOUS INFORMATION

I. RELEVANT ANATOMY OF THE HEAD AND NECK

1. BLOOD SUPPLY TO THE TONSIL:
   a. Facial artery → tonsillar branch (most important).
   → ascending palatine branch
   b. Lingual artery → dorsal lingual artery
   c. Internal Maxillary artery → descending palatine and greater palatine arteries
   d. Ascending pharyngeal artery

2. BLOOD SUPPLY TO THE ADENOIDS:
   a. Facial artery → ascending palatine branch
   b. Ascending pharyngeal artery
   c. Internal Maxillary artery → pharyngeal branch
   d. Thyro-cervical trunk → ascending cervical branch

3. There are three dehiscences or weak spots through which an esophageal diverticulum can take place:
   a. Killian's dehiscence = between the cricopharyngeus and thyropharyngeus muscles.
   b. Lamier Hackeman's Space = between the circular and longitudinal fibers of the esophagus.
   c. Killian-Jameison Space = between the cricopharyngeus and the circular fibers of the esophagus.

4. CRANIAL NERVE CENTRAL CONNECTION:

<u>I Nerve</u> = subcallosal, hippocampal gyrus, uncus area. This first cranial nerve receives crossed and uncrossed fibers.

<u>III Nerve</u> = (a) Motor nucleus (also known as lateral nucleus, medial nucleus of Perlia) → extraocular muscles and levator palpebral superioris.
= (b) Edinger-Wesphal nucleus (parasympathetic nucleus, anterior medial nucleus) → ciliary ganglion → sphincter of iris and ciliary muscles.

<u>IV Nerve</u> = Motor nucleus (Crossed fibers only) → extra-ocular muscle.

<u>VI Nerve</u> = Motor nucleus (Uncrossed fibers only) → extra-ocular muscle.

<u>V Nerve</u> = (a) Semilunar ganglion (main sensory nucleus). (Gasserian ganglion) → somatic sensory fibers.
= (b) Mesencephalic nucleus → deep sense
= (c) Motor nucleus (crossed and uncrossed fibers) → for example, masticator muscles, tensor tympani, tensor palati muscle and anterior belly of the digastric muscle.

<u>VII Nerve</u> = (a) Motor Nucleus (crossed for lower face, crossed and uncrossed for upper face)
= (b) Superior salivary nucleus (nervus intermedius) ——→ parasympathetic secretory to submaxillary and lacrimal glands.
= (c) Tractus solitarius nucleus (geniculate ganglion ——→ taste and sensation).

<u>VIII Nerve</u> = Cochlear dorsal and ventral nuclei, vestibular, superior, spinal, medial, and lateral nuclei.

<u>IX Nerve</u> = (a) Ambiguus nucleus (motor) ——→ stylopharyngeus inferior salivatory nucleus ——→ Jacobson's nerve ——→ otic ganglion ——→ parotid gland. Tractus solitarius nucleus ——→ inferior ganglion (petrosal) ——→ deep sense and taste.
= (b) Sensory nucleus of the V nerve ——→ superior ganglion (jugular) ——→ somatic sensation.

<u>X Nerve</u> = (a) Nucleus Ambiguus (motor) ——→ soft palate and pharyngeal muscle.
= (b) (Nucleus Ambiguus ——→ XI Nerve bulbar portion ——→ joins the X nerve ——→ recurrent laryngeal nerve ——→ intrinsic laryngeal muscles).
= (c) Dorsal motor nucleus (parasympathetic) ——→ secretory fibers, regulates the heart rate and gastric peristalsis.
= (d) Sensory nucleus of V nerve ——→ jugular ganglion (superior) ——→ somatic sensation ——→ meningeal branch and auricular branch (Arnold's nerve).
= (e) Tractus solitarius nucleus ——→ nodose ganglion (inferior) ——→ taste and deep sensation.

<u>XI Nerve</u> = (a) Nucleus Ambiguus ——→ internal or medullary or bulbar branch ——→ joins the X nerve just outside the base of skull ——→ recurrent laryngeal nerve.
= (b) C_1 to C_6 ——→ external or spinal branch ——→ trapezius and sternocleidomastoid muscle.

<u>XII Nerve</u> = Hypoglossal nucleus ——→ intrinsic muscles of the tongue.

5. Cavernous sinus and superior orbital fissure syndromes - See Chapter 18. The superior orbital fissure transmits the ophthalmic vein, a branch of the middle meningeal artery, III nerve, IV nerve, frontal nerve of V_1, lacrimal nerve of V_1, nasociliary nerve of V_1 and VI. The inferior orbital fissure transmits the zygomatic nerve and sphenopalatine twigs to the lacrimal gland.

6. a. Superior constrictor muscle spans from the median raphe and the pharyngeal tubercle of the occipital bone to the pterygomandibular ligament, mandible and medial pterygoid plate.
   b. Medial constrictor muscle spans from the median raphe to the hyoid bone and stylohyoid ligament.

c. Inferior constrictor muscle spans from the median raphe to the oblique line of the thyroid cartilage, cricoid, and cricothyroid muscle.

7. The Uvula has five muscles:
   a. Palatopharyngeus (pharynx to soft palate)
   b. Palatoglossus (tongue to soft palate)
   c. Muscle uvula (posterior nasal spine to soft palate)
   d. Tensor palati (sphenoid, medial pterygoid plate, eustachian tube to soft palate).
   e. Levator palati (petrous, superior constrictor muscle, eustachian tube to soft palate).

8. The pterygomandibular raphe is between the buccinator and the superior constrictor muscles.

9. a. The ciliary ganglion is a parasympathetic ganglion. It receives preganglionic parasympathetic fibers from the Edinger-Westphal nucleus. The synapses are within the ganglion. The post-ganglionic fibers go to the ciliary muscles and the iris sphincter. It also receives the post-ganglionic sympathetic fibers on its way to the vessels within the eye. There is no sympathetic synapse within this ganglion. The nasociliary branch of V_1 carries sensation back to the central nervous system via the ganglion. There is no synapse for this sensory innervation within the ciliary ganglion.

b. The sphenopalatine ganglion is a parasympathetic ganglion. It receives its preganglionic parasympathetic fibers via the greater superficial petrosal nerve from the superior salivatory nucleus. The post-ganglionic fibers innervate the lacrimal gland via the zygomatic nerve. Sensory nerves of V_2 pass through it without any synapses. The sympathetic post-ganglionic nerve also pass through it without synapse.

c. The submandibular ganglion also has synapses for the parasympathetic. The preganglionic fibers are from the superior salivatory nucleus via the chorda tympani. The post-ganglionic parasympathetic fibers go to the submaxillary gland. The sensory fibers are V_3 and the post-ganglionic sympathetic fibers from the facial artery pass through it without synapses.

d. The otic ganglion also has synapses for the parasympathetics. The preganglionic fibers are mainly from the inferior salivatory nucleus via the Jacobson's nerve (branch of the IX nerve). A small contribution is from the superior salivatory nucleus via the lesser superficial petrosal nerve (branch of the VII nerve). The sensory branch of V_3 and the postganglionic sympathetic from the middle meningeal artery pass through this ganglion without synapses.

10. Foramina of the base of the skull and their contents - See Chapter 11.

11. The skull is made of cartilaginous as well as membranous bone. The cartilaginous bone contributes to:

a. occipital
b. sphenoid
c. ethmoid
d. mastoid
e. petrous

The membranous bone contributes to:

a. sphenoid
b. parietal
c. frontal
d. lacrimal
e. nasal bones
f. maxilla
g. mandible
h. palate
i. zygoma
j. premaxilla
k. tympanic ring
l. squamosa
m. vomer
n. bony modilus

12. The orbital walls are made up of maxillary bone, frontal bone, ethmoid bone, zygomatic bone, sphenoid bone and lacrimal bone. The lacrimal gland is in the zygomatic process of the frontal bone while the sac is in a fossa bound by the lacrimal bone and the frontal process of the maxilla. The zygoma has four processes:

a. frontal
b. maxillary
c. towards the temporal bone
d. to greater wing of the sphenoid

The maxilla has four processes:

a. frontal
b. zygomatic
c. palatine
d. alveolar

The mandible is the only facial bone capable of pathological fractures.

13. Eighty-five percent of superior thyroid arteries are derived from the external carotid artery while 15% of them are derived directly from the common carotid artery.

14. REFERRED OTOLGIA:

Hypopharynx = via jugular ganglion and Arnold's nerve of X.
Oral Tongue = via Gasserian ganglion and auriculotemporal nerve.
Base of Tongue = via petrosal ganglion and Jacobson's nerve.

15. RETROMOLAR TRIGONE:

Lateral (oblique line from the body of the mandible to the coronoid process)

Medial (extension of alveolar ridge to the coronoid process)

× Internal Alveolar nerve

Molar tooth

16. The true cord is 1.7 mm. thick

17. The parapharyngeal space is bound:
laterally by the mandible
medially by the buccopharyngeal fascia and the superior constrictor muscles.
superiorly by the base of the skull
inferiorly by the carotid artery

The great vessels, IX, X, XI, XII nerves are within it. The most common tumor within this are the neurogenic tumors.

18. The jugular foramen is bound by the occipital bone medially and the temporal bone laterally.

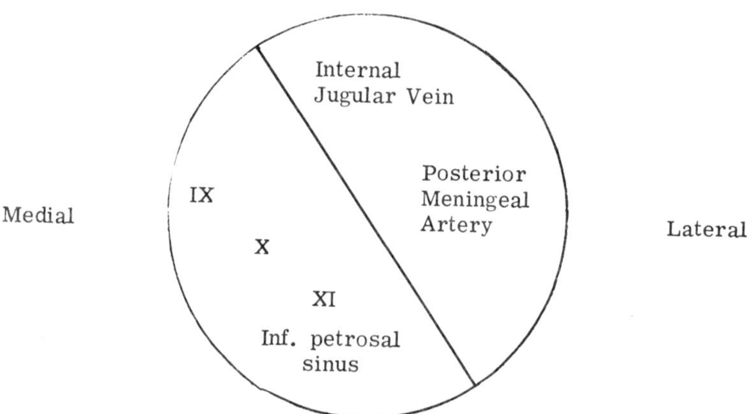

19. Scalenus anticus: anterior tubercle of transverse process of $C_{3,4,5,6}$ to first rib.

Scalenus medius: posterior tubercle of transverse process of $C_{1,2,3,4,5,6,7}$ to first rib.

Scalenus posticus: posterior tubercle of transverse process of $C_{4,5,6}$ to second rib.

20. Branches of the external carotid artery are:

a. superior thyroid artery which gives off the infrahyoid artery, superior laryngeal artery, sternomastoid branch, the crico-thyroid branch, a few glandular branches.

b. Lingual artery which gives off the suprahyoid artery, the dorsalis linguae branches and a sublingual branch.

c. the facial artery which gives off the ascending palatine artery, the tonsillar artery, glandular branches, submental artery, the inferior labial artery as well as the superior labial artery.

d. The occipital artery which gives off muscular branches to the surrounding muscles, descending branch, a meningeal branch, mastoid branch, auricular branch, and terminal occipital branches.

e. The posterior auricular artery which gives off stylomastoid artery, auricular branch, and the occipital branch.

f. The ascending pharyngeal artery which gives off pharyngeal branches, a small meningeal branch, and the inferior tympanic artery.

g. The superficial temporal artery which gives off auricular branches, small parotid branches, the transverse facial artery, the middle temporal artery, the zygomatic branch, the anterior branch and the posterior branch.

h. Maxillary artery which gives off the deep auricular artery, the anterior tympanic artery, the middle meningeal artery, the accessory meningeal artery, pterygoid branches, the buccal artery, the infraorbital artery, the greater palatine artery, the artery of the pterygoid canal, the pharyngeal branch and the sphenopalatine artery.

II. HISTOLOGY AND PATHOLOGY

As in the previous section, it is not the intent of this chapter to cover histology and pathology of the head and neck. It merely highlights the areas that may be appropriate in this type of synopsis.

1. LINING EPITHELIUM:

Middle ear	= non-ciliated cuboidal epithelium in general, though in the area near the eustachian tube orifice, the epithelium may be ciliated cuboidal.
Eustachian tube	= pseudostratified ciliated columnar epithelium with goblet cells.
Mastoid and epitympanum	= pavement epithelium without cilia.
Endolymphatic duct and proximal portion of the sac.	= villous and lined by columnar epithelium
Distal sac	= smooth and lined by cuboidal epithelium

NOSE:

a. Lower 2/3 of the septum lateral wall below the superior turbinate.	= respiratory epithelium (pseudostratified ciliated, columnar epithelium with irregular basal cells and goblet cells) (Schneiderian epithelium).
b. Upper 1/2 of the septum lateral wall above superior turbinate and "roof" of the nose.	= pseudostratified, non-ciliated, columnar epithelium with serous glands of Bowman. Bipolar olfactory cells as well as supporting and basal cells.
c. Vestibule	= stratified squamous epithelium with some glands.

NASOPHARYNX:

a. upper 1/2	= ciliated columnar
b. lower 1/2	= non-keratinizing epidermoid epithelium.

Paranasal sinuses and nasolacrimal duct	= respiratory epithelium
Between the oral pharynx and nasopharynx	= transitional cells
Oropharynx and laryngo-pharynx	= stratified squamous epithelium
Palatine tonsils	= squamous epithelium
Adenoid	= ciliated columnar epithelium
Lingual tonsil	= squamous epithelium (striated muscular fibers are usually seen in the specimen)

LARYNX:

a. true cord, false cord, upper 2/3 of epiglottis, aryepiglottic folds.	= non-keratinizing stratified squamous epithelium
b. the rest	= pseudostratified ciliated columnar epithelium

(Mucous glands are found in the ventricle, saccule, posterior surface of the epiglottis, and margin of the aryepiglottic folds).

Trachea and bronchi	= pseudostratified ciliated columnar epithelium with goblet cells
Upper 2/3 of the esophagus	= stratified squamous epithelium with inner circular muscular layer and outer longitudinal muscular layer
Lower 1/3 of the esophagus	= villous type of columnar epithelium with the same muscular layers.

2. Antoni Type A: This arrangement is found in neurogenic tumors. The cells are arranged in palisade or picket fencelike arrangements with the formation of the so-called Verocay bodies. These cells are delicately intertwined with connective tissues and reticular fibrils.

Antoni Type B: This has a less orderly architectural formation. The Schwann cells are haphazardly dispersed within the loose reticular fibrils and small cystic spaces. This is also found in neurogenic tumors. (Neurogenic tumor is the most frequently found benign primary tumor in the parapharyngeal spaces).

3. Learn to differentiate between hemangioma, pyogenic granuloma and hemangiopericytoma.

4. AMELOBLASTOMA: (See Chapter 17) Histologically, it consists of a meshwork of interlacing wide strands and island of epithelial tumor cells in a moderately cellular connective tissue stroma. The periphery is lined with palisading large cells, columnar or cuboidal.

5. Warthin-Finkeldey giant cells are found in the lymphoid tissues in measles.

6. Actinomyces are frequently found in tonsillar specimen. These are considered saprophytes with little clinical significance.

7. Chordoma (neuroectodermal cell origin) has physaliferous cells. Chordoma is not radiosensitive.

8. Granular cell myoblastoma can give rise to pseudoepitheliomatous hyperplasia in the larynx. Three percent of granular cell myoblastoma progress to malignancy. (In order of decreasing frequency of involvement: tongue, skin, breast, subcutaneous tissues, respiratory tract).

9. INVERTED PAPILLOMA: (Schneiderian papilloma, transitional cell papilloma, Ewing's papilloma or Cylindrical cell papilloma) The cells are rich in glycogen. Thirteen percent of nasal inverted papilloma progress to malignancy; even the histologically benign category is locally invasive. It usually arises from the lateral nasal wall rather than from the septum. Treatment of choice is wide excision through a lateral rhinotomy approach.

10. Mixed tumor is the most common parotid tumor in the general population, next is the mucoepidermoid tumor. Seventy-five percent of mucoepidermoid tumors are clinically benign. In children, mucoepidermoid tumors or lymphangioma are more common than mixed tumor in the parotid.

11. Rhinoscleroma has Mikulicz's cells and Russell fuchsinophile bodies. It can also give rise to pseudoepitheliomatous hyperplasia of the larynx. The treatment of choice is presently sulfonamides and antibiotics (streptomycin or tetracycline). The causative agent is Klebsiella rhinoscleromatis (von Frisch's bacillus). The primary site is the anterior nares. There are 3 stages in this disease: 1st: atrophic, 2nd: nodular, 3rd: stenotic.

12. The Reed-Sternberg cell is found in Hodgkin's Disease but not in lymphosarcoma or reticulum cell sarcoma.

13. Tympanosclerosis is a hyaline-fibro-sclerotic lesion due to a nonspecific degenerative inflammatory process.

14. Children with Idiopathic Respiratory Distress Syndrome (Hyaline Membrane Disease) lack a surface active material called surfactant. The major component of surfactant is alpha-lecithin.

15. Some etiologies for hypocalcemia:
Hypoparathyroidism
Malabsorption
Renal failure
Acute pancreatitis
Hypoproteinemia

Hypercalcemia:
Hyperparathyroidism
Milk-alkali syndrome
Vitamin D intoxication
Sarcoidosis
Multiple myeloma
Metastatic diseases

Increased alkaline phosphatase activity implies:

a. Osteoblastic activity
b. Liver disease
c. Paget's disease
d. Fracture
e. Osteosarcomas
f. Carcinoma of the prostate
g. Metabolic bone diseases

16. Thyroid adenoma may present as a calcified mass in the neck. Papillary carcinoma of the thyroid may have "psammoma bodies". Medullary carcinoma of the thyroid gland has amyloid deposits and is thyrocalcitonia producing.

17. In fibrous dysplasia, the female is much more frequently afflicted than the male. The maxilla is the most frequently involved bone in the head and neck area, the next being the mandible, followed by the frontal bone. If the alkaline phosphatase level is increased in fibrous dysplasia, there may be early malignant changes.

18. Rhabdomyosarcoma is most commonly located in the orbit. Its cells are rich in glycogen content.

19. NOMA: gangrenous stomatitis - usually starts at the mucous membrane of the corner of the mouth or cheek and spreads to involve the entire lip or cheek. This is usually found in debilitated children. The micro-organisms found are: borrelia, staphylococci and anaerobic streptococci.

20. The most common benign tumor of the tonsil is squamous papilloma. Some investigators think this is precancerous.

21. PEMPHIGUS: This is an uncommon disease characterized by bullae and erosions of skin, mucous membrane, acantholysis, chemical alterations in blood and high mortality rate. The etiology is unknown. This disease affects all races but with a higher incidence in the Jewish population. The age of onset is between 40 and 60 years old. There are intercellular attachments. Nikolski's sign is present. (Firm pressure on top of an intact blister results in extension at the edges).

PEMPHIGOID: This is a chronic bullous disease of unknown etiology. The bullae are smaller, more tense and rupture less easily. Involvement of the mouth is less severe and less frequent than Pemphigus. The mortality rate is considerably lower. The bullae are subepidermal and acantholysis is absent.

22. Cherubism presents with painless, symmetrical swelling of the posterior mandible and rami. Radiologically, it shows well-defined multilocular radiolucencies sometimes containing displaced teeth. There is a familial tendency. Pathologically, giant cell reparative granuloma with hemosiderin deposits are noted. There is no bone formation and no evidence of fibrous dysplasia. It is a self-limiting disease which ceases as the child reaches puberty. Regression of the lesions and reshaping of the bone may leave minimal disfigurement.

23. RELAPSING POLYCHONDRITIS: (See Chapter 11). It can give rise to sensorineural hearing loss. There is an increased urinary acid mucopolysaccharide content.

24. MIKULICZ'S DISEASE: (See Chapter 14). There is an increased incidence of lymphoma and macroglobulinemia among these patients.

25. The most common submaxillary gland malignancy is "Adenocystic carcinoma".

26. Hereditary lipoid proteinosis most commonly affects the larynx; next (in order of decreasing frequencies) are mastoid, tongue, thyroid and nose.

27. The normal sweat chloride is less than 50 mEq per liter, the normal zinc level is 90 mg%.

28. Patients with mucoviscidosis often secrete trypsin in the stool.

29. The lymphatic drainage of the palate is towards the retropharyngeal nodes, subdigastric nodes and subparotid nodes.

30. Halisteresis = osteomalacia.

31. Ptyalism = excessive salivation.

32. Lead poisoning is characterized by abrupt onset of colic, constipation or diarrhea, anorexia, weakness, paralysis, coma and convulsions. The erythrocytes show basophilic stippling. The lead level is usually greater than 0.08 mg per 100 gm of whole blood. The urinary level is 0.15 mg per liter. There is also increased delta-amino-levulinic acid and coproporphyrin III in the urine as well as glycosuria. Radiologically there are linear radio-opacifications parallel to the growing bone or circling the ossification centers.

33. Localized compact osteoma is most common in the frontal sinus. Localized cancellous osteoma is more frequently found in the maxillary and ethmoid sinuses. Fibrous dysplasia is most commonly found in the maxillary sinus.

34. Hyperostosis frontalis interna is a form of localized dysplasia limited to the inner table of the frontal bone and occurring mainly in elderly females. Headache may be associated with it. Obesity, dizziness, psychological disturbances and inverted sleep rhythm may be seen. (The constellation of these findings is known as Morgagni-Stewart-Morel Syndrome).

35. HISTIOCYTOSIS X: (Lipoid dystrophies) (involves reticulo-endothelial system, skin, and skeleton).

<u>Types:</u>
Letterer-Siwe Disease: Affects infants and young children. Pyrexia, splenomegaly, hepatomegaly, lymphadenopathy, skeletal lesions, purpuric rash, secondary hypochromic anemia, usually fatal.

Hand-Schüller-Christian Disease: This is a less severe and more chronic form in children and young adults. Exophthalmos, diabetes insipidus secondary to involvement of the sphenoid is characteristic of this disease. 10% of these patients have triad consisting of diabetes inspidus, exophthalmos, and skull lesion. This disease carries a 30% mortality rate. Two percent of the patients present with seventh nerve weakness. Another finding is polyps in the external auditory canal. The treatment of choice is radiation.

Eosinophilic Granuloma: This is the least severe and it also is found in children and young adults. It is characterized by localized skeletal lesions of the temporal and frontal bones. Otological manifestation may include otorrhea, granulation tissues in the external auditory canal and facial weakness. The treatment is excision and curettage, steroids, and possibly radiation. This disease carries a good prognosis.

36. MUCORMYCOSIS: (See Chapter 11). It is caused by rhinocerebral phycomycosis.

37. Paralysis of the recurrent laryngeal nerve and the superior laryngeal nerve will cause a vocal cord to be in a cadaveric position. Paralysis of the recurrent laryngeal nerve alone will give rise to vocal cord in a paramedial position.

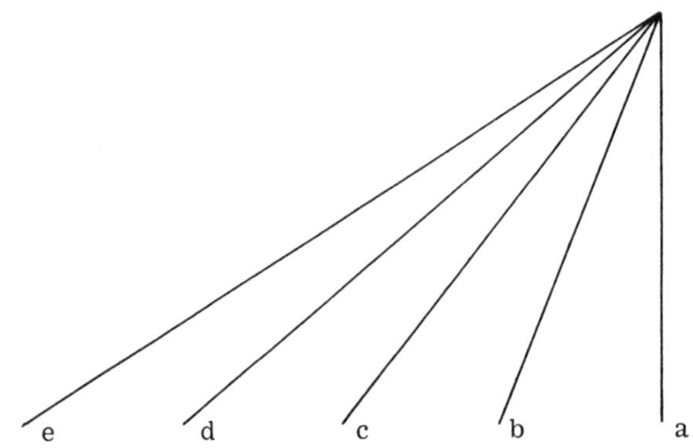

a-b = 3.5 mm	a = median position
a-c = 7 mm	b = paramedian position
a-d = 13.5 mm	c = cadaveric position or intermediate position
a-e = 19 mm	d = gentle abduction
	e = abduction

a = phonation b = whisper c = cadaveric d = quiet respiration e = deep inspiration

Ephemeral adductor paralysis is the same as mogiphonia which is stage fright aphonia. (For more complete discussion of paralysis of the recurrent laryngeal nerve, See Chapter 12).

38. The carotid body is more sensitive to changes in oxygen tension than to changes in carbon dioxide tension, while the respiratory center is more sensitive to carbon dioxide changes than to oxygen changes. Hypoxemia is defined as pO_2 below 40 mm Hg.

39. The least common type of tracheal-esophageal fistula and atresia of the esophagus is one in which the upper end of the esophagus forms a fistula with the trachea while the lower end of the esophagus is not connected to the upper end of the esophagus nor to the trachea, it is a blind pouch. For more discussion of T-E fistula, see Chapter 13.

40. The cricoid is the most common origin of cartilaginous tumor of the larynx.

41. Sodium buriate crystals are found in gout.

42. False positive serology may occur in:

a. malaria
b. leprosy
c. lupus
d. collagen disease in general
e. rheumatoid arthritis
f. measles
g. smallpox
h. hepatitis
i. infectious mononucleosis

False positive heterophile may occur in:

a. Serum sickness
b. Rheumatoid arthritis
c. Hodgkin's disease
d. Brucellosis
e. Hepatitis

43. Actinomycosis is treated with penicillin and tetracycline. Blastomycosis is treated with stilbamidine.

44. Olfactory neuroepithelioma = malignant tumor of the olfactory mucous membrane; peak age is 11-20 years old. Treatment is primary surgical excision and radiation for residual tumor.

45. Acanthosis nigricans is an uncommon dermatosis characterized by hyperpigmentation and epidermal hypertrophy. The malignant form is associated with internal cancer primarily adenocarcinoma. The benign juvenile form may be associated with metabolic disorders. Involvement is usually bilateral and symmetrical and exhibits a predilection for flexural and intertriginous areas.

46. The VIII nerve is covered with astrocytes and glial cells up to the entrance of the internal acoustic canal. Within the canal, the VIII nerve is covered with Schwann cells. Acoustic neurinoma arises from Schwann's cells and therefore theoretically acoustic neurinoma arises from within the internal auditory canal.

47. In order to be carcinocidal, the temperature for cryosurgery needs to be at least -160° to -180°C.

48. Desmoid tumors are most commonly found in the abdominal wall and extremities. They are locally destructive and the treatment of choice is wide excision. Recurrence rates varies from 40-70%.

49. The triad of coughing, choking, and cyanosis during feeding implies that the child has tracheo-esophageal fistula.

50. Etiologies for caseating necrosis include:
- a. tularemia
- b. brucellosis (20% of patients with brucellosis present with hearing loss as well).
- c. Tbc or atypical Tbc
- d. fungus

51. Atrophic rhinitis is caused by klebsiella ozena. Rhinosporosis is caused by rhinosporosis sebeeri or rhinosporosis kinealyi.

52. Calcified stylohyoid ligament occurs in 4% of the population.

53. Certain viruses have been incriminated as causing certain diseases:

RNA viruses = Picornavirus (enterovirus and rhinovirus)
Reovirus
Arbovirus (encephalitis, yellow fever, dengue fever)
Myxovirus (measles, mumps, flu, croup)

DNA viruses = Papovavirus (papilloma of nose, pharynx, and larynx)
Adenovirus (URI)
Herpes (zoster, simplex, cytomegalovirus)
Poxvirus

54. Most acquired choanal atresias are believed to be a result of tonsillectomy and adenoidectomy.

55. Keratotic papilloma = wart

56. Leukoplakia displays:
- a. parakeratosis
- b. hyperkeratosis
- c. dyskeratosis
- d. no pleomorphism
- e. no anaplasia
- f. no desmoplasia

57. Definition:

Metaplasia = change from one cell type to another
Anaplasia = reverting to more primitive cell type
Desmoplasia = connective tissue reaction to tumor
Keratoacanthosis = large acanthoma
Pleomorphic = occurrence in more than one form, existence in more than one morphological type of cells
Acanthosis = increased thickness of prickle cell layer
Parakeratosis = the nuclei migrated to the surface
Dyskeratosis = the normal maturation sequence is disrupted and hence keratin is displaced in the wrong layer, e.g. in the prickle cell layer.
Hyperkeratosis = increased keratin layer, e.g. this is found in pachydermal laryngis.

58. By dividing the suprahyoid muscles, as in the "hyoid-drop", the larynx can be dropped by about 4 cm.

59. Brucellosis can be caused by brucellosis melitensis or brucellosis abortus. It is usually transmitted by milk or by animals. The prognosis is good. Twenty percent of patients have sensori-neural hearing loss.

60. Nevus: Intra-epithelial = benign
Junctional = premalignant
Intradermal = benign
Blue nevus = benign
mixed nevus = benign

61. Craniopharyngioma arises from Rathke's pouch area. The symptoms include decreased vision, primary optic atrophy, bitemporal hemianopsia, hypopituitary function, enlargement of the sella turcica.

62. Congenital esophageal stenosis is most common at the junction between the middle and distal 1/3 of the esophagus. It is best treated with dilatation.

63. TUBE FEEDING SYNDROME: Tube feeding syndrome usually results from too high a protein intake as well as too high a caloric intake. This results in excess osmotic load. This is usually accompanied by too little water intake. Consequently, dehydration ensues leading to hypernatremia, hyperchloremia and azotemia. This is further compounded by negative nitrogen balance in these patients. In response to this stress, the kidney compensates by excreting concentrated urine to preserve water. Since little water is excreted, sodium and chloride are also retained causing further hypernatremia and hyperchloremia. Further,in the presence of high protein intake without adequate caloric intake, there is an increase in urea production leading to solid diuresis and dehydration. This pathophysiological state will lead to mental deterioration, fever, tachycardia, neuromuscular irritability and hyperreflexia. This most common complication from this syndrome is pneumonia finally resulting in coma and death.

The treatment is to rapidly decrease the protein and solute load and to increase fluid intake intravenously. The patient should be followed closely, along with daily electrolyte assay. Over-aggressive treatment can lead to water intoxication. In a normal person receiving tube feeding, no more than 70 gm per liter of protein and 1/2 a calorie per ml of tube feeding should be administered. The urine osmolality should be kept below 500 mOsm per liter. The normal intake should be about 1 gm to 1.5 gm of protein per kilogram per day for an individual. The normal serum osmolality should range between 285 and 310 mOsm per liter.

Incidentally, diarrhea is occasionally noted with this syndrome.

64. Adequate urinary volume includes:
   a. 10 drops per minute
   b. 30 cc per hour
   c. 700 cc per day

65. During an emergency in which an air embolism is suspected, the patient should be placed with the left side down.

66. Acidosis and vomiting can result from starvation after tonsillectomy in children. Treatment of this would be to encourage the intake of "sweets".

67. The symptoms of cardiac tamponade are:
   a. low cardiac output
   b. muffled heart sounds
   c. increased central venous pressure
   d. decreased amplitude on EKG
   e. definitive diagnosis made by pericardiocentesis

68. A tear in the middle fossa dura will "seal" rapidly because of the adjacent arachnoid mesh rich in fibroblasts. The posterior fossa is in the basal cistern which is an arachnoid-free region and hence a dura tear in the posterior fossa does not seal as rapidly.

69. The complications of cholesteatoma in decreasing order of frequency are:
   a. fistula
   b. extradural or perisinus abscess
   c. serous or suppurative labyrinthitis
   d. facial paralysis
   e. meningitis
   f. brain abscess
   g. sigmoid thrombophlebitis
   h. subperiosteal abscess

70. The fenestration operation restores hearing but lacks the transformer and lever mechanism, thus leaves an unrestored conductive hearing loss of about 35dB. Failure from the fenestration operation occurs within two years. If the hearing results are sustained for two years, it is most likely that it will be sustained forever. The osseous closure of the fenestration is rare if enchondralization as well as irrigation to remove the bone dust is done during the operation.

71. a. Mucopolysaccharide content is increased in exophthalmic tissues as well as in hypothyroidism.
   b. Chondroitin sulfate is found in urine in Hurler's syndrome.
   c. The cells of inverted papilloma have an increased glycogen content.
   d. Hypothyroid cells also have an increased hyaluronic acid content.
   e. The patients with oculo-pharyngeal syndrome have an increased cellular content of creatinine phosphokinase.
   f. Rhabdomyosarcoma cells have increased glycogen content.
   g. Relapsing polychondritis patients have an increased urinary content of mucopolysaccharide.
   h. Trypsin is found in the stool of patients with mucoviscidosis.

72. CARCINOMA OF THE TONGUE: Ninety-five percent of malignancies of the tongue are epidermoid. Malignant lesions of the oral tongue are three times as common as those of the pharyngeal tongue.

Among lesions of the oral tongue, the postero-lateral border is the most frequent site. The middle 1/3 of the tongue is more frequently involved with malignancies than the anterior 1/3.

73. NASOPHARYNGEAL CARCINOMA: due to its location, quite frequently presents first with a neck mass. Another common symptom is "blocked" ear secondary to serous otitis media.

74. The site of the "unknown" primary for a metastatic node in order of decreasing frequency is: nasopharynx, base of tongue, pyriform sinus.

75. THE TOLUIDINE BLUE TEST: It stains mitotic lesions, mucin, food particles and exudates a royal blue. It does not reveal submucosal extensions. Technique:

- a. Rinse mouth well
- b. Paint with 2% aqueous solution of Toluidine Blue
- c. Wait 30 seconds
- d. Rinse with warm water or 1% acetic acid to remove excess dye.
- e. The positive areas are stained a royal blue.

76. Calcium gluconate = 9% free calcium (Dosage: 12 to 15 gm a day)
Calcium Chloride = 27% free calcium (irritating to the stomach)
Calcium lactate = 13% free calcium (Dosage: 10 to 12 gm a day)

77. 50% of myxedema patients have reversible sensori-neural hearing loss.

78. Amyloidosis gives a positive crystal violet stain.

79. Adenocystic carcinoma constitutes 6% of all salivary gland tumors.

80. T99 scan will reveal Warthin's tumor as a "hot" nodule.

81. Papilloma of the oral cavity is most frequently seen in the faucial region. Some physicians consider them premalignant.

82. The incidence of carcinoma of the esophagus is increased in patients with:

- a. achalasia
- b. oculopharyngeal syndrome
- c. caustic burns
- d. Plummer-Vinson syndrome
- e. Pernicious anemia

83. HERPANGINA: <u>Etiology</u> - Coxsackie A, characterized by minute vesicles in the anterior pillars of the fauces.

84. In achalasia, aspiration pneumonitis is a frequent complication. Prior to esophagoscopy, it is wise to first pass an NG tube to remove the retained esophageal contents.

85. Leiomyoma is the most common benign tumor of the esophagus.

86. SCLERODERMA: This is a disease of unknown etiology perhaps secondary to some immune mechanism related to the connective tissues. The most common site within the gastrointestinal tract is the esophagus and small bowel. The upper esophagus is not usually involved. This disease is more prevalent in females than in males. Physiological abnormalities include decreased motility of the esophagus and esophagitis. Pathologically the mucosa and the submucosa are involved; however, the longitudinal muscles are seldom involved. A typical barium swallow will reveal a flaccid, dilated esophagus which is similar to that of achalasia.

87. DERMATOMYOSITIS: This is a nonsuppurative, nonhemorrhagic type of polymyositis in which cutaneous and muscle changes are noted. In the muscle, inflammatory reaction followed by granulation tissue invasion and hyaline degeneration is noted. The skin changes are nonspecific. Dysphagia occurs in most of the so-called collagen disorders but it is encountered most frequently in dermatomyositis (60% of patients with dermatomyositis complain of dysphagia). Unlike scleroderma, there is no esophagitis in dermatomyositis. Decreased esophageal motility is present in both disorders.

	Dermatomyositis	Scleroderma
Dysphagia	Pharyngeal	Sternal
Nasal regurgitation	Frequent	Absent
Stage of disease	Severe muscle disease	Widespread surface disease
Remissions	With steroids	None
Complications	Rare	Esophagitis, herniation
Findings at Esophagoscopy	Normal	Esophageal ulceration
X-ray	Loss of peristalsis	Loss of peristalsis
Motility	Decreased	Decreased
Site of maximum involvement in the esophagus	Upper 1/3	Lower 2/3

88. Sites of carcinoma of the head and neck in order of decreasing frequenty: Lip, Tongue, Floor of mouth, Tonsil, Larynx.

89. The advantages of surgical resection followed by radiation:
   a. Without prior irradiation, a frozen section, when obtained, is more reliable.
   b. Better wound healing.

   The disadvantages:
   a. An operated field has decreased blood supply and consequently, poor oxygenation. This condition renders the tumor less radiosensitive.
   b. Since there is poorer blood supply, the patient is more susceptible to radionecrosis.

The advantages of pre-operative radiation:

a. Since an unoperated field is better vascularized, the tumor is more radiosensitive.

b. Pre-operative radiation does not convert an inoperable lesion into an operable one. However, it does help to sterilize submucosal inapparent pseudopod involvement, making the planned margin of resection a safer one.

The disadvantages:

a. Unreliable frozen section

b. Decreased healing potential

90. The most commonly encountered malignancy in children is malignant lymphoma. A proper work up should include a histological diagnosis, limits of the primary lesion, chest PA and lateral x-rays, IVP and bone marrow study. The overall prognosis is about 30%. Lymphoma can be staged as follows:

Stage I: localized

Stage II: limited to above the diaphragm without systemic symptoms.

Stage III: diffuse disease

91. SEASONAL ALLERGIES:

Early Spring	=	Trees
Late Spring	=	Grasses
Fall	=	Ragweed

92. There are 2 types of Asthma:

a. Intrinsic, which usually manifests itself after age 30. It is non-seasonal. It is correlated with infection.

b. Extrinsic, which manifests itself before age 30. It is seasonal.

93. HISTAMINE:

1. Histamine is found in mast cells, platelets, leukocytes and the parietal cell region of the stomach.
2. It:
   a. contracts smooth muscles.
   b. increases dilatation and permeability of capillaries and venules.
   c. dilates arterioles and venules via a direct action on the musculature.
   d. contracts larger vessels.
   e. stimulates exocrine glands.
   f. increases gastric secretion.
3. Anti-histamine (e.g. Benadryl) is not effective against unreleased histamine.

94. SEROTONIN:

a. Serotonin is found in platelets, cerebral tissues and the mucosa of the gastrointestinal tract. It is not found in the mast cells in man.

b. It increases capillary permeability.

c. It contracts smooth muscles.

95. KININS: These are active polypeptides in blood during certain hypersensitivity reactions.

a. Kallidin I (Bradykinin) is found in plasma and increases capillary permeability, causes smooth muscle contraction and vasodilatation. It is formed by the action of enzymes on plasma globulin.
b. Kallidin II is a decapeptide. It has similar properties as Kallidin I but is formed by different enzymes. The enzyme may be Kallikrein.

Complement: This is a group of serum proteins which react sequentially during certain Antigen-Antibody reactions. Currently, 9 components of the human complement have been described, some of which have been purified and characterized.

(Epinephrine, Ephedrine, Isuprel, Neosynephrine, Anti-histamine, Steroid - see Chapter 28: Medications).

If both parents are allergic, there is a 76% chance of the offspring being allergic. Fifty percent of allergic patients have a (+) family history.

96. AURICULAR TRAUMA: Hematoma of the auricle secondary to trauma accumulates between the cartilage and the perichondrium. This lesion needs to be drained and stented to prevent reaccumulation. Late cases require contour carving of the cartilage.

Frostbite produces 3 stages of physiological changes:

a. vasoconstriction with increased capillary permeability
b. vasodilation
c. clumping of red blood cells

Frostbite of the ears should be treated by warming the part with soaks just above the body temperature and then the area may be left to dry, surgically clean. Overzealous warming may cause unnecessary vasodilation and clumping of the red blood cells. Anticoagulants may be administered. The gangrenous portion which develops may be considerably less on the inside than appears on the surface. Treatment, therefore, is to let the natural separation take place, to conserve as much tissue as possible prior to considering reconstruction surgically.

97. UMBO BLEBS: Benign idiopathic thin wall blebs containing a thin lipoid fluid, asymptomatic and resolves spontaneously. It occurs 1 in 364 examinations of tympanic membranes.

98. "Onion-skin" effect is the term used to refer to areas of lytic bone absorption expansion of cortex and subperiosteal new bone formation in x-ray of Ewing's tumor. Ewing's tumor is a primary malignancy beginning in bone marrow.

99. GLOMUS TUMORS: 50% arise from the jugular bulb but can arise from Arnold's nerve (auricular branch of X) tympanic branch of IX (Jacobson's nerve). Chief cells are noted to be arranged in nests and cords with abundant endothelial lined vascular channels.

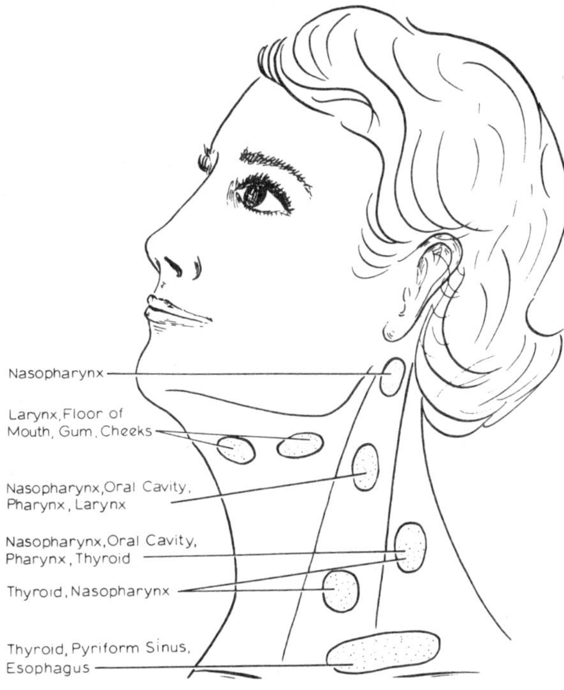

Figure 31-1. Lymphatic Drainage

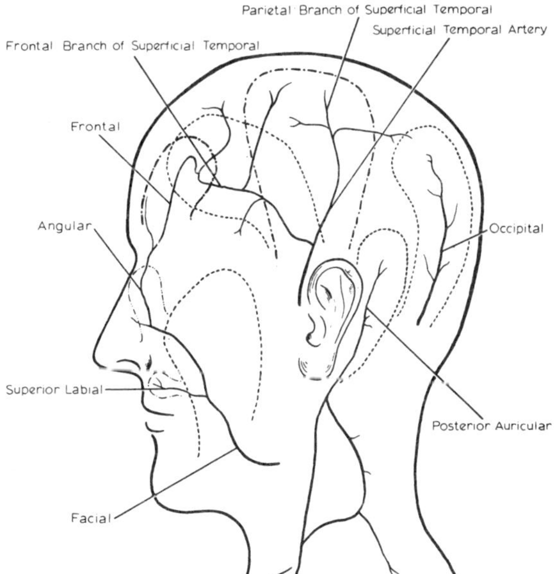

Figure 31-2. Pedicled Flaps of the Head with their Blood Supply

100. Proctor, B.: Archives Otolaryngology 97:8, 1973.
With every swallow the tensor veli palatini opens the tubal opening. As the middle ear is aerated, the tensor tympani regulates the degree of tension of the tympanic membrane. This synergism of action is made possible by a common innervation via otic ganglion.

101. Derlacki, E.: Archives Otolaryngology 97:177, 1973.
Primary cholesteatomas originating in the petrous pyramid are investigated usually because of a facial palsy of gradual onset and progression. There is usually a homolateral profound sensorineural deafness and a loss of caloric response. Patient's age is usually between 35 and 55 years.

102. Cundy, R. et al.: Archives Otolaryngology 98:131-133, 1973.
Nasopharyngeal carcinoma invasion into adjacent areas and structures is well known. Bony destruction commonly occurs in the floor of the sphenoid sinuses. The foramen lacerum, carotid canal, and foramen ovale are passageways most often used for extension into the cranium - occasionally the eustachian tube. Metastases to the temporal bone generally arise from hematogenous spread.

Enchondral bone is more resistant to neoplasm than periosteal bone and thus, labyrinthine and cochlea invasion is rare.

103. Bruce, M. et al.: Archives Otolaryngology 98:322-324, 1973.
Branham's sign - When a major afferent vessel is occluded, mean arterial pressure rises abruptly, heart rate then decreases.

104. Fechner, R.: Archives Otolaryngology 99:234, 1974.
10% of patients with inverted papillomas may have cancer either when they first present or after several resections for inverted papilloma.

105. Montgomery, W.: Archives Otolaryngology 99:255-260, 1974.
Three methods of gaining extra length for a primary anastomosis of the trachea in order to avoid excessive tension on the suture line:

1. Superior mobilization of the distal trachea from the thorax.
2. Incising the annular ligaments between the tracheal rings.
3. Release of the larynx or hyoid bone from its upper muscular attachments.

106. Sessions, R. et al.: Archives of Otolaryngology 99:261, 1974.
Epstein-Barr virus is transmitted orally and is etiologically related to infectious mononucleosis, carcinoma of the nasopharynx and possibly Burkitt's lymphoma.

107. Conley, J.: Archives Otolaryngology 99:315-319, 1974.
Melanoma of the mucous membranes of the head and neck originates in the oral cavity about 50% of the time. However, melanoma of the tongue is very rare.

108. Schmidt, P.: Archives Otolaryngology 99:402-405, 1974.
An intranasal meningoencephalocele is usually situated medially to the middle turbinate as it enters the nose through the cribriform plate.
Compression of the jugular veins will cause swelling of a meningoencephalocele-Furstenberg's sign.

109. Ward, P. et al.: Laryngoscope 79:1295-1306, 1969.
Fibrous dysplasia is most common in the maxilla.

110. Goepfert, H. et al.: Archives Otolaryngology 100:8-10, 1974.
Squamous cell carcinoma is the most frequent malignant tumor of the nasal vestibule. Radiation therapy is usually the primary treatment with surgery able to salvage most radiation failures.

111. Phipatanakul, C.: Archives Otolaryngology 100:109-112, 1974.
Association of bronchial asthma and paranasal sinusitis:
1. Bacterial seeding of the lung from mucopurulent drainage of sinuses.
2. Hypersensitivity to bacterial products in sinuses.
3. Reflex bronchospasm through the sympathetic nervous system. Common sympathetic fibers from sphenopalatine ganglion pass via carotid plexus to the cervical ganglia and the tracheobronchial musculature.

112. Nadol, J.: Archives Otolaryngology 100:273-278, 1974.
Hennebert's sign; (+) fistula sign with intact tympanic membrane and no apparent inflammatory ear disease. Due to saccular dilatation in syphilis with adherence to stapes footplate.

113. Alexander, F.: Laryngoscope 73:537-546, 1963.
Mucoceles are the most common expanding lesion of the sphenoid sinus.

114. Bailey, B.: Archives Otolaryngology 101:1-5, 1975.
Olfactory neuroblastoma is best treated by a combination of surgery and radiation therapy.

115. Luetje, C.: Archives Otolaryngology 101:11-14, 1975.
Extranodal presentation in head and neck non-Hodgkin's lymphoma occurs in Waldeyer's ring about 50% of the time.

116. Conley, J.: Archives Otolaryngology 101:39-41, 1975.
In parotid gland malignancies, the incidence of node metastases in patients with facial nerve involvement is 60%.

117. Randall, G. et al.: Archives Otolaryngology 101:63-66, 1975.
"Pseudosarcoma" of larynx and oropharynx is a pleomorphic variant of an epidermoid carcinoma and not a benign connective tissue response. Ogura suggests it should be called Spindle Cell Carcinoma.

118. Morgenstein, K.: Archives Otolaryngology 101:157-159, 1975.
In post-traumatic laryngeal reconstruction, the keys are a subglottic area with a stable cricoid cartilage or graft and a mucosa-lined airway.

119. Gadlage, R.: Archives Otolaryngology 101:422-425, 1975.
Vidian nerve has parasympathetic fibers that innervate nasal mucous glands and blood vessels. These fibers control the mucous secretions, but only partially effect vasodilatation. Thus a vidian neurectomy is best indicated for profuse rhinorrhea, not nasal congestion.

120. Dellon, A. et al.: Archives Otolaryngology 101:465-466, 1975.
Exfoliated cells from head and neck cancer rarely pass into the bronchial tree. A solitary nodule with positive cytology from bronchial washings more likely represents a second primary in the lung.

121. Rybak, L.: Archives Otolaryngology 101:710, 1975.
Multiple endocrine neoplasia - Type 2- Medullary carcinoma of the thyroid associated with parathyroid adenoma and pheochromocytoma.

122. Pease, G. et al.: Archives Otolaryngology 101:761-762, 1975.
Osteogenic sarcoma of the mandible is the most common primary malignant tumor of the mandible.

123. Sessions, D. et al.: Laryngoscope 83:890-897, 1973.
Treatment - Embryonal Rhabdomyosarcoma
1. As wide a surgical resection as possible
2. Primary area is irradiated 5000-6000 rads
3. Concomitant with radiation therapy, Actinomycin D and vincristine are given followed by maintenance vincristine and cyclophosphamide

124. Miyamoto, R. et al.: Laryngoscope 83:890-897, 1973.
Thyroid gland is the most common site of metastatic hypernephroma in the head and neck and hypernephroma is the most common neoplasm which metastasizes to the thyroid gland.

125. McWilliams, B. et al.: Laryngoscope 83:1745-1753, 1973.
Vocal cord nodules are the most common laryngeal pathology occurring with velopharyngeal insufficiency.

126. Abramson, M.: Laryngoscope 83:1764-1768, 1973.
3 forms of treatment for parotid duct injury:
1. Primary anastomosis
2. Suppression of parotid secretions
3. Diversion of salivary flow into the oral cavity

127. Cook, T. et al.: Laryngoscope 83:1802-1809, 1973.
Nasal - pulmonary reflex accounts for the observation that chronic nasal obstruction, especially nasal packs, decreases pulmonary compliance and increases pulmonary resistance.

128. Wertz, M.: Laryngoscope 84:507-521, 1974.
Incidence of carcinomatous change in lingual thyroid is about 5%. This change is usually associated with prolonged stimulation of the quantitatively deficient gland.

129. Thawley, S.: Laryngoscope 84:1445-1453, 1974.
Boerhaave's Syndrome - spontaneous esophageal rupture secondary to severe vomiting. 90% of tears occur on the left side approximately 2-3 cm proximal to the gastroesophageal junction.

130. Work, W. et al.: Laryngoscope 84:1748-1755, 1974.
Neurogenic tumors account for about 1/3 of lesions of the parapharyngeal space.

131. Pollock, R.: Laryngoscope 84:2113-2118, 1974.
Treatment of malignant hyperthermia
1. Discontinuation of the anesthetic agent
2. 100% Oxygen
3. Procaine amide and sodium bicarbonate
4. Hypothermia including ice packing

Facial nerve is injured in about 25% of longitudinal temporal bone fractures, and is the delayed type. In transverse fractures, the facial nerve is affected in about 50% and is of immediate onset.

132. To work up a bleeding disorder the following steps are taken:
A. History: A complete medical history should be taken stressing the following points.
a. Prior surgical procedures. If the patient has undergone a prior surgical procedure without significant hemorrhage, this is often the best indication of normal hemostatic function. More attention should be given to prolonged bleeding requiring transfusions following minor procedures.
b. Medications and toxins. One should ascertain whether the patient is taking any medication particularly heparin, coumadin, acetylsalicylic acid, etc. and exposure to toxins at work or at home.
c. Family history of bleeding. This is of particular importance in congenital defects although a small percentage of defects have no positive family history of bleeding.
d. Spontaneous hemorrhage.
e. Prolonged bleeding with minor trauma.
B. Physical examination: A complete physical examination with particular attention to:
a. Purpuras
b. Hemarthroses
c. Hepatomegaly
d. Splenomegaly
C. Laboratory Studies: The following chart is a synopsis of laboratory values usually found in the various coagulation defects.

Defect	Platelets	Bleeding Time	PTT	Pro Time	TGT
I	N	UN	I	I	N
II	N	N	I	I	N
V	N	N	I	I	mild PD
VII	N	N	N	I	N
VIII	N	N	I	N	PD
IX	N	N	I	N	SD
X	N	N	I	I	SD

Defect	Platelets	Bleeding Time	PTT	Pro Time	TGT
XI	N	N	I	N	mild SD and PD
XII	N	N	I	N	mild SD and PD
XIII	N	N	N	N	N

N=normal I=increased UN=usually normal PD=plasma defect
SD=serum defect

As a routine for patients undergoing surgical procedures the following tests may be performed. [The test (f) is not used as a screening test].

a. Hemoglobin, Hematocrit: to rule out anemia from unsus-suspected bleeding or chronic disease.

b. White blood count with differential: to rule out leukemia, infectious diseases, etc.

c. Partial Thromboplastin Time (PTT): tests for all the coagulation factors except IV, VII and XII. Normal value is 30 to 45 seconds (definitely abnormal if over 50 seconds).

Consists of adding commercially prepared partial thromboplastin to the patient's plasma in the presence of calcium.

d. Prothrombin Time (Pro Time): tests for Factors II, VII, IX and X. Consists of adding whole thromboplastin to the patient's plasma in the presence of calcium.

Normal value is 11 to 13 seconds.

e. Platelet Count: Normal value 100,000-450,000 per mm^3 depending on method.

Bleeding problems usually do not occur unless the platelet count is below 50-60,000 per mm^3.

The PTT and the Prothrombin time will detect over 90% of the coagulation defects. Combined with the other tests and a careful history and physical examination, defects in hemostasis should be detected with only rare exceptions.

f. Thromboplastin Generation Test (TGT): This test consists of substituting the patient's plasma or serum as one of the reagents in the following equation:

$$\text{Absorbed Plasma (plasma treated with } Al(OH)_3) + \text{Platelets} + \text{Serum} \xrightarrow{Ca(Cl)_2} \text{Blood Thromboplastin}$$

(*see preceding chart for interpretation of this test).

For example: If a patient demonstrated normal platelets, bleeding time, and Pro Time but showed increased PTT, he can be deficient in either Factor VIII or IX.

If Factor VIII is deficient:

$$\text{Patient's plasma} + \text{normal platelets} + \text{normal serum} \xrightarrow{Ca(Cl)_2} \text{deficient thromboplastin}$$

$$\text{Normal plasma} + \text{normal platelets} + \text{patient's serum} \xrightarrow{Ca(Cl)_2} \text{normal thromboplastin}$$

If Factor IX is deficient:

Patient's plasma + normal platelets + normal serum $\xrightarrow{Ca(Cl)2}$ normal thromboplastin

Normal plasma + normal platelets + patient's serum $\xrightarrow{Ca(Cl)2}$ deficient thromboplastin

If the platelets are abnormal:

Normal plasma + patient's platelets + normal serum $\xrightarrow{Ca(Cl)2}$ deficient thromboplastin

Platelet count is normal in thrombopathia and abnormal in thrombocytopenia.

g. Tests for Specific Factors: A definitive diagnosis for each of the factor deficiencies can be made by assaying for each factor. These tests are particularly helpful when the preceding table fails to give the diagnosis e.g. fails to differentiate between deficiency in Factor XI and that of XII. Factor assays are extremely specialized and are beyond the scope of this book.

Treatment:

When a deficiency is detected using the preceding screening tests or when there is a strong suspicion of hemostatic abnormalities from the history and/or physical examination, a hematologist should be consulted for the management of the patient. Before any treatment is instituted, blood should be drawn for laboratory studies. In the rare instance when the patient is hemorrhaging due to an unsuspected disorder the following guidelines may be used:

1. First choice of treatment: Fresh whole blood (less than 2-3 hours old if possible). This contains all the necessary factors needed to produce hemostasis in the bleeding patient if given in adequate amounts.

2. Second choice of treatment: Fresh frozen plasma (has all factors except platelets).

3. Third choice of treatment: Bank (stored) blood. This lacks I, V, VIII and platelets.

4. Fourth choice of treatment: Stored plasma.

III. When preparing for an oral examination, it is helpful for the candidate to be familiar with the history, physical findings, radiological findings, and pathological findings of a few common disease entities. It is also appropriate for him to know prognosis, and certain statistics discussed in the recent literature. Some of the clinical disease entities are:

1. A lump in the neck - Is this infectious, cystic, or a hard tumor? ?TB, fungal diseases, cat scratch fever, lymphoma, thyroid disease may be implicated. Is a barium swallow necessary? Cervical spine films? Is this a mass with an unknown primary malignancy (nasopharynx, base of tongue, and pyriform sinus)?

2. Evaluating a child with airway problem; Is it congenital? Is it vascular? is it pharyngeal or laryngeal? Is it secondary to a foreign body?

3. The etiologies for a nasal septum perforation.

4. Paralysis of the vocal cord - a work-up may include complete blood count, urinalysis, chest and cervical spine x-rays, barium swallow, lumbar puncture, glucose tolerance test, ESR, neurological consultation, all x-rays, etc. What is Ortner's syndrome? What does the EKG show? Is there any thyroid disease? Does sarcoidosis enter the list of differential diagnoses?

5. Massive facial fracture - emergency room management and definitive surgical care.

6. Sinusitis - acute sinusitis as well as chronic sinusitis, able to read x-rays adequately, able to treat the acute problems as well as the long term problems.

7. Tinnitus - character of the tinnitus, is it pulsatile? what brought it on? duration, hearing loss, vertigo, complete neurological and otolaryngological examination. Do acoustic trauma, glomus tumor, acoustic neurinoma enter into the list of differential diagnoses? Be prepared to order the necessary tests to further evaluate a patient with tinnitus, be prepared to justify ordering the particular test or tests. Be prepared also to discuss the technique of how some of the tests are done and the interpretation of some of the tests, for example, ABLB, Bekesy.

8. Vertigo - the history and character of the vertigo are very important. Definition of vertigo, dizziness, lightheadedness, etc. is important. Be prepared to work-up the patient with dizziness not only from an otological standpoint, but perhaps from a cardiovascular, endocrine, allergic and neurological standpoint. Here again, be discriminate in what tests you order and be able to describe the technique as well as the results.

9. Chronic otitis media - immediate management as well as long term management.

10. Sudden hearing loss - be familiar with the current concepts and literature on the etiology and management of this disease entity.

11. Malignancies of the various otolaryngological anatomical sites.

12. Management of a conductive hearing loss not necessarily secondary to otosclerosis - complications of middle ear surgery.

13. Facial nerve palsies of various etiologies: management, different electrical testings.

14. Nasal obstruction in children - choanal polyp, allergic polyps, enlarged adenoid, angiofibroma, fibroma, deviated septum, allergy, choanal atresia, foreign body, tumor, etc.

15. Prepare to discuss progressive hearing loss and vertigo in children and in an adult, Meniere's disease, acoustic neurinoma, meningioma, congenital syphilis, suppurative labyrinthitis, cholesteatoma, ototoxicity, Cogan's syndrome, otosclerosis, eosinophilic granuloma, perilymphatic fistula, vascular, viral, and functional hearing loss. What are the syndromes that can give hearing loss and vertigo? (See Chapter 6).

16. Prepare to discuss metabolic and electrolyte disorders in postoperative patients. The following points may be used to help in your preparation:

a. The daily fluid requirement is 2200 cc. per 24 hours.

b. The daily output of fluid is about 700 cc. through respiration, 1200 cc. in the urine, 100 cc. through perspiration if the patient has no fever, and 200 cc. in the feces.

c. The daily caloric need ranges from 1800 calories to 3000 calories depending on the metabolic rate.

d. During surgery, when the skin incision is made:
(1) catechols, growth hormones and cortisol levels are increased leading to an increase in serum glucose, glucogenesis, glucagon level and a decrease in insulin receptor sites.
(2) there is an increase in ADH leading to decreased urinary output.

e. Symptoms of water intoxication are lethargy, seizure activities and coma. (Serum sodium in the range of 115-120 mEq per litre.) Water intoxication can lead to congestive heart failure, decreased glomerular flow rate and renal failure.

f. SIADH (Syndrome of Inappropriate ADH) can be caused by diabinese, Atromid, Vincristine, Cytoxan, Demerol and morphine sulfate. The findings are low serum, increased urinary sodium and increased urine osmolality (greater than 300 mOsm.).

g. Metabolic acidosis can be caused by lactic acidosis which can be secondary to excessive ethanolic intake, obstructive pulmonary disease, sepsis, DBI and Diamox. Sepsis is a common cause of lactic acidosis in postoperative patients.

h. Metabolic alkalosis can be caused by vomiting, NG tube suction, decreased extracellular fluid volume, decreased chloride and potassium, increased aldosterone levels and by diuretics. One of the treatments is replacement of chloride.

i. Hyperosmolar Coma (i.e., greater than 340 mOsm/litre; the normal value is 285-290 mOsm/litre) is a condition that can be caused by Dilantin, steroids, thiozide diuretics, myocardial infarction and stroke. The serum sodium, BUN and blood sugar are elevated. In spite of elevated serum glucose, there is no ketoacidosis.

j. Normal serum values:

Na = 140
K = 4
Cl = 95-105
HCO_3 = 28

Normal arterial blood gases:

pO_2	=	95-100	pH	= 7.4
pCO_2	=	40	Oxygen saturation	= 97-100%

k. Weight loss, decreased serum albumin and decreased total iron binding capacity are indications of malnutrition in a postoperative patient. A decrease in caloric intake leads to ketosis which in turn leads to decreased urinary excretion of uric acid which can cause gout symptoms. (Remember that 1000 cc. of 5% dextrose and water IV solution has only 200 calories.)

CHAPTER 32

MULTIPLE CHOICE QUIZ

Answers are not given so as to offer the reader an opportunity to pursue each topic further. The editor feels that a question taken as an end in itself is of less educational value than when it is used as a "spring-board" to explore the whole subject.

1. Embryologically, melanomas are said to arise from:
   A. Neurocrest cells
   B. Ectodermal cells
   C. Entodermal cells
   D. Mesodermal cells
   E. None of the above

2. Pseudoepithelial hyperplasia can be caused by:
   A. Blastomycosis
   B. Granular cell myoblastoma
   C. Blastomycosis and granular cell myoblastoma
   D. Sarcoid
   E. None of the above

3. Physiologists believe that the cilia of the Schneiderian mucosa:
   A. Beat approximately 100 beats per second
   B. Are stationary
   C. Beat approximately 8 to 10 beats per second
   D. Have secretory function as well
   E. Are permanently damaged by 4% cocaine solution

4. Reverting to primitive cell type is called:
   A. Dyskeratosis
   B. Parakeratosis
   C. Acanthosis
   D. Anaplasia
   E. Metaplasia

5. Statistics have shown that:
   A. 60% of parotid tumors are benign and 50% of the submaxillary tumors are malignant
   B. 50% of parotid and submaxillary tumors are benign
   C. 80% of parotid tumors are benign and 50% of submaxillary tumors are malignant
   D. 80% of parotid and submaxillary tumors are benign
   E. Acinic cell carcinomas of the parotid are usually located in the deep lobe

6. The most common parotid lesion in children is:
   A. Mixed tumor
   B. Lymphangioma
   C. Lymphoma
   D. Mucoepidermoid carcinoma
   E. Warthin's tumor

7. Warthin's tumor of the parotid is most common in:
   A. The tail of the parotid in females over 60 years old
   B. The tail of the parotid in males over 60 years old
   C. The superficial lobe, equally distributed in both sexes
   D. The deep lobe in females
   E. Young adult males

8. Pleomorphic adenoma of the salivary glands consists of:
   A. Ductal elements only
   B. Predominance of lymphocytes
   C. Epithelial and myoepithelial elements
   D. Cartilage rest cells
   E. None of the above

9. The most common etiology for a neck mass in an adult is:
   A. Infectious
   B. Branchial cleft cyst
   C. Primary benign tumor
   D. Metastasis
   E. Neurolemmoma

10. The stylopharyngeus is innervated by:
   A. X
   B. XI (bulbar root)
   C. VII
   D. Mandibular division of V
   E. IX

11. The most common site of orbital floor fracture is:
   A. Anteromedial
   B. Anterolateral
   C. Posteromedial
   D. Posterolateral
   E. Variable

12. The most common type of zygomatic fracture is:
   A. Arch fracture without displacement
   B. Trimalar fracture
   C. Body fracture without rotation
   D. Arch fracture with displacement
   E. Body fracture with rotation

13. In order of frequencies, one of the following is correct:
   A. Condylar, body, angle, symphysis, alveolar F(x)
   B. Condylar, ramus, symphysis, coronoid F(x)
   C. Body, angle, ramus, symphysis F(x)
   D. Symphysis, body, angle, coronoid F(x)
   E. Condylar, alveolar, symphysis, body F(x)

14. In equivocal mandibular fracture, measuring the angle of the mandible is a helpful hint. The angle of a young child between 5 and 10 years old is approximately:
   A. 90°
   B. 110°
   C. 175°
   D. 140°
   E. About the same as an edentulous patient

15. Criteria for supraglottic laryngectomy in a supraglottic lesion include all <u>except</u>:
   A. Lesion does not come within 5 cm. of the foramen cecum
   B. Lesion does not include the anterior commissure
   C. Lesion does not involve either arytenoid
   D. Lesion does not involve the apex of the pyriform sinus
   E. Lesion does not involve the postcricoid area

16. Sloughing of pedicle flaps is usually due to:
   A. Tissue edema
   B. Poor vascular supply
   C. Constricting dressings
   D. Radiated receptor site
   E. Infection

17. One of the following has been found to be deficient in patients with juvenile papilloma:
    A. Fe
    B. Mg
    C. Zn
    D. Gamma globulin
    E. Viral antibody

18. One type of hemangioma does not usually regress:
    A. A hemangioma that grows aggressively during the first year of life
    B. The cavernous type
    C. The capillary type
    D. Subglottic hemangioma
    E. Spider hemangioma

19. The most common type of T-E fistula and esophageal atresia is:
    A. The upper esophagus is connected with the trachea while the lower segment ends in a blind pouch
    B. Both upper and lower esophageal segments connect with the trachea
    C. Neither segment connects with the trachea
    D. The upper esophagus ends in a blind pouch, the lower esophagus is connected with the trachea
    E. Completely variable

20. The least common type of T-E fistula and esophageal atresia is:
    A. The upper esophagus is connected with the trachea while the lower segment ends in a blind pouch
    B. Both upper and lower esophageal segments connect with the trachea
    C. Neither segment connects with the trachea
    D. The upper esophagus ends in a blind pouch, the lower esophagus is connected with the trachea
    E. Completely variable

21. Each of the following situations suggests a central lesion <u>except:</u>
    A. Gaze nystagmus
    B. Nylen-Aschan Type II positional nystagmus
    C. Symmetrical opticokinetic nystagmus
    D. Nylen-Aschan Type I positional nystagmus
    E. Fixation accentuates nystagmus or fixation fails to suppress nystagmus

22. The foramen of Huschke:
    A. Is in the vicinity of the fissure of Santorini
    B. Transmits the chorda tympani nerve
    C. Transmits sympathetic fibers
    D. Transmits parasympathetic fibers
    E. Transmits both sympathetic and parasympathetic fibers

23. The most common congenital pulmonary abnormality is found in the:
    A. Right lower lobe
    B. Right middle lobe
    C. Right upper lobe
    D. Left upper lobe
    E. Left lower lobe

24. In a normal adult, which one of the following situations is correct?
    A. The carotid body is more sensitive to oxygen tension than to CO_2 tension; the respiratory center is more sensitive to CO_2 tension than to oxygen tension, the carotid sinus has a regulatory function on blood pressure.
    B. The carotid body has a regulatory function on blood pressure, the respiratory center is more sensitive to oxygen tension than to CO_2 tension, the carotid sinus is more sensitive to oxygen tension than to CO_2 tension.
    C. The carotid body is more sensitive to CO_2 tension than to oxygen tension, the respiratory center is more sensitive to CO_2 tension than to oxygen tension, the carotid sinus has a regulatory function on blood pressure.
    D. The carotid body is more sensitive to oxygen tension than to CO_2 tension, the respiratory center is more sensitive to oxygen tension than to CO_2 tension, the carotid sinus has a regulatory function on blood pressure.
    E. The carotid body is equally sensitive to oxygen tension and CO_2 tension while the carotid sinus has a regulatory function on blood pressure.

25. Among the local anesthetic agents listed, the most toxic dose for a 70 Kg adult is:
    A. 100 cc of 0.5% Procaine infiltration
    B. 20 cc of 2% Xylocaine infiltration
    C. 5 cc of 4% Cocaine topically
    D. 10 cc of 2% Tetracaine infiltration
    E. 20 cc of 2% Carbocaine infiltration

26. A 40-year-old white male presents with a midline neck mass. Biopsy reveals a tumor showing calcification and the presence of psammoma bodies histologically. The most likely diagnosis is:
    A. Calcified tubercle
    B. Papillary carcinoma of the thyroid
    C. Medullary carcinoma of the thyroid
    D. Hashimoto's thyroiditis
    E. Thyroid cyst

27. Medullary carcinoma of the thyroid is believed to:
    A. Be thyrocalcitonin-producing
    B. Have dense stroma with amyloid deposition and to be thyrocalcitonin-producing
    C. Have scattered calcifications
    D. Have psammoma bodies
    E. Have none of the above

28. Embryologically, carotid body tumors are believed to arise from:
    A. Neurocrest cells
    B. Ectodermal cells
    C. Entodermal cells
    D. Mesodermal cells
    E. Epithelial and myoepithelial cells

29. Doubling the amplitude of vibration would cause a:
A. 10 dB increase in intensity
B. 6 dB increase in intensity
C. 50 dB increase in intensity
D. 27 dB increase in intensity
E. 30 dB increase in intensity

30. All of the following are equivalents except:
A. 0 db at 1000 Hz
B. 10^{-16} watts per sq cm
C. 0.0002 dynes per sq cm
D. 0.0002 microbar
E. 10^{-12} watts per sq cm

31. The combination of the tympanic membrane footplate transformer mechanism and the lever mechanism amplifies sound by:
A. 10 dB
B. 50 dB
C. 30 dB
D. 25 dB
E. 15 dB

32. The area of the footplate is:
A. 3.5 sq mm
B. 2 sq mm
C. 5 sq mm
D. variable
E. 1 sq mm

33. The area of the round window is:
A. 3.5 sq mm
B. 2 sq mm
C. 5 sq mm
D. variable
E. 1 sq mm

34. Mikulicz's disease is commonly associated with an increased incidence of:
A. Lymphoma
B. Macroglobulinemia
C. Hypoglobulinemia
D. Lymphoma and macroglobulinemia
E. Lymphoma and hypoglobulinemia

35. The most common malignant tumor of the submaxillary gland is:
A. Adenocystic carcinoma
B. Squamous cell carcinoma
C. Mucoepidermoid carcinoma
D. Malignant mixed tumor
E. Lymphoma

36. Brooke's tumor is:
A. Of squamous cell origin
B. Of ductal cell origin
C. Of basal cell origin
D. A cartilaginous tumor
E. Highly malignant

37. A 65-year-old edentulous male suffered a bilateral telescoping subcondylar fracture. This is best treated by:
A. Intermaxillary fixation with the help of gunning splints
B. Bilateral open reduction with intermaxillary fixation for six weeks postoperatively

C. Unilateral open reduction with fixation postoperatively for three weeks
D. Bilateral open reduction and no fixation postoperatively
E. Unilateral open reduction with fixation postoperatively for six weeks

38. The first antibody made by an infant is of the:
A. IgA group
B. IgE group
C. IgG group
D. IgM group
E. None of the above

39. Hay fever individuals have an excessive amount of:
A. IgE antibodies
B. IgA antibodies
C. IgM antibodies
D. IgG antibodies
E. IgA and IgG antibodies

40. The most common site of accessory salivary gland tumor is the:
A. Soft palate
B. Hard palate
C. Sublingual area
D. Buccal mucosa
E. Posterior pharyngeal wall

41. The Galen anastomosis is the anastomosis between the:
A. IX and X nerves in the pharyngeal plexus
B. Lesser superficial petrosal nerve and the sympathetic fibers
C. Right and left superior laryngeal nerves
D. Superior laryngeal nerve and the recurrent laryngeal nerve
E. Superior thyroid artery and the inferior thyroid artery

42. Among the anatomical sites listed, hereditary lipoid proteinosis most commonly affects:
A. Tongue
B. Thyroid
C. Larynx
D. Mastoid air cells
E. Nose

43. Normal sweat chloride is:
A. Between 50 mEq per liter and 100 mEq per liter
B. 120 mEq per liter
C. Less than 50 mEq per liter
D. 75 mEq per liter
E. 150 mEq per liter

44. All of the following are considered adequate urine output for a patient <u>except</u>:
A. 1200 cc per 24 hours
B. 10 drops per minute
C. 30 cc per hour
D. 30 drops per minute
E. None of the above

45. Leukoplakia has all of the following <u>except</u>:
A. Parakeratosis
B. Hyperkeratosis
C. Desmoplasia
D. Dyskeratosis
E. Whitish in color

46. A 50-year-old Negro female presents with facial paralysis and a parotid mass. Biopsy of her mediastinum would reveal a mass which would have one of the following histologic characteristics:
A. Schaumann's bodies
B. Mikulicz's cells
C. Verocay bodies
D. Warthin-Finkelday cells
E. Phylasiferous cells

47. A 35-year-old white female presents with episodic vertigo, unilateral severe sensorineural hearing loss, unilateral tinnitus. Further audiometric examination revealed a high SISI score and a Type II Bekesy. A Silverstein labyrinthotomy would reveal a fluid containing all of the following except:
A. Succinate dehydrogenase
B. Malic dehydrogenase
C. Diaphorases
D. Potassium concentration of 150 mEq per liter
E. Na concentration of 150 mEq per liter

48. A 43-year-old mother gave birth to a 9-pound girl. The child is mentally retarded and of short stature. At 15 years of age she still has not shown signs of frontal sinus development. This syndrome is often associated with:
A. Conductive hearing loss
B. Abnormal E chromosomes
C. Fishlike mouth
D. Acute leukemia
E. Macroglobulinemia

49. A 12-year-old boy has recurrent pneumonitis, associated with eosinophilia. A question of parasitic involvement was raised. This has been referred to as:
A. Adie's syndrome
B. Loeffler's syndrome
C. Kartagener's syndrome
D. Wallenberg's syndrome
E. Right middle lobe syndrome

50. A 36-year-old white male has a long history of chronic suppurative otitis media. Two days ago he developed pain over the mastoid region with "picket fence" spiking fever. He is lethargic and toxic. Which of the signs would most likely be elicited?
A. Kernig's sign
B. Brudzinski's sign
C. Hennebert's sign
D. Wartenberg's sign
E. Griesinger's sign

51. Subclavian steal syndrome is associated with all of the following except:
A. Nuchal rigidity
B. Intermittent vertigo
C. Blurred vision
D. Occipital headache
E. Pain in the upper extremity

52. A 50-year-old French Canadian lady presents with ptosis and dysphagia. Family history revealed that her mother died of esophageal carcinoma and at least two-thirds of her relatives have had similar symptoms for varying durations. She most probably has:

A. Ocular pharyngeal syndrome
B. Plummer-Vinson syndrome
C. Patterson-Kelly syndrome
D. Achalasia
E. Scleroderma

53. A 36-year-old lady was diagnosed as having a frontal lobe tumor. Among other symptoms, she has anosmia, ipsilateral optic atrophy, and contralateral papilledema. This constellation of symptoms has been referred to as:
A. Avellis' syndrome
B. Tapia syndrome
C. Vernet syndrome
D. Foster-Kennedy syndrome
E. Collet-Sicard syndrome

54. A 6-year-old girl is noted to have low set ears, large ear lobes, possible ossicular deformity, web neck, short stature and renal symptoms. Her chromosome abnormality is:
A. XXY
B. XO
C. Trisomy 21
D. Trisomy 13
E. Trisomy 18

55. A 7-year-old Israeli boy is noted to have low set ears, to have probable ossicular deformity, and to be of short stature. The geneticist concluded that the patient has a polysaccharide metabolic problem which is inherited autosomal recessively. Among other findings, one of the following will be noted:
A. Polydipsia, polyuria
B. Hypoglycemia
C. Chondroitin sulfate in the urine
D. Trypsin in the stool
E. Calcification of the sella

56. Apert's syndrome (acrocephalosyndactyly) has all of the following characteristics <u>except</u>:
A. Autosomal recessive
B. Hearing loss present at birth
C. Conductive hearing loss
D. Patent cochlear aqueduct
E. Flat audiometric pattern

57. All of the following syndromes are associated with hearing loss and renal abnormalities <u>except</u>:
A. Apert's syndrome
B. Well's syndrome
C. Turner's syndrome
D. Leopard syndrome
E. Fanconi syndrome

58. A 3-year-old white male is noted to have severe sensorineural hearing loss, retinitis pigmentosa, obesity and diabetes. This is believed to be autosomal recessive. The most likely diagnosis is:
A. Usher's syndrome
B. Apert's syndrome
C. Alstrom's syndrome
D. Waardenberg's syndrome
E. Wallenberg's syndrome

59. Identify A, B, C, D, E, F. (Figure 32-1)

A. ____________ D. ____________
B. ____________ E. ____________
C. ____________ F. ____________

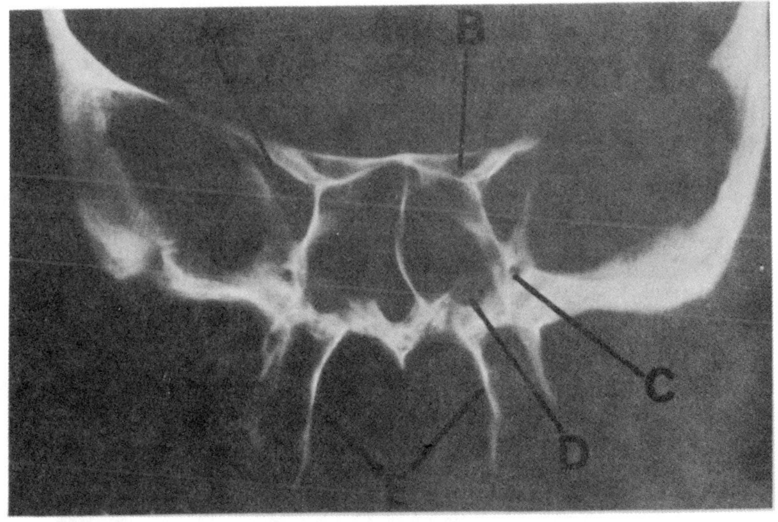

FIGURE 32-1.

60. Identify A and B. (Figure 32-2)

A. ____________
B. ____________

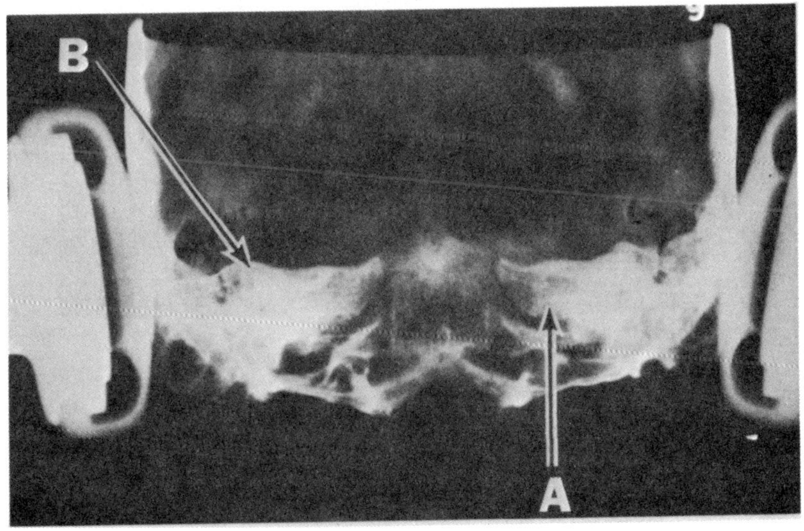

FIGURE 32-2.

61. Identify A and B. (Figure 32-3)
A. ______________________
B. ______________________

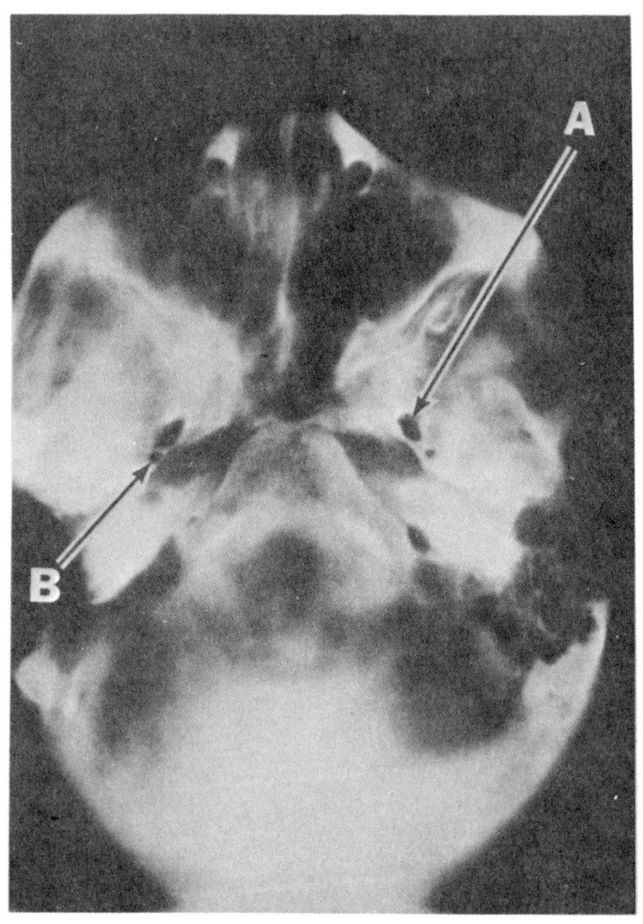

FIGURE 32-3.

62. The auricle is mainly supplied by:
A. Postauricular and facial arteries
B. Postauricular artery and superficial temporal artery
C. Occipital and postauricular arteries
D. Occipital, postauricular and facial arteries
E. Anterior tympanic and posterior tympanic arteries

63. A 10-year-old white girl presents with a sudden onset of fever, loss of appetite, dysphagia, pharyngitis, mild abdominal pain, and nausea and vomiting. Vesiculopapular lesions measuring 1-2 mm in diameter are present on the oral mucosa. These lesions soon would break down giving rise to grayish-yellow ulcers. The disease is thought to be caused by:
A. Virus, Herpex simplex
B. Vincent's organisms
C. Haemophilus influenzae
D. Coxsackie virus
E. Measles

64. Theoretically a patient with ossicular discontinuity with an intact tympanic membrane will present with a conductive loss of about:
A. 45 dB
B. 30 dB
C. 60 dB
D. 85 dB
E. 50 dB

65. The most frequent cause of death in acute otitis media is:
A. Sigmoid sinus thrombosis
B. Meningitis
C. Temporal lobe abscess
D. Cerebellar abscess
E. Brain abscess in general

66. Other than coalescent mastoiditis, the most common complication of acute otitis media is:
A. Subdural abscess
B. Meningitis
C. Sigmoid sinus thrombosis
D. Extradural abscess
E. Temporal lobe abscess

67. Other than meningitis, the most common cause of death in acute otitis media is:
A. Lateral sinus thrombophlebitis
B. Temporal lobe abscess
C. Cerebellar abscess
D. Extradural abscess
E. Subdural abscess

68. A 50-year-old white male presents with a suppurative left ear for 10 days. His temperature has spiked to 103° twice a day for the past four days. His hemoglobin is 10.5 gm%. He appears emaciated; palpation of the mastoid process reveals edema and pain of this area. The most likely diagnosis is:
A. Mastoiditis
B. Lateral sinus thrombosis
C. Subdural abscess
D. Meningitis
E. None of these

69. A 45-year-old white, right-handed male developed right mastoiditis secondary to chronic otitis media. Culture grew pseudomonas. In spite of aggressive treatment with geopenicillin and gentamicin, he developed severe headache, Jacksonian convulsions, rise in blood pressure and slowing of the pulse rate. The neurologist entertained the diagnosis of right temporal lobe abscess. Besides other symptoms, he most probably would have:
A. Ataxia
B. Aphasia
C. Paresis and numbness of the left side
D. Spontaneous nystagmus
E. All of the above

70. A 20-year-old diabetic developed a fulminating coalescent mastoiditis. In this age group, the chances of having pneumatization of the petrous pyramid is:
A. 10%
B. 30%
C. 50%
D. 75%
E. 90%

71. A Pancoast's tumor of the lung is one:
A. Located in the right middle lobe
B. Located in the apex
C. Of "oat cell" type
D. Of "alveolar cell" type
E. Can be of any cell type

72. A 27-year-old girl developed a slow-growing nontender mass in the parapharyngeal space. This mass can be palpated in the lateral pharyngeal wall as well as behind the angle of the mandible. The most likely pathological diagnosis is:
A. Neurolemmoma
B. Mixed tumor
C. Fibroma
D. Leiomyoma
E. Lymphoma

73. In order of decreasing frequencies, it is generally agreed that the incidence of carcinoma is:
A. Lip, larynx, tongue, tonsil
B. Larynx, tongue, tonsil, lip
C. Lip, tonsil, larynx, tongue
D. Larynx, floor of mouth, tongue, tonsil
E. Lip, tongue, floor of mouth, tonsil, larynx

74. A 20-year-old female developed a very slowly enlarging left malar region. A routine laboratory work-up revealed elevated serum alkaline phosphatase, with normal Ca and P. One of the following situations is most likely:
A. Increased osteoblastic activity
B. Malignant degeneration
C. Increased osteoclastic activity
D. Increased osteoblastic and osteoclastic activity
E. Part of the usual profile of this disease entity

75. Squamous cell carcinoma has been reported in the auricle, external auditory canal and middle ear. Among these regions the incidence of carcinoma of the middle ear is:
A. 70%
B. 50%
C. 30%
D. 10%
E. 2%

76. A 60-year-old alcoholic developed a squamous cell carcinoma of the hard palate. The primary and early site of lymphatic drainage would be:
A. Subdigastric
B. Retropharyngeal
C. Submaxillary
D. Subparotid
E. High jugular chain

77. An 80-year-old male has multiple areas of senile keratosis. He is concerned and consulted an otolaryngologist regarding the chances of malignant degeneration. A well-informed otolaryngologist would give an estimated figure of:
A. 1% malignant degeneration rate
B. 5% malignant degeneration rate
C. 10% malignant degeneration rate
D. 20% malignant degeneration rate
E. 50% malignant degeneration rate

78. A 32-year-old white male presents with multiple cysts of the jaw and multiple basal cell carcinomas of the skin. X-ray shows abnormal ribs and abnormal metacarpals. This condition is:
A. Autosomal recessive
B. Autosomal dominant
C. Nonhereditary
D. Associated with xeroderma pigmentosa
E. Sex-linked recessive

79. Carcinoma of the nasopharynx often involves:
A. The node of Rouvier
B. The node of Delphian
C. The node of Krause
D. All of these
E. None of these

80. A 50-year-old male presents with unilateral left nasal obstruction and left facial swelling. The Ohngren's line is used to:
A. Stage the tumor
B. Correlate site of tumor and its aggressiveness
C. Classify metastasis
D. Classify the histological nature of the tumor
E. None of the above

81. A student of head and neck oncology should be aware of the lymphatics. It has been demonstrated that certain regions have richer lymphatic drainage than others. In order of decreasing amount of lymphatics, the following is correct:
A. Pyriform sinus, base of tongue, supraglottic, subglottic
B. Base of tongue, pyriform sinus, supraglottic, subglottic

C. Pyriform sinus, subglottic, supraglottic, glottic
D. Transglottic, subglottic, supraglottic, glottic
E. Post cricoid, pyriform sinus, supraglottic, subglottic

82. Referred otalgia is frequently encountered in an otolaryngology practice. Referred pain from a base of tongue lesion involves the:
A. Gasserian ganglion
B. Petrosal ganglion
C. Sphenopalatine ganglion
D. Otic ganglion
E. Nodose ganglion

83. A 50-year-old male with a left false cord squamous cell carcinoma is undergoing pulmonary function testing as a preoperative work-up. The vital capacity is:
A. The same as tidal volume
B. The sum of tidal volume and inspiratory reserve volume
C. The sum of tidal volume and residual volume
D. The sum of tidal volume, inspiratory reserve volume and expiratory reserve volume
E. The same as inspiratory capacity

84. A 60-year-old Southern male has worked on a cotton plantation and in a cotton plant for the past 40 years. He was admitted to a hospital recently for chronic cough and pulmonary insufficiency. X-ray showed scattered diffuse infiltrates and emphysematous changes. This condition has been referred to as:
A. Bagassosis
B. Bysinosis
C. Berylliosis
D. Anthracosis
E. Sarcoidosis

85. The SISI test is characterized by all of the following <u>except:</u>
A. SISI score higher than 60% in sensory hearing loss
B. Lone SISI score in typical neural lesions
C. The test is performed at 20 dB above threshold
D. The test is performed at 2000 Hz
E. The test can be used in both unilateral hearing loss and bilateral hearing loss

86. The Tone Decay Test is characterized by all of the following <u>except:</u>
A. Performed at 20 dB above threshold
B. A tone decay of 40 dB suggests a neural pathology
C. The score is the number of dB increase that is needed to maintain the tone for 60 seconds
D. Can be performed at any frequency
E. Patients with Meniere's disease usually do not have a high tone decay score

87. Interaural attenuation is about:
A. 15 dB
B. 20 dB
C. 30 dB
D. 50 dB
E. 70 dB

88. Identify A and B: (Figure 32-4)
A. ____________________
B. ____________________

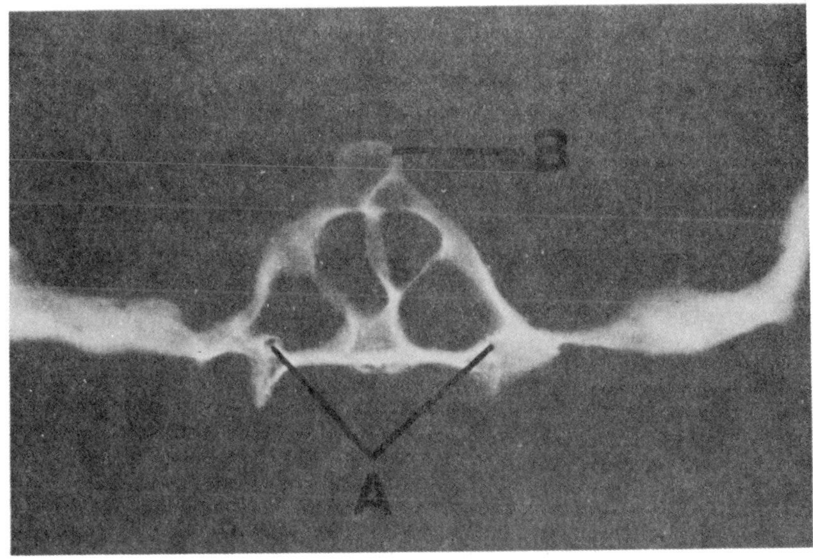

FIGURE 32-4.

89. A 30-year-old female is being evaluated by an otolaryngologic allergist for seasonal "sneezing, allergic rhinitis, watery eyes and itchy nose". Her symptoms are present mainly in the spring. She is most likely allergic to:
A. Ragweed
B. Grass pollen
C. Tree pollen
D. Mold
E. All of these

90. During the process of anaphylactic shock, the following take place <u>except</u>:
A. Peripheral vasodilatation
B. Release of histamine
C. Injury to the vascular endothelium
D. Intravascular coagulation
E. Smooth muscle contraction

91. Antihistamine is prescribed by many otolaryngologists for allergic and vasomotor rhinitis. The mechanism of action of this medication:
A. Inhibits the formation of histamine
B. Hydrolyzes histamine
C. Competes with histamine for the tissue sites
D. Is antiinflammatory
E. Is unknown

92. Glucocorticoids have been used by many otolaryngologists for many "allergic" states. The rationale for this practice embraces all the following except:
A. Anti-inflammatory
B. Alters the antibody-antigen reaction
C. Releases enzymes that metabolize histamine
D. Retards the formation of histamine in the mast cells
E. Suppresses tissue edema

93. A young otolaryngologist is performing a mastoid-tympanoplasty under general anesthesia utilizing halothane. A safe amount of 1% Xylocaine with 1:100,000 epinephrine for infiltration would be no more than:
A. 1 cc
B. 5 cc
C. 10 cc
D. 30 cc
E. 50 cc

94. The muscles involved in the function of the eustachian tube include all of the following except:
A. Tensor tympani
B. Tensor palatini
C. Levator palatini
D. Salpingopharyngeus
E. Salpingopalatus

95. A 19-year-old college student presents with peritonsillar abscess. His trismus is particularly due to involvement of:
A. External pterygoid muscle
B. Internal pterygoid muscle
C. Masseter muscle
D. Buccinator muscle
E. Palatoglossus and palatopharyngeus muscles

96. The middle thyroid artery is derived from:
A. Thyrocervical trunk
B. External carotid artery
C. Superior thyroid artery
D. Inferior thyroid artery
E. None of these

97. The jugular foramen is bounded by the:
A. Occipital bone only
B. Temporal bone only
C. Sphenoid bone only
D. Occipital bone medially and temporal bone laterally
E. Sphenoid bone medially and temporal bone laterally

98. All of the following, except one, pass through the jugular foramen:
A. Inferior petrosal sinus
B. IX
C. X
D. Posterior meningeal artery
E. XII

99. The facial nerve trunk can be located:
A. Medial to the styloid process
B. 6-8 mm medial to the petrotympanic fissure
C. 6-8 mm inferior to the petrotympanic fissure
D. 6-8 mm inferomedial to the tympanomastoid fissure
E. Superior to the tragal cartilage

100. A 35-year-old female with a past history of heavy smoking presents with intermittent hemoptysis. The most likely diagnosis is:
    A. Bronchiectasis
    B. Bronchial adenoma
    C. Tracheobronchitis
    D. Tuberculosis
    E. Mitral stenosis

101. The blood supply of the esophagus includes all except:
    A. Inferior thyroid artery
    B. Internal mammary artery
    C. Intercostal artery
    D. Left gastric artery
    E. Left inferior phrenic artery

102. The most common site of esophageal carcinoma is:
    A. Upper 1/3
    B. Middle 1/3
    C. Lower 1/3
    D. Cervical
    E. Esophagogastric junction

103. Anomaly of the great vessels is one of the common etiologies of dysphagia and/or dyspnea. The most frequent type of these is:
    A. Anomalous innominate artery
    B. Double aortic arch
    C. Anomalous subclavian artery
    D. Right aortic arch
    E. Pulmonary artery compression

104. A 30-year-old Negro male presents with dysphagia. Thorough diagnostic studies reveal a posterior mediastinal tumor. The most likely preoperative diagnosis would be:
    A. Dermoid or teratoma
    B. Lymphoma
    C. Bronchial cyst
    D. Pericardial cyst
    E. Neurolemmoma

105. Which one of the following is correct?
    A. Right middle lobe has 3 segments, right lower lobe has 4 segments
    B. Left upper lobe has 3 segments, left lower lobe has 4 segments, right upper lobe has 2 segments
    C. Right upper lobe has 3 segments, right lower lobe has 5 segments, left upper lobe has 4 segments
    D. Left lower lobe has 3 segments and right middle lobe has 3 segments
    E. Right lower lobe has 4 segments and left lower lobe has 4 segments

106. The PTT test measures all the factors listed in:
A. VII, VIII, IX, X, XI, XII
B. V, VIII, IX, X, XI, XII
C. V, VII, IX, X
D. VII, VIII, X, XI, XII
E. V, IX, X, XI, XII

107. Christmas Disease or Hemophilia B is:
A. Autosomal recessive and lack of factor IX
B. Sex-linked recessive and lack of factor IX
C. Autosomal recessive and lack of factor XI
D. Sex-linked recessive and lack of factor XI
E. Sex-linked recessive and lack of factor VIII

108. A 20 Kg boy underwent tonsillectomy and adenoidectomy. The estimated blood loss was 500 cc. This represents:
A. 35% of his blood volume; he should require transfusion therapy
B. 35% of his blood volume; he should require no transfusion therapy
C. 20% of his blood volume; he should require transfusion therapy
D. 20% of his blood volume; he should require no transfusion therapy
E. 15% of his blood volume; he should require no transfusion therapy

109. Chloromycetin:
A. Is bacteriocidal and it disrupts the cell wall
B. Is bacteriostatic and it disrupts the cell wall
C. Is bacteriocidal and it disrupts protein synthesis
D. Is bacteriostatic and it disrupts protein synthesis
E. Disrupts the cell membrane

110. Inner ear congenital anomalies have been classified by otologic histopathologists. The Schiebe type demonstrates:
A. Complete bony and membranous degeneration
B. Incomplete bony and membranous degeneration
C. Membranous cochlear and saccular degeneration
D. Membranous vestibular aplasia
E. Membranous cochlear aplasia

111. Inner ear anomaly secondary to maternal rubella is most similar to the type classified as:
A. Michel
B. Mundini-Alexander
C. Schiebe
D. Bing-Siebermann
E. Alexander

112. An otolaryngologist counseling the parents of a congenitally deaf child was asked the frequency of a "deaf" gene in the general population. The answer should be one in:
A. 100 people carries a recessive deaf gene
B. 50 people carries a recessive deaf gene
C. 25 people carries a recessive deaf gene
D. 8 people carries a recessive deaf gene
E. 4 people carries a recessive deaf gene

113. A 43-year-old mother gave birth to a 9 pound girl. The child is mentally retarded and of short stature. At 15 years of age she still has not shown signs of frontal sinus development. This syndrome is due to:
A. Abnormal G group chromosomes
B. Abnormal E group chromosomes
C. Patau's syndrome
D. XO
E. Trisomy 17

114. A young expectant housewife contracted rubella in the first trimester. She is frightened and consulted the obstetrician regarding the wisdom of a therapeutic abortion. Among weighing the chances of other anomalies, the obstetrician wants to know the risk of hearing loss in this newborn. It is:
A. 75%
B. 50%
C. 40%
D. 20%
E. 10%

115. An ataxic 30-year-old male died of renal failure. At autopsy he was noted to have cystic kidneys, angioma of the cerebellum and scattered petechiae of the skin. This condition has been referred to as:
A. Rendu-Osler-Weber
B. Sturge-Weber syndrome
C. Neurofibromatosis
D. Hippel-Lindau Disease
E. Stevens-Johnson syndrome

116. Jervell-Lang-Nielson syndrome includes all of the following characteristics <u>except</u>:
A. Autosomal recessive
B. Bilateral deafness
C. Renal failure
D. Recurrent syncope
E. Abnormal EKG's

117. A mentally retarded 10-year-old child is noted to have mixed hearing loss, exophthalmos, parrot-beaked nose, small maxilla and mandibular prognathism. This syndrome is autosomal dominant and is called:
A. Crouzon's disease
B. Treacher-Collins's disease
C. Mohr's syndrome
D. Pendred's syndrome
E. Pierre-Robin syndrome

118. Trautmann's Triangle is:
A. Formed by the 3 semicircular canals
B. Formed by the superior petrosal sinus, sigmoid sinus and the bony labyrinth
C. Formed by the tegmen and the sigmoid sinus
D. Formed by the spine of Henle, temporal line and posterior osseous external auditory canal
E. Formed by the superior petrosal sinus, inferior petrosal sinus and the sigmoid sinus

119. Identify A and B. (Figure 32-5)
A. ______________________
B. ______________________

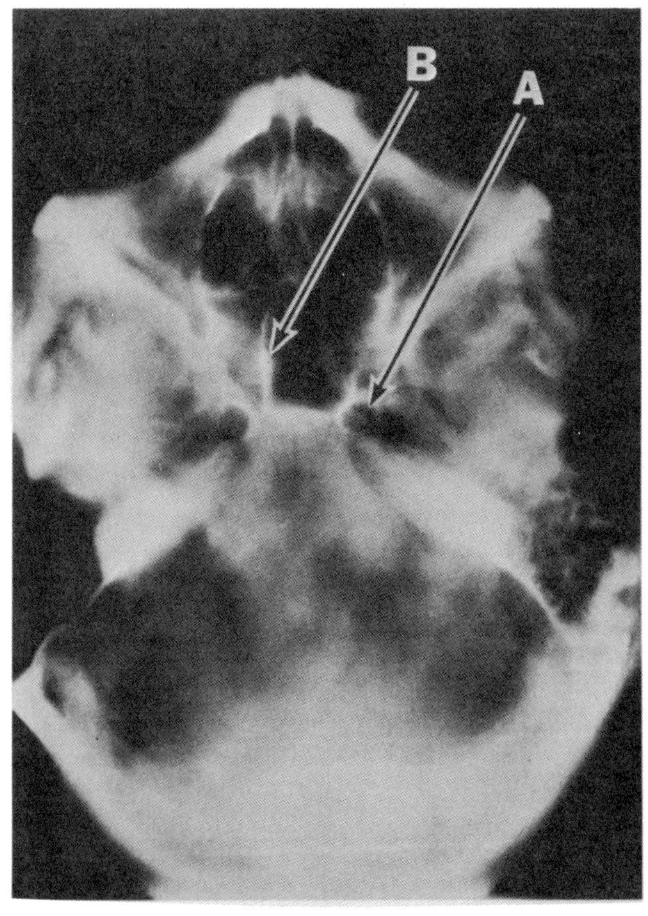

FIGURE 32-5.

120. Muscles attached to the temporal bone include all of the following <u>except</u>:
   A. Posterior digastric muscle
   B. Temporal muscle
   C. Longus capitis muscle
   D. Sternocleidomastoid muscle
   E. Trapezius muscle

121. All of the following are attached to the malleus <u>except</u>:
   A. Lateral malleal ligament
   B. Superior malleal ligament
   C. Anterior malleal ligament
   D. Posterior malleal ligament
   E. Tensor tympani tendon

122. The works of Bruce Proctor demonstrated that there are:
   A. 5 malleal folds and 4 incudal folds
   B. 4 malleal folds and 4 incudal folds
   C. 4 malleal folds and 3 incudal folds
   D. 5 malleal folds and 5 incudal folds
   E. 3 malleal folds and 2 incudal folds

123. The anterior pouch of von Troltsch is between the:
   A. Pars flaccida and superior malleal fold
   B. Pars tensa and anterior malleal fold
   C. Pars tensa and anterior malleal ligament
   D. Pars flaccida and anterior malleal ligament
   E. Short process of the malleus and chorda tympani

124. Prussak's space is bounded by:
   A. Lateral malleal fold, superior malleal ligament, neck of malleus and Shrapnell's membrane
   B. Pars flaccida and anterior malleal fold
   C. Pars tensa and anterior malleal fold
   D. Lateral malleal fold, lateral process of the malleus, the neck of the malleus and Shrapnell's membrane
   E. Lateral malleal fold, lateral process of the malleus, the long process of the malleus and pars tensa

125. The blood supply of the middle ear and mastoid includes all of the following <u>except</u>:
   A. Caroticotympanic artery
   B. Middle meningeal artery
   C. Stylomastoid artery
   D. Deep auricular artery
   E. Ascending pharyngeal artery

126. Russell bodies are found in:
   A. Rhinoscleroma
   B. Rhinosporosis
   C. Ameloblastoma
   D. Acoustic neurinoma
   E. Papillary carcinoma of the thyroid

127. A 40-year-old male presents with recurrent papilloma of the left nasal fossa. He reportedly had 2 previous intranasal surgical excisions. Biopsy report indicated it to be inverting papilloma. In counseling the patient regarding surgical therapy, the otolaryngologist was asked about the risk of this lesion turning malignant. The answer is:
A. 0.1%
B. 4%
C. 13%
D. 20%
E. 50%

128. The cells described in the lesion of #128 are rich in:
A. Lipids
B. Hyaluronic acids
C. Chondroitin sulfate
D. Glycogen
E. None of these

129. A young patient is noted to have dysphagia, regurgitation, but no dyspnea. Barium swallow and angiography revealed an indentation of the posterior esophagus. This condition could be:
A. Double aortic arch
B. Anomalous innominate artery
C. Dysphagia lusoria
D. Scleroderma
E. Barrett syndrome

130. A 10-year-old boy was brought to see an otolaryngologist because of unilateral ptosis since birth. However, upon opening the lower jaw to the contralateral side, the ptotic lid is elevated. A paternal uncle has the same symptoms. This pattern of symptomatology has been referred to as:
A. Marcus Gunn's syndrome
B. Horner's syndrome
C. Wartenberg's syndrome
D. Melkerson's syndrome
E. Richard-Rendell's syndrome

131. The axillary sheath is an extension of:
A. Superficial layer of the deep fascia
B. Visceral fascia
C. Pretracheal fascia
D. Prevertebral fascia
E. None of the above

132. In studying achondroplastic dwarfs, it is of interest to determine the derivation of the various bones. All of the following <u>except</u> one are membranous bone:
A. Sphenoid
B. Frontal
C. Mandible
D. Zygoma
E. Mastoid process

133. A 16-year-old girl was hit in the left eye by a golf ball. She suffered a left "blowout" fracture that necessitated surgical correction. At the time of surgery, it is not only important to know the anatomical landmarks but the nerves and vessels associated with each landmark. The superior orbital fissure transmits all of the following <u>except</u>:

A. III
B. IV
C. VI
D. V second division
E. Ophthalmic vein

134. Congenital esophageal stenosis is a very rare condition. It is most commonly located at the:
A. Cervical esophagus and treated with surgery
B. Cervical esophagus and treated with dilatation
C. Junction of the middle and distal thirds and best treated with dilatation
D. Esophagogastric junction and best treated with surgery
E. Esophagogastric junction and best treated with dilatation

135. An otolaryngology resident rotating through a large facial deformity clinic will see more patients having a:
A. Cleft lip with cleft palate than having a cleft lip alone
B. Cleft lip than having a cleft palate
C. Cleft palate than having a cleft lip and cleft palate
D. Cleft lip than having cleft lip with cleft palate
E. Cleft palate than having a cleft lip

136. A 45-year-old male was admitted by the internist to the hospital because of ascites, diarrhea, asthma-like symptoms and episodic flushing. He was also noted to be hoarse and on physical examination a mass was noted on the right true cord. He has a past history of having an intra-abdominal tumor removed. This tumor of the larynx was biopsied and was not a squamous cell carcinoma. This tumor most likely secretes:
A. Epinephrine
B. Norepinephrine
C. Thyrocalcitonin
D. Serotonin
E. Histamine

137. A nine-year-old girl was noted to have multiple recurrent upper respiratory and lower respiratory infections. She has had 3 nasal polypectomies in the past. She is treated with high protein-low fat diet with supplementary water soluble vitamins and pancreatic extracts. One of the following describes her condition:
A. Autosomal recessive inheritance
B. Elevated trypsin
C. Serotonin noted in the stool in 10 to 15% of this disease
D. Chondroitin sulfate can be measured in the urine
E. None of the above

138. A six-year-old girl was referred to an otolaryngologist because of hearing loss. Audiometric studies revealed a 40 dB conductive loss in the left ear. She was also noted to have downward sloping palpebral fissures, depressed cheek bones, deformed pinnas, receding chin and large fish-like mouth. She has:
A. Crouzon's disease
B. Pierre-Robin syndrome
C. Franceschetti syndrome
D. Mohr syndrome
E. None of these

139. A 65-year-old refugee from Cuba seeks the help of an otolaryngologist because of nasal crusting and nasal obstruction. On examination he was noted to have atrophic rhinitis. One of the organisms causing this condition is:
   A. Klebsiella ozaenae
   B. Klebsiella pneumoniae
   C. Klebsiella rhinoscleromatis
   D. Rhinosporidium seeberi
   E. Rhinosporidium kinealyi

140. Nasal physiologists believe that the pH of the nose is:
   A. 7.3 and it secretes 1000 cc per 24 hours
   B. 7.5 and it secretes 1000 cc per 24 hours
   C. 7.3 and it secretes 500 cc per 24 hours
   D. 7.5 and it secretes 500 cc per 24 hours
   E. 7.4 and it secretes 500 cc per 24 hours

141. A 35-year-old female presents with vague vertiginous symptoms and abnormal articulation. She was noted to have spontaneous nystagmus, scanning speech, and intention tremor and mild ataxia. A likely diagnosis is:
   A. Myasthenia gravis
   B. Amyotrophic lateral sclerosis
   C. Multiple sclerosis
   D. Bulbar polio
   E. Wallenberg syndrome

142. Oro-antral fistulas are encountered in both an otolaryngologic and an oral surgical practice. The tooth most commonly incriminated for this pathological entity is:
   A. Canine
   B. First premolar
   C. Second premolar
   D. First molar
   E. Second molar

143. The parasympathetic secretory fibers to the parotid are carried by:
   A. Greater superficial petrosal nerve
   B. Chorda tympani
   C. Auriculotemporal nerve
   D. Branches of V (second division)
   E. None of the above

144. The solitary tract nucleus is the nucleus of:
   A. Secretory fibers to the lacrimal gland
   B. Secretory fibers to the salivary glands
   C. Taste fibers of VII
   D. Taste fibers of IX
   E. Taste fibers of VII and IX

145. The Edinger-Westphal nucleus is the:
   A. Motor nucleus of III
   B. Parasympathetic nucleus of III
   C. Motor nucleus of V
   D. Sensory nucleus of V
   E. Secretory nucleus of IX

146. The innervation of the intrinsic laryngeal muscles is from the:
   A. Glossopharyngeal nerve
   B. Vagus nerve
   C. Bulbar portion of the accessory nerve
   D. Cervical portion of the accessory nerve
   E. Recurrent laryngeal nerve only

147. Cavernous sinus thrombosis is more often than not a fatal complication of ethmoiditis. The following structures except one are in intimate relationship with this sinus:
   A. Internal carotid artery
   B. Ophthalmic artery
   C. II nerve
   D. III nerve
   E. V nerve

148. All of the following except one constitute the muscles of the uvula:
   A. Palatoglossus
   B. Muscle uvula
   C. Tensor palati
   D. Levator palati
   E. Stylopharyngeus

149. The pterygomandibular raphe is made up of the:
   A. Medial and lateral pterygoid muscles
   B. Buccinator and the superior constrictor muscles
   C. Middle constrictor muscle and the posterior pharyngeal wall
   D. Superior constrictor muscle and the posterior pharyngeal wall
   E. Superior and middle constrictor muscles

150. The anterior and posterior ethmoidal foramina are located within the:
   A. Frontal bone
   B. Ethmoid bone
   C. Sphenoid bone
   D. Lacrimal bone
   E. Nasal bone

151. The blood supply of the nasopharyngeal tonsil includes all of the following except:
   A. Ascending palatine artery
   B. Ascending pharyngeal artery
   C. Internal maxillary artery
   D. Thyrocervical trunk
   E. Lingual artery

152. The tonsils are supplied by many vessels, but the main blood supply is from:
   A. Facial artery
   B. Lingual artery
   C. Internal maxillary artery
   D. Ascending pharyngeal artery
   E. None of these

153. Zenker's diverticulum is one of the causes of dysphagia. It commonly occurs at the so-called Killian's dehiscence. This area of weakness is between:
   A. Cricopharyngeus and the muscles of the esophagus
   B. Cricopharyngeus and the inferior constrictor
   C. Cricopharyngeus and thyropharyngeus muscles
   D. The middle and inferior constrictors
   E. None of the above

154. A 45-year-old female gives a history of recurrent parotid swelling with mild pain. Examination revealed an inflamed Stensen's duct. No opaque calculus was identified. Sialography revealed chronic sialectasis. Culture of the ductal orifice during an exacerbation would most likely yield:
   A. Beta hemolytic streptococcus, group A
   B. Streptococcus viridans
   C. Staphylococcus albus
   D. Staphylococcus aureus
   E. Pneumococcus

155. An otolaryngologist was asked to see a newborn with a "cat-like" cry. He appeared to be microcephalic with cleft lip and palate. He had mild inspiratory stridor which the otolaryngologist diagnosed as laryngomalacia. This constellation of symptoms is due to abnormality of:
   A. B group of chromosomes
   B. D group of chromosomes
   C. E group of chromosomes
   D. G group of chromsomes
   E. None of these

156. It is not infrequent for a pathologist to notice Trichinella within muscle tissues. Certain percentage of routine autopsies have yielded this finding. This figure is estimated to be:
   A. 1%
   B. 5%
   C. 15%
   D. 30%
   E. 50%

157. The greater cornu of the hyoid bone is believed to be derived from the:
   A. 1st branchial arch
   B. 2nd branchial arch
   C. 3rd branchial arch
   D. 4th branchial arch
   E. 5th branchial arch

158. The thymus gland is believed to be derived from the:
   A. 2nd branchial arch
   B. 2nd branchial pouch
   C. 3rd branchial arch
   D. 3rd branchial pouch
   E. 4th branchial arch

159. The oral tongue is a (n):
   A. Ectodermal derivative
   B. Entodermal derivative
   C. Mesodermal derivative
   D. Ectodermal and mesodermal derivative
   E. Entodermal and mesodermal derivative

160. The inferior turbinate is believed to be derived from:
A. 1st ethmoturbinal
B. 2nd ethmoturbinal
C. 3rd ethmoturbinal
D. Nasoturbinal
E. Maxilloturbinal

161. Certain parts of the temporal bone are derived from cartilage while other parts are membranous bone. All of the following are membranous bone <u>except</u>:
A. Petrous pyramid
B. Squamosa
C. Tympanic ring
D. Osseous canal
E. Bony modiolus

162. The concha is derived from the:
A. 1st branchial arch
B. 1st branchial groove
C. 2nd branchial arch
D. 2nd branchial groove
E. 2nd branchial pouch

163. The first part of the membranous labyrinth to appear is the:
A. Cochlea
B. Saccule
C. Utricle
D. Endolymphatic duct
E. Cochlear aqueduct

164. A 12-year-old white male presents with recurrent suppuration from his left ear and exophthalmos. Examination revealed a normal tympanic membrane with polyps in the osseous external auditory canal. Mastoid x-ray was unremarkable though some "punched out" lesions were noted in the occipital and parietal regions. Upon closer questioning he was found to have diabetes insipidus. The most likely diagnosis is:
A. Neurofibromatosis
B. Hand-Schuller-Christian disease
C. Pituitary adenoma
D. "Canal" cholesteatoma
E. Polyostotic fibrous dysplasia

165. The pre-epiglottic space is an important anatomical landmark in regard to the spread of laryngeal carcinoma. It is bounded by all of the following <u>except</u>:
A. Vallecula
B. Hyoid bone
C. Thyrohyoid membrane
D. Hyo-epiglottic ligament
E. Pharyngo-epiglottic ligament

166. The most common cause of chronic laryngeal stenosis is:
A. Trauma
B. High tracheotomy
C. Congenital
D. Tuberculosis
E. Syphilis

167. A 60-year-old depressed lady drank "Drano" in a suicidal attempt. Fortunately, she was brought to the emergency room less than one hour after ingestion. On esophagoscopy definite burns were ascertained. The esophagus is weakest:
A. One hour after ingestion
B. First 48 hours after ingestion

C. First week after ingestion
D. Second week after ingestion
E. Fourth week after ingestion

168. A 60-year-old heavy smoker gave a history of one month's hoarseness. Examination revealed a fungating, warty, well differentiated squamous cell carcinoma of the left true cord. The anterior commissure is clear. The cord is somewhat fixed. No lymphadenopathy was noted. The diagnosis of verrucous carcinoma was made histologically. This should be treated with:
A. Radiation
B. Radiation and laryngectomy
C. Laryngectomy
D. Hemilaryngectomy
E. Hemilaryngectomy and left radical neck dissection

169. Congenital laryngeal cyst is most frequently found in:
A. Epiglottis
B. Aryepiglottic folds
C. Glottis
D. Subglottis
E. Variable

170. Upon phonation, indirect laryngoscopy revealed incomplete closure of the posterior larynx. One of the following intrinsic muscles is paralyzed:
A. Interarytenoid muscle
B. Lateral cricoarytenoid muscle
C. Thyroarytenoid muscle
D. Cricothyroid muscle
E. Posterior cricoarytenoid muscle

171. The myoelastic theory of voice production states that:
A. The effective force setting the cords into vibration is the infraglottic air pressure. This pressure in turn acts on the true cords which are first approximated and tensed by the laryngeal muscles
B. Vibrations of the true cords are a direct result of the active muscle contractions
C. Vibrations of the true cords are a direct result of the infraglottic air pressure and they are independent of laryngeal muscles
D. The vibratory frequency of the vocal cords is the result of a cerebellar induced nerve impulse
E. Auditory feedback monitors voice production

172. Infectious mononucleosis has been associated with the following <u>except</u>:
A. Ruptured spleen
B. Guillain-Barré
C. Hepatomegaly
D. Exophthalmos
E. Paul-Bunnell test

173. A diabetic mother gave birth to a premature baby who developed severe respiratory distress. The baby was treated with humidiified oxygen. In view of an otherwise negative physical examination, the most likely diagnosis was idiopathic respiratory distress syndrome. The pulmonary tissues in this disease lack:
A. Creatinine phosphokinase
B. α-lecithin (alpha-lecithin)
C. Acid mucopolysaccharides
D. Trypsin
E. None of these

174. Cupulolithiasis is an entity believed to be due to:
A. Dislodgement of the statoconia of the saccule to the horizontal canal
B. Dislodgement of the statoconia of the saccule to the posterior canal
C. Dislodgement of the statoconia of the utricle to the horizontal canal
D. Dislodgement of the statoconia of the utricle to the posterior canal
E. Free floating statoconia in all 3 semicircular canals

175. Isolated otosclerosis of the footplate is encountered approximately:
A. 50%
B. 30%
C. 10%
D. 5%
E. 1%

176. The mother of a family of 4 has clinical otosclerosis. All 4 children are in the first decade. What are the chances of the children having clinical otosclerosis ultimately? The father is asymptomatic:
A. 75%
B. 60%
C. 50%
D. 20%
E. 5%

177. The maximum output of a 512 tuning fork is:
A. 50 dB
B. 60 dB
C. 70 dB
D. 80 dB
E. 90 dB

178. The maximum increase in pressure occurs when the sound has a wave-length "x" times that of the length of the external auditory canal. The value of "x" is:
A. 1
B. 2
C. 3
D. 4
E. 10

179. Streptomycin sulfate has successfully been used to treat bilateral incapacitating Meniere's disease. Which part of the membranous labyrinth is most sensitive to this medication?
A. Endolymphatic duct and sac
B. Semicircular canals
C. Saccule
D. Utricle
E. Cochlea

180. A 32-year-old man has a 2 month history of hoarseness. Direct laryngoscopy revealed a mass in the left posterior larynx on the true cord. Biopsy is as shown. This lesion is considered to have a potential for malignant degeneration. The incidence for this has been estimated to be:
A. 0.5%
B. 1%
C. 3%
D. 10%
E. 15%

181. Anosmia has been associated with all except one of the following:
A. Turner's syndrome
B. Kalman's syndrome
C. Foster-Kennedy syndrome
D. Atrophic rhinitis
E. Vitamin E deficiency

182. Etiologies for macroglossia include all of the following except:
A. Myxedema
B. Amyloidosis
C. Behcet's syndrome
D. von Gierke's disease
E. Tertiary syphilis

183. All of the following diseases may have sensorineural hearing loss except:
A. Brucellosis
B. Myxedema
C. Wilson's disease
D. Trichinosis
E. Relapsing polychondritis

184. The most comfortable and healthy environment is:
A. 50% humidity at 70-75° F
B. 70% humidity at 70-75° F
C. 30% humidity at 70-75° F
D. 10% humidity at 80° F
E. None of these

185. The following statements are consistent with Ewald's Laws except:
A. The horizontal canal is maximally stimulated by ampullo-petal flow
B. The posterior canal is maximally stimulated by ampullo-fugal flow
C. When a labyrinth is maximally stimulated, it elicits nystagmus toward itself
D. The superior canal is maximally stimulated by ampullo-fugal flow
E. The utricle and saccule are maximally stimulated by ampullo-petal flow

186. A 42-year-old female presents with bilateral sensorineural hearing loss, saddle nose, tender auricle and hoarseness. Among other findings she may be noted to have:
A. Increase in urinary chondroitin sulfate
B. Increase in urinary acid mucopolysaccharide
C. Increase in glycogen content in the pathological cells
D. Increase in mucopolysaccharides in the subepithelial tissues
E. Increase in amount of trypsin in her stool

187. A 20-year-old boy was noted to have cafe au lait spots throughout his trunk and extremities. He has multiple subcutaneous nodules and has elevated diastolic blood pressures. At the age of 15 he was operated upon for intussusception. There is a definite positive family history for similar disorders. His hypertension is most likely secondary to:
A. Pheochromocytoma
B. Renal disease
C. Early onset arteriosclerotic vascular disease
D. Insensitive carotid sinus apparatus
E. Unknown etiology

188. The membranous labyrinth is derived from:
A. Ectoderm
B. Mesoderm
C. Entoderm
D. Ectoderm and mesoderm
E. Ectoderm and entoderm

189. The Reinke's space in the larynx is:
A. Located in the ventricle
B. Similar to the pre-epiglottic space
C. Perpendicular to the long axis of the true cord
D. Limited above and below by the linea arcuata
E. Situated between the deeper elastic layer and thyroarytenoid muscle

190. A 32-year-old lady underwent an uneventful stapedectomy. She experienced mild dizziness and sensorineural hearing loss for the first 7 days postoperatively. The most likely diagnosis and treatment is:
A. Fistula of the oval window, surgical exploration
B. Granuloma, surgical exploration
C. Granuloma, conservative management
D. Serous labyrinthitis, surgical exploration
E. Serous labyrinthitis, conservative management

191. A 50-year-old lady has bilateral sensorineural hearing loss. Her audiogram shows a flat curve. Her hearing loss is considered to be socially useful if the hearing loss in the speech frequencies is less than:
A. 15 dB
B. 25 dB
C. 30 dB
D. 45 dB
E. 60 dB

192. A right-handed, 35-year-old lady underwent labyrinthectomy in the left ear for unilateral incapacitating Meniere's disease with no useful auditory function. Compensation for this loss of its impulses takes place in the:
A. Ipsilateral vestibular nuclei
B. Cerebellum
C. Median longitudinal fasciculus
D. Reticular formation
E. Contralateral labyrinth

193. Patients with Louis-Bar syndrome have symptoms which include ataxia, oculocutaneous telangiectasia and:
A. Situs inversus
B. Phenylketonuria
C. Sinopulmonary infections
D. Sensorineural deafness
E. Convulsive disorder

194. The most frequently encountered malignant tumor of the nose and paranasal sinuses is:
A. Adenocarcinoma and adenoid cystic carcinoma
B. Squamous cell carcinoma
C. Chondrosarcoma and sarcoma
D. Mixed tumor
E. None of the above

195. A 60-year-old male developed convulsion, unconsciousness, chest pain and hypotension after maxillary sinus irrigation. This suggests the following diagnosis and the first step in therapy is:
A. Septicemia, antibiotics
B. Cocaine reaction, intravenous valium
C. Air embolism, place patient in the recumbent position with the left side down
D. Air embolism, place patient in the recumbent position with the right side down
E. Maxillary artery thrombosis, anticoagulation

196. Submaxillary calculi can be visualized by x-ray in:
A. 10% of the cases
B. 25% of the cases
C. 50% of the cases
D. 75% of the cases
E. 90% of the cases

197. The most common benign intramural tumor of the esophagus is:
A. Angioma
B. Fibroma
C. Leiomyoma
D. Lipoma
E. Neurolemmoma

198. Esophageal perforation due to passage of a Bougie tip is best prevented by:
A. Use of antispasmodic drug prior to dilatation
B. Dilatation through an esophagoscope
C. Use of general anesthesia
D. Use of a swallowed thread as a guide
E. Use of lubricant on the dilator

199. A 40-year-old lady presented with a 1x2 cm. nontender, slowly enlarging mass in the infra-auricular area. Should this mass be located in the superficial lobe, the initial surgical treatment would be:
A. Enucleation
B. Superficial parotidectomy
C. Total parotidectomy with preservation of facial nerve
D. Total parotidectomy with facial nerve
E. Incisional biopsy for permanent section

200. A 60-year-old male presented with an ulcerating lesion measuring $1\frac{1}{2}$ cm in diameter in the concha of the left auricle. Examination under the microscope revealed that this lesion barely extended into the cartilaginous canal. Middle ear and mastoid were normal. No neck node was palpated. Biopsy revealed this to be a squamous cell carcinoma. The proper course of management would be:
A. Preoperative radiation followed by en-bloc partial temporal bone resection (leaving the stapes and facial nerve intact) and parotidectomy
B. Preoperative radiation followed by partial temporal bone resection (leaving stapes and facial nerve intact)
C. Radiation therapy only
D. Parotidectomy and partial temporal bone resection (leaving stapes and facial nerve intact)
E. Auriculectomy and excision of cartilaginous canal

201. A 55-year-old healthy male developed a squamous cell carcinoma of the medial wall of the left pyriform sinus, not involving the apex. This lesion also extended to the left lingual surface of the epiglottis. The base of the tongue was determined to be free of tumor. No metastatic node was palpated. The proper course of action would be:
A. Radiation therapy for cure
B. Preoperative radiation therapy followed by total laryngopharyngectomy
C. Preoperative radiation therapy followed by supraglottic laryngopharyngectomy and left radical neck dissection en-bloc
D. Preoperative radiation followed by total laryngopharyngectomy and left radical neck dissection en-bloc
E. Supraglottic laryngopharyngectomy and left radical neck dissection en-bloc

202. A 35-year-old male presented with hoarseness for 3 months. He smokes one pack a day for the past 15 years. Indirect laryngoscopy revealed a 3 mm lesion on the left true cord, middle third. The rest of the ENT examination was unremarkable. Direct laryngoscopy and excisional biopsy were done. Pathology report revealed this to be a granular cell myoblastoma and that the margins were not clear of tumor. The proper management would include:
A. Close follow-up
B. Hemilaryngectomy
C. Total laryngectomy
D. Re-excisional biopsy with microscopic laryngoscopy
E. Cordectomy

203. A 40-year-old healthy male presented with unilateral nasal obstruction. Examination revealed papilloma-like growth in the left nasal fossa. The rest of the ENT examination was unremarkable. Sinus x-rays showed involvement of the left maxillary sinus and erosion of the left nasomaxillary wall. The biopsy was reported as inverting papilloma. The proper course of action should be:

A. Intranasal resection of papilloma and Caldwell-Luc
B. Lateral rhinotomy and partial maxillectomy
C. Lateral rhinotomy, removal of naso-antral wall and Caldwell-Luc if necessary
D. Maxillectomy
E. Partial maxillectomy

204. A 40-year-old female presented with a pulsatile, nontender, slowly growing mass in the left upper neck. The rest of the ENT and general examination was negative. Carotid angiography shows an "egg-shell" appearing mass displacing the internal carotid artery laterally and widening the bifurcation. The course of action should be:

A. Resection of the tumor in total only if it can be done without sacrificing the internal carotid artery
B. Resection of the tumor in total even if resection of the internal carotid artery is necessary
C. Radiation
D. Preoperative radiation and resection of the tumor in total even if the internal carotid artery has to be sacrificed
E. Preoperative radiation and resection of the tumor in total only if the internal carotid artery can be spared

INDEX